Cancer Drug Discovery and Development

Series Editor
Beverly A. Teicher
Bethesda, MD, USA

More information about this series at http://www.springer.com/series/7625

John Pollard • Nicola Curtin
Editors

Targeting the DNA Damage Response for Anti-Cancer Therapy

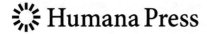 Humana Press

Editors
John Pollard
Vertex Pharmaceuticals (Europe) Ltd
Abingdon, Oxfordshire, UK

Nicola Curtin
Northern Institute for Cancer Research
Medical School
Newcastle University
Newcastle upon Tyne, UK

Newcastle University Institute for Ageing
Medical School
Newcastle University
Newcastle upon Tyne, UK

ISSN 2196-9906   ISSN 2196-9914   (electronic)
Cancer Drug Discovery and Development
ISBN 978-3-030-09336-5   ISBN 978-3-319-75836-7   (eBook)
https://doi.org/10.1007/978-3-319-75836-7

Contents

1   **Targeting DNA Repair in Anti-Cancer Treatments**.   1
Thomas Helleday

2   **The DNA Damage Response: Roles in Cancer Etiology
and Treatment**   11
Laura R. Butler, Oren Gilad, and Eric J. Brown

3   **Control of DNA Replication by ATR**.   35
Emilio Lecona and Oscar Fernández-Capetillo

4   **Targeting ATR for Cancer Therapy: Profile and Expectations
for ATR Inhibitors**   63
Nicola Curtin and John Pollard

5   **Targeting ATR for Cancer Therapy:
ATR-Targeted Drug Candidates**   99
Magnus T. Dillon and Kevin J. Harrington

6   **ATM: Its Recruitment, Activation, Signalling and Contribution
to Tumour Suppression**.   129
Atsushi Shibata and Penny Jeggo

7   **Pre-clinical Profile and Expectations for Pharmacological
ATM Inhibition**   155
Anika M. Weber and Anderson J. Ryan

8   **Targeting ATM for Cancer Therapy: Prospects
for Drugging ATM**.   185
Ian Hickson, Kurt G. Pike, and Stephen T. Durant

9   **Targeting CHK1 for Cancer Therapy: Rationale, Progress
and Prospects**.   209
David A. Gillespie

10 **Preclinical Profiles and Contexts for CHK1
    and CHK2 Inhibitors** 241
    Ian Collins and Michelle D. Garrett

11 **Clinical Development of CHK1 Inhibitors** 277
    Alvaro Ingles Garces and Udai Banerji

12 **Established and Emerging Roles of the DNA-Dependent
    Protein Kinase Catalytic Subunit (DNA-PKcs)** 315
    Edward J. Bartlett and Susan P. Lees-Miller

13 **Targeting DNA-PK as a Therapeutic Approach in Oncology** 339
    Celine Cano, Suzannah J. Harnor, Elaine Willmore,
    and Stephen R. Wedge

14 **Dbait: A New Concept of DNA Repair Pathways Inhibitor
    from Bench to Bedside** 359
    Marie Dutreix, Flavien Devun, Nirmitha Herath,
    and Patricia Noguiez-Hellin

15 **Alternative Non-homologous End-Joining: Mechanisms
    and Targeting Strategies in Cancer** 375
    Pratik Nagaria and Feyruz V. Rassool

About the Editors 401

Contributors

Udai Banerji Drug Development Unit, The Institute of Cancer Research and The Royal Marsden, London, UK

Edward J. Bartlett Department of Biochemistry and Molecular Biology and Robson DNA Science Centre, Arnie Charbonneau Cancer Institute, University of Calgary, Calgary, AB, Canada

Sir William Dunn School of Pathology, University of Oxford, Oxford, England, UK

Eric J. Brown Department of Cancer Biology, Abramson Family Cancer Research Institute, Perelman School of Medicine, University of Pennsylvania, Philadelphia, PA, USA

Laura R. Butler Atrin Pharmaceuticals, Pennsylvania Biotechnology Center, Doylestown, PA, USA

Celine Cano Northern Institute for Cancer Research, School of Chemistry, Newcastle University, Newcastle upon Tyne, UK

Ian Collins Cancer Research UK Cancer Therapeutics Unit at The Institute of Cancer Research, London, UK

Nicola Curtin Northern Institute for Cancer Research, Medical School, Newcastle University, Newcastle upon Tyne, UK

Newcastle University Institute for Ageing, Medical School, Newcastle University, Newcastle upon Tyne, UK

Flavien Devun Institut Curie, PSL Research University, CNRS, INSERM, UMR 3347, Orsay, France

Université Paris Sud, Université Paris-Saclay, CNRS, INSERM, UMR 3347, Orsay, France

DNA Therapeutics, Genopole, Evry, France

Magnus T. Dillon The Institute of Cancer Research, London, UK

The Royal Marsden NHS Foundation Trust, London, UK

Stephen T. Durant Oncology IMED Biotech Unit, Innovative Medicines and Early Development, AstraZeneca, Cambridge, UK

Marie Dutreix Institut Curie, PSL Research University, CNRS, INSERM, UMR 3347, Orsay, France

Université Paris Sud, Université Paris-Saclay, CNRS, INSERM, UMR 3347, Orsay, France

Oscar Fernández-Capetillo Genomic Instability Group, Spanish National Cancer Research Centre (CNIO), Madrid, Spain

Science for Life Laboratory, Division of Genome Biology, Department of Medical Biochemistry and Biophysics, Karolinska Institute, Stockholm, Sweden

Michelle D. Garrett School of Biosciences, University of Kent, Kent, UK

Oren Gilad Atrin Pharmaceuticals, Pennsylvania Biotechnology Center, Doylestown, PA, USA

David A. Gillespie Institute of Biomedical Technologies, Canary Islands Centre for Biomedical Research, Faculty of Medicine, University of La Laguna, Tenerife, Spain

Suzannah J. Harnor Northern Institute for Cancer Research, Newcastle University, School of Chemistry, Newcastle upon Tyne, UK

Kevin J. Harrington The Institute of Cancer Research, London, UK

The Royal Marsden NHS Foundation Trust, London, UK

Thomas Helleday Science for Life Laboratory, Division of Translational Medicine and Chemical Biology, Department of Medical Biochemistry and Biophysics, Karolinska Institutet, Stockholm, Sweden

Nirmitha Herath Institut Curie, PSL Research University, CNRS, INSERM, UMR 3347, Orsay, France

Université Paris Sud, Université Paris-Saclay, CNRS, INSERM, UMR 3347, Orsay, France

DNA Therapeutics, Genopole, Evry, France

Ian Hickson Northern Institute for Cancer Research (NICR), Newcastle University, Newcastle, UK

Alvaro Ingles Garces Drug Development Unit, The Institute of Cancer Research and The Royal Marsden, London, UK

Penny Jeggo Genome Damage and Stability Centre, Life Sciences, University of Sussex, Brighton, UK

Emilio Lecona Genomic Instability Group, Spanish National Cancer Research Centre (CNIO), Madrid, Spain

Susan P. Lees-Miller Department of Biochemistry and Molecular Biology and Robson DNA Science Centre, Arnie Charbonneau Cancer Institute, University of Calgary, Calgary, AB, Canada

Pratik Nagaria Department of Radiation Oncology and Marlene and Stewart Greenebaum Comprehensive Cancer Center, University of Maryland School of Medicine, Baltimore, MD, USA

BioReliance Corporation, A MilliporeSigma Company, Rockville, MD, USA

Patricia Noguiez-Hellin Institut Curie, PSL Research University, CNRS, INSERM, UMR 3347, Orsay, France

Université Paris Sud, Université Paris-Saclay, CNRS, INSERM, UMR 3347, Orsay, France

DNA Therapeutics, Genopole, Evry, France

Kurt G. Pike Oncology IMED Biotech Unit, Innovative Medicines and Early Development, AstraZeneca, Cambridge, UK

John Pollard Vertex Pharmaceuticals (Europe) Ltd, Abingdon, Oxfordshire, UK

Feyruz V. Rassool Department of Radiation Oncology and Marlene and Stewart Greenebaum Comprehensive Cancer Center, University of Maryland School of Medicine, Baltimore, MD, USA

Anderson J. Ryan Cancer Research UK and Medical Research Council Oxford Institute for Radiation Oncology, The Department of Oncology, University of Oxford, Oxford, UK

Atsushi Shibata Eduction and Research Support Centre, Graduate School of Medicine, Gunma University, Maebashi, Gunma, Japan

Anika M. Weber Cancer Research UK and Medical Research Council Oxford Institute for Radiation Oncology, The Department of Oncology, University of Oxford, Oxford, UK

Stephen R. Wedge Northern Institute for Cancer Research, Medical School, Newcastle University, Newcastle upon Tyne, UK

Elaine Willmore Northern Institute for Cancer Research, Medical School, Newcastle University, Newcastle upon Tyne, UK

Chapter 1
Targeting DNA Repair in Anti-Cancer Treatments

Thomas Helleday

Abstract Treatment of cancer started long before the emergence of modern pharmaceuticals, and over the decades, mankind has tried just about everything to battle this disease. Besides surgery, only a handful of treatments have stood the test of time: ionizing radiation, discovered by Wilhelm Röntgen, and chemotherapy treatments, discovered serendipitously in the release of mustard gas following the bombing of an American cargo ship in Bari (Italy) during the Second World War. Antimetabolites and natural products were also found to have potent anti-cancer effects and much later it was discovered that all the anti-cancer drugs share the same target: DNA. Hence, there is overwhelming evidence that causing DNA damage is an effective way of treating cancer.

DNA was for a long time thought to be highly stable, a prevailing view until Tomas Lindahl discovered the spontaneous decay of DNA (Lindahl and Andersson 1972; Lindahl and Nyberg 1974). As DNA is indispensable for life, Dr. Lindahl hypothesized that there must be a way to repair the DNA and subsequently he identified the first DNA repair protein, a uracil DNA glycosylase (Lindahl 1974). For this discovery he got the 2015 Nobel Prize in Chemistry, which he shared with Drs. Paul Modrich and Aziz Sancar for their discoveries of other DNA repair pathways. Over the years, hundreds of DNA repair proteins have been identified and their individual role has been studied in great biochemical detail (Hoeijmakers 2001).

Although DNA damaging agents dramatically improved cancer survival rates and prolonged life, it was evident early on that cancers relapsed and developed resistance. For clinicians it was clear that the cancer cells somehow escaped the

COI statement: the author is listed inventor of numerous patents targeting DNA repair in cancers and recieves royalty from PARP inhibitor sales.

T. Helleday (✉)
Science for Life Laboratory, Division of Translational Medicine and Chemical Biology,
Department of Medical Biochemistry and Biophysics, Karolinska Institutet,
Stockholm, Sweden
e-mail: thomas.helleday@scilifelab.se

treatments and a likely mechanism was by improving their ability to repair DNA. Hence, a way to decrease the DNA repair capacity of cancer cells has been on the agenda for a long time to improve cancer treatment, in particular in the radiation oncology field. The big issue has always been how to selectively sensitize the cancer cells and not the non-transformed cells?

Keywords DNA repair · DNA damage response · Synthetic lethality · Replication stress

1.1 PARP Inhibitors to Targeted DNA Repair

Finding a way to target DNA repair did not take such a long time. Just a few years after Dr. Lindahl's discovery of base excision repair, Dr. Barbara Durkatcz, in Dr. Shall's laboratory, discovered that poly(ADP-ribose)polymerase (PARP) was critical to complete the DNA excision repair process (Durkacz et al. 1980). The work was facilitated by the earlier discovery by Dr. Shall of the first PARP inhibitor, benzamide (Shall 1975), later improved to 3-aminobenzamide (Purnell and Whish 1980). One of the most important discoveries using the PARP inhibitors was that these caused an increase in sister chromatid exchange (Oikawa et al. 1980). This original report from Sugimura's laboratory was the first of many investigating the involvement of PARP in homologous recombination in a number of different organisms, and in 1995 Tomas Lindahl described PARP as the master regulator of homologous recombination (Lindahl et al. 1995). The finding that homologous recombination-defective cells were highly sensitive to PARP inhibitors was likely delayed due to a lack of highly potent PARP inhibitors. The first very potent PARP inhibitor was generated by the late Dr. Roger Griffin and co-workers at Newcastle University (Griffin et al. 1995). These PARP inhibitors potentiated the effects of different anti-cancer drugs such as temozolomide not only in cancer cells (Boulton et al. 1995), but also in healthy cells, and so may require dose reductions of the chemotherapy (Plummer et al. 2013).

The big breakthrough for PARP inhibitors was in 2003, when the groups of Dr. Thomas Helleday from the University of Sheffield and Dr. Nicola Curtin from Newcastle collaboratively demonstrated that potent PARP inhibitors effectively kill homologous recombination defective cancers, such as those defective in the breast cancer susceptibility gene 2 (BRCA2) (Helleday 2003). This was later published together with the groups of Drs. Ashworth and Jackson (Bryant et al. 2005; Farmer et al. 2005), the latter group using the highly potent PARP inhibitor olaparib, developed by the company KuDOS Pharmaceuticals Ltd. (Farmer et al. 2005). Olaparib is the active ingredient in the first-ever FDA approved DNA repair inhibitor, which was for the treatment of BRCA mutated ovarian cancer.

The use of PARP inhibitors to selectively kill homologous recombination defective cancers received a lot of attention as normal cells were largely protected from their toxic effects, and patients receiving PARP inhibitors exhibited mild side effects as compared to traditional chemotherapy treatments. Previously, yeast geneticists had suggested to exploit liabilities in the mutated cancers using the concept of synthetic lethality, to identify novel treatment options (Hartwell et al. 1997). This was first exemplified using PARP inhibitors in BRCA mutated cancers. Although many BRCA mutated patients benefit from PARP inhibitors, most relapse with PARP inhibitor resistant cancers (Fong et al. 2009). Also, many patients with mutations in genes other than BRCA respond to treatment, making it difficult to identify responding patient cohorts.

1.2 Limits to the Synthetic Lethal Approach of Targeting Cancer

Following the PARP-BRCA paradigm much attention has been focussed on the identification of novel synthetic lethal interactions in cancer. From a DNA repair perspective it was very fortunate that cancers turn out to have many more mutations in DNA repair genes than initially anticipated, suggesting a plethora of possibilities to identify new synthetic lethal interactions. Now, a decade later, and after much research on this not only from academic laboratories, but also from industry, we are in a position to be able to determine if this strategy has been successful. Unfortunately, there has yet to be a similar example of a strong synthetic lethal approach, such as PARP-BRCA, working in the clinical setting. The advocates for synthetic lethality would probably argue that there hasn't been sufficient time or effort for thorough evaluation, given that the first PARP inhibitor (olaparib/Lynparza™) was approved only a few years ago. There are several reasons for this strategy not to work as effectively as it could have done. First, there is large intra-tumour heterogeneity in cancers (Gerlinger et al. 2012) and hence there are likely cancer clones that do not harbour the targeted mutation. One reason for the success of PARP inhibitors in BRCA mutated ovarian cancers could well be that the mutation stem from a germline mutation present in all cells. Secondly, additional mutations in the BRCA gene itself (Sakai et al. 2008) or loss of 53BP1 gene expression (Bunting et al. 2010) for instance, can result in PARP inhibitor resistance. Thirdly, the synthetic lethal screens have mostly been conducted using RNAi approaches and transient loss of a protein rarely completely phenocopies the effect of an inhibited enzyme. Also, some DNA repair inhibitors exert their effect by protein trapping or other edgetic perturbations. Finally, the most important caveat to progressing the targeting of DNA repair is the lack of DNA repair inhibitors. Today, several hundred DNA repair proteins are described, but we lack high quality small molecule probes to study the inhibitory effect of the vast majority of these. Although there are now numerous small molecules described to target various DNA repair proteins (Curtin 2012; Helleday et al. 2008), unfortunately the development of these inhibitors has largely been carried out in absence of medicinal chemistry competence and most of the described small molecules are pan-assay interference compounds (PAINS) (Baell and Walters 2014) of little or no use to understanding mechanism of action. A more concerted effort is needed to identify additional small molecule inhibitors of DNA repair proteins.

1.3 Combining Chemotherapy Treatment with DNA Repair Inhibitors

With the risk of increasing normal tissue toxicity, the prevailing strategy used for DNA repair inhibitors has been to combine them with standard of care chemotherapy treatments. Clinically, this may initially sound like an attractive model, in particular if the standard of care treatment has tolerable side effects. Many trials have been conducted and in general, it appears that those with a clear underlying mechanism of action have been more successful than those without basic science input. There are two overall strategies, either to (1) increase the amount of DNA damage by inhibiting the repair or (2) exploit defects in the DNA damage response, such as loss of functional p53, to target the remaining checkpoint proteins (such as CHK1) required to prevent cells entering mitosis with DNA damage (Ma et al. 2010). The latter strategy has a clear mechanistic rationale and has had some success in the clinic, while the former is limited to only a few success stories. It is probable that the reason for chemotherapy regimens to fail is unlikely to be their inability to cause a sufficient amount of DNA damage, but likely that the cells have defence mechanisms beyond DNA, making them insensitive to treatment. As such just increasing the amount of DNA damage in this scenario may not make a lot of difference in some tumors. Success in the clinic will likely improve through the incorporation of scientific rationale into the design of clinical trials such as genetic or molecular markers of sensitivity or rational combinations with drugs that block orthogonal survival pathways.

1.4 Exploiting the Inherent High Level of DNA Damage in Cancers; Replication Stress

Cancer cells have a high level of inherent DNA damage, which can be caused by loss of DNA repair pathways, hypoxia, oxidative damage or replication stress (Helleday 2008). Since high levels of DNA damage are ubiquitous in cancers, this could be an interesting approach that is not limited to genotype. A fundamental discovery was of the existence of oncogene-induced replication stress in cancer (Bartkova et al. 2005; Bartkova et al. 2006; Di Micco et al. 2006; Gorgoulis et al. 2005; Halazonetis et al. 2008), which can be caused by oncogene-induced dNTP deprivation (Bester et al. 2011) or transcriptional collisions (Jones et al. 2013).

One of the key enzymes dealing with replication stress is ATR and accordingly it has been demonstrated that specific ATR inhibitors selectively kill cancers with replication stress (Murga et al. 2011; Toledo et al. 2011). Currently, the DNA repair field is focussing on understanding the molecular mechanisms of oncogene-induced replication stress and how this can be exploited for treatments, and several in depth reviews on this topic can be found in this volume.

Cancer cells typically lose redox homeostasis and suffer from an increased level of reactive oxygen species (ROS), which has previously been exploited in cancer treatment by targeting metabolic pathways (Gorrini et al. 2013). In cancer cells, it has been demonstrated that the MTH1 protein is required to prevent ROS from causing DNA damage by sanitizing the dNTP pool, and through targeting MTH1 with small molecule inhibitors selective killing of but not non-transformed cells could be achieved (Gad et al. 2014; Huber et al. 2014). There will likely be more targeted approaches, such as ATR and MTH1, which will emerge in the future and can be used to target the cancer phenotype more generally. In general, understanding the molecular mechanisms on how inhibitors work will be challanging as protein loss rarely recapitulate the effect of inhibitors. Furthermore, different inhibitors commonly disrupt different edges in the network, resulting in that different inhibitors show differential efficiency on killing cancer cells, which is the case for instance for PARP or MTH1 inhibitors.

1.5 Future Challenges in Targeting DNA Repair for Cancer Treatments

Causing DNA damage is a highly effective way of killing cancer cells and we have just started to do this in a more intelligent way, by exploiting specific DNA repair inhibitors. We are certainly not in for an easy ride, since cancer cells have a number of different DNA repair pathways inactivated or over-activated and there are likely many possibilities for cancer cells to adapt to a changed environment (such as a targeted DNA repair inhibitor treatment). More and more proteins involved in DNA repair and the DNA damage response are constantly being reported, and soon there will be >1000 proteins with described roles in these processes. In this situation, there are likely redundancies and possibilities for a cancer cell to rewire the network and gain resistance to a specific DNA repair inhibitor. Hence, success is likely going to emerge from combination treatments. In line with this, combination of Wee1 and PARP inhibitors or ATR and CHK1 inhibitors (Sanjiv et al. 2016) are promising. The foreseeable future path to success will likely reside in the exploitation of more DNA repair inhibitor combinations, which has much promise.

A future challenge in the development of DNA repair inhibitors is the complexity of the underlying biology and that protein loss often gives a different phenotype to protein inhibition. In this context, it is important to point out that even today the underlying mechanism for PARP inhibitors selectively killing BRCA defective cells is still not resolved (Helleday 2011). Interestingly, the inhibitory activity to PARP1 is not even correlated with the killing effect of BRCA defective cells, but is explained by the ability of the inhibitors to trap PARP1 onto DNA (Murai et al. 2012). However, there is currently no biochemical explanation of how PARP inhibitors actually trap PARP1 onto DNA. Similarly, the first reported MTH1 small molecule inhibitors have been criticised as there is a possibility to generate an MTH1 enzymatic inhibitor that does not kill cancer cells (Petrocchi et al. 2016; Warpman Berglund et al. 2016). More recent research demonstrates that MTH1 is able to bind and activate proteins critical for establishing mitosis and the ability of compounds to break these protein interactions appear important to also cause toxicity to cancer cells. Hence, it appears that the MTH1 protein is not just a simple enzyme with a single biochemical activity and thus compounds that interact with MTH1 in diverse ways can result in distinct phenotypes. Clearly, more basic research is required to be able to in detail explain how both PARP and MTH1 inhibitors work.

When it comes to targeting oncogenic kinases it is often sufficient to impair a single activity of the protein to achieve anti-cancer properties, which facilitates industrial drug development. Since PARP, MTH1 and likely other proteins involved in DNA repair also have structural properties and relevant unknown protein interactions it is likely that the discovery of small molecule inhibitors to these proteins will be complex. Potentially, more open collaborative efforts are needed between industry and academia to ensure a full understanding of the DNA repair proteins and processes can translate to effective targeted therapies.

In conclusion, we are at the beginning of a new era in targeting DNA repair for cancer treatment, and collaborative efforts are likely required to unveil the complexity of this disease and to ultimately expose and exploit its vulnerabilities.

Acknowledgements I thank Sean Rudd for helpful input. The laboratory is mainly funded by Knut and Alice Wallenberg Foundation, the Swedish Research Council, the European Research Council, Swedish Cancer Society, the Swedish Children's Cancer Foundation, the Strategic Research Foundation, the Swedish Pain Relief Foundation, AFA foundation, and the Torsten and Ragnar Söderberg Foundation.

References

Baell J, Walters MA (2014) Chemistry: chemical con artists foil drug discovery. Nature 513: 481–483

Bartkova J, Horejsi Z, Koed K, Kramer A, Tort F, Zieger K, Guldberg P, Sehested M, Nesland JM, Lukas C, Orntoft T, Lukas J, Bartek J (2005) DNA damage response as a candidate anti-cancer barrier in early human tumorigenesis. Nature 434:864–870

Bartkova J, Rezaei N, Liontos M, Karakaidos P, Kletsas D, Issaeva N, Vassiliou LV, Kolettas E, Niforou K, Zoumpourlis VC, Takaoka M, Nakagawa H, Tort F, Fugger K, Johansson F, Sehested M, Andersen CL, Dyrskjot L, Orntoft T, Lukas J et al (2006) Oncogene-induced senescence is part of the tumorigenesis barrier imposed by DNA damage checkpoints. Nature 444:633–637

Bester AC, Roniger M, Oren YS, Im MM, Sarni D, Chaoat M, Bensimon A, Zamir G, Shewach DS, Kerem B (2011) Nucleotide deficiency promotes genomic instability in early stages of cancer development. Cell 145:435–446

Boulton S, Pemberton LC, Porteous JK, Curtin NJ, Griffin RJ, Golding BT, Durkacz BW (1995) Potentiation of temozolomide-induced cytotoxicity: a comparative study of the biological effects of poly(ADP-ribose) polymerase inhibitors. Br J Cancer 72:849–856. Order

Bryant HE, Schultz N, Thomas HD, Parker KM, Flower D, Lopez E, Kyle S, Meuth M, Curtin NJ, Helleday T (2005) Specific killing of BRCA2-deficient tumours with inhibitors of poly(ADP-ribose)polymerase. Nature 434:913–917

Bunting SF, Callen E, Wong N, Chen HT, Polato F, Gunn A, Bothmer A, Feldhahn N, Fernandez-Capetillo O, Cao L, Xu X, Deng CX, Finkel T, Nussenzweig M, Stark JM, Nussenzweig A (2010) 53BP1 inhibits homologous recombination in Brca1-deficient cells by blocking resection of DNA breaks. Cell 141:243–254

Curtin NJ (2012) DNA repair dysregulation from cancer driver to therapeutic target. Nat Rev Cancer 12:801–817

Di Micco R, Fumagalli M, Cicalese A, Piccinin S, Gasparini P, Luise C, Schurra C, Garre M, Nuciforo PG, Bensimon A, Maestro R, Pelicci PG, d'Adda di Fagagna F (2006) Oncogene-induced senescence is a DNA damage response triggered by DNA hyper-replication. Nature 444:638–642

Durkacz BW, Omidiji O, Gray DA, Shall S (1980) (ADP-ribose)n participates in DNA excision repair. Nature 283:593–596

Farmer H, McCabe N, Lord CJ, Tutt AN, Johnson DA, Richardson TB, Santarosa M, Dillon KJ, Hickson I, Knights C, Martin NM, Jackson SP, Smith GC, Ashworth A (2005) Targeting the DNA repair defect in BRCA mutant cells as a therapeutic strategy. Nature 434:917–921

Fong PC, Boss DS, Yap TA, Tutt A, Wu P, Mergui-Roelvink M, Mortimer P, Swaisland H, Lau A, O'Connor MJ, Ashworth A, Carmichael J, Kaye SB, Schellens JH, de Bono JS (2009) Inhibition of poly(ADP-Ribose) polymerase in tumors from BRCA mutation carriers. N Engl J Med 361:123–134

Gad H, Koolmeister T, Jemth AS, Eshtad S, Jacques SA, Strom CE, Svensson LM, Schultz N, Lundback T, Einarsdottir BO, Saleh A, Gokturk C, Baranczewski P, Svensson R, Berntsson RP, Gustafsson R, Stromberg K, Sanjiv K, Jacques-Cordonnier MC, Desroses M et al (2014) MTH1 inhibition eradicates cancer by preventing sanitation of the dNTP pool. Nature 508:215–221

Gerlinger M, Rowan AJ, Horswell S, Larkin J, Endesfelder D, Gronroos E, Martinez P, Matthews N, Stewart A, Tarpey P, Varela I, Phillimore B, Begum S, McDonald NQ, Butler A, Jones D, Raine K, Latimer C, Santos CR, Nohadani M et al (2012) Intratumor heterogeneity and branched evolution revealed by multiregion sequencing. N Engl J Med 366:883–892

Gorgoulis VG, Vassiliou LV, Karakaidos P, Zacharatos P, Kotsinas A, Liloglou T, Venere M, Ditullio RA Jr, Kastrinakis NG, Levy B, Kletsas D, Yoneta A, Herlyn M, Kittas C, Halazonetis TD (2005) Activation of the DNA damage checkpoint and genomic instability in human pre-cancerous lesions. Nature 434:907–913

Gorrini C, Harris IS, Mak TW (2013) Modulation of oxidative stress as an anticancer strategy. Nat Rev Drug Discov 12:931–947

Griffin RJ, Pemberton LC, Rhodes D, Bleasdale C, Bowman K, Calvert AH, Curtin NJ, Durkacz BW, Newell DR, Porteous JK et al (1995) Novel potent inhibitors of the DNA repair enzyme poly(ADP-ribose)polymerase (PARP). Anticancer Drug Des 10:507–514

Halazonetis TD, Gorgoulis VG, Bartek J (2008) An oncogene-induced DNA damage model for cancer development. Science 319:1352–1355

Hartwell LH, Szankasi P, Roberts CJ, Murray AW, Friend SH (1997) Integrating genetic approaches into the discovery of anticancer drugs. Science 278:1064–1068

Helleday T (2003) Use of rnai inhibiting parp activtiy for the manufacture of a medicament for the treatment of cancer. patent WO 2005012524r A1

Helleday T (2008) Amplifying tumour-specific replication lesions by DNA repair inhibitors–a new era in targeted cancer therapy. Eur J Cancer 44(7):921–927

Helleday T (2011) The underlying mechanism for the PARP and BRCA synthetic lethality: clearing up the misunderstandings. Mol Oncol 5:387–393

Helleday T, Petermann E, Lundin C, Hodgson B, Sharma RA (2008) DNA repair pathways as targets for cancer therapy. Nat Rev Cancer 8:193–204

Hoeijmakers JH (2001) Genome maintenance mechanisms for preventing cancer. Nature 411:366–374

Huber KV, Salah E, Radic B, Gridling M, Elkins JM, Stukalov A, Jemth AS, Gokturk C, Sanjiv K, Stromberg K, Pham T, Berglund UW, Colinge J, Bennett KL, Loizou JI, Helleday T, Knapp S, Superti-Furga G (2014) Stereospecific targeting of MTH1 by (S)-crizotinib as an anticancer strategy. Nature 508:222–227

Jones RM, Mortusewicz O, Afzal I, Lorvellec M, Garcia P, Helleday T, Petermann E (2013) Increased replication initiation and conflicts with transcription underlie Cyclin E-induced replication stress. Oncogene 32:3744–3753

Lindahl T (1974) An N-glycosidase from Escherichia coli that releases free uracil from DNA containing deaminated cytosine residues. Proc Natl Acad Sci U S A 71:3649–3653

Lindahl T, Andersson A (1972) Rate of chain breakage at apurinic sites in double-stranded deoxyribonucleic acid. Biochemistry 11:3618–3623

Lindahl T, Nyberg B (1974) Heat-induced deamination of cytosine residues in deoxyribonucleic acid. Biochemistry 13:3405–3410

Lindahl T, Satoh MS, Poirier GG, Klungland A (1995) Post-translational modification of poly(ADP-ribose) polymerase induced by DNA strand breaks. Trends Biochem Sci 20:405–411

Ma CX, Janetka JW, Piwnica-Worms H (2010) Death by releasing the breaks: CHK1 inhibitors as cancer therapeutics. Trends Mol Med 17:88–96

Murai J, Huang SY, Das BB, Renaud A, Zhang Y, Doroshow JH, Ji J, Takeda S, Pommier Y (2012) Trapping of PARP1 and PARP2 by Clinical PARP Inhibitors. Cancer Res 72:5588–5599

Murga M, Campaner S, Lopez-Contreras AJ, Toledo LI, Soria R, Montana MF, D'Artista L, Schleker T, Guerra C, Garcia E, Barbacid M, Hidalgo M, Amati B, Fernandez-Capetillo O (2011) Exploiting oncogene-induced replicative stress for the selective killing of Myc-driven tumors. Nat Struct Mol Biol 18:1331–1335

Oikawa A, Tohda H, Kanai M, Miwa M, Sugimura T (1980) Inhibitors of poly(adenosine diphosphate ribose) polymerase induce sister chromatid exchanges. Biochem Biophys Res Commun 97:1311–1316

Petrocchi A, Leo E, Reyna NJ, Hamilton MM, Shi X, Parker CA, Mseeh F, Bardenhagen JP, Leonard P, Cross JB, Huang S, Jiang Y, Cardozo M, Draetta G, Marszalek JR, Toniatti C, Jones P, Lewis RT (2016) Identification of potent and selective MTH1 inhibitors. Bioorg Med Chem Lett 26:1503–1507

Plummer R, Lorigan P, Steven N, Scott L, Middleton MR, Wilson RH, Mulligan E, Curtin N, Wang D, Dewji R, Abbattista A, Gallo J, Calvert H (2013) A phase II study of the potent PARP inhibitor, Rucaparib (PF-01367338, AG014699), with temozolomide in patients with metastatic melanoma demonstrating evidence of chemopotentiation. Cancer Chemother Pharmacol 71:1191–1199

Purnell MR, Whish WJ (1980) Novel inhibitors of poly(ADP-ribose) synthetase. Biochem J 185:775–777

Sakai W, Swisher EM, Karlan BY, Agarwal MK, Higgins J, Friedman C, Villegas E, Jacquemont C, Farrugia DJ, Couch FJ, Urban N, Taniguchi T (2008) Secondary mutations as a mechanism of cisplatin resistance in BRCA2-mutated cancers. Nature 451:1116–1120

Sanjiv K, Hagenkort A, Calderon-Montano JM, Koolmeister T, Reaper PM, Mortusewicz O, Jacques SA, Kuiper RV, Schultz N, Scobie M, Charlton PA, Pollard JR, Berglund UW, Altun M, Helleday T (2016) Cancer-specific synthetic lethality between ATR and CHK1 kinase activities. Cell Rep 14:298–309

Shall S (1975) Proceedings: experimental manipulation of the specific activity of poly(ADP-ribose) polymerase. J Biochem 77:2

Toledo LI, Murga M, Zur R, Soria R, Rodriguez A, Martinez S, Oyarzabal J, Pastor J, Bischoff JR, Fernandez-Capetillo O (2011) A cell-based screen identifies ATR inhibitors with synthetic lethal properties for cancer-associated mutations. Nat Struct Mol Biol 18:721–727

Warpman Berglund U, Sanjiv K, Gad H, Kalderen C, Koolmeister T, Pham T, Gokturk C, Jafari R, Maddalo G, Seashore-Ludlow B, Chernobrovkin A, Manoilov A, Pateras IS, Rasti A, Jemth AS, Almlof I, Loseva O, Visnes T, Einarsdottir BO, Gaugaz FZ et al (2016) Validation and development of MTH1 inhibitors for treatment of cancer. Ann Oncol 27:2275–2283

Chapter 2
The DNA Damage Response: Roles in Cancer Etiology and Treatment

Laura R. Butler, Oren Gilad, and Eric J. Brown

Abstract Cancer is one of the highest causes of morbidity and mortality worldwide. Traditional chemotherapeutics are associated with toxic side effects due to a lack of specificity for cancer cells. A new and rapidly expanding class of drugs known as targeted therapeutics are being developed that have high therapeutic potential with less severe side effects in comparison to conventional chemotherapeutics. Targeted therapeutics are aimed at defects found in cancer cells that are not present in the highly-proliferative cells of normal tissues. These defects include dys regulated oncogenes and DNA repair defects that cause cells to rely heavily on the DNA damage response (DDR) and checkpoint signaling. This association indicates that the DDR may include promising targets for targeted therapeutics. Examples of such therapeutics currently under investigation and in clinical use are described here, including inhibitors of PARP, DNA-PKcs and the ATR-CHK1 signaling pathway. Targeted therapeutics not only offer the promise of killing cancers with reduced side effects, but are well suited to use in combination with other therapeutics to increase efficacy and kill cancers before drug-resistance can occur.

Keywords Targeted therapeutics · Synthetic lethality · DNA damage response · HR deficiency · Chemotherapeutic resistance · Oncogenic stress · Checkpoint inhibition · Replication stress · ATR/ATM/DNA-PK/PARP/p53/BRCA

L. R. Butler · O. Gilad
Atrin Pharmaceuticals, Pennsylvania Biotechnology Center, Doylestown, PA, USA
e-mail: laura.butler@atrinpharma.com; oren.gilad@atrinpharma.com

E. J. Brown (✉)
Department of Cancer Biology, Abramson Family Cancer Research Institute, Perelman School of Medicine, University of Pennsylvania, Philadelphia, PA, USA
e-mail: brownej@upenn.edu

© Springer International Publishing AG, part of Springer Nature 2018
J. Pollard, N. Curtin (eds.), *Targeting the DNA Damage Response for Anti-Cancer Therapy*, Cancer Drug Discovery and Development, https://doi.org/10.1007/978-3-319-75836-7_2

2.1   Problems Associated with Current Chemo- and Radiotherapies

Chemotherapy is the most common form of treatment for cancer. Chemotherapies poison all dividing cells, leading to cell death or growth inhibition. Because cell division is key to the pathologies caused by cancer, cancer cells are exquisitely sensitive to chemotherapeutics. Unfortunately, while chemotherapeutics have proven to be extremely effective in killing cancer cells, they are also toxic to dividing cells in normal healthy tissues of the body, such as cells of the immune system, gut, and hair follicles, which underlies the common side effects of neutropenia, anemia, diarrhea, vomiting and hair loss (NIH 2015). Notably, the toxic nature of these compounds, and the essential functions of affected normal tissues, limits the doses these drugs can be administered at, thereby also constraining their therapeutic efficacy and ultimately fostering the acquisition of resistance.

Cancers are heterogeneous and constantly evolving. However, the administration of chemotherapeutics accelerates this process of evolution. The reason most chemotherapeutics are toxic to dividing cells is because they cause DNA damage (Siddick 2002; Hurley 2002). While this damage leads to the death of some cancer cells, it concomitantly increases the mutation rate of the surviving fraction of cancer cells as well as putting them under selection pressure to tolerate a variety of stress conditions that would normally not be possible. Acquired abilities include the loss of programed cell death pathways that are invoked by DNA damage and that are the ultimate means by which chemotherapies operate. Thus, most cancers ultimately develop resistance to chemotherapeutics.

One opportunity to overcome the development of chemotherapeutic resistance falls squarely on targeting the means by which resistance is acquired. Since most chemotherapeutics are at least initially effective, targeting resistance would appear to be an obvious approach to increasing benefit. However, preventing the development of resistance, while simultaneously administering compounds that cause the genetic changes needed to acquire resistance, has its challenges. An alternative approach is to use fundamentally distinct second-line therapies after chemotherapeutic resistance has been acquired. Ideally, these second-line therapies would include treatments that selectively kill cells that have lost the "checkpoint" mechanisms that promote cell death when DNA is damaged.

In addition to toxic side-effects during treatment, chemotherapeutics sometimes cause therapy-related cancers. These secondary cancers are caused by the genetic mutations and deletions in normal cells generated during chemotherapeutic treatment, the most common of which being acute myeloid leukemia (AML) and myelodysplastic syndrome (MDS) (American Cancer Society 2014; Curtis et al. 2006). Therapy-related cancers arising from chemotherapeutic alkylating agents have proven difficult to treat and are associated with poor outcomes. In summary, while chemotherapeutics can be efficacious at treating some cancers, at least initially, the high toxicities, the development of drug resistance and the occurrence of therapy-related cancers demonstrate the need for better and more selective targeted cancer treatments.

2.2   The Promise of Targeted Cancer Treatment

Targeted cancer therapies differ from conventional chemotherapeutics in that they inhibit the proteins and pathways that are either dysregulated in cancer or rendered more important by such dysregulation. Because the alterations being targeted are better associated with the cancer than normal tissues, these treatment strategies will putatively suffer fewer consequences than chemotherapeutics. Importantly, decreased toxicity in normal tissues may make such treatments less dose-limited. Indeed, patient studies and in silico modeling of the evolution of antibiotic resistance predict that higher initial kill rates suppress the acquisition of resistance, highlighting the potential benefit of higher dosing for anti-cancer drugs.

In addition, targeted treatments do not damage DNA directly. Although some treatments may ultimately indirectly cause DNA damage (e.g., PARP, ATR, CHK1 and WEE1 inhibition), this damage may be more confined and less likely to foster cancer evolution than the damage caused by chemotherapeutics. These qualities also delay the acquisition of resistance. Finally, while therapy-related cancers pose an unknown risk factor, such outcomes may occur less frequently with targeted agents than with chemo- and radiation-therapy due to greater cancer selectivity.

The first generation of targeted therapies focused on pathways that cancer cells rely on for growth or survival. These cancer drivers include mutations or amplified expression of oncogenes, the cellular counterparts of genes originally identified as cell growth regulators in oncogenic viruses. The value of targeting growth factor signaling pathways has been demonstrated by inhibition of BCR-ABL with Gleevec for treating CML (An et al. 2010), EML4-ALK with Crizotinib in non-small cell lung cancers (Kwak et al. 2010), and BRAF (V600E) with Vemurafanib in melanomas (Flaherty et al. 2010; Sosman et al. 2012). These approaches have varied widely in success, from long-term remission to response times as short as three months. The key problem with these therapies is the ability of cells to rewire their original dependence on certain pathways to compensatory ones, which are then amplified. The ability to accomplish such a shift in growth factor dependence dictates the efficacy of these treatments.

A fundamentally distinct approach has focused on inhibiting pathways that cancer cells rely upon indirectly through alterations in other networks. This approach, known as synthetic lethality, was originally a genetic tool used to test the assignment of genes to specific pathways and define compensatory pathways in model organisms. Using this tool, when two genes are deleted, the result reflects whether they operate in the same pathway (epistatic) or in distinct compensatory pathways (synthetic lethal) as described in Fig. 2.1.

The promise of applying this approach to cancer treatment is clear. Mutations associated with cancer can cause an increased, or essential, reliance on other pathways that compensate for problems arising from these mutations. By targeting these compensatory networks, one can kill the cancer cells specifically. Such therapies are tolerated by non-cancer cells by virtue of the alternate primary pathway remaining intact. Specific gain-of-function oncogenic mutations are among these cancer-associated mutations because they invoke stress responses to signaling

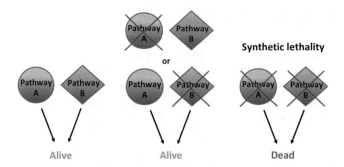

Fig. 2.1 Synthetic lethality. Knocking out either pathway alone does not affect the viability of the cells, but knocking out both pathways results in cell death and thus causes synthetic lethality

pathway perturbations. In addition, deleterious cancer-associated mutations, ones that eliminate safeguards that prevent cells from undergoing uncontrolled cell growth or induce apoptosis (tumor suppressor genes), can be targeted by synthetic lethal approaches, based similarly on associated changes in cellular function. Remarkably, some of the pathways most relied upon due to oncogenic and tumor suppressor gene mutations are involved in the DNA damage response (DDR). Notably, specific DNA repair and cell cycle checkpoint genes that operate within the DDR are frequently mutated in cancer and these mutations create their own dependencies on compensatory DDR genes. In summary, the proteins involved in the DDR are excellent drug targets for the treatment of a broad spectrum of cancers since they enable the exploitation of synthetic lethality.

2.3 The DNA Damage Response (DDR)

DNA can be damaged by a wide range of both endogenous and exogenous sources including reactive oxygen species, ultraviolet light, ionizing radiation, chemical agents, and as a result of other cellular processes. DNA double strand breaks (DSBs) are one of the most toxic DNA lesions a cell can encounter and are repaired by two main pathways: homologous recombination (HR) and non-homologous end-joining (NHEJ) (Fig. 2.2). HR uses the homologous sequence on the sister chromatid as a template to faithfully repair damaged DNA, as a result HR can only occur in the late-S and G2 phases of the cell cycle when a second copy of DNA is present. NHEJ has no such requirement, and as such can function throughout the cell cycle, re-ligating broken DNA ends in an error-prone process that can result in the loss of genetic information.

Repair by HR is initiated by MRE11-RAD50-NBS1 (MRN) and Ct-BP interacting protein (CtIP) mediated end resection. The broken DNA is resected generating 3′ ssDNA overhangs that become coated with Replication Protein A (RPA). RPA is subsequently replaced by RAD51, in a BRCA2 dependent manner, mediating strand

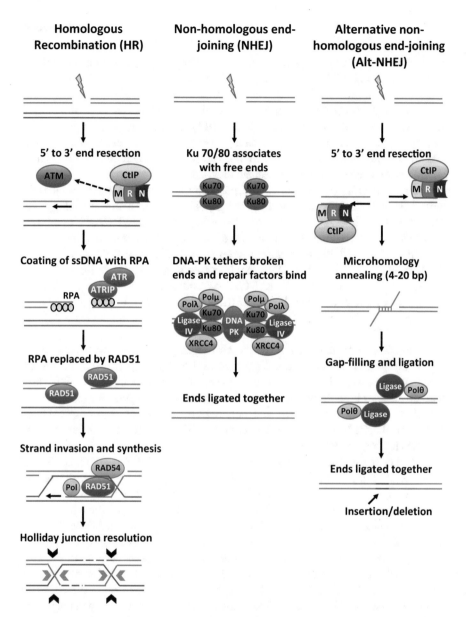

Fig. 2.2 The DNA damage response. *Homologous recombination (HR)* begins with signaling of the DSB in which ATM plays an early role. 5′–3′ end resection by MRN-CtIP is followed by coating of the ssDNA with RPA which triggers checkpoint initiation by ATR. RPA is displaced by RAD51, which along with RAD54 initiates strand exchange and homology search. Polymerases use the homologous sequence as a template to synthesize new DNA, resulting in the formation of cross-over structures (Holliday junctions) that are cleaved by resolvases at the end of the HR pathway. *Non-homologous end joining (NHEJ)* begins with association of the Ku70/80 heterodimer on the broken DNA ends which mediates binding of other repair factors, including DNA-PK which tethers the broken ends, and polymerases μ and λ which work together with ligase IV and XRCC4 to fill in the gaps and join the DNA ends. *Alternative non-homologous end-joining (alt-NHEJ)* begins with small-scale resection of the broken ends by MRN-CtIP, the resected ends then anneal at regions of microhomology where polymerase θ works together with ligases to fill and seal the gap, often resulting in insertions or deletions

invasion and homology search. Once the homologous sequence has been identified, new complementary DNA is synthesized by DNA polymerases. During HR cross-over structures known as Holliday junctions are formed between the invading strand and template DNA. These structures are resolved by resolvases MUS81-EME1, SLX1-SLX4 and GEN1 (Matos and West 2014). RAD54 plays multiple roles in HR, promoting chromatin remodeling prior to end processing, aiding RAD51mediated strand invasion and homology search, and finally stimulating MUS81-EME1 resolvase activity (Mazin et al. 2010).

The second DSB repair pathway, NHEJ, can either directly ligate blunt DNA ends or ligate ends with very short overhangs, but does not require homology. The KU70/80 heterodimer is rapidly recruited to broken DNA ends, DNA-PKcs binds to the KU70/80 heterodimer to become the active DNA-PK complex (Gottlieb and Jackson 1993). DNA-PK is important in tethering the broken DNA ends together (Graham et al. 2016), while DNA polymerases μ and λ, DNA ligase IV and XRCC4 are also recruited to the KU70/80 heterodimer, leading to gap-filling and ligation to complete the repair by NHEJ (Chang et al. 2017). In some cases where limited resection is required DNA-PK can bind and activate the nuclease Artemis (Ma et al. 2002).

In the absence of functional NHEJ, a third repair pathway known as alternative NHEJ (alt-NHEJ) or micro-homology mediated end-joining (MMEJ) can repair DSBs. While classical NHEJ has no requirement for homology, alt-NHEJ uses 4–20 bp of microhomology. Alt-NHEJ relies on different enzymes for resection and gap-filling utilizing MRN, CtIP and polymerase θ, and not requiring KU70/80 (Chang et al. 2017). Classical and alternative NHEJ can result in insertions and deletions leading to mutation.

The phosphatidylinositol 3-kinase-related kinases (PIKKs) ATM, ATR and DNA-PK play important signaling functions in the repair pathways, with overlapping roles in checkpoint activation. ATM is activated in the initial stages of the DSB response, prior to repair pathway choice, triggering a signaling cascade to instigate repair and checkpoint activation. ATR is activated by single-stranded DNA (ssDNA) that arises at single stranded breaks, stalled replication forks or upon resection at DSBs, protecting stalled forks and also stimulating checkpoint activation. Whereas DNA-PK plays a more pathway-specific role, being activated in the early stages of NHEJ where it functions in end-tethering and recruitment of other NHEJ repair factors (Branzei and Foiani 2008). These kinases are critical for checkpoint signaling and DNA repair, their roles are discussed in more detail later in the chapter.

The choice of repair pathway is influenced by the interplay between cell cycle phase and the balance of repair factors at the break. Chromatin compaction varies throughout the cell cycle and this, together with the absence or presence of sister chromatids and cell cycle regulated expression of repair factors plays a huge part in determining the pathway used for repair, with NHEJ repairing DSBs in G1, HR favored in late S/G2 and NHEJ dominating again in G2 (Branzei and Foiani 2008; Kakarougkas and Jeggo 2014). Another determining factor is the balance and competition of repair factors at the break, while 53BP1 has been shown to inhibit end resection (thus promoting NHEJ over HR), this inhibition can be overcome by BRCA1 which aids in the removal of 53BP1 to allow resection, stimulating HR

(Bunting et al. 2010). The DDR is a complex process involving multiple pathways coordinated by many proteins, as such these repair pathways and associated checkpoint signaling are frequently attenuated in cancer cells, providing the basis for many treatment strategies as discussed throughout this chapter.

2.4   Oncogenes Cause Genomic Instability and DDR Activation

Many proto-oncogenes function in signaling pathways to promote cellular proliferation. Alterations that cause increased expression or activity of these genes convert these normal growth regulators into "oncogenes", which aberrantly drive cellular proliferation and tumor development. Common oncogenes include MYC and mutated forms of the RAS family. As a transcription factor, MYC overexpression causes unregulated expression of genes that promote cell proliferation. The RAS family of proteins are small GTPase signaling factors that short-circuit growth factor regulated signaling when mutated and locked in the GTP-bound active state. MYC amplification is observed in 50–70% of all tumors (Nilsson and Cleveland 2003; Vita and Henriksson 2006), and ~30% of all cancers harbor mutations in the RAS family of oncogenes (Fernandez-Medarde and Santos 2011).

Oncogene expression produces what is known as "oncogenic stress", a vague description of the effects of dysregulation of pro-growth signaling pathways. More specifically, the hyperactivation of one component of the multifocal signaling network normally generated by growth factor receptor engagement leads to imbalances in metabolites and proteins, which negatively impact normal cellular growth and homeostasis. The effects of such imbalances include proteotoxic and genotoxic stresses, which subsequently cause the activation of numerous stress response pathways as countermeasures. For example, oncogene expression, while initially inducing a period of hyperproliferation, ultimately causes the activation of the DDR and oncogene-induced senescence (OIS). However, dysregulation of these processes allows bypass of OIS and continued proliferation of the cancer cells (Bartkova et al. 2005; Bartkova et al. 2006; Di Micco et al. 2006; Gorgoulis et al. 2005), even with persistent DNA damage. Indeed, activating mutations in RAS and overexpression of MYC have long been known to trigger genomic instability, as characterized by gross chromosomal aberrations and gene amplification (Denko et al. 1994; Felsher and Bishop 1999). Oncogenic stress promotes the formation of DNA double strand breaks (DSBs), and a large fraction of these result from the collapse of stalled replication forks (Zeman and Cimprich 2014). Replication fork stalling can result from a variety of mechanisms, including deoxynucleotide (dNTP) depletion (Bester et al. 2011), unrepaired base lesions (Waters et al. 2009), mis-incorporated ribonucleotides (Williams et al. 2016), reactive oxygen species (ROS) (Branzei and Foiani 2010), aberrant DNA secondary structures (such as hairpins, triplex and quadruplex DNA) (Boyer et al. 2013), and premature origin firing before the DNA synthetic machinery can be fully expressed and employed (Toledo et al. 2013).

Oncogenic stress has been found to increase DNA breakage at common fragile sites (CFS) (Bartkova et al. 2005; Gorgoulis et al. 2005), and 20–50% of cancer-related chromosomal translocations and deletions contain breakpoints associated with these sites (Dillon et al. 2010; Bignell et al. 2010). CFS are detected as gaps or breaks in metaphase chromosomes following treatments that cause replicative stress (Glover et al. 1984). By preventing M phase entry under replication stress, the ATR-CHK1 checkpoint signaling pathway is integral to averting chromosome breaks at these fragile sites (Glover et al. 1984; Brown and Baltimore 2000; Brown and Baltimore 2003; Casper et al. 2002). Breakage of these sites is strongly correlated with the escape of cells with under-replicated DNA into M phase (Casper et al. 2002). It has been proposed that the breakage and repair of these fragile sites results in a significant fraction of cancer-associated chromosomal re-arrangements and loss of heterozygosity (LOH) and that this is due to the replicative stress generated by oncogene expression (Dillon et al. 2010; Bignell et al. 2010; Halazonetis et al. 2008). Notably, however, most cancer-associated breakpoints are not in CFS and the mechanisms underlying breakage at these other sites are yet to be defined.

2.5 Tumor Suppression Through Checkpoint Activation and DNA Repair

While oncogenes activate pathways that drive cancer progression, another set of genes, known as tumor suppressors, limit tumor initiation and progression through their involvement in cell cycle checkpoints and DNA repair. Loss or attenuation of the function of these genes can disrupt normal regulatory pathways, akin to the effects of oncogenes, and foster cancer progression.

DSBs and are sensed by the MRE11-RAD50-NBS1 (MRN) complex (Lavin 2007). The MRN complex activates the kinase ATM (ataxia telangiectasia mutated), which phosphorylates a number of proteins triggering a signaling cascade that leads to the recruitment of important downstream factors for the repair of DSBs and checkpoint activation. One of the earliest events in the DSB signaling pathway is the phosphorylation of the histone variant H2AX by ATM (Rogakou et al. 1998). MDC1 (mediator of DNA damage checkpoint protein 1) binds to the phosphorylated H2AX (γH2AX) and is also itself phosphorylated by ATM (Stewart et al. 2003). The ubiquitin ligase RNF8 (RING-finger-containing nuclear factor 8) binds to phosphorylated MDC1 (Kolas et al. 2007) and initiates a signaling cascade that involves recruitment of downstream proteins via generation and binding of ubiquitin conjugates, ultimately leading to the localization of BRCA1 (breast cancer susceptibility gene 1), 53BP1 (p53 binding protein 1), and co-factors required for the repair of the double stranded break (Mailand et al. 2007) (Fig. 2.3).

ATM phosphorylates hundreds of substrates in response to DNA damage (Matsuoka et al. 2007; Shiloh and Ziv 2013). While a number of these phosphorylation events are important for initiating DNA repair events, ATM also plays a crucial role in activating cell cycle checkpoints in response to DNA damage. ATM activity

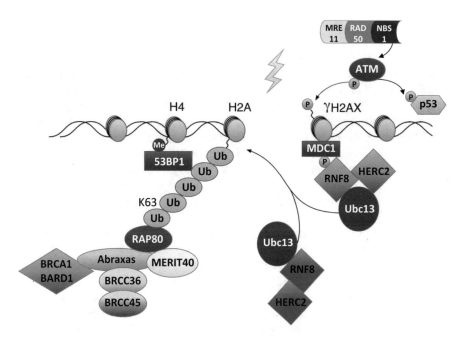

Fig. 2.3 DNA double stand break (DSB) signaling. DSBs are sensed by the MRE11/RAD50/ NBS1 (MRN) complex which phosphorylates ATM, leading to the downstream phosphorylation of an array of proteins including p53, H2AX and MDC1. MDC1 binds to γH2AX where it recruits the E3 ubiquitin ligase RNF8. RNF8 interacts with the E2 ubiquitin-conjugating enzyme UBC13 to begin building K63-linked ubiquitin chains on histones surrounding the DSB, a second ubiquitin ligase, RNF168, works together with UBC13 to amplify theses chains. A third ubiquitin ligase, HERC2, stabilizes the interactions between RNF8/RNF168 and UBC13. RAP80 binds to the K63-linked ubiquitin chains allowing recruitment of the BRCA1 A complex (RAP80, Abraxas, BRCA1, MERIT40, BRCC36 and BRCC45). BRCA1 is critical for repair of DSBs by homologous recombination. 53BP1 is important in the repair of DSBs by non-homologous end-joining and is recruited to DSBs in a manner dependent on both RNF8/RNF168 ubiquitination and H4K20me2

leads to the stabilization and activation of p53 through both direct and indirect phosphorylation events, resulting in activation of the G1/S-phase cell cycle checkpoint regulation and p53-mediated apoptosis (Shiloh and Ziv 2013). p53 co-ordinates checkpoint activation and apoptosis by controlling the cellular transcriptome. The key p53-regulated event that halts G1/S-phase progression is the increase in p21 expression. p21 is a cyclin-dependent kinase inhibitor that prevents G1/S transition by suppressing Cyclin E (CCNE)- and Cyclin A (CCNA)-associated CDK2 activities (Harper et al. 1995). When excessive DNA damage is generated, or normal levels of damage are left unrepaired, apoptotic pathways can be triggered by p53-dependent transcription of the Bcl-2 family of genes that promote apoptosis (PUMA, BAK, and BAX). p53 can also function to induce apoptosis in a transcription-independent manner causing permeabilization of the mitochondrial membrane and release of cytochrome c (Kiraz et al. 2016). Due to its myriad roles in DNA repair, cell cycle regulation, and apoptosis, p53 is considered one of the most important tumor suppressor genes, a status confirmed by the fact that it is the most commonly altered gene in human cancers, with mutation or loss of p53 in more than 50% of all cancers (Hollstein et al. 1991). Germline p53 mutation results in Li-Fraumeni syndrome, a syndrome associated with a high risk of early onset and multiple malignancies (Malkin et al. 1990). With critical roles in the DSB DNA damage response, ATM and MRN are also important tumor suppressors. Germline heterozygous ATM mutations cause Ataxia Telangiectasia, while germline mutations in NBS1 (part of the MRN complex) result in Nijmegen breakage syndrome, diseases characterized by neurologic disorders and an increased predisposition to cancer. High frequencies of somatic ATM mutations have been observed in lymphoid malignancies (Gumy-Pause et al. 2004), while somatic mutations in the components of the MRN complex have also been observed at lower levels in multiple cancer types (Regal et al. 2013; Varon et al. 2001).

It is well established that germline mutations in the DNA damage repair genes BRCA1 and BRCA2 are associated with hereditary predisposition to breast, ovarian, prostate and pancreatic cancers. BRCA1 and BRCA2 play important yet distinct roles in the repair of DSBs by homologous recombination. BRCA1 is recruited to DSBs via the RNF8/RNF168 generated K63-linked ubiquitin chains which are bound by RAP80, a central component of the BRCA1-A complex. While the BRCA1-A complex is responsible for the recruitment of BRCA1 to DSBs, the BRCA1-B, C and BRCA1-PALB2-BRCA2 complexes are important for the diverse roles of BRCA1 in the DSB response as described in Fig. 2.4. PALB2 interacts with and bridges BRCA1 and BRCA2 (Sy et al. 2009; Xia et al. 2006), BRCA2 in turn binds RAD51, an important repair factor required for strand invasion during homologous recombination (Baumann and West 1998). The BRCA1-B complex is comprised of BRCA1, BACH1 and TOPBP1 and influences the S-phase checkpoint (Gong et al. 2010) and the Fanconi Anemia pathway for the repair of inter-strand crosslinks (ICLs) (Litman et al. 2005). In the BRCA1-C complex BRCA1 interacts with CtIP and MRN, mediating end resection (Chen et al. 2008), an essential process required for the repair of DSBs by homologous recombination.

Hereditary mutations in the BRCA genes are considered autosomal dominant as only one copy of the mutated allele needs to be inherited to confer an increased cancer risk. A somatic mutation in the second allele is required for disease progression. The estimated prevalence of BRCA1 and BRCA2 mutation carriers is 0.07–0.22% in the general population (Anglian Breast Cancer Study Group 2000), with about 2.4% of patients with breast cancer possessing a BRCA mutation (although this number varies and is considerably higher for the Ashkenazi Jewish population) (Malone et al. 2006). Somatic mutations, copy number variations or epigenetic silencing of the BRCA or other HR genes have been detected in approximately half of all high grade serous ovarian cancer cases (Cancer Genome Atlas Research Network 2011), demonstrating the importance of dysregulation of the HR pathway in these cancers. Besides breast and ovarian cancers, mutations in HR genes have also been observed in various other cancers including PALB2 in pancreatic cancer (Waddell et al. 2015) and BRCA1 in lung cancers (Marsit et al. 2004).

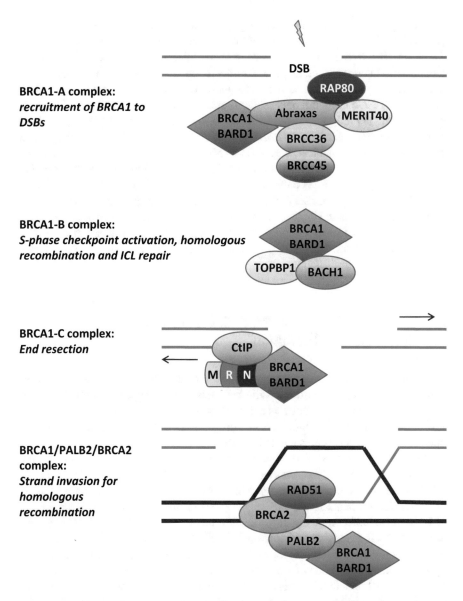

BRCA1-A complex:
recruitment of BRCA1 to DSBs

BRCA1-B complex:
S-phase checkpoint activation, homologous recombination and ICL repair

BRCA1-C complex:
End resection

BRCA1/PALB2/BRCA2 complex:
Strand invasion for homologous recombination

Fig. 2.4 BRCA1 complexes. BRCA1-A complex is responsible for recruitment of BRCA1 to DSBs, RAP80 binds to the RNF8-RNF168 generated polyubiquitin chains at DSBs, Abraxas acts as a scaffold protein bringing together the other components of the BRCA1-A complex (BRCA1, MERIT40, BRCC36 and BRCC45). The BRCA1-B complex, comprised of BRCA1, BACH1 and TOPBP1, has multiple roles including S-phase checkpoint activation, homologous recombination and interstrand crosslink repair. The BRCA1-C complex (BRCA1, CIP and MRN) plays a key role in mediating end resection, preparing the DNA for strand invasion, a process enabled by the BRCA1/PALB2/BRCA2 complex for the repair of DSBs by homologous recombination

Although deleterious mutations in any one component of the HR pathway may be infrequent, the combined frequency of loss-of-function in this pathway can be high. The term "BRCAness" was coined to describe alterations that cause homologous repair defects (Turner et al. 2004) and refers to the similarity in phenotype of these mutations, resulting in responsiveness to similar therapeutic approaches, e.g., PARP inhibition. "BRCAness" not only relates to mutations in well-established HR genes, but also their altered expression. In addition, mutations in other genes have been shown to cause susceptibility to PARP inhibition or platinum therapy, although their role in HR may be unclear, e.g. PTEN (Mendes-Pereira et al. 2009; Lord and Ashworth 2016). Thus, looking for defects in a specific functional pathway rather than mutations in individual pathway components could allow for faster assessment of synthetic lethal approaches and a more rapid advance in applying such treatments to the clinic. Defects in HR force tumor cells to rely on the more error prone repair pathways, driving further mutation in the cancer cells (Zamborszky et al. 2017). This leads to further dys regulation of normal cellular processes, driving tumor development and proliferation.

2.6   Targeting HR and ATM Deficiencies with PARP and DNA-PK Inhibition

Deficiencies in DNA repair pathways render cancer cells susceptible to therapies that would normally trigger these pathways, causing tumor-specific synthetic lethality as the cancer cells cannot repair the damage, ultimately triggering cell death. PARP and DNA-PKcs inhibitors are two drug classes that have recently been developed to target cancers with such deficiencies.

PARP inhibitors have displayed excellent efficacy in BRCA1/2 mutant ovarian cancers (Bryant et al. 2005; Farmer et al. 2005; Leung et al. 2011). PARP (poly-ADP-ribose polymerase) is an enzyme involved in the early stages of base excision repair (BER) and single strand break repair (SSBR), one model to explain the activity of PARP inhibitors is trapping of the inactive enzyme on the damaged DNA leading to replication fork stalling and subsequent DSB formation. Thus, in the context of HR deficiency there is persistence of DNA lesions that would normally be repaired by HR, causing cytotoxicity (Murai et al. 2012). This synthetic lethal approach has led to the development of a series of PARP inhibitors that are now in clinical trials, with Olaparib representing the first PARP inhibitor that was approved by the European Medicines Agency and the US Food and Drug Administration (FDA) in 2014 for the treatment of BRCA1/2 mutant ovarian cancers and FDA approval for BRCA1/2-deficient breast cancers in January of 2018. Olaparib was joined by two additional PARP inhibitors, rucaparib and nirarparib, in FDA approval for BRCA1/2-deficient ovarian cancer in 2016 and 2017, respectively.

While suppression of NHEJ by 53BP1 deletion or DNA-PK inhibition has been shown to restore HR function and resistance to PARP inhibition in BRCA mutated cells (Bouwman et al. 2010; Patel et al. 2011), it has also been shown that suppression of NHEJ can exacerbate the effects of HR deficiency, indicating some overlapping compensatory functions of these repair pathways (Couedel et al. 2004). DNA-PK is activated by DSBs, phosphorylating a range of substrates including CHK2 (Li and Stern 2005) and H2AX (Stiff et al. 2004), which are also phosphorylated by ATM. While ATM is important in initiating DNA resection for repair of DSBs by HR, DNA-PK is integral to repair of DSBs by NHEJ. Therefore it is not surprising, given their vital roles in the respective HR and NHEJ DSB repair pathways, that deletion of ATM and DNA-PK are embryonic lethal in mice (Gurley and Kemp 2001). Furthermore, it has been shown that ATM defective cells are unable to repair DSBs when DNA-PK is inhibited, and that inhibition of DNA-PK in mice bearing ATM defective lymphomas display prolonged survival (Riabinska et al. 2013), thus demonstrating the potential clinical benefit of treating patients with ATM deficient tumors with DNA-PK targeted therapies.

2.7 Targeting Oncogenic Stress, ATM-p53 Loss, and HR Deficiency with ATR, CHK1 and WEE1 Inhibitors

The common cancer-associated defects outlined above resulting in oncogenic stress and failure of the DDR provide an excellent mechanism for specific targeting of cancer cells by abrogating the S-G2-M checkpoints. While ATM and DNA-PK are important in the repair of DSBs, ATR is integral to the protection of single-stranded DNA (ssDNA). Single stranded DNA is generated at stalled replication forks and at sites of end resection, which are formed during the repair of DSBs. Upon being exposed, ssDNA is rapidly coated by the nucleoprotein RPA, and this nucleoprotein filament is bound by the interdependent ATRIP-ATR complex (Zou and Elledge 2003) (Fig. 2.5).

ATR initiates the intra-S and G2/M checkpoints by activating the downstream kinase CHK1 (Liu et al. 2000), CHK1 in turn phosphorylates CDC25A, leading to its degradation (Sorensen et al. 2003; Zhao et al. 2002; Mailand et al. 2000). The phosphatase CDC25A plays an important role in checkpoint initiation by removing the inhibitory phosphorylation within the ATP triphosphate-interacting regions of CDK2 (Mailand et al. 2000; Welburn et al. 2007; Falck et al. 2001; Atherton-Fessler et al. 1994) and CDK1 (Atherton-Fessler et al. 1994; Norbury et al. 1991; Strausfeld et al. 1991), initiating the intra-S and G2/M checkpoints respectively (regulation of the cell cycle is described in more detail in Fig. 2.6). Activation of the intra-S checkpoint suppresses inappropriate origin firing (Feijoo et al. 2001; Merrick et al. 2004; Santocanale and Diffley 1998), allowing time for damage repair and restart of stalled or collapsed replication forks, while the G2/M checkpoint prevents inappropriate entry of cells with incompletely-replicated DNA or resected DSBs into mitosis (Kastan and Bartek 2004). Thus, activation of the checkpoints prevents inappropriate proliferation and counters the negative effects of oncogenic stress.

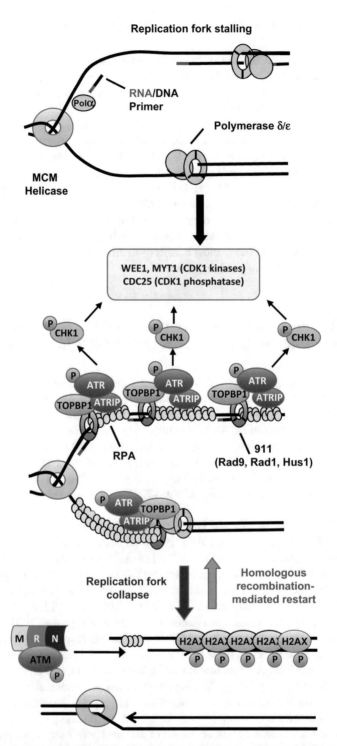

Fig. 2.5 Replication fork collapse. Replication fork stalling occurs when the DNA polymerase becomes uncoupled from MCM helicase leading to the exposure of single stranded DNA (ssDNA). The single stranded DNA becomes coated with RPA which is bound by ATR-ATRIP.

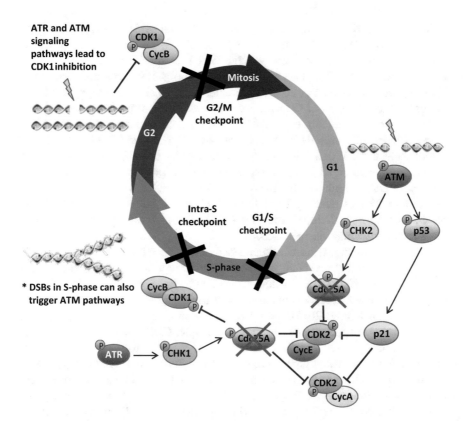

Fig. 2.6 The roles of ATM and ATR in checkpoint activation. DSBs in G1 lead to activation to ATM. ATM phosphorylates CHK2 which in turn phosphorylates CDC25A leading to its degradation. The phosphatase CDC25A is no longer able to remove the inhibitory phosphorylation of CDK2, thereby preventing activation of the CDK2-Cyclin E and CDK2-Cyclin A complexes and thus preventing progression from G1 to S-phase. ATM also activates p53 both directly and indirectly, leading to increased transcription of p21 which also suppresses CDK2-associated activities as well as triggering apoptosis. In S-phase stalled replication forks trigger ATR, leading to CHK1 phosphorylation and activation, which ultimately drives the degradation of CDC25A and the inhibition of CDK2 by WEE1 and MYT1. Inhibition of CDK2-Cyclin E and CDK2-Cyclin A enforces the intra-S checkpoint. Furthermore, DSBs occurring in S-phase can also trigger ATM-regulated pathways, contributing to cell cycle delay and apoptosis. In G2 the concerted efforts of ATR and ATM in response to DSBs results in inhibition of the CDK1-Cyclin B complex triggering the G2/M checkpoint

◀

Fig. 2.5 (continued) The 911 complex is also loaded onto the RPA coated ssDNA recruiting the ATR activator TOPBP1. Activated ATR phosphorylates CHK1 kinase which initiates checkpoint activation by regulating the activity of the downstream kinases WEE1 and MYT1 and the phosphatase CDC25A. Checkpoint activation allows time for resolution of the stalled fork before replication can continue. In some circumstances, such as loss of ATR activity, replication forks collapse into DSBs, triggering repair by homologous recombination before replication restart can occur

The ATR-CHK1 pathway not only controls the cell cycle checkpoints through degradation of CDC25A but also affects the inhibitory phosphorylation of CDK1 and CDK2 by regulating the activity of the WEE1 kinase. CDK1/2 are phosphorylated on Thr14 by WEE1 (Parker and Piwnica-Worms 1992) and both Thr14 and Tyr15 by MYT1 (Booher et al. 1997; Mueller et al. 1995), these phosphorylation events lead to inhibition of CDK1/2 activity by reducing affinity for their peptide/protein susbtrates (Welburn et al. 2007). CHK1 is able to phosphorylate WEE1 on Ser549, which increases the interaction between WEE1 and the 14-3-3 proteins, greatly enhancing WEE1's inhibitory kinase activity towards CDK1 (Lee et al. 2001). In an additional layer of regulation CHK1 phosphorylation of CDC25 increases CDC25 binding by the 14-3-3 complex, which leads to cytoplasmic retention of CDC25 thus reducing its ability to dephosphorylate and activate CDK1 in the nucleus (Chen et al. 2003). Thus, the ATR-CHK1 pathway regulates checkpoint initiation through multiple mechanisms.

In addition to triggering checkpoint activation the ATR-CHK1 pathway also plays an important role in stabilizing the replication fork. The main proposed mechanisms by which ATR-CHK1 mediates fork stabilization are the regulation of repair enzymes including helicases, nucleases and translocases and prevention of S-M phase transition (Cortez 2015). Indeed, in several respects, cell cycle regulation and fork stabilization appear to be linked. For example, CDK1 activity stimulates the interaction of nucleases MUS81-EME1 with SLX1-SLX4, forming a complex that promotes the coordinated processing of Holliday junctions in G2/M (Wyatt et al. 2013). These nucleases have also been found to cleave stalled replication forks generated by inhibition of ATR (Ragland et al. 2013; Couch et al. 2013) or WEE1 (Beck et al. 2012; Dominguez-Kelly et al. 2011), which causes replication fork collapse into DSBs. Notably, inhibition of CDK1 activity by WEE1 in S-phase prevents premature formation of the SLX4-MUS81 complex, thus preventing inappropriate cleavage of replication intermediates in this phase of the cell cycle (Duda et al. 2016). CDK1-Cyclin B (CCNB), AURKA and PLK1function in a positive feedback loop that has also been implicated in fork collapse upon inhibition of ATR, with the premature activation of PLK1 proposed to promote replisome disassembly (Ragland et al. 2013). In addition, it is well established that elevated CDK2 activity can cause premature firing of replication origins, before sufficient E2F-driven expression of a complete complement of replication factors can be attained, and cause more rapid depletion of nucleotide pools. These events can cause an increase in replication fork stalling and dependence on ATR, CHK1 and WEE1 for stability. Thus, inhibition of ATR-CHK1-mediated checkpoint activity in the context of oncogenic signaling permits the premature initiation of signaling events that ultimately disrupt DNA replication and destabilize the replication fork. Although traditionally it is considered that ATR and CHK1 mediate fork protection through checkpoint activation and downstream events, other evidence accumulated over the past two decades implies roles for these kinases in preventing fork collapse by additional more direct means. A notable example of this is the phosphorylation of the annealing helicase SMARCAL1 by ATR, which restricts its fork regression activity thus preventing aberrant fork collapse (Couch et al. 2013). ATR also plays a role in the repair of inter-strand crosslinks (ICLs), structures that can cause fork stalling, by phosphory-lating FANCI and promoting monoubiquitination of FANCD2 (Andreassen et al. 2004; Ishiai et al. 2008), a crucial step in the repair of ICLs. Therefore, current evidence indicates that the mechanism of DNA breakage following ATR inhibi-tion may depend on multiple conditions, including: the events that cause ATR activation; the activation state of the AURKA-PLK1-CDK1 kinase circuit; and the rate of reformation of the replication fork by homologous recombination after fork collapse into DSBs.

In light of the mechanism of fork collapse driven by ATR, CHK1 and WEE1 inhibition several opportunities exist for selective cancer targeting. One opportunity is synthetic lethal interaction of oncogenic stress with such inhibition. As discussed earlier, oncogenic stress triggers replication stress, causing cancer cells to activate and rely on ATR for fork stability (Halazonetis et al. 2008). Therefore it follows that disruption of fork stability by inhibition of ATR, CHK1 or WEE1 will be detrimen-tal to these cells, as has been demonstrated by the synthetic lethal interaction of ATR suppression in RAS and MYC transformed cancers (Gilad et al. 2010; Murga et al. 2011; Schoppy et al. 2012; Toledo et al. 2011) and CHK1 inhibition in MYC driven lymphomas (Murga et al. 2011; Ferrao et al. 2012).

Another opportunity for synthetic lethal interaction is represented by the poten-tial for targeting HR defective cancers with ATR/CHK1 inhibitors. Similar to their sensitivity to platinum therapy and PARP inhibitors, HR-deficient tumors are also sensitive to ATR/CHK1 inhibition (Kim et al. 2016; Krajewska et al. 2015). Conflicting reports exist regarding the effects of ATR inhibition on HR, with some demonstrating that a loss of ATR activity results in reduction of HR (Prevo et al. 2012; Yazinski et al. 2017; Sorensen et al. 2005) while others indicate an increase in markers of HR in response to ATR inhibition (Chanoux et al. 2009). Nevertheless, it is clear that inhibition of the ATR/CHK1 pathway results in fork collapse and DSB formation (Brown and Baltimore 2003; Toledo et al. 2011; Fokas et al. 2012; Cortez 2015), and that HR-deficient tumors are susceptible to this treatment. Presumably, this increased susceptibility is due either to epistatic hypomorph sensi-tivity caused by further impedance of residual HR activity by ATR/CHK1 inhibi-tion, or to increased persistence of ATRi/CHKi-mediated DSBs due to delayed reformation of the replication fork structure by HR (Chanoux et al. 2009).

Although PARP inhibition has proven effective in the treatment of BRCA1/2 mutant ovarian cancers, PARPi resistance is typically acquired within months of treatment (Audeh et al. 2010; Chiarugi 2012). However, even though the mechanism of resis-tance to PARPi and platinum treatment most often involves the reacquisition of HR function; cisplatin and PARPi-resistant tumors remain susceptible to ATR/CHK1 inhi-bition (Yazinski et al. 2017; Mohni et al. 2015). This may be the product of synthetic lethality with oncogenic stress that is also present in these cells. Thus ATR/CHK1 inhibition could be an effective co-treatment with platinum and PARPi therapies, as demonstrated in the treatment of BRCA-mutant ovarian cancers (Kim et al. 2016), or could be useful as follow-up treatment after platinum/PARPi resistance is acquired.

ATRi/CHK1i also causes synthetic lethality with ATM and p53 deficiency (Reaper et al. 2011). ATM is important in the early stages of HR resection and together with p53 inactivation of the G1/S phase cell cycle checkpoint (Shiloh and Ziv 2013). Therefore, ATM/p53 deficiency in combination with ATRi/CHK1i causes nearly complete abrogation of the DNA damage response checkpoint function, allowing S-phase breaks to pass through M-phase, and to move once again into S-phase due to ATM-p53 checkpoint loss. This dysregulation of the cell cycle checkpoints and failure to engage HR allows cells to accumulate massive amounts of unrepaired DNA damage ultimately resulting in cell death (Reaper et al. 2011). Given the potential for ATR/CHK1 inhibitors to target cancers exhibiting oncogenic stress and/or HR deficiencies, such drugs have a very high therapeutic potential for targeting a large number and broad spectrum of cancers. Furthermore, the synthetic lethality of ATR inhibition with the described defects observed in cancer cells supports the observation that non-cancer cells may tolerate ATR inhibition, thus increasing the therapeutic benefit of this treatment strategy.

2.8   Future Areas of Research

The advancement in our knowledge of the genetic defects exhibited by different cancers and the emergence of targeted therapies that exploit such defects, demonstrate an important and necessary change to the way we view and treat cancers. As we now enter the era of personalized medicine, a key area of future research will be to define the best treatment strategies based on the mutation spectrum of each cancer. DNA repair defects in cancers represent vulnerability with high potential for exploitation using DNA repair inhibitors for treatment. It is possible that combinations of cancer-associated mutations will predict the benefit of treating with one DNA damage repair inhibitor over another, or the best combinations of these targeted therapies.

Although a solid understanding of the way in which specific cancer-associated defects can be targeted is being developed, there is an urgent need for bioinformatics and systems biology to enhance this understanding and to aid in the identification of cancers that will be susceptible to particular therapies. By combining our wealth of knowledge on cancer-specific defects, as well as enhanced identification of susceptible cancers and improved targeted therapies, a significant increase in the efficacy of cancer treatments, with fewer toxic side effects, is within reach. Therefore, targeted therapies will provide an enormous benefit to cancer patients.

Acknowledgments We would like to thank our support from the National Cancer Institute of the National Institutes of Health under award numbers: R41CA203436 (LB, OG, EJB) and 1R01CA189743 (EJB). Additional funding was provided through the Ben Franklin Technology Partners of Southeastern PA, an initiative of the Pennsylvania Department of Community and Economic Development funded by the Ben Franklin Technology Development Authority (LB, OG), the Pennsylvania Department of Health (EJB), The Basser Center for BRCA Research (EJB), and the Abramson Family Cancer Research Institute (EJB).

References

American Cancer Society 2014 Second cancers in adults. 12/11/14 [cited 2016 11/14/16]; Available from: http://www.cancer.org/acs/groups/cid/documents/webcontent/002043-pdf.pdf

An X et al (2010) BCR-ABL tyrosine kinase inhibitors in the treatment of Philadelphia chromosome positive chronic myeloid leukemia: a review. Leuk Res 34(10):1255–1268

Andreassen PR, D'Andrea AD, Taniguchi T (2004) ATR couples FANCD2 monoubiquitination to the DNA-damage response. Genes Dev 18(16):1958–1963

Anglian Breast Cancer Study Group (2000) Prevalence and penetrance of BRCA1 and BRCA2 mutations in a population-based series of breast cancer cases. Br J Cancer 83(10):1301–1308

Atherton-Fessler S et al (1994) Cell cycle regulation of the p34cdc2 inhibitory kinases. Mol Biol Cell 5(9):989–1001

Audeh MW et al (2010) Oral poly(ADP-ribose) polymerase inhibitor olaparib in patients with BRCA1 or BRCA2 mutations and recurrent ovarian cancer: a proof-of-concept trial. Lancet 376(9737):245–251

Bartkova J et al (2005) DNA damage response as a candidate anti-cancer barrier in early human tumorigenesis. Nature 434(7035):864–870

Bartkova J et al (2006) Oncogene-induced senescence is part of the tumorigenesis barrier imposed by DNA damage checkpoints. Nature 444(7119):633–637

Baumann P, West SC (1998) Role of the human RAD51 protein in homologous recombination and double-stranded-break repair. Trends Biochem Sci 23(7):247–251

Beck H et al (2012) Cyclin-dependent kinase suppression by WEE1 kinase protects the genome through control of replication initiation and nucleotide consumption. Mol Cell Biol 32(20):4226–4236

Bester AC et al (2011) Nucleotide deficiency promotes genomic instability in early stages of cancer development. Cell 145(3):435–446

Bignell GR et al (2010) Signatures of mutation and selection in the cancer genome. Nature 463(7283):893–898

Booher RN, Holman PS, Fattaey A (1997) Human Myt1 is a cell cycle-regulated kinase that inhibits Cdc2 but not Cdk2 activity. J Biol Chem 272(35):22300–22306

Bouwman P et al (2010) 53BP1 loss rescues BRCA1 deficiency and is associated with triple-negative and BRCA-mutated breast cancers. Nat Struct Mol Biol 17(6):688–695

Boyer AS et al (2013) The human specialized DNA polymerases and non-B DNA: vital relationships to preserve genome integrity. J Mol Biol 425(23):4767–4781

Branzei D, Foiani M (2008) Regulation of DNA repair throughout the cell cycle. Nat Rev Mol Cell Biol 9(4):297–308

Branzei D, Foiani M (2010) Maintaining genome stability at the replication fork. Nat Rev Mol Cell Biol 11(3):208–219

Brown EJ, Baltimore D (2000) ATR disruption leads to chromosomal fragmentation and early embryonic lethality. Genes Dev 14(4):397–402

Brown EJ, Baltimore D (2003) Essential and dispensable roles of ATR in cell cycle arrest and genome maintenance. Genes Dev 17(5):615–628

Bryant HE et al (2005) Specific killing of BRCA2-deficient tumours with inhibitors of poly(ADP-ribose) polymerase. Nature 434(7035):913–917

Bunting SF et al (2010) 53BP1 inhibits homologous recombination in Brca1-deficient cells by blocking resection of DNA breaks. Cell 141(2):243–254

Cancer Genome Atlas Research Network (2011) Integrated genomic analyses of ovarian carcinoma. Nature 474(7353):609–615

Casper AM et al (2002) ATR regulates fragile site stability. Cell 111(6):779–789

Chang HHY et al (2017) Non-homologous DNA end joining and alternative pathways to double-strand break repair. Nat Rev Mol Cell Biol 18(8):495–506

Chanoux RA et al (2009) ATR and H2AX cooperate in maintaining genome stability under replication stress. J Biol Chem 284(9):5994–6003

Chen MS, Ryan CE, Piwnica-Worms H (2003) Chk1 kinase negatively regulates mitotic function of Cdc25A phosphatase through 14-3-3 binding. Mol Cell Biol 23(21):7488–7497

Chen L et al (2008) Cell cycle-dependent complex formation of BRCA1.CtIP.MRN is important for DNA double-strand break repair. J Biol Chem 283(12):7713–7720

Chiarugi A (2012) A snapshot of chemoresistance to PARP inhibitors. Trends Pharmacol Sci 33(1):42–48

Cortez D (2015) Preventing replication fork collapse to maintain genome integrity. DNA Repair (Amst) 32:149–157

Couch FB et al (2013) ATR phosphorylates SMARCAL1 to prevent replication fork collapse. Genes Dev 27(14):1610–1623

Couedel C et al (2004) Collaboration of homologous recombination and nonhomologous end-joining factors for the survival and integrity of mice and cells. Genes Dev 18(11):1293–1304

Curtis RE, Freedman DM, Ron E, LAG R, Hacker DG, Edwards BK, Tucker MA, Fraumeni JF Jr (2006) New malignancies among cancer survivors: SEER cancer registries, 1973–2000. NIH: National Cancer Institute, Bethesda, MD

Denko NC et al (1994) The human Ha-ras oncogene induces genomic instability in murine fibroblasts within one cell cycle. Proc Natl Acad Sci U S A 91(11):5124–5128

Di Micco R et al (2006) Oncogene-induced senescence is a DNA damage response triggered by DNA hyper-replication. Nature 444(7119):638–642

Dillon LW, Burrow AA, Wang YH (2010) DNA instability at chromosomal fragile sites in cancer. Curr Genomics 11(5):326–337

Dominguez-Kelly R et al (2011) Wee1 controls genomic stability during replication by regulating the Mus81-Eme1 endonuclease. J Cell Biol 194(4):567–579

Duda H et al (2016) A mechanism for controlled breakage of under-replicated chromosomes during mitosis. Dev Cell 39(6):740–755

Falck J et al (2001) The ATM-Chk2-Cdc25A checkpoint pathway guards against radioresistant DNA synthesis. Nature 410(6830):842–847

Farmer H et al (2005) Targeting the DNA repair defect in BRCA mutant cells as a therapeutic strategy. Nature 434(7035):917–921

Feijoo C et al (2001) Activation of mammalian Chk1 during DNA replication arrest: a role for Chk1 in the intra-S phase checkpoint monitoring replication origin firing. J Cell Biol 154(5):913–923

Felsher DW, Bishop JM (1999) Transient excess of MYC activity can elicit genomic instability and tumorigenesis. Proc Natl Acad Sci U S A 96(7):3940–3944

Fernandez-Medarde A, Santos E (2011) Ras in cancer and developmental diseases. Genes Cancer 2(3):344–358

Ferrao PT et al (2012) Efficacy of CHK inhibitors as single agents in MYC-driven lymphoma cells. Oncogene 31(13):1661–1672

Flaherty KT et al (2010) Inhibition of mutated, activated BRAF in metastatic melanoma. N Engl J Med 363(9):809–819

Fokas E et al (2012) Targeting ATR in vivo using the novel inhibitor VE-822 results in selective sensitization of pancreatic tumors to radiation. Cell Death Dis 3:e441

Gilad O et al (2010) Combining ATR suppression with oncogenic Ras synergistically increases genomic instability, causing synthetic lethality or tumorigenesis in a dosage-dependent manner. Cancer Res 70(23):9693–9702

Glover TW et al (1984) DNA polymerase alpha inhibition by aphidicolin induces gaps and breaks at common fragile sites in human chromosomes. Hum Genet 67(2):136–142

Gong Z et al (2010) BACH1/FANCJ acts with TopBP1 and participates early in DNA replication checkpoint control. Mol Cell 37(3):438–446

Gorgoulis VG et al (2005) Activation of the DNA damage checkpoint and genomic instability in human precancerous lesions. Nature 434(7035):907–913

Gottlieb TM, Jackson SP (1993) The DNA-dependent protein kinase: requirement for DNA ends and association with Ku antigen. Cell 72(1):131–142

Graham TG, Walter JC, Loparo JJ (2016) Two-stage synapsis of DNA ends during non-homologous end joining. Mol Cell 61(6):850–858

Gumy-Pause F, Wacker P, Sappino AP (2004) ATM gene and lymphoid malignancies. Leukemia 18(2):238–242

Gurley KE, Kemp CJ (2001) Synthetic lethality between mutation in Atm and DNA-PK(cs) during murine embryogenesis. Curr Biol 11(3):191–194

Halazonetis TD, Gorgoulis VG, Bartek J (2008) An oncogene-induced DNA damage model for cancer development. Science 319(5868):1352–1355

Harper JW et al (1995) Inhibition of cyclin-dependent kinases by p21. Mol Biol Cell 6(4):387–400

Hollstein M et al (1991) p53 mutations in human cancers. Science 253(5015):49–53

Hurley LH (2002) DNA and its associated processes as targets for cancer therapy. Nat Rev Cancer 2(3):188–200

Ishiai M et al (2008) FANCI phosphorylation functions as a molecular switch to turn on the Fanconi anemia pathway. Nat Struct Mol Biol 15(11):1138–1146

Kakarougkas A, Jeggo PA (2014) DNA DSB repair pathway choice: an orchestrated handover mechanism. Br J Radiol 87(1035):20130685

Kastan MB, Bartek J (2004) Cell-cycle checkpoints and cancer. Nature 432(7015):316–323

Kim H et al (2016) Targeting the ATR/CHK1 Axis with PARP inhibition results in tumor regression in BRCA-mutant ovarian cancer models. Clin Cancer Res 23(12):3097–3108

Kiraz Y et al (2016) Major apoptotic mechanisms and genes involved in apoptosis. Tumour Biol 37(7):8471–8486

Kolas NK et al (2007) Orchestration of the DNA-damage response by the RNF8 ubiquitin ligase. Science 318(5856):1637–1640

Krajewska M et al (2015) ATR inhibition preferentially targets homologous recombination-deficient tumor cells. Oncogene 34(26):3474–3481

Kwak EL et al (2010) Anaplastic lymphoma kinase inhibition in non-small-cell lung cancer. N Engl J Med 363(18):1693–1703

Lavin MF (2007) ATM and the Mre11 complex combine to recognize and signal DNA double-strand breaks. Oncogene 26(56):7749–7758

Lee J, Kumagai A, Dunphy WG (2001) Positive regulation of Wee1 by Chk1 and 14-3-3 proteins. Mol Biol Cell 12(3):551–563

Leung M et al (2011) Poly(ADP-ribose) polymerase-1 inhibition: preclinical and clinical development of synthetic lethality. Mol Med 17(7–8):854–862

Li J, Stern DF (2005) Regulation of CHK2 by DNA-dependent protein kinase. J Biol Chem 280(12):12041–12050

Litman R et al (2005) BACH1 is critical for homologous recombination and appears to be the Fanconi anemia gene product FANCJ. Cancer Cell 8(3):255–265

Liu Q et al (2000) Chk1 is an essential kinase that is regulated by Atr and required for the G(2)/M DNA damage checkpoint. Genes Dev 14(12):1448–1459

Lord CJ, Ashworth A (2016) BRCAness revisited. Nat Rev Cancer 16(2):110–120

Ma Y et al (2002) Hairpin opening and overhang processing by an Artemis/DNA-dependent protein kinase complex in nonhomologous end joining and V(D)J recombination. Cell 108(6):781–794

Mailand N et al (2000) Rapid destruction of human Cdc25A in response to DNA damage. Science 288(5470):1425–1429

Mailand N et al (2007) RNF8 ubiquitylates histones at DNA double-strand breaks and promotes assembly of repair proteins. Cell 131(5):887–900

Malkin D et al (1990) Germ line p53 mutations in a familial syndrome of breast cancer, sarcomas, and other neoplasms. Science 250(4985):1233–1238

Malone KE et al (2006) Prevalence and predictors of BRCA1 and BRCA2 mutations in a population-based study of breast cancer in white and black American women ages 35 to 64 years. Cancer Res 66(16):8297–8308

Marsit CJ et al (2004) Inactivation of the Fanconi anemia/BRCA pathway in lung and oral cancers: implications for treatment and survival. Oncogene 23(4):1000–1004

Matos J, West SC (2014) Holliday junction resolution: regulation in space and time. DNA Repair (Amst) 19:176–181

Matsuoka S et al (2007) ATM and ATR substrate analysis reveals extensive protein networks responsive to DNA damage. Science 316(5828):1160–1166

Mazin AV et al (2010) Rad54, the motor of homologous recombination. DNA Repair (Amst) 9(3):286–302

Mendes-Pereira AM et al (2009) Synthetic lethal targeting of PTEN mutant cells with PARP inhibitors. EMBO Mol Med 1(6–7):315–322

Merrick CJ, Jackson D, Diffley JF (2004) Visualization of altered replication dynamics after DNA damage in human cells. J Biol Chem 279(19):20067–20075

Mohni KN et al (2015) A synthetic lethal screen identifies DNA repair pathways that sensitize cancer cells to combined ATR inhibition and cisplatin treatments. PLoS One 10(5):e0125482

Mueller PR et al (1995) Myt1: a membrane-associated inhibitory kinase that phosphorylates Cdc2 on both threonine-14 and tyrosine-15. Science 270(5233):86–90

Murai J et al (2012) Trapping of PARP1 and PARP2 by Clinical PARP Inhibitors. Cancer Res 72(21):5588–5599

Murga M et al (2011) Exploiting oncogene-induced replicative stress for the selective killing of Myc-driven tumors. Nat Struct Mol Biol 18(12):1331–1335

NIH 2015 National cancer institite–side effects. 04/29/15 [cited 2016 11/14/16]; Available from: https://www.cancer.gov/about-cancer/treatment/side-effects

Nilsson JA, Cleveland JL (2003) Myc pathways provoking cell suicide and cancer. Oncogene 22(56):9007–9021

Norbury C, Blow J, Nurse P (1991) Regulatory phosphorylation of the p34cdc2 protein kinase in vertebrates. EMBO J 10(11):3321–3329

Parker LL, Piwnica-Worms H (1992) Inactivation of the p34cdc2-cyclin B complex by the human WEE1 tyrosine kinase. Science 257(5078):1955–1957

Patel AG, Sarkaria JN, Kaufmann SH (2011) Nonhomologous end joining drives poly(ADP-ribose) polymerase (PARP) inhibitor lethality in homologous recombination-deficient cells. Proc Natl Acad Sci U S A 108(8):3406–3411

Prevo R et al (2012) The novel ATR inhibitor VE-821 increases sensitivity of pancreatic cancer cells to radiation and chemotherapy. Cancer Biol Ther 13(11):1072–1081

Ragland RL et al (2013) RNF4 and PLK1 are required for replication fork collapse in ATR-deficient cells. Genes Dev 27(20):2259–2273

Reaper PM et al (2011) Selective killing of ATM- or p53-deficient cancer cells through inhibition of ATR. Nat Chem Biol 7(7):428–430

Regal JA et al (2013) Disease-associated MRE11 mutants impact ATM/ATR DNA damage signaling by distinct mechanisms. Hum Mol Genet 22(25):5146–5159

Riabinska A et al (2013) Therapeutic targeting of a robust non-oncogene addiction to PRKDC in ATM-defective tumors. Sci Transl Med 5(189):189ra78

Rogakou EP et al (1998) DNA double-stranded breaks induce histone H2AX phosphorylation on serine 139. J Biol Chem 273(10):5858–5868

Santocanale C, Diffley JF (1998) A Mec1- and Rad53-dependent checkpoint controls late-firing origins of DNA replication. Nature 395(6702):615–618

Schoppy DW et al (2012) Oncogenic stress sensitizes murine cancers to hypomorphic suppression of ATR. J Clin Invest 122(1):241–252

Shiloh Y, Ziv Y (2013) The ATM protein kinase: regulating the cellular response to genotoxic stress, and more. Nat Rev Mol Cell Biol 14(4):197–210

Siddick ZH (2002) The cancer handbook. In: Mechanisms of action of cancerchemotherapeutic agents: DNA-interactive alkylating agents and antitumour platinum-based drugs, 1st edn. John Wiley & Sons, Ltd, Hoboken, New Jersey

Sorensen CS et al (2003) Chk1 regulates the S phase checkpoint by coupling the physiological turnover and ionizing radiation-induced accelerated proteolysis of Cdc25A. Cancer Cell 3(3):247–258

Sorensen CS et al (2005) The cell-cycle checkpoint kinase Chk1 is required for mammalian homologous recombination repair. Nat Cell Biol 7(2):195–201

Sosman JA et al (2012) Survival in BRAF V600-mutant advanced melanoma treated with vemurafenib. N Engl J Med 366(8):707–714

Stewart GS et al (2003) MDC1 is a mediator of the mammalian DNA damage checkpoint. Nature 421(6926):961–966

Stiff T et al (2004) ATM and DNA-PK function redundantly to phosphorylate H2AX after exposure to ionizing radiation. Cancer Res 64(7):2390–2396

Strausfeld U et al (1991) Dephosphorylation and activation of a p34cdc2/cyclin B complex in vitro by human CDC25 protein. Nature 351(6323):242–245

Sy SM, Huen MS, Chen J (2009) PALB2 is an integral component of the BRCA complex required for homologous recombination repair. Proc Natl Acad Sci U S A 106(17):7155–7160

Toledo LI et al (2011) A cell-based screen identifies ATR inhibitors with synthetic lethal properties for cancer-associated mutations. Nat Struct Mol Biol 18(6):721–727

Toledo LI et al (2013) ATR prohibits replication catastrophe by preventing global exhaustion of RPA. Cell 155(5):1088–1103

Turner N, Tutt A, Ashworth A (2004) Hallmarks of 'BRCAness' in sporadic cancers. Nat Rev Cancer 4(10):814–819

Varon R et al (2001) Mutations in the nijmegen breakage syndrome gene (NBS1) in childhood acute lymphoblastic leukemia (ALL). Cancer Res 61(9):3570–3572

Vita M, Henriksson M (2006) The Myc oncoprotein as a therapeutic target for human cancer. Semin Cancer Biol 16(4):318–330

Waddell N et al (2015) Whole genomes redefine the mutational landscape of pancreatic cancer. Nature 518(7540):495–501

Waters LS et al (2009) Eukaryotic translesion polymerases and their roles and regulation in DNA damage tolerance. Microbiol Mol Biol Rev 73(1):134–154

Welburn JP et al (2007) How tyrosine 15 phosphorylation inhibits the activity of cyclin-dependent kinase 2-cyclin A. J Biol Chem 282(5):3173–3181

Williams JS, Lujan SA, Kunkel TA (2016) Processing ribonucleotides incorporated during eukaryotic DNA replication. Nat Rev Mol Cell Biol 17(6):350–363

Wyatt HD et al (2013) Coordinated actions of SLX1-SLX4 and MUS81-EME1 for Holliday junction resolution in human cells. Mol Cell 52(2):234–247

Xia B et al (2006) Control of BRCA2 cellular and clinical functions by a nuclear partner, PALB2. Mol Cell 22(6):719–729

Yazinski SA et al (2017) ATR inhibition disrupts rewired homologous recombination and fork protection pathways in PARP inhibitor-resistant BRCA-deficient cancer cells. Genes Dev 31(3):318–332

Zamborszky J et al (2017) Loss of BRCA1 or BRCA2 markedly increases the rate of base substitution mutagenesis and has distinct effects on genomic deletions. Oncogene 36(6):746–755

Zeman MK, Cimprich KA (2014) Causes and consequences of replication stress. Nat Cell Biol 16(1):2–9

Zhao H, Watkins JL, Piwnica-Worms H (2002) Disruption of the checkpoint kinase 1/cell division cycle 25A pathway abrogates ionizing radiation-induced S and G2 checkpoints. Proc Natl Acad Sci U S A 99(23):14795–14800

Zou L, Elledge SJ (2003) Sensing DNA damage through ATRIP recognition of RPA-ssDNA complexes. Science 300(5625):1542–1548

Chapter 3
Control of DNA Replication by ATR

Emilio Lecona and Oscar Fernández-Capetillo

Abstract DNA replication needs to be carefully controlled to prevent genomic instability and ensure cellular fitness. ATR is a PI3K-like kinase and is a central factor supervising the correct completion of DNA replication. The recruitment, activation and specific substrate recognition of ATR is tightly regulated to promote differential responses at a local (fork), regional (replication factory) and global (nucleus) level. Both during normal S phase or in response to the stalling of replication forks, ATR is responsible for fork stabilization and repair, as well as checkpoint activation together with its substrate, the CHK1 kinase. Malignant transformation is accompanied by oncogenic mutations that promote unscheduled entry into S phase and an increase in problems during DNA replication. This renders cancer cells particularly dependent on a proficient replication stress response for their survival, making the ATR-CHK1 pathway an attractive target for cancer treatment. In this chapter, we review the mechanisms of ATR activation, its downstream effects, and the functions of this pathway in cancer.

Keywords ATR · CHK1 · DNA replication · Replication stress · Cancer

E. Lecona
Genomic Instability Group, Spanish National Cancer Research Centre (CNIO),
Madrid 28029, Spain
e-mail: elecona@cnio.es

O. Fernández-Capetillo (✉)
Genomic Instability Group, Spanish National Cancer Research Centre (CNIO),
Madrid 28029, Spain

Science for Life Laboratory, Division of Genome Biology, Department of Medical
Biochemistry and Biophysics, Karolinska Institute, S-171 21 Stockholm, Sweden
e-mail: ofernandez@cnio.es

© Springer International Publishing AG, part of Springer Nature 2018   35
J. Pollard, N. Curtin (eds.), *Targeting the DNA Damage Response
for Anti-Cancer Therapy*, Cancer Drug Discovery and Development,
https://doi.org/10.1007/978-3-319-75836-7_3

3.1   Introduction

Every cell cycle the genetic information contained in the DNA needs to be copied and transmitted to the daughter cells. The DNA replication machinery encounters many challenges due to the damage inflicted by both endogenous and exogenous sources that can hamper the faithful copy of the DNA. The presence of damage is sensed by the cells through the DNA damage response (DDR) machinery that activates specific checkpoints in different phases of the cell cycle. These checkpoints stop the progression through the cell cycle to allow for DNA repair. At higher levels of DNA damage, or on certain cell types, the activation of the checkpoint leads to the induction of apoptosis, preventing the accumulation of potentially harmful cells. Initial studies in yeast revealed the existence of genes that code for proteins necessary to respond to problems during DNA replication. The inactivation of these genes prevents the arrest of the cell cycle induced by agents that affect DNA replication, such as hydroxyurea. As a consequence, damaged cells progress through mitosis, accumulate toxic levels of genomic instability and die (Weinert et al. 1994). One of these checkpoint genes was Mec1, encoding for a kinase that was later identified as ATR in mammals (Cimprich et al. 1996).

ATR is a member of the PI3K-related kinase family that also includes ATM, DNA-PKcs, SMG-1 and mTOR (Lovejoy and Cortez 2009). ATR, ATM and DNA-PKcs are the main effectors of the DDR (Berti and Vindigni 2016). The hierarchical model of the DDR establishes that specific lesions in the DNA are recognized by distinct protein sensors that lead to the activation of the effector kinases, thereby eliciting the repair by the appropriate mechanisms. Accordingly, DNA double strand breaks (DSB) activate ATM or DNA-PKcs, while alterations in the progression of replication forks lead to the activation of ATR. ATR is the main player in the response to problems arising during DNA replication that are collectively known as replication stress, making it essential for normal DNA replication and also during the response to agents that can challenge the progression of the replication fork such as DNA polymerase inhibitors, nucleotide analogues or UV light. A very elaborate mechanism of recruitment and activation of ATR leads to the phosphorylation and activation of its main target, the CHK1 kinase. CHK1 is also essential and responsible for the modulation of DNA replication and the cell cycle in the presence of replication stress. Thus, the deletion of both ATR and CHK1 is embryonic lethal. Over the last two decades our knowledge of the biology of ATR has vastly increased. Here we summarize our current understanding of the recruitment and activation of ATR and how its signalling is necessary to ensure correct DNA replication and is deregulated in cancer.

3.2   ATR Is a PI3K-Related Kinase (PIKK)

All PIKK members share a common domain organization (Baretic and Williams 2014) (Fig. 3.1). The N-terminal region is composed by HEAT repeats and is variable in length. The first set of repeats shows a superhelical organization and displays distinct configurations in the different PIKKs, protruding away from the catalytic core in the C-terminus. In ATR, this region has been proven to be essential since it constitutes the interaction domain for ATRIP (ATR Interacting Protein), the partner of ATR (see below). Additionally, a mutation in the HEAT repeats at S1333 results in a hyperactive kinase (Luzwick et al. 2014). The repeats at the N-terminal region are followed by the FAT domain, composed of additional helical HEAT repeats that are highly conserved in the PIKK family (Fig. 3.1). The analysis of the structure of the FAT domain in mTOR and DNA-PKcs has revealed that this domain wraps half of the kinase domain, providing structural support (Yang et al. 2013; Sibanda et al. 2010). Although the sequence is not conserved in the PI3K family, a similar helical region is also found in the other members of the family, suggesting a conserved function for this region. Next, we find the catalytic domain (Fig. 3.1) that is composed of two lobes (N and C), similar to a canonical kinase domain. This kinase domain is also homologous to the PI3K kinase domain (Walker et al. 1999), although it lacks the ability to phosphorylate lipids and only targets proteins. The inability of PIKK proteins to act on lipids is due to the presence of three insertions within the C-lobe of their catalytic domains. The last of these insertions is the FATC (C-terminal FAT) domain (Fig. 3.1), which is highly conserved in all PIKKs and constitutes an integral part of the catalytic core. Again, although the FATC domain is not conserved in the PI3K family it has been shown that a similar structure is found as part of the PI3K kinase domain. Right before the FATC domain there is a variable region that shows low conservation within the PIKK family of proteins. This region has been shown to be very important for the activity of ATM, ATR and DNA-PKcs and thus it was termed PIKK regulatory domain (PRD) (Mordes et al. 2008a, Sun et al. 2007) (Fig. 3.1). The equivalent region in mTOR is known as the negative regulatory domain, since its deletion yields a super-active enzyme (Sekulic et al. 2000). In the case of ATR, the PRD mediates the binding to TOPBP1, one of the essential regulators of the activation of ATR (Mordes et al. 2008a).

The conservation of the catalytic domain in the PIKK family results in a very similar target sequence for all the members of the family. ATR, ATM, SMG-1 and DNA-PK preferentially act on Ser and Thr residues followed by a Gln (S/T-Q motif)

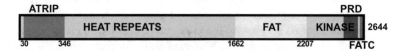

Fig. 3.1 Domain organization of ATR. There are three main domains in ATR. First, the HEAT repeats where the interaction domain with ATRIP is found. Then the FAT domain that gives structural support to the kinase domain. Last, the kinase domain includes the PIKK regulatory domain (PRD) responsible for the binding of TOPBP1 and the FATC domain

(Matsuoka et al. 2007), while mTOR phosphorylates Ser and Thr residues followed by a Pro or a hydrophobic residue (Kang et al. 2013). This shared target sequence raises the question about how the different PIKK phosphorylate specific targets. The activation of PIKK, and in particular ATR, is established in three steps: first, the generation of specific lesions leads to their recruitment to damage sites, and this recruitment is mediated by distinct partners that sense the specific stimuli; second, once they are re-localized to the sites of activation, PIKK require the interaction with additional proteins that act as activators to achieve full enzymatic capacity; last, the phosphorylation of some of their key substrates is dependent on the presence of specific proteins or adaptors, that direct the catalytic activity of the PIKK. In the next sections we will describe the mechanisms that recruit, activate and direct the action of ATR during replication stress.

3.3   ATR Activation

3.3.1   First Step: ssDNA Recruits the ATR-ATRIP Complex

The initial studies on ATR and its yeast homologues focused on the search for substrates that also form part of the checkpoint. In 1999 the Carr lab described the interaction of Rad26 with Rad3 (ATR) in *S. pombe* (Edwards et al. 1999). Interestingly, Rad3/ATR was shown to phosphorylate Rad26 independent from other checkpoint proteins. Later, several studies revealed that Rad26 and its homologue in *S. cerevisiae*, Dcd2, were essential for the activation of the checkpoint and the phosphorylation of the targets of Rad3/Mec1/ATR (Paciotti et al. 2000; Rouse and Jackson 2000). The work of the Elledge lab led to the identification of the homologue of Rad26/Dcd2 in humans, ATRIP. This work also demonstrated that the stability of ATR and ATRIP is compromised in the absence of their partner, suggesting the formation of a stable ATR-ATRIP complex (Cortez et al. 2001). Immunoprecipitation experiments confirmed that most of ATR present in a cell is associated with ATRIP and ATR-ATRIP works as a complex in the checkpoint response (Zou and Elledge 2003).

The establishment of ATR-ATRIP as a complex also helped to elucidate the mechanism of recruitment that leads to the activation of ATR in response to problems during DNA replication. Classical studies had shown that many different types of DNA damage activated ATR, including telomere deprotection, DSB or agents that affect DNA replication. However, the activation of ATR by these stimuli is not always direct, which made it difficult to determine the common ground to all these situations. In all cases the activation of ATR relies on the presence of ssDNA. In response to DSB, the activation of ATR is secondary to ATM-dependent end-resection of DNA ends that generates ssDNA stretches. In contrast, during DNA replication the stalling of replication forks directly leads to the formation of ssDNA, followed by recruitment of ATR and its activation (Fig. 3.2). In a similar way, agents that create barriers to the progress of replication forks lead to an accumulation of ssDNA that is sensed by ATR and has

Fig. 3.2 Recruitment and activation of ATR. Stepwise mechanism for the activation of ATR. (**a**) The block of a replication fork accumulates ssDNA and creates an ssDNA-dsDNA junction. (**b**) ssDNA loads RPA that brings ATR-ATRIP through the interaction with ATRIP. The ssDNA-dsDNA junction is bound by RAD17-RFC that loads the 9-1-1 clamp. (**c**) The 9-1-1 clamp together with ATRIP recruit TOPBP1 to activate ATR

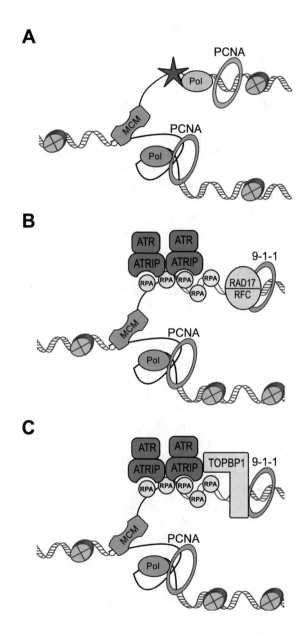

been defined as the main feature of replication stress (Fig. 3.2). Thus, the ATR-ATRIP complex is key to maintain and repair replication forks during every S phase, making it essential for cell division and survival.

How does the ATR-ATRIP complex sense the presence of ssDNA? The presence of ssDNA is highly dangerous in a cell, and it is quickly protected by the ssDNA binding protein complex RPA (Fig. 3.2b). RPA directly interacts with and recruits

ATRIP, and the extent of ATRIP recruitment is dependent on the length of the ssDNA stretch (Zou and Elledge 2003). The biochemical dissection of the interaction of the ATR-ATRIP complex with ssDNA-RPA revealed two different regions in ATRIP that mediate the binding to ATR and RPA: a short region in the C-terminus of ATRIP binds to the N-terminal HEAT repeats in ATR, and the N-terminus of ATRIP is responsible for the interaction with RPA (Ball et al. 2005). Additionally, ATRIP presents a coiled-coil domain right after the RPA binding region that induces the oligomerization of the complex independent of its activation (Ball and Cortez 2005). The recruitment of ATR-ATRIP to ssDNA requires both the interaction with RPA and the oligomerization domain in ATRIP, suggesting that the loading of the complex on chromatin is cooperative (Ball and Cortez 2005). The formation of ssDNA-RPA patches constitutes the signal that recruits the ATR-ATRIP kinase to stalled forks or DSB (Fig. 3.2b). However, full activation of ATR cannot be achieved by its sole recruitment to ssDNA and requires additional components.

3.3.2 Second Step: TOPBP1 Is Necessary for Full Activation of ATR-ATRIP

The formation of the ATR-ATRIP complex is conserved across species and the employment of model systems helped to dissect the mechanisms of activation of this kinase. *In vitro* studies with *Xenopus* ATR-ATRIP revealed that binding to ssDNA cannot trigger the full activation of the kinase (Kumagai et al. 2004). The activation of ATR-ATRIP is stronger in the presence of DNA structures that combine ssDNA stretches and dsDNA, resembling stalled replication forks (Kumagai et al. 2004) (Fig. 3.2). Further studies identified TOPBP1 as the key factor to stimulate the activity of ATR-ATRIP (Kumagai et al. 2006) (Fig. 3.2c). TOPBP1 has multiple roles in chromatin, however it is essential for the loading of core components of the replisome such as the GINS complex or the leading strand DNA polymerase POLE. It is composed of multiple BRCT repeats (9 in mammals and *Xenopus*, 4 in yeast) and it acts as a scaffold to recruit and bring together multiple proteins (Wardlaw et al. 2014). The BRCT repeats are usually organized in pairs that mediate the recognition of phosphorylated factors. In addition to DNA replication, TOPBP1 also regulates transcription and the DNA damage response through the interaction with multiple partners mediated by specific BRCT domains.

In the case of ATR-ATRIP, a region of TOPBP1 located between BRCT6 and BRCT7 is sufficient to trigger the activation of ATR-ATRIP, the ATR activation domain (AAD) (Kumagai et al. 2006). In *S. cerevisiae* and *S. pombe* an AAD region is found in the C-terminal region of the protein, although the sequence shows low conservation to the mammalian AAD (Lin et al. 2012; Mordes et al. 2008b). The ectopic addition of the AAD elicits a powerful activation of ATR-ATRIP independent of the presence of damage in *Xenopus* egg extracts (Kumagai et al. 2006), as does the fusion of the AAD to PCNA or H2B in chicken cells (Delacroix et al. 2007). The fusion of the AAD to a fragment of the estrogen receptor generated a system that can activate/deactivate ATR-ATRIP at will through the addition of an inert derivative of tamoxifen (Toledo et al. 2011). As to how TOPBP1 stimulates ATR activity, TOPBP1 interacts with both ATR and ATRIP (Fig. 3.2c). First, TOPBP1 needs to bind to a region next to the coiled-coil domain in ATRIP to activate ATR; second the PRD domain in ATR is also necessary for the interaction with the BRCT7-8 in TOPBP1, and for the stimulation of the activity of ATR-ATRIP (Mordes et al. 2008a). Further, biochemical analysis of the phosphorylation of CHK1 by ATR-ATRIP confirmed that TOPBP1 and the recruitment of ATR-ATRIP by RPA cooperate to achieve optimal activity of the complex (Choi et al. 2010). Thus, TOPBP1 establishes multiple contacts with ATR-ATRIP and strongly increases the kinase activity of the complex within chromatin. Consequently, their contact must be exquisitely controlled. How is thus the action of TOPBP1 on ATR-ATRIP regulated?

Stalled replication forks or resected DSBs generate a specific DNA structure containing a dsDNA-ssDNA junction. The presence of RPA covering the ssDNA not only recruits the ATR-ATRIP complex but it also brings the clamp loader RAD17-RFC to the junctions (Fig. 3.2b). Then, RAD17-RFC catalyzes the loading of the RAD9-HUS1-RAD1 clamp (9-1-1) onto the junctions (Fig. 3.2b). The N-terminal region of RAD9 forms a heterotrimeric complex with HUS1 and RAD1, creating a ring-shaped structure that is similar to PCNA (Broustas and Lieberman 2012; Parrilla-Castellar et al. 2004). The C-terminus of RAD9 is heavily phosphorylated, showing both constitutive and DNA damage-induced modifications, but only the phosphorylation at S387 is required for the activation of ATR-ATRIP (Delacroix et al. 2007; Lee et al. 2007). This residue is conserved in vertebrate homologs of RAD9 and shows constitutive phosphorylation (St Onge et al. 2003). TOPBP1 directly binds phosphorylated S387 in RAD9 through its BRCT1-2 domains and this interaction is required to recruit TOPBP1 to dsDNA-ssDNA junctions (Delacroix et al. 2007; Lee et al. 2007) (Fig. 3.2c). As a result, TOPBP1 can contact and activate ATR-ATRIP, leading to the efficient phosphorylation of its substrates, mainly CHK1. In addition, ATR-ATRIP is autophosphorylated at S1989 within the FAT domain and the phosphorylation at this serine residue is recognized by the BRCT7-8 domains in TOPBP1 (Liu et al. 2011). This phosphorylation enhances the effect of TOPBP1 on ATR-ATRIP.

Although the 9-1-1 clamp is the main mediator of the activation of ATR-ATRIP by TOPBP1 in the presence of replication stress, there are additional factors that also contribute to this process. The MRN complex (MRE11, RAD50, NBS1) plays a role in the activation of ATM by DSB. During the DDR the MRN complex also interacts with TOPBP1 leading to its recruitment to DSB and the activation of ATR-ATRIP (Yoo et al. 2009). However, the regulation of the ATR-ATRIP complex by MRN is not limited to the response to DSB. Studies in *Xenopus* egg extracts have shown that MRN is necessary for the initial recruitment of TOPBP1 to structures resembling stalled replication forks through the interaction of MRE11 with the BRCT3-6 domains in TOPBP1 (Duursma et al. 2013; Lee and Dunphy 2013). Then, TOPBP1 is transferred to the 9-1-1 complex that is required for the stimulation of ATR-ATRIP by TOPBP1 (Duursma et al. 2013). Another regulator of the function of the 9-1-1 clamp and TOPBP1 was recently discovered. RHINO associates stoichiometrically with 9-1-1 and also interacts with TOPBP1. Although it is not necessary for the recruitment of either factor, the presence of RHINO further stimulates the action of ATR-ATRIP on CHK1 (Cotta-Ramusino et al. 2011; Lindsey-Boltz et al. 2015).

The activation of ATR-ATRIP is a multi-step process that depends on the presence of ssDNA adjacent to an ssDNA-dsDNA junction. The binding of RPA to ssDNA has two functions: on the one hand, it directly recruits ATR-ATRIP; on the other hand, it promotes the loading of the 9-1-1 clamp on the junction. The 9-1-1 clamp, in a complex with RHINO and in cooperation with MRN, mediates the recruitment of TOPBP1, the activator of ATR-ATRIP. Nevertheless, even though all of the above leads to an active ATR, the phosphorylation of its target kinase CHK1, the key checkpoint transducer or the ATR-dependent signalling cascade, demands one additional step.

3.3.3   Third Step: CLASPIN Is an Adaptor for CHK1 Phosphorylation

Although there are many substrates of ATR-ATRIP, its local recruitment and activation at sites of replication stress precludes a wide action of this kinase leading to an unscheduled activation of checkpoint responses. In addition, the phosphorylation and activation of CHK1 occur on chromatin, promoting its dissociation to trigger cellular responses (Smits et al. 2006). Central to this process, CLASPIN regulates both the phosphorylation of CHK1 and its eviction. CLASPIN was first identified in *Xenopus* egg extracts as a factor binding to CHK1 and required for its phosphorylation and activation in the presence of oligonucleotides that mimic replication stress (Kumagai and Dunphy 2000). Later studies confirmed that both the phosphorylation of CHK1 by ATR-ATRIP and its own auto-phosphorylation are stimulated by CLASPIN (Kumagai et al. 2004). Further, while TOPBP1 is a general activator of ATR-ATRIP, CLASPIN is specifically required for the phosphorylation of CHK1, even if ATR-ATRIP is fully active (Liu et al. 2006). Accordingly, it has been proposed that CLASPIN acts as an adaptor between ATR-ATRIP and CHK1.

The mechanism of action of CLASPIN on CHK1 is complex and highly regulated (Fig. 3.3). CLASPIN presents several conserved repeats that are phosphorylated upon induction of replication stress, either directly by ATR-ATRIP or by other kinases dependent on ATR-ATRIP (Chini and Chen 2006; Jeong et al. 2003; Kumagai and Dunphy 2003) (Fig. 3.3b). A specific region in the N-terminus of CHK1, close to the catalytic domain, recognizes this phosphorylation and establishes a damage dependent interaction between CLASPIN and CHK1 (Chini and Chen 2006; Jeong et al. 2003; Kumagai and Dunphy 2003) (Fig. 3.3b). This interaction is established at replication stress sites thanks to a multifactorial recruitment of CLASPIN mediated by its binding to ATR-ATRIP, the TIMELESS-TIPIN complex bound to RPA, and phosphorylated AND-1 (a target of ATR itself) (Chini and Chen 2003; Hao et al. 2015; Kemp et al. 2010) (Fig. 3.3a). Once bound to CLASPIN,

Fig. 3.3 Phosphorylation
of CHK1 by ATR-ATRIP.
(**a**) CLASPIN is recruited
to stalled replication forks
through the interaction
with multiple factors:
TIMELESS-TIPIN,
AND-1 and ATR-
ATRIP. CLASPIN is
phosphorylated by
ATR-ATRIP (**b**). CHK1
interacts with
phosphorylated CLASPIN
and is phosphorylated by
ATR-ATRIP

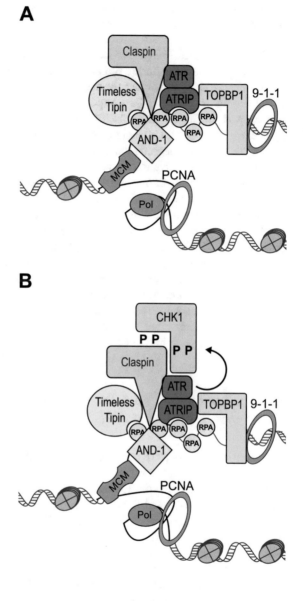

CHK1 is phosphorylated by ATR at S345 and S317 and also phosphorylates itself at S296, leading to its dissociation from CLASPIN and eviction from chromatin (Jeong et al. 2003; Smits et al. 2006) (Fig. 3.3b). Accordingly, the phosphorylated and active form of CHK1 is not accumulated at sites of damage and is found throughout the nucleus. Actually, the immobilization of CHK1 on chromatin impairs the activation of the checkpoint (Smits et al. 2006). Of note, ATM-dependent phosphorylation of CHK2, which occurs at sites of DSBs (in a CLASPIN-independent manner) is also followed by the diffusion of the activated kinase throughout the nucleoplasm (Lukas et al. 2003).

The levels of CLASPIN are modulated during the cell cycle to ensure that CHK1 activation only happens during S and G2/M phases (Chini and Chen 2003). There are two mechanisms that induce the degradation of CLASPIN. During G1, the APC-CDH1 complex induces the ubiquitination of CLASPIN and its degradation (Faustrup et al. 2009), while the SCF-βTrCP E3 ligase ubiquitinates CLASPIN upon entry into mitosis (Mailand et al. 2006; Mamely et al. 2006; Peschiaroli et al. 2006). Further, the degradation of CLASPIN induced by SCF-βTrCP is also necessary for the inactivation of the replication stress response through the loss of CHK1 activity that allows the progression into mitosis (Mailand et al. 2006; Mamely et al. 2006; Peschiaroli et al. 2006). Several deubiquitinases have been shown to act on CLASPIN to counteract the effect of SCF-βTrCP and prolong the activation of CHK1 in the presence of replication stress, including USP7, USP20 and USP29 (Faustrup et al. 2009; Martin et al. 2015; Yuan et al. 2014; Zhu et al. 2014).

Given the central role of CHK1 in the activation of the checkpoint during unperturbed DNA replication and after stress, CLASPIN is a key mediator of the response to replication stress. Acting as a specific adaptor for CHK1, CLASPIN converts a local response mediated by ATR-ATRIP into a nuclear activation of the checkpoint machinery that prevents the firing of new origins of replication and blocks the progression into mitosis.

3.3.4 Fine Tuning: Post-Translational Modifications Regulate the Activation of ATR-ATRIP

The process of ATR-ATRIP activation is subjected to additional layers of regulation through different post-translational modifications deposited on, or recognized by ATRIP. First, there are two activities that favour the binding of ATRIP to RPA: the ubiquitination of RPA and the deacetylation of ATRIP. PRP19 is a E3 ubiquitin ligase that forms a complex with CDC5L, PRL1 and SPF27 and takes part in the regulation of splicing. The complex was shown to interact with RPA bound to ssDNA and ubiquitinate RPA32 and RPA70. The K63-linked ubiquitin chains in RPA favour the recruitment of ATR-ATRIP through the interaction with ATRIP (Marechal et al. 2014). The K32 in ATRIP, a residue within its RPA binding region, is deacetylated by SIRT2 in the presence of replication stress. This deacetylation also promotes its interaction with RPA, leading to increased recruitment and activation of ATR-ATRIP (Zhang et al. 2016).

Second, SUMOylation also contributes to different steps in the activation of ATR-ATRIP. Recent evidence suggests that functionally related proteins are SUMOylated together in the same pathway to elicit a coordinated response (Psakhye and Jentsch 2012). Interestingly, the replisome is a SUMO rich environment (Lopez-Contreras et al. 2013) and replication stress has been shown to induce global changes in SUMOylation that target many proteins in the replisome

(Bursomanno et al. 2015; Xiao et al. 2015). In agreement with this model, ATRIP is SUMOylated at K234 and K289 by SUMO2/3, promoting its interaction with many proteins in the replication stress response, including ATR, RPA, TOPBP1 and the MRN complex, and contributing to ATR-ATRIP activation (Wu et al. 2014). Additionally, the SUMO ligase PIAS3 enhances the autophosphorylation of ATR through a yet undetermined mechanism (Wu and Zou 2016). Thus, the activation of ATR-ATRIP is subject to the modulation by different modifications, most of which are likely not essential individually but which collectively contribute to modulate the strength of the checkpoint response.

In summary, a multi-layered mechanism of activation of ATR-ATRIP ensures that this cytostatic/cytotoxic response is properly controlled to safeguard the stability of replication forks.

3.4   Local, Regional and Global Checkpoint Functions of ATR-ATRIP

It is clear that ATR-ATRIP is required during both unperturbed DNA replication and in the response to replication stress. How can ATR-ATRIP exert a differential control under distinct situations? Recent evidence shows that the function of ATR-ATRIP can be established in three levels: a local function that protects individual replication forks; a regional regulation of origin firing within each replication factory to ensure DNA replication; and a global checkpoint action to control DNA replication and cell cycle progression through the activation of CHK1 (Fig. 3.4). While the local and regional roles of ATR-ATRIP are activated during each S phase, the global checkpoint activation requires the presence of strong replication stress.

3.4.1   Local Action of ATR-ATRIP on Replication Forks

Regarding the local function of ATR-ATRIP, it has been shown that mild replication stress that slows fork progression but does not accumulate ssDNA induces the loading and activation of ATR-ATRIP, with no other downstream effectors being activated (Koundrioukoff et al. 2013). Further, a phosphoproteomic analysis in yeast revealed that ATR is activated during S phase, leading to the phosphorylation of a specific set of target proteins, different from the substrates targeted by ATR during replication stress (Bastos de Oliveira et al. 2015). The activation of ATR-ATRIP is especially relevant in early S phase, when it limits the accumulation of ssDNA (Buisson et al. 2015). The accumulation of excessive levels of replication stress is highly dangerous for the cell, since it can exhaust the pool of RPA and thus lead to the exposure of unprotected ssDNA which seems to be the signal for the nucleolytic degradation of stalled replication forks (Toledo et al. 2013). Thus, one of the main functions of ATR-ATRIP during DNA replication is to limit the accumulation of ssDNA. How is this protection achieved? Although it was initially proposed that

ATR-ATRIP stabilizes the replisome in the presence of stressing factors, it has been shown that the arrest of the replication forks does not induce the disassembly of the replisome (Dungrawala et al. 2015). Instead ATR-ATRIP works through the protection of the fork itself, stabilizing its structure and recruiting factors that protect the fork from degradation and promote its restart when the problems are fixed (Berti and Vindigni 2016; Dungrawala et al. 2015) (Fig. 3.4, top left).

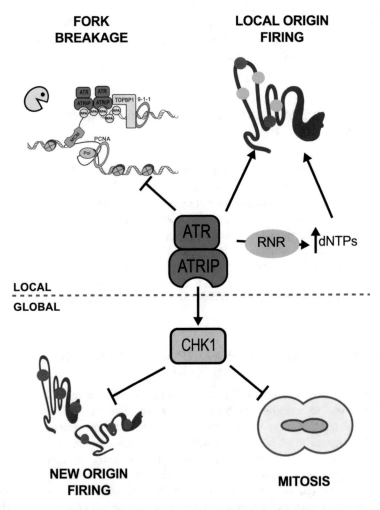

Fig. 3.4 Local and global actions of ATR-ATRIP. The activation of ATR-ATRIP regulates DNA replication locally (*top*): ATR-ATRIP protects stalled replication fork from their breakage (*top left*) and it also stimulates local origin firing and the supply of nucleotides for the completion of DNA replication (*top right*). At the global level ATR-ATRIP exerts its actions through the activation of CHK1 (*bottom*). By diverse mechanisms CHK1 blocks new origin firing (*bottom left*) and entry into mitosis (*bottom right*)

There are several factors that account for the protection of the fork by ATR-ATRIP. First, the phosphorylation of RPA by ATR-ATRIP recruits PALB2 to replication stress sites (Murphy et al. 2014), leading to the binding of BRCA2 that protects forks from Mre11 mediated degradation (Schlacher et al. 2011). Second, FANCD2 is also recruited to forks in the presence of replication stress through an ATR-ATRIP-dependent interaction with the MCM helicase (Lossaint et al. 2013). Similar to BRCA2, FANCD2 also contributes to the protection of stalled replication forks (Schlacher et al. 2012). Third, ATR-ATRIP also stimulates the recruitment of helicases that take part in the restoration and restart of the fork by different mechanisms. Among them, SMARCAL1 is phosphorylated by ATR-ATRIP, stimulating its binding to stalled forks through the interaction with RPA, where it prevents the collapse of the forks (Ciccia et al. 2009; Couch et al. 2013; Yuan et al. 2009). The RECQ helicases BLM and WRN also contribute to the stabilization and restart of stalled forks and are direct targets of ATR-ATRIP (Davies et al. 2007; Pichierri et al. 2003).

While the action of ATR-ATRIP in the replication fork prevents its collapse and the generation of deleterious double strand breaks, it is not sufficient to ensure DNA replication. Additional regulation of the function of replication factories needs to be established to allow the timely completion of the S phase.

3.4.2 Regional Modulation of Replication Factories

During DNA replication initiation only a subset of origins that have been licensed are actually fired, while a number of origins where the MCM helicase is loaded remain "dormant" (Blow et al. 2011). When a replication fork encounters a problem that stops its progression, the nearby dormant origins are fired to help complete the replication of this region (Ge et al. 2007; Ibarra et al. 2008) (Fig. 3.4, top right). This is not a global mechanism and it seems to be restricted to the factories that are already active, while the activation of ATR-ATRIP and CHK1 induces a global block of new origin firing (Ge and Blow 2010).

Different mechanisms have been proposed for the firing of the dormant origins that are close to stalled replication forks. On one hand, when the speed of the forks is reduced it takes longer to complete replication of a given area, allowing time for the firing of additional licensed origins. Alternatively, ATR-ATRIP phosphorylates several core DNA replication factors such as MCM complex members that could help in the firing of origins nearby the site of replication stress (Cortez et al. 2004; Yoo et al. 2004), although it is not clear how ATR-ATRIP could connect to the dormant origins. A recent study has put forward a role for FANCI in stimulating the firing of dormant origins in the presence of mild replication stress through a direct interaction with the MCM helicase (Chen et al. 2015). When the levels of replication stress increase the activation of ATR-ATRIP leads to the phosphorylation of FANCI, shifting its function to promote replication fork restart (Chen et al. 2015). The relevance of dormant origins during unperturbed S phase and in the presence of mild stress is demonstrated by the sensitivity to agents that generate replication stress, observed when the levels of MCM components are reduced, limiting the number of licensed origins (Blow et al. 2011; Ibarra et al. 2008).

In addition to the regulation of proteins involved in DNA replication, ATR has a more direct way to influence DNA replication. The regional regulation of origin firing within a given replication factory requires an increased supply of nucleotides for the progression of newly fired origins. A connection between the activation of ATR and the synthesis of nucleotides has been clearly established (Fig. 3.4, top right). In S. *cerevisiae* a small protein, Sml1, inhibits the ribonucleotide reductase (RNR), the rate limiting enzyme in the synthesis of nucleotides (Zhang et al. 2007; Zhao et al. 1998). Sml1 is phosphorylated by Mec1/ATR leading to its degradation and enhancing the production of nucleotides (Zhao et al. 2001). However, there is no true mammalian orthologue of Sml1 and the mechanisms by which Sml1 binds the RNR are not conserved (Specks et al. 2015). In mammals, ATR-ATRIP indirectly regulates the activity of the ribonucleotide reductase by several pathways such as the stabilization of E2F1 that activates the transcription of RNR2, the small subunit of the enzyme (Buisson et al. 2015; Zhang et al. 2009), and directly prevents the degradation of RNR proteins by the proteasome (D'Angiolella et al. 2012). Regardless of how ATR stimulates the RNR, this pathway is also an essential branch of ATR signalling in mammals and a RNR2 transgenic mice doubles the median lifespan of ATR hypomorphic mice suffering from accelerating ageing (Lopez-Contreras et al. 2015; Murga et al. 2009). A proper supply of nucleotides facilitates the process of DNA replication and is particularly helpful in conditions of replication stress. In fact, an extra supply of nucleotides reduces the levels of replication stress induced by oncogenes (Bester et al. 2011) or reprogramming factors (Ruiz et al. 2015). Together with the regulation of the firing of dormant origins, the increased levels of ribonucleotide reductase support the response to replication problems within the context of a replication factory.

3.4.3   Global Regulation of DNA Replication and the Cell Cycle

There are two main global functions for the checkpoint activated by ATR that are exerted through CHK1: first, the cell cycle arrest to prevent progression into mitosis with unreplicated DNA; and second, the inhibition of DNA replication to prevent RPA exhaustion (Smits and Gillespie 2015) (Fig. 3.4, bottom). Entry into mitosis is driven by CDK1 activity. Wee1-dependent phosphorylation of CDK1 at T14 and Y15 inhibits its activity and is counteracted by the CDC25 family of phosphatases (CDC25A, B and C) (Lindqvist et al. 2009). CHK1 prevents the activation of CDK1 by interfering with the CDC25 family through different mechanisms. The phosphorylation of CDC25A induces its degradation (Chen et al. 2003;

Mailand et al. 2000) while the phosphorylation of both CDC25A and CDC25C results in binding by the 14-3-3 proteins that blocks their activity (Chen et al. 2003; Peng et al. 1997). Additionally, CHK1 also phosphorylates Wee1 stimulating the phosphorylation of CDK1 (Lee et al. 2001). Together, CHK1 favours CDK1 inhibitory phosphorylations to enforce the inhibition of the entry into mitosis (Fig. 3.4, bottom right).

Besides entry into mitosis, the replication stress response can also globally affect origin firing (Fig. 3.4, bottom left). After the MCM helicase is loaded at the origins of DNA replication, the formation of an active helicase requires the incorporation of the GINS complex and CDC45 (Hills and Diffley 2014). The loading of CDC45 on chromatin requires the association of TOPBP1 and TRESLIN, which is dependent on the phosphorylation of TRESLIN by S-phase CDK (Boos et al. 2011; Kumagai et al. 2011). Additionally, the DDK (Cdc7/Dbf4) kinase also contributes to CDC45 loading and origin firing (Hills and Diffley 2014). CHK1 controls origin firing both in unperturbed conditions and after replication stress through two different mechanisms. On one hand, CHK1 controls the activity of CDK2 by modulating the stability of CDC25A, similar to its action on CDK1. During an unperturbed S phase, the accumulation of CHK1 limits the activity of CDK2 and controls the firing of additional origins of replication (Maya-Mendoza et al. 2007; Petermann et al. 2010; Syljuasen et al. 2005). However, it is unclear how CHK1 can elicit a specific inhibitory action on CDK2 at origins of replication while allowing for high CDK2 activity elsewhere in the nucleus. A more direct action of CHK1 on origin firing is established through the phosphorylation of TRESLIN that blocks the interaction with TOPBP1, impairing the loading of CDC45 (Boos et al. 2011; Guo et al. 2015). In the presence of replication stress or DNA damage, the strong activation of CHK1 blocks three activities required for origin firing: first, it leads to CDC25A degradation and CDK2 inhibition (Petermann et al. 2010); second, it phosphorylates TRESLIN and blocks the loading of CDC45 (Boos et al. 2011; Guo et al. 2015); third, CHK1 reduces the activity of the DDK kinase, possibly by the phosphorylation of DBF4 (Heffernan et al. 2007).

The different levels of action of ATR-ATRIP and CHK1 illustrate the flexibility of the replication stress response pathway. ATR and CHK1 are necessary for normal S phase through a local action on the stabilization of the stalled replication forks and the modulation of new origin firing that ensures complete DNA replication. In unperturbed conditions or after mild replication stress the activation of the ATR-CHK1 pathway needs to be controlled to prevent the full activation of the checkpoint. When strong problems arise during S phase, the signal is then transmitted to the whole nucleus through the action of CHK1 that stops DNA replication and blocks entry into mitosis. The mechanisms that drive the gradual activation of the ATR-CHK1 pathway have not been elucidated yet. Given their central role in the control of DNA replication and the maintenance of genome instability, it is no surprise that ATR and CHK1 play a prominent role in the development of diseases such as cancer or aging.

3.5 Functions of ATR and CHK1 in Cancer

3.5.1 ATR and CHK1 Are Essential

Given the function of ATR and CHK1 as checkpoint proteins, it was initially hypothesized that they would act as tumour suppressors, similar to mutations in ATM. However, the absence of ATR or CHK1 is lethal at the cellular and the organism level (Brown and Baltimore 2000; de Klein et al. 2000; Liu et al. 2000; Takai et al. 2000). While heterozygous mice are viable and fertile, the absence of ATR or CHK1 results in early embryonic lethality. In both cases the lethality is due to the combination of two factors: first, the lack of ATR or CHK1 prevents fork stabilization and repair leading to ssDNA accumulation and RPA exhaustion; second, in the absence of these proteins there is no cell cycle arrest at G2/M. Therefore, cells that have accumulated damage in S phase are then forced to enter mitosis and die by mitotic catastrophe (Brown and Baltimore 2000; Takai et al. 2000).

Further supporting that ATR or CHK1 cannot be catalogued as tumour suppressors, mice bearing a heterozygous deletion of ATR or CHK1 show only a modest increase in tumour incidence (Brown and Baltimore 2000; Liu et al. 2000). Moreover, deleterious mutations in either gene are not particularly recurrent in cancer, and only one mutation in ATR has been related to familiar cancer (Tanaka et al. 2012), although neither the impact nor the relevance of this mutation have been clarified. Rather than being lost, ATR and CHK1 expression seems to be gained in tumours. For instance, a recent analysis of more than 1000 ovarian cancers revealed recurrent CHK1 amplifications (Krajewska et al. 2015), and increased CHK1 levels have been reported across various tumours (Derenzini et al. 2015; Sarmento et al. 2015). The reason for tumours to select for high ATR/CHK1 levels is that their elevated endogenous levels of replication stress make them particularly reliant on the RS-response (similar to the concept of oncogene addition), which constitutes the basis for the potential use of ATR and CHK1 inhibitors in cancer therapy (Lecona and Fernandez-Capetillo 2014). Supporting this concept, CHK1 overexpression facilitates transformation by oncogenes, through reducing oncogene-induced RS (Lopez-Contreras et al. 2012). Unexpectedly, the actual data support that ATR and CHK1 are oncogenes rather than tumour suppressors.

Whereas the genetic deletion of ATR is cell lethal, there is a synonymous mutation that compromises ATR mRNA splicing leading to the human hereditary Seckel syndrome (O'Driscoll et al. 2003). In this syndrome a severe reduction of ATR levels is observed together with dwarfism, microcephaly and other developmental defects. Additional mutations in ATR and also in ATRIP have been found in patients that share the main features of the Seckel syndrome, confirming that the overarching cause for the phenotype is the lack of ATR-ATRIP function during S phase (Ogi et al. 2012).

A mouse model for the Seckel syndrome further confirmed that ATR is not a tumour suppressor. In this syndrome the expression of ATR is severely compromised, leading to much lower ATR levels than in the ATR heterozygous mice. This strong reduction in ATR, rather than promoting tumour formation, protects ATR-Seckel mice were from tumorigenesis induced by several oncogenes (see below). The generation of a humanized version of the ATR gene bearing the Seckel syndrome mutation recapitulated many of the features of the human disease (Murga et al. 2009), including the dwarfism and craniofacial abnormalities that originally named the disease as "bird-headed dwarfism". Seckel mice presented high levels of replication stress during embryonic development, but premature aging in the adult. These observations led to the proposal of the concept of "Intrauterine Programming of Ageing": the velocity at which mammals age is influenced by stresses they suffer during embryogenesis (Fernandez-Capetillo 2010). As mentioned, and in contrast to other syndromes associated with genome instability, Seckel mice are not tumour prone (Murga et al. 2009). What is more, the reduced levels of ATR in this model prevented the formation of tumours induced by oncogenes such as MYC or MLL-ENL, and was synthetic lethal with the loss of tumour suppressors like P53 (Murga et al. 2009, 2011; Schoppy et al. 2012).

In summary, and contrary to initial thoughts, the ATR/CHK1 axis cannot be catalogued as a tumour suppressor but rather as an oncogene that favours the growth of malignant cells. What then is the role of the ATR-CHK1 pathway during malignant transformation?

3.5.2 Malignant Transformation Generates Replication Stress

Oncogenic events that drive malignant transformation frequently promote a promiscuous S-phase entry, leading cells to replicate their DNA when they are not ready, and thus generating replication stress and DNA damage (Fig. 3.5a). The persistent accumulation of replication stress ultimately generates DNA breaks and activates the ATM/p53 DDR, which constitutes the basis of the "oncogene-induced DNA damage" model of cancer progression (Halazonetis et al. 2008). While oncogene activation can generate replication stress through multiple mechanisms, all of them are signalled through the ATR axis (Fig. 3.5a).

As described above, the licensing of back-up DNA replication origins is necessary to prevent replication stress. Counter-intuitively, overexpression of CYCLIN E reduces the number of replication origins licensed during G1, as does reducing the levels of components of the MCM helicase (Bagley et al. 2012; Ekholm-Reed et al. 2004; Pruitt et al. 2007; Shima et al. 2007). Interestingly, MCM hypomorphism in mice is slightly cancer-prone, arguing that the genomic instability generated by moderate levels of replication stress could lead to cancer (Bagley et al. 2012; Pruitt et al. 2007; Shima et al. 2007). In contrast to CYCLIN E, the overexpression of other oncogenes such as MYC or RAS has an opposite effect and increases replication origin firing, which has been proposed to lead to replication stress due to the exhaustion of dNTP pools (Bartkova et al. 2006; Bester et al. 2011; Di Micco

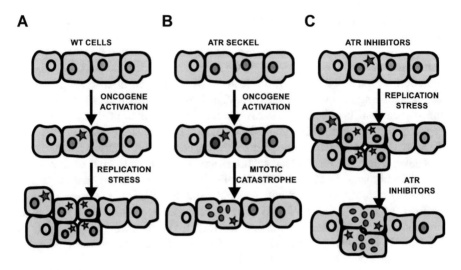

Fig. 3.5 Replication stress during malignant transformation. (**a**) In normal cells, oncogene activation (red star) increases the levels of replication stress (red nucleus). Transformed cells rely on the ATR pathway to proliferate in the presence of this replication stress. (**b**) A reduced activity of ATR is not compatible with malignant transformation. In ATR Seckel mice, there is an increase in basal levels of replication stress (red nucleus). The activation of an oncogene (red star) accumulates toxic levels of damage that lead to mitotic catastrophe. (**c**) After malignant transformation the treatment with ATR inhibitors increases replication stress to toxic levels and pushes cancer cells into mitosis. This combined effect induces specific cancer cell death

et al. 2006; Dominguez-Sola et al. 2007; Jones et al. 2013). In support of this, an extra supply of nucleosides has been shown to limit genomic instability induced by oncogenes (Bester et al. 2011) or reprogramming factors (Ruiz et al. 2015).

In addition to exhausting dNTP pools, an increased origin firing can also provoke a higher number of replication-transcription collisions. These collisions induce fork stalling (Jones et al. 2013) and are thought to be a major cause of genome instability, particularly at common fragile sites (Helmrich et al. 2013). Among others, the formation of RNA-DNA hybrids called R-loops have been shown to lead to replication-transcription collisions and participate in the induction of replication stress (Aguilera and Garcia-Muse 2012). It is possible that oncogene-induced replication stress involves several of these pathways, such as altering the number of licensed origins, affecting the dNTP pools and promoting the formation of R-loops by stimulating widespread transcription.

As mentioned above, moderate levels of replication stress can lead to genomic instability and cancer (Hanahan and Weinberg 2011). However, replication stress is a pathological condition and it can lead to cell death above a tolerable threshold (Lecona and Fernandez-Capetillo 2014). In this context, the replication stress response can play the role of an oncogene, by limiting the levels of replication stress in cancer cells and thus promoting cell viability.

3.5.3   The Replication Stress Response Favours Malignant Transformation

The toxic consequences of replication stress could constitute a barrier for cellular transformation. In this context, an increased activity of the ATR-CHK1 pathway should play the role of an oncogene and facilitate oncogenic transformation. Accordingly, a higher dose of CHK1 facilitates transformation with Ras and E1A by reducing the amount of RS-induced by the oncogenes and thus limiting the toxicity of the transformation process (Lopez-Contreras et al. 2012). Actually, the expression of ATR and CHK1 is frequently upregulated in cancer and this effect is due, at least in part, to the fact that these genes are regulated during the cell cycle. Additionally, CHK1 is also under the direct control of different oncogenes such as Myc, E2F or c-fos (Hoglund et al. 2011, Schulze et al. 2014; Verlinden et al. 2007).

Besides CHK1, and as mentioned, an increased supply of nucleotides is an alternative method to reduce replication stress (Bester et al. 2011; Lopez-Contreras et al. 2012) and could also favour the survival of cells after oncogene activation. In this context, an upregulation of the levels of the ribonucleotide reductase is frequently found in human cancers (Aye et al. 2015). Further, the expression of RRM2 is also controlled during the cell cycle by E2F (Aye et al. 2015) and is increased by oncogenes like Myc (Bester et al. 2011). As a whole, the presence of replication stress is the price that cancer cells pay for their fast proliferation. In order to deal with this replication stress transformed cells select for the overexpression of factors that can buffer this stress.

The overall picture that emerges from these studies is that the same transcription factors that promote S-phase entry e.g. MYC, E2F, also promote the expression of factors that limit replication stress such as CHK1 or the RNR. In analogy to the "oncogene-addiction" model, this renders tumours highly dependent on a proficient ATR/CHK1 response, and is the basis for the use of ATR/CHK1 inhibitors in cancer.

3.5.4   Targeting the Replication Stress Response in Cancer

The fact that cellular transformation requires a proficient replication stress response can be used to design treatments to specifically kill cancer cells. Blocking the action of ATR or CHK1 could be especially deleterious for cells with altered DNA replication that heavily rely on their action to prevent entry into mitosis with unreplicated DNA, causing widespread DNA damage (Ruiz et al. 2016). Accordingly, and as mentioned above, the deleterious effects of reduced ATR activity are further aggravated by the loss of the tumour suppressor p53 (Ruzankina et al. 2009; Toledo et al. 2011) or by the expression of oncogenes such as Myc or MLL-ENL (Murga et al. 2011; Schoppy et al. 2012) (Fig. 3.5b). In addition to cancers that show an impaired control of DNA replication, the absence of other checkpoint proteins also makes cells heavily depend on the action of ATR. In this sense reduced levels of ATR are also synthetic lethal with the deletion of ATM (Murga et al. 2009).

Regarding the translation of these findings to the clinic, independent strategies have been employed to develop selective ATR inhibitors (Charrier et al. 2011; Foote et al. 2013; Reaper et al. 2011; Toledo et al. 2011). The use of these inhibitors has confirmed that the unscheduled entry into S-phase of cancer cells induced by the overexpression of oncogenes like CYCLIN E or the deletion of tumour suppressors like p53, as well as the loss of ATM render these cells particularly sensitive to the ATR inhibitors (Reaper et al. 2011; Toledo et al. 2011) (Fig. 3.5c).

DNA replication was one of the first targets in the development of modern chemotherapy. In 1948 Sydney Farber described the use of anti-folates that target nucleotide metabolism to treat children leukemia (Farber and Diamond 1948). We now know that this treatment is likely working through the generation of replication stress in cancer cells. In this context, ATR inhibitors are a revisited version of this strategy. The advantage of these ATR inhibitors is that, in addition to inducing replication stress, they also promote mitotic entry, thereby leading to major segregation problems (Ruiz et al. 2016) (Fig. 3.5c). The design, development and applications of these inhibitors will be the subject of the next chapters.

3.6 Concluding Remarks

The response to DNA damage is essential to safeguard genome integrity. Many different agents, both extrinsic and intrinsic, pose a threat to the cells and the DNA damage response has evolved different mechanisms to face these challenges. Regarding replication stress, ATR and CHK1 are the key components of the cellular response, the activity of which is essential to safeguard genome integrity during every S-phase. Nevertheless, the presence of higher levels of replication stress in cancer cells, due to the effect of oncogenes, renders them particularly dependent on the ATR/CHK1 response. To what extent these ideas will translate into treatments of clinical efficacy remains to be seen, and will likely be addressed in the coming decade.

References

Aguilera A, Garcia-Muse T (2012) R loops: from transcription byproducts to threats to genome stability. Mol Cell 46:115–124

Aye Y, Li M, Long MJ, Weiss RS (2015) Ribonucleotide reductase and cancer: biological mechanisms and targeted therapies. Oncogene 34:2011–2021

Bagley BN, Keane TM, Maklakova VI, Marshall JG, Lester RA, Cancel MM, Paulsen AR, Bendzick LE, Been RA, Kogan SC, Cormier RT, Kendziorski C, Adams DJ, Collier LS (2012) A dominantly acting murine allele of Mcm4 causes chromosomal abnormalities and promotes tumorigenesis. PLoS Genet 8:e1003034

Ball HL, Cortez D (2005) ATRIP oligomerization is required for ATR-dependent checkpoint signaling. J Biol Chem 280:31390–31396

Ball HL, Myers JS, Cortez D (2005) ATRIP binding to replication protein A-single-stranded DNA promotes ATR-ATRIP localization but is dispensable for Chk1 phosphorylation. Mol Biol Cell 16:2372–2381

Baretic D, Williams RL (2014) PIKKs – the solenoid nest where partners and kinases meet. Curr Opin Struct Biol 29:134–142

Bartkova J, Rezaei N, Liontos M, Karakaidos P, Kletsas D, Issaeva N, Vassiliou LV, Kolettas E, Niforou K, Zoumpourlis VC, Takaoka M, Nakagawa H, Tort F, Fugger K, Johansson F, Sehested M, Andersen CL, Dyrskjot L, Orntoft T, Lukas J, Kittas C, Helleday T, Halazonetis TD, Bartek J, Gorgoulis VG (2006) Oncogene-induced senescence is part of the tumorigenesis barrier imposed by DNA damage checkpoints. Nature 444:633–637

Bastos de Oliveira FM, Kim D, Cussiol JR, Das J, Jeong MC, Doerfler L, Schmidt KH, Yu H, Smolka MB (2015) Phosphoproteomics reveals distinct modes of Mec1/ATR signaling during DNA replication. Mol Cell 57:1124–1132

Berti M, Vindigni A (2016) Replication stress: getting back on track. Nat Struct Mol Biol 23:103–109

Bester AC, Roniger M, Oren YS, Im MM, Sarni D, Chaoat M, Bensimon A, Zamir G, Shewach DS, Kerem B (2011) Nucleotide deficiency promotes genomic instability in early stages of cancer development. Cell 145:435–446

Blow JJ, GE XQ, Jackson DA (2011) How dormant origins promote complete genome replication. Trends Biochem Sci 36:405–414

Boos D, Sanchez-Pulido L, Rappas M, Pearl LH, Oliver AW, Ponting CP, Diffley JF (2011) Regulation of DNA replication through Sld3-Dpb11 interaction is conserved from yeast to humans. Curr Biol 21:1152–1157

Broustas CG, Lieberman HB (2012) Contributions of Rad9 to tumorigenesis. J Cell Biochem 113:742–751

Brown EJ, Baltimore D (2000) ATR disruption leads to chromosomal fragmentation and early embryonic lethality. Genes Dev 14:397–402

Buisson R, Boisvert JL, Benes CH, Zou L (2015) Distinct but concerted roles of ATR, DNA-PK, and Chk1 in countering replication stress during S phase. Mol Cell 59:1011–1024

Bursomanno S, Beli P, Khan AM, Minocherhomji S, Wagner SA, Bekker-Jensen S, Mailand N, Choudhary C, Hickson ID, Liu Y (2015) Proteome-wide analysis of SUMO2 targets in response to pathological DNA replication stress in human cells. DNA Repair (Amst) 25:84–96

Charrier JD, Durrant SJ, Golec JM, Kay DP, Knegtel RM, Maccormick S, Mortimore M, O'donnell ME, Pinder JL, Reaper PM, Rutherford AP, Wang PS, Young SC, Pollard JR (2011) Discovery of potent and selective inhibitors of ataxia telangiectasia mutated and Rad3 related (ATR) protein kinase as potential anticancer agents. J Med Chem 54:2320–2330

Chen MS, Ryan CE, Piwnica-Worms H (2003) Chk1 kinase negatively regulates mitotic function of Cdc25A phosphatase through 14-3-3 binding. Mol Cell Biol 23:7488–7497

Chen YH, Jones MJ, Yin Y, Crist SB, Colnaghi L, Sims RJ 3rd, Rothenberg E, Jallepalli PV, Huang TT (2015) ATR-mediated phosphorylation of FANCI regulates dormant origin firing in response to replication stress. Mol Cell 58:323–338

Chini CC, Chen J (2003) Human Claspin is required for replication checkpoint control. J Biol Chem 278:30057–30062

Chini CC, Chen J (2006) Repeated phosphopeptide motifs in human Claspin are phosphorylated by Chk1 and mediate Claspin function. J Biol Chem 281:33276–33282

Choi JH, Lindsey-Boltz LA, Kemp M, Mason AC, Wold MS, Sancar A (2010) Reconstitution of RPA-covered single-stranded DNA-activated ATR-Chk1 signaling. Proc Natl Acad Sci U S A 107:13660–13665

Ciccia A, Bredemeyer AL, Sowa ME, Terret ME, Jallepalli PV, Harper JW, Elledge SJ (2009) The SIOD disorder protein SMARCAL1 is an RPA-interacting protein involved in replication fork restart. Genes Dev 23:2415–2425

Cimprich KA, Shin TB, Keith CT, Schreiber SL (1996) cDNA cloning and gene mapping of a candidate human cell cycle checkpoint protein. Proc Natl Acad Sci U S A 93:2850–2855

Cortez D, Guntuku S, Qin J, Elledge SJ (2001) ATR and ATRIP: partners in checkpoint signaling. Science 294:1713–1716

Cortez D, Glick G, Elledge SJ (2004) Minichromosome maintenance proteins are direct targets of the ATM and ATR checkpoint kinases. Proc Natl Acad Sci U S A 101:10078–10083

Cotta-Ramusino C, McDonald ER 3rd, Hurov K, Sowa ME, Harper JW, Elledge SJ (2011) A DNA damage response screen identifies RHINO, a 9-1-1 and TopBP1 interacting protein required for ATR signaling. Science 332:1313–1317

Couch FB, Bansbach CE, Driscoll R, Luzwick JW, Glick GG, Betous R, Carroll CM, Jung SY, Qin J, Cimprich KA, Cortez D (2013) ATR phosphorylates SMARCAL1 to prevent replication fork collapse. Genes Dev 27:1610–1623

D'Angiolella V, Donato V, Forrester FM, Jeong YT, Pellacani C, Kudo Y, Saraf A, Florens L, Washburn MP, Pagano M (2012) Cyclin F-mediated degradation of ribonucleotide reductase M2 controls genome integrity and DNA repair. Cell 149:1023–1034

Davies SL, North PS, Hickson ID (2007) Role for BLM in replication-fork restart and suppression of origin firing after replicative stress. Nat Struct Mol Biol 14:677–679

de Klein A, Muijtjens M, Van Os R, Verhoeven Y, Smit B, Carr AM, Lehmann AR, Hoeijmakers JH (2000) Targeted disruption of the cell-cycle checkpoint gene ATR leads to early embryonic lethality in mice. Curr Biol 10:479–482

Delacroix S, Wagner JM, Kobayashi M, Yamamoto K, Karnitz LM (2007) The Rad9-Hus1-Rad1 (9-1-1) clamp activates checkpoint signaling via TopBP1. Genes Dev 21:1472–1477

Derenzini E, Agostinelli C, Imbrogno E, Iacobucci I, Casadei B, Brighenti E, Righi S, Fuligni F, Ghelli Luserna Di Rora A, Ferrari A, Martinelli G, Pileri S, Zinzani PL (2015) Constitutive activation of the DNA damage response pathway as a novel therapeutic target in diffuse large B-cell lymphoma. Oncotarget 6:6553–6569

Di Micco R, Fumagalli M, Cicalese A, Piccinin S, Gasparini P, Luise C, Schurra C, Garre M, Nuciforo PG, Bensimon A, Maestro R, Pelicci PG, d'Adda Di Fagagna F (2006) Oncogene-induced senescence is a DNA damage response triggered by DNA hyper-replication. Nature 444:638–642

Dominguez-Sola D, Ying CY, Grandori C, Ruggiero L, Chen B, Li M, Galloway DA, Gu W, Gautier J, Dalla-Favera R (2007) Non-transcriptional control of DNA replication by c-Myc. Nature 448:445–451

Dungrawala H, Rose KL, Bhat KP, Mohni KN, Glick GG, Couch FB, Cortez D (2015) The replication checkpoint prevents two types of fork collapse without regulating replisome stability. Mol Cell 59:998–1010

Duursma AM, Driscoll R, Elias JE, Cimprich KA (2013) A role for the MRN complex in ATR activation via TOPBP1 recruitment. Mol Cell 50:116–122

Edwards RJ, Bentley NJ, Carr AM (1999) A Rad3-Rad26 complex responds to DNA damage independently of other checkpoint proteins. Nat Cell Biol 1:393–398

Ekholm-Reed S, Mendez J, Tedesco D, Zetterberg A, Stillman B, Reed SI (2004) Deregulation of cyclin E in human cells interferes with prereplication complex assembly. J Cell Biol 165:789–800

Farber S, Diamond LK (1948) Temporary remissions in acute leukemia in children produced by folic acid antagonist, 4-aminopteroyl-glutamic acid. N Engl J Med 238:787–793

Faustrup H, Bekker-Jensen S, Bartek J, Lukas J, Mailand N (2009) USP7 counteracts SCFbetaTrCP-but not APCCdh1-mediated proteolysis of Claspin. J Cell Biol 184:13–19

Fernandez-Capetillo O (2010) Intrauterine programming of ageing. EMBO Rep 11:32–36

Foote KM, Blades K, Cronin A, Fillery S, Guichard SS, Hassall L, Hickson I, Jacq X, Jewsbury PJ, McGuire TM, Nissink JW, Odedra R, Page K, Perkins P, Suleman A, Tam K, Thommes P, Broadhurst R, Wood C (2013) Discovery of 4-{4-[(3R)-3-Methylmorpholin-4-yl]-6-[1-(methylsulfonyl)cyclopropyl]pyrimidin-2-y 1}-1H-indole (AZ20): a potent and selective inhibitor of ATR protein kinase with monotherapy in vivo antitumor activity. J Med Chem 56:2125–2138

Ge XQ, Blow JJ (2010) Chk1 inhibits replication factory activation but allows dormant origin firing in existing factories. J Cell Biol 191:1285–1297

Ge XQ, Jackson DA, Blow JJ (2007) Dormant origins licensed by excess Mcm2-7 are required for human cells to survive replicative stress. Genes Dev 21:3331–3341

Guo C, Kumagai A, Schlacher K, Shevchenko A, Shevchenko A, Dunphy WG (2015) Interaction of Chk1 with Treslin negatively regulates the initiation of chromosomal DNA replication. Mol Cell 57:492–505

Halazonetis TD, Gorgoulis VG, Bartek J (2008) An oncogene-induced DNA damage model for cancer development. Science 319:1352–1355

Hanahan D, Weinberg RA (2011) Hallmarks of cancer: the next generation. Cell 144:646–674

Hao J, de Renty C, Li Y, Xiao H, Kemp MG, Han Z, Depamphilis ML, Zhu W (2015) And-1 coordinates with Claspin for efficient Chk1 activation in response to replication stress. EMBO J 34:2096–2110

Heffernan TP, Unsal-Kacmaz K, Heinloth AN, Simpson DA, Paules RS, Sancar A, Cordeiro-Stone M, Kaufman WK (2007) Cdc7-Dbf4 and the human S checkpoint response to UVC. J Biol Chem 282:9458–9468

Helmrich A, Ballarino M, Nudler E, Tora L (2013) Transcription-replication encounters, consequences and genomic instability. Nat Struct Mol Biol 20:412–418

Hills SA, Diffley JF (2014) DNA replication and oncogene-induced replicative stress. Curr Biol 24:R435–R444

Hoglund A, Nilsson LM, Muralidharan SV, Hasvold LA, Merta P, Rudelius M, Nikolova V, Keller U, Nilsson JA (2011) Therapeutic implications for the induced levels of Chk1 in Myc-expressing cancer cells. Clin Cancer Res 17:7067–7079

Ibarra A, Schwob E, Mendez J (2008) Excess MCM proteins protect human cells from replicative stress by licensing backup origins of replication. Proc Natl Acad Sci U S A 105:8956–8961

Jeong SY, Kumagai A, Lee J, Dunphy WG (2003) Phosphorylated Claspin interacts with a phosphate-binding site in the kinase domain of Chk1 during ATR-mediated activation. J Biol Chem 278:46782–46788

Jones RM, Mortusewicz O, Afzal I, Lorvellec M, Garcia P, Helleday T, Petermann E (2013) Increased replication initiation and conflicts with transcription underlie cyclin E-induced replication stress. Oncogene 32:3744–3753

Kang SA, Pacold ME, Cervantes CL, Lim D, Lou HJ, Ottina K, Gray NS, Turk BE, Yaffe MB, Sabatini DM (2013) mTORC1 phosphorylation sites encode their sensitivity to starvation and rapamycin. Science 341:1236566

Kemp MG, Akan Z, Yilmaz S, Grillo M, Smith-Roe SL, Kang TH, Cordeiro-Stone M, Kaufmann WK, Abraham RT, Sancar A, Unsal-Kacmaz K (2010) Tipin-replication protein A interaction mediates Chk1 phosphorylation by ATR in response to genotoxic stress. J Biol Chem 285:16562–16571

Koundrioukoff S, Carignon S, Techer H, Letessier A, Brison O, Debatisse M (2013) Stepwise activation of the ATR signaling pathway upon increasing replication stress impacts fragile site integrity. PLoS Genet 9:e1003643

Krajewska M, Fehrmann RS, Schoonen PM, Labib S, de Vries EG, Franke L, Van Vugt MA (2015) ATR inhibition preferentially targets homologous recombination-deficient tumor cells. Oncogene 34:3474–3481

Kumagai A, Dunphy WG (2000) Claspin, a novel protein required for the activation of Chk1 during a DNA replication checkpoint response in Xenopus egg extracts. Mol Cell 6:839–849

Kumagai A, Dunphy WG (2003) Repeated phosphopeptide motifs in Claspin mediate the regulated binding of Chk1. Nat Cell Biol 5:161–165

Kumagai A, Kim SM, Dunphy WG (2004) Claspin and the activated form of ATR-ATRIP collaborate in the activation of Chk1. J Biol Chem 279:49599–49608

Kumagai A, Lee J, Yoo HY, Dunphy WG (2006) TopBP1 activates the ATR-ATRIP complex. Cell 124:943–955

Kumagai A, Shevchenko A, Shevchenko A, Dunphy WG (2011) Direct regulation of Treslin by cyclin-dependent kinase is essential for the onset of DNA replication. J Cell Biol 193:995–1007

Lecona E, Fernandez-Capetillo O (2014) Replication stress and cancer: it takes two to tango. Exp Cell Res 329:26–34

Lee J, Dunphy WG (2013) The Mre11-Rad50-Nbs1 (MRN) complex has a specific role in the activation of Chk1 in response to stalled replication forks. Mol Biol Cell 24:1343–1353

Lee J, Kumagai A, Dunphy WG (2001) Positive regulation of Wee1 by Chk1 and 14-3-3 proteins. Mol Biol Cell 12:551–563

Lee J, Kumagai A, Dunphy WG (2007) The Rad9-Hus1-Rad1 checkpoint clamp regulates interaction of TopBP1 with ATR. J Biol Chem 282:28036–28044

Lin SJ, Wardlaw CP, Morishita T, Miyabe I, Chahwan C, Caspari T, Schmidt U, Carr AM, Garcia V (2012) The Rad4(TopBP1) ATR-activation domain functions in G1/S phase in a chromatin-dependent manner. PLoS Genet 8:e1002801

Lindqvist A, Rodriguez-Bravo V, Medema RH (2009) The decision to enter mitosis: feedback and redundancy in the mitotic entry network. J Cell Biol 185:193–202

Lindsey-Boltz LA, Kemp MG, Capp C, Sancar A (2015) RHINO forms a stoichiometric complex with the 9-1-1 checkpoint clamp and mediates ATR-Chk1 signaling. Cell Cycle 14:99–108

Liu Q, Guntuku S, Cui XS, Matsuoka S, Cortez D, Tamai K, Luo G, Carattini-Rivera S, Demayo F, Bradley A, Donehower LA, Elledge SJ (2000) Chk1 is an essential kinase that is regulated by ATR and required for the G(2)/M DNA damage checkpoint. Genes Dev 14:1448–1459

Liu S, Bekker-Jensen S, Mailand N, Lukas C, Bartek J, Lukas J (2006) Claspin operates downstream of TopBP1 to direct ATR signaling towards Chk1 activation. Mol Cell Biol 26:6056–6064

Liu S, Shiotani B, Lahiri M, Marechal A, Tse A, Leung CC, Glover JN, Yang XH, Zou L (2011) ATR autophosphorylation as a molecular switch for checkpoint activation. Mol Cell 43:192–202

Lopez-Contreras AJ, Gutierrez-Martinez P, Specks J, Rodrigo-Perez S, Fernandez-Capetillo O (2012) An extra allele of Chk1 limits oncogene-induced replicative stress and promotes transformation. J Exp Med 209:455–461

Lopez-Contreras AJ, Ruppen I, Nieto-Soler M, Murga M, Rodriguez-Acebes S, Remeseiro S, Rodrigo-Perez S, Rojas AM, Mendez J, Munoz J, Fernandez-Capetillo O (2013) A proteomic characterization of factors enriched at nascent DNA molecules. Cell Rep 3:1105–1116

Lopez-Contreras AJ, Specks J, Barlow JH, Ambrogio C, Desler C, Vikingsson S, Rodrigo-Perez S, Green H, Rasmussen LJ, Murga M, Nussenzweig A, Fernandez-Capetillo O (2015) Increased Rrm2 gene dosage reduces fragile site breakage and prolongs survival of ATR mutant mice. Genes Dev 29:690–695

Lossaint G, Larroque M, Ribeyre C, Bec N, Larroque C, Decaillet C, Gari K, Constantinou A (2013) FANCD2 binds MCM proteins and controls replisome function upon activation of s phase checkpoint signaling. Mol Cell 51:678–690

Lovejoy CA, Cortez D (2009) Common mechanisms of PIKK regulation. DNA Repair (Amst) 8:1004–1008

Lukas C, Falck J, Bartkova J, Bartek J, Lukas J (2003) Distinct spatiotemporal dynamics of mammalian checkpoint regulators induced by DNA damage. Nat Cell Biol 5:255–260

Luzwick JW, Nam EA, Zhao R, Cortez D (2014) Mutation of serine 1333 in the ATR HEAT repeats creates a hyperactive kinase. PLoS One 9:e99397

Mailand N, Falck J, Lukas C, Syljuasen RG, Welcker M, Bartek J, Lukas J (2000) Rapid destruction of human Cdc25A in response to DNA damage. Science 288:1425–1429

Mailand N, Bekker-Jensen S, Bartek J, Lukas J (2006) Destruction of Claspin by SCFbetaTrCP restrains Chk1 activation and facilitates recovery from genotoxic stress. Mol Cell 23:307–318

Mamely I, van Vugt MA, Smits VA, Semple JI, Lemmens B, Perrakis A, Medema RH, Freire R (2006) Polo-like kinase-1 controls proteasome-dependent degradation of Claspin during checkpoint recovery. Curr Biol 16:1950–1955

Marechal A, Li JM, Ji XY, Wu CS, Yazinski SA, Nguyen HD, Liu S, Jimenez AE, Jin J, Zou L (2014) PRP19 transforms into a sensor of RPA-ssDNA after DNA damage and drives ATR activation via a ubiquitin-mediated circuitry. Mol Cell 53:235–246

Martin Y, Cabrera E, Amoedo H, Hernandez-Perez S, Dominguez-Kelly R, Freire R (2015) USP29 controls the stability of checkpoint adaptor Claspin by deubiquitination. Oncogene 34:1058–1063

Matsuoka S, Ballif BA, Smogorzewska A, Mcdonald ER 3rd, Hurov KE, Luo J, Bakalarski CE, Zhao Z, Solimini N, Lerenthal Y, Shiloh Y, Gygi SP, Elledge SJ (2007) ATM and ATR substrate analysis reveals extensive protein networks responsive to DNA damage. Science 316:1160–1166

Maya-Mendoza A, Petermann E, Gillespie DA, Caldecott KW, Jackson DA (2007) Chk1 regulates the density of active replication origins during the vertebrate S phase. EMBO J 26: 2719–2731

Mordes DA, Glick GG, Zhao R, Cortez D (2008a) TopBP1 activates ATR through ATRIP and a PIKK regulatory domain. Genes Dev 22:1478–1489

Mordes DA, Nam EA, Cortez D (2008b) Dpb11 activates the Mec1-Ddc2 complex. Proc Natl Acad Sci U S A 105:18730–18734

Murga M, Bunting S, Montana MF, Soria R, Mulero F, Canamero M, Lee Y, Mckinnon PJ, Nussenzweig A, Fernandez-Capetillo O (2009) A mouse model of ATR-Seckel shows embryonic replicative stress and accelerated aging. Nat Genet 41:891–898

Murga M, Campaner S, Lopez-Contreras AJ, Toledo LI, Soria R, Montana MF, D'Artista L, Schleker T, Guerra C, Garcia E, Barbacid M, Hidalgo M, Amati B, Fernandez-Capetillo O (2011) Exploiting oncogene-induced replicative stress for the selective killing of Myc-driven tumors. Nat Struct Mol Biol 18:1331–1335

Murphy AK, Fitzgerald M, Ro T, Kim JH, Rabinowitsch AI, Chowdhury D, Schildkraut CL, Borowiec JA (2014) Phosphorylated RPA recruits PALB2 to stalled DNA replication forks to facilitate fork recovery. J Cell Biol 206:493–507

O'Driscoll M, Ruiz-Perez VL, Woods CG, Jeggo PA, Goodship JA (2003) A splicing mutation affecting expression of ataxia-telangiectasia and Rad3-related protein (ATR) results in Seckel syndrome. Nat Genet 33:497–501

Ogi T, Walker S, Stiff T, Hobson E, Limsirichaikul S, Carpenter G, Prescott K, Suri M, Byrd PJ, Matsuse M, Mitsutake N, Nakazawa Y, Vasudevan P, Barrow M, Stewart GS, Taylor AM, O'Driscoll M, Jeggo PA (2012) Identification of the first ATRIP-deficient patient and novel mutations in ATR define a clinical spectrum for ATR-ATRIP Seckel syndrome. PLoS Genet 8:e1002945

Paciotti V, Clerici M, Lucchini G, Longhese MP (2000) The checkpoint protein Ddc2, functionally related to S. pombe Rad26, interacts with Mec1 and is regulated by Mec1-dependent phosphorylation in budding yeast. Genes Dev 14:2046–2059

Parrilla-Castellar ER, Arlander SJ, Karnitz L (2004) Dial 9-1-1 for DNA damage: the Rad9-Hus1-Rad1 (9-1-1) clamp complex. DNA Repair (Amst) 3:1009–1014

Peng CY, Graves PR, Thoma RS, Wu Z, Shaw AS, Piwnica-Worms H (1997) Mitotic and G2 checkpoint control: regulation of 14-3-3 protein binding by phosphorylation of Cdc25C on serine-216. Science 277:1501–1505

Peschiaroli A, Dorrello NV, Guardavaccaro D, Venere M, Halazonetis T, Sherman NE, Pagano M (2006) SCFbetaTrCP-mediated degradation of Claspin regulates recovery from the DNA replication checkpoint response. Mol Cell 23:319–329

Petermann E, Woodcock M, Helleday T (2010) Chk1 promotes replication fork progression by controlling replication initiation. Proc Natl Acad Sci U S A 107:16090–16095

Pichierri P, Rosselli F, Franchitto A (2003) Werner's syndrome protein is phosphorylated in an ATR/ATM-dependent manner following replication arrest and DNA damage induced during the S phase of the cell cycle. Oncogene 22:1491–1500

Pruitt SC, Bailey KJ, Freeland A (2007) Reduced Mcm2 expression results in severe stem/progenitor cell deficiency and cancer. Stem Cells 25:3121–3132

Psakhye I, Jentsch S (2012) Protein group modification and synergy in the SUMO pathway as exemplified in DNA repair. Cell 151:807–820

Reaper PM, Griffiths MR, Long JM, Charrier JD, Maccormick S, Charlton PA, Golec JM, Pollard JR (2011) Selective killing of ATM- or p53-deficient cancer cells through inhibition of ATR. Nat Chem Biol 7:428–430

Rouse J, Jackson SP (2000) LCD1: an essential gene involved in checkpoint control and regulation of the MEC1 signalling pathway in Saccharomyces cerevisiae. EMBO J 19:5801–5812

Ruiz S, Lopez-Contreras AJ, Gabut M, Marion RM, Gutierrez-Martinez P, Bua S, Ramirez O, Olalde I, Rodrigo-Perez S, Li H, Marques-Bonet T, Serrano M, Blasco MA, Batada NN, Fernandez-Capetillo O (2015) Limiting replication stress during somatic cell reprogramming reduces genomic instability in induced pluripotent stem cells. Nat Commun 6:8036

Ruiz S, Mayor-Ruiz C, Lafarga V, Murga M, Vega-Sandino M, Ortega S, Fernandez-Capetillo O (2016) A genome-wide CRISPR screen identifies CDC25A as a determinant of sensitivity to ATR inhibitors. Mol Cell 62(2):307–313

Ruzankina Y, Schoppy DW, Asare A, Clark CE, Vonderheide RH, Brown EJ (2009) Tissue regenerative delays and synthetic lethality in adult mice after combined deletion of ATR and Trp53. Nat Genet 41:1144–1149

Sarmento LM, Povoa V, Nascimento R, Real G, Antunes I, Martins LR, Moita C, Alves PM, Abecasis M, Moita LF, Parkhouse RM, Meijerink JP, Barata JT (2015) CHK1 overexpression in T-cell acute lymphoblastic leukemia is essential for proliferation and survival by preventing excessive replication stress. Oncogene 34:2978–2990

Schlacher K, Christ N, Siaud N, Egashira A, Wu H, Jasin M (2011) Double-strand break repair-independent role for BRCA2 in blocking stalled replication fork degradation by MRE11. Cell 145:529–542

Schlacher K, Wu H, Jasin M (2012) A distinct replication fork protection pathway connects Fanconi anemia tumor suppressors to RAD51-BRCA1/2. Cancer Cell 22:106–116

Schoppy DW, Ragland RL, Gilad O, Shastri N, Peters AA, Murga M, Fernandez-Capetillo O, Diehl JA, Brown EJ (2012) Oncogenic stress sensitizes murine cancers to hypomorphic suppression of ATR. J Clin Invest 122:241–252

Schulze J, Lopez-Contreras AJ, Uluckan O, Grana-Castro O, Fernandez-Capetillo O, Wagner EF (2014) Fos-dependent induction of Chk1 protects osteoblasts from replication stress. Cell Cycle 13:1980–1986

Sekulic A, Hudson CC, Homme JL, Yin P, Otterness DM, Karnitz LM, Abraham RT (2000) A direct linkage between the phosphoinositide 3-kinase-AKT signaling pathway and the mammalian target of rapamycin in mitogen-stimulated and transformed cells. Cancer Res 60:3504–3513

Shima N, Alcaraz A, Liachko I, Buske TR, Andrews CA, Munroe RJ, Hartford SA, Tye BK, Schimenti JC (2007) A viable allele of Mcm4 causes chromosome instability and mammary adenocarcinomas in mice. Nat Genet 39:93–98

Sibanda BL, Chirgadze DY, Blundell TL (2010) Crystal structure of DNA-PKcs reveals a large open-ring cradle comprised of HEAT repeats. Nature 463:118–121

Smits VA, Gillespie DA (2015) DNA damage control: regulation and functions of checkpoint kinase 1. FEBS J 282:3681–3692

Smits VA, Reaper PM, Jackson SP (2006) Rapid PIKK-dependent release of Chk1 from chromatin promotes the DNA-damage checkpoint response. Curr Biol 16:150–159

Specks J, Lecona E, Lopez-Contreras AJ, Fernandez-Capetillo O (2015) A single conserved residue mediates binding of the ribonucleotide reductase catalytic subunit RRM1 to RRM2 and is essential for mouse development. Mol Cell Biol 35:2910–2917

St Onge RP, Besley BD, Pelley JL, Davey S (2003) A role for the phosphorylation of hRad9 in checkpoint signaling. J Biol Chem 278:26620–26628

Sun Y, Xu Y, Roy K, Price BD (2007) DNA damage-induced acetylation of lysine 3016 of ATM activates ATM kinase activity. Mol Cell Biol 27:8502–8509

Syljuasen RG, Sorensen CS, Hansen LT, Fugger K, Lundin C, Johansson F, Helleday T, Sehested M, Lukas J, Bartek J (2005) Inhibition of human Chk1 causes increased initiation of DNA replication, phosphorylation of ATR targets, and DNA breakage. Mol Cell Biol 25:3553–3562

Takai H, Tominaga K, Motoyama N, Minamishima YA, Nagahama H, Tsukiyama T, Ikeda K, Nakayama K, Nakanishi M, Nakayama K (2000) Aberrant cell cycle checkpoint function and early embryonic death in Chk1(−/−) mice. Genes Dev 14:1439–1447

Tanaka A, Weinel S, Nagy N, O'Driscoll M, Lai-Cheong JE, Kulp-Shorten CL, Knable A, Carpenter G, Fisher SA, Hiragun M, Yanase Y, Hide M, Callen J, Mcgrath JA (2012) Germline mutation in ATR in autosomal- dominant oropharyngeal cancer syndrome. Am J Hum Genet 90:511–517

Toledo LI, Murga M, Zur R, Soria R, Rodriguez A, Martinez S, Oyarzabal J, Pastor J, Bischoff JR, Fernandez-Capetillo O (2011) A cell-based screen identifies ATR inhibitors with synthetic lethal properties for cancer-associated mutations. Nat Struct Mol Biol 18:721–727

Toledo LI, Altmeyer M, Rask MB, Lukas C, Larsen DH, Povlsen LK, Bekker-Jensen S, Mailand N, Bartek J, Lukas J (2013) ATR prohibits replication catastrophe by preventing global exhaustion of RPA. Cell 155:1088–1103

Verlinden L, Vanden Bempt I, Eelen G, Drijkoningen M, Verlinden I, Marchal K, de Wolf-Peeters C, Christiaens MR, Michiels L, Bouillon R, Verstuyf A (2007) The E2F-regulated gene Chk1 is highly expressed in triple-negative estrogen receptor /progesterone receptor /HER-2 breast carcinomas. Cancer Res 67:6574–6581

Walker EH, Perisic O, Ried C, Stephens L, Williams RL (1999) Structural insights into phosphoinositide 3-kinase catalysis and signalling. Nature 402:313–320

Wardlaw CP, Carr AM, Oliver AW (2014) TopBP1: A BRCT-scaffold protein functioning in multiple cellular pathways. DNA Repair (Amst) 22:165–174

Weinert TA, Kiser GL, Hartwell LH (1994) Mitotic checkpoint genes in budding yeast and the dependence of mitosis on DNA replication and repair. Genes Dev 8:652–665

Wu CS, Zou L (2016) The SUMO (small ubiquitin-like modifier) ligase PIAS3 primes ATR for checkpoint activation. J Biol Chem 291:279–290

Wu CS, Ouyang J, Mori E, Nguyen HD, Marechal A, Hallet A, Chen DJ, Zou L (2014) SUMOylation of ATRIP potentiates DNA damage signaling by boosting multiple protein interactions in the ATR pathway. Genes Dev 28:1472–1484

Xiao Z, Chang JG, Hendriks IA, Sigurethsson JO, Olsen JV, Vertegaal AC (2015) System-wide analysis of SUMOylation dynamics in response to replication stress reveals novel small ubiquitin-like modified target proteins and acceptor lysines relevant for genome stability. Mol Cell Proteomics 14:1419–1434

Yang H, Rudge DG, Koos JD, Vaidialingam B, Yang HJ, Pavletich NP (2013) mTOR kinase structure, mechanism and regulation. Nature 497:217–223

Yoo HY, Shevchenko A, Shevchenko A, Dunphy WG (2004) Mcm2 is a direct substrate of ATM and ATR during DNA damage and DNA replication checkpoint responses. J Biol Chem 279:53353–53364

Yoo HY, Kumagai A, Shevchenko A, Shevchenko A, Dunphy WG (2009) The Mre11-Rad50-Nbs1 complex mediates activation of TopBP1 by ATM. Mol Biol Cell 20:2351–2360

Yuan J, Ghosal G, Chen J (2009) The annealing helicase HARP protects stalled replication forks. Genes Dev 23:2394–2399

Yuan J, Luo K, Deng M, Li Y, Yin P, Gao B, Fang Y, Wu P, Liu T, Lou Z (2014) HERC2-USP20 axis regulates DNA damage checkpoint through Claspin. Nucleic Acids Res 42:13110–13121

Zhang Z, Yang K, Chen CC, Feser J, Huang M (2007) Role of the C terminus of the ribonucleotide reductase large subunit in enzyme regeneration and its inhibition by Sml1. Proc Natl Acad Sci U S A 104:2217–2222

Zhang YW, Jones TL, Martin SE, Caplen NJ, Pommier Y (2009) Implication of checkpoint kinase-dependent up-regulation of ribonucleotide reductase R2 in DNA damage response. J Biol Chem 284:18085–18095

Zhang H, Head PE, Daddacha W, Park SH, Li X, Pan Y, Madden MZ, Duong DM, Xie M, Yu B, Warren MD, Liu EA, Dhere VR, Li C, Pradilla I, Torres MA, Wang Y, Dynan WS, Doetsch PW, Deng X, Seyfried NT, Gius D, Yu DS (2016) ATRIP deacetylation by SIRT2 drives ATR checkpoint activation by promoting binding to RPA-ssDNA. Cell Rep 14:1435–1447

Zhao X, Muller EG, Rothstein R (1998) A suppressor of two essential checkpoint genes identifies a novel protein that negatively affects dNTP pools. Mol Cell 2:329–340

Zhao X, Chabes A, Domkin V, Thelander L, Rothstein R (2001) The ribonucleotide reductase inhibitor Sml1 is a new target of the Mec1/Rad53 kinase cascade during growth and in response to DNA damage. EMBO J 20:3544–3553

Zhu M, Zhao H, Liao J, Xu X (2014) HERC2/USP20 coordinates CHK1 activation by modulating CLASPIN stability. Nucleic Acids Res 42:13074–13081

Zou L, Elledge SJ (2003) Sensing DNA damage through ATRIP recognition of RPA-ssDNA complexes. Science 300:1542–1548

Chapter 4
Targeting ATR for Cancer Therapy: Profile and Expectations for ATR Inhibitors

Nicola Curtin and John Pollard

Abstract ATR is a highly versatile player in the DNA damage response (DDR) that signals DNA damage via CHK1 phosphorylation to the S and G2/M cell cycle checkpoints and to promote DNA repair. It is activated by ssDNA, principally occurring due to replication stress that is caused by unrepaired endogenous DNA damage or induced by a variety of anticancer chemotherapy and ionizing radiation. Since an almost ubiquitous feature of cancer cells is loss of G1 control, e.g., through p53 mutation, it is thought that their greater dependence on S and G2/M checkpoint function may render them more susceptible to ATR inhibition. ATR promotes homologous recombination DNA repair and inter-strand cross-link repair. Impairment of ATR function by genetic means or with inhibitors increases the sensitivity of cells to a wide variety of DNA damaging chemotherapy and radiotherapy, with the greatest sensitization observed with gemcitabine and cisplatin. Early inhibitors developed in the 1990s were weak and non-specific but the encouraging data led to the development of more potent and specific inhibitors. We review here the pre-clinical chemo- and radiosensitisation data obtained with these inhibitors that has led to the entry into clinical trial, the potential to combine ATR inhibitors with other DNA repair modulators, and identification of single-agent ATR inhibitor cytotoxicity in cells with activated oncogenes and particular defects in the DDR that may result in greater replication stress or dependence on ATR for survival.

N. Curtin
Northern Institute for Cancer Research, Medical School, Newcastle University, Newcastle upon Tyne, UK

Newcastle University Institute for Ageing, Medical School, Newcastle University, Newcastle upon Tyne, UK
e-mail: nicola.curtin@newcastle.ac.uk

J. Pollard (✉)
Vertex Pharmaceuticals (Europe) Ltd, Abingdon, Oxfordshire, UK
e-mail: john_pollard@vrtx.com

© Springer International Publishing AG, part of Springer Nature 2018
J. Pollard, N. Curtin (eds.), *Targeting the DNA Damage Response for Anti-Cancer Therapy*, Cancer Drug Discovery and Development, https://doi.org/10.1007/978-3-319-75836-7_4

Keywords Ataxia Telangiectasia Mutated and RAD3 related (ATR) · ATR inhibitor
· Cell cycle checkpoint · Replication stress · DNA repair

4.1 Role of ATR in the DNA Damage Response

The DNA damage response (DDR) is a beautifully orchestrated system of DNA damage sensors, transducers and effectors that signal damage for repair and to cell cycle checkpoints to prevent the damage from becoming fixed and transferred to the next generation. Forty years ago DNA was thought to be very stable but Tomas Lindahl found that it was actually being damaged at an astonishing rate, one that would be incompatible with life unless it was also continuously being repaired at a similar rate. In 2015 the Nobel Prize for Chemistry was awarded to Tomas Lindahl, Paul Modrich and Aziz Sancar for their pioneering work on DNA repair (Cleaver 2016). By far and away the most common lesions are single base damage and single strand breaks (SSBs), forming at the rate of 10,000–100,000 lesions per cell/day (Lindahl 1993) and largely due to reactive oxygen species (ROS) resulting from normal metabolism. Whilst these lesions are generally repaired quickly, in replicating cells the rate of repair may not be fast enough to stop the single strand lesions from encountering the advancing replication fork. When this happens the helicase and replication machinery, which are core components of the replication fork, become uncoupled resulting in regions of single stranded DNA (ssDNA). This event has been termed replication stress (RS, recently reviewed in (Taylor and Lindsay 2016)). The impact of this is either stalled replication or the collapse of the fork to reveal a single-ended double strand break (DSB). In addition to unresolved DNA damage from oxidative stress, RS can arise from a number of other events. These include exposure to various exogenous DNA damaging agents such as ultraviolet light (UV), ionizing radiation (IR) and many commonly used cancer chemotherapies. Expression of oncogenes that induce unscheduled proliferation can also lead to RS. This arises when the rate of replication induced by the oncogene is not matched by the metabolic capacity of the cell and the pool of nucleotides required to extend the DNA chain is exhausted. Furthermore, RS can arise from the replication of difficult to copy or fragile regions of the DNA and from highly transcribed regions of DNA, where the transcription and replication machinery can compete for the same region of DNA (Gaillard et al. 2015). Ataxia Telangiectasia Mutated and Rad3-related (ATR) is a vital sensor of RS and a variety of other DNA lesions that generate regions of single-stranded DNA (ssDNA) in double stranded DNA (dsDNA). ATR is critical to cell cycle arrest at the S and G2 checkpoints as well as initiation of DNA repair (Fig. 4.1), as described below. ATR is a member of the PI-3K like family of kinases (PIKKs), which include Ataxia Telangiectasia Mutated (ATM) and DNA-PK$_{CS}$ (DNA-dependent protein kinase catalytic subunit) (Durocher and Jackson 2001), protein kinases that are also involved in the DDR. Many of the phosphorylation substrates of ATR are also common to ATM, and the two are both

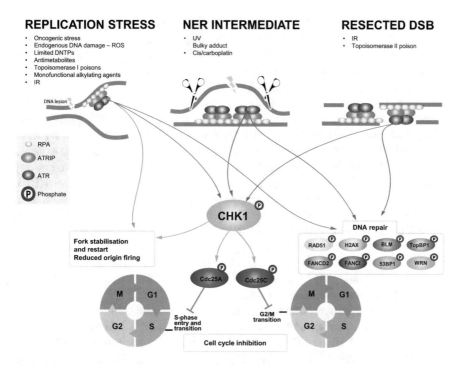

Fig. 4.1 ATR is an apical mediator of the DDR, recruited to regions of ssDNA within dsDNA. The ATR—ATRIP complex is recruited to regions of RPA coated ssDNA within dsDNA that arise at sites of RS and as intermediates during nucleotide excision repair and following resection of DNA DSBs. Once activated, ATR phosphorylates numerous substrates the most important of which is CHK1. This sets off a phosphorylation cascade to coordinate several important cell functions including the arrest of cell cycle by activation of intra-S and G2/M checkpoints, regulation of origin firing, stabilisation of replication forks, and the repair of DNA lesions

involved in the response to DSBs. There is also crosstalk between the two PIKKs. In response to DNA damage ATM and ATR phosphorylate many proteins that are involved in DNA replication, recombination and repair, and cell cycle regulation (Matsuoka et al. 2007).

ssDNA formed at sites of RS is a highly unstable structure that is readily dissected by exonucleases. To prevent this, replication protein A (RPA) is rapidly recruited to ssDNA where it both protects the DNA from exonuclease activity but also acts to recruit proteins that enable the cell to stabilize the stalled fork and repair the damaged DNA. Foremost amongst these is the ATR-interacting protein (ATRIP). ATRIP in-turn recruits ATR (Zou and Elledge 2003; Itakura et al. 2004; Dart et al. 2004). RPA has been shown to activate ATR, and the longer the length of ssDNA the greater the level of ATR activation, supporting the theory that multiple RPA molecules bind the ssDNA to activate ATR (Choi et al. 2010). In the absence of ATR, stalled replication forks collapse resulting in the formation of lethal DSBs and unprotected origins fire, creating increased levels of ssDNA, depleting the RPA pool and ultimately resulting in replication-based catastrophe (Toledo et al. 2013).

The ATR-ATRIP complex is further regulated by a number of other proteins including TopBP1 (Lindsey-Boltz and Sancar 2011), which is recruited to the junction of ssDNA and dsDNA via an interaction with the DNA damage specific RAD9-RAD1-HUS1 clamp (known as 9-1-1). Assembly of this multi-protein complex leads to full activation of the protein kinase activity of ATR.

The activation of ATR is not limited to RS, other cellular events can lead to the generation of ssDNA, which is the catalyst for formation of the ATR protein complex. Such events include generation of intermediates formed during the repair of damaged DNA by the DSB repair, mismatch repair (MMR) and nucleotide excision repair (NER) pathways. DSBs, such as those caused by IR may be repaired by any one of four pathways: Non-homologous end joining (NHEJ), alternative NHEJ, homologous recombination repair (HRR) or single-strand annealing (reviewed in (Mlasenov et al. 2016)). Of these the only pathway that preserves the DNA sequence as well as restoring DNA integrity is HRR, with which ATR is intimately connected, as it uses the sister chromatid as a template for repair. An obligatory early step in HRR is the processing of the DNA DSB by end resection to generate a $3'$ overhang. End resection is achieved by a number of steps: CtIP, which is an ATR phosphorylation target, recruits the MRN complex (composed of Mre11, Rad50 and Nbs1). MRE11 has $3'$-$5'$ exonuclease activity and initiates end resection, which is continued by EXO 1 following its recruitment by CtIP. The DNA2/BLM complex then unwinds the DNA and the DNA2 component completes end resection. RPA coats the ssDNA to recruit ATRIP and ATR (Fig. 4.1) (Shiotani and Zou 2009; Symington and Gautier 2011).

MMR acts on DNA lesions caused by insertion or deletion loops resulting from replication errors and mismatches in the DNA base-pairs that often occur due to alkylating mutagens (Fang et al. 1993). One of the primary events during MMR is formation of Mut protein complexes (MutSα, Sβ and MutLα) and nuclease excision of the aberrant bases. This reveals ssDNA that is subsequently coated by RPA (Genschel and Modrich 2009), leading to the recruitment of ATR. It is thought that Mut complexes act as scaffolds for proteins involved in DNA repair and checkpoint activation, such as ATR (Liu et al. 2010). In keeping with this, depletion of MSH2 (a component of the MutSα complex) by siRNA blocks ATR activity (Wang and Qin 2003); MMR-proficient cells form ATR foci following DNA alkylation, in contrast to MMR-deficient cells (Caporali et al. 2004); and MSH3 (a component of the MutSβ complex) binds hairpin loops in RPA-coated ssDNA to recruit ATRIP and activate ATR (Burdova et al. 2015). Furthermore, the G2 arrest associated with the repair of the mismatch repair (MMR) substrate, 6-thioguanine, has been shown to be ATR dependent (Yamane et al. 2004). Another common source of DNA damage is UV and environmental chemicals that form DNA distorting adducts, these are repaired by nucleotide excision repair (NER). At sites of damage a number of protein complexes are formed that include the DNA-damage binding (DDB) complexes DDB1 and DDB2 and the XPC-Rad23B complex. These in turn recruit exonuclease activities such as ERCC1 that excise 20–30 nucleotides of DNA around the damage site on one of the strands of DNA, leaving a portion of ssDNA as a template for repair by polymerase activities (Sibghatullah et al. 1989).

Once activated at regions of RPA coated ssDNA, ATR can phosphorylate a very long list of putative substrates and although the molecular consequences for many of these are yet to be determined it is clear that they control a number of important cellular functions that include promotion of cell survival, arrest of replication and cell cycle, stabilisation of the stalled fork and repair of the damaged DNA (Myers et al. 2009). These events are described in more detail below.

4.1.1 ATR Signaling to Regulate DNA Replication and Cell Cycle Progression

The best characterized substrate for ATR is the checkpoint kinase CHK1. ATR mediates CHK1 activation by phosphorylation at residues S317 and S345, both of which are required for CHK1 activation (Zhao and Piwnica-Worms 2001). Phosphorylation of CHK1^{ser345} by ATR is often used as a marker of ATR activity (Peasland et al. 2011; Liu et al. 2000; Parsels et al. 2011). Upon phosphorylation at both these residues CHK1 becomes active, triggering autophosphorylation at serine 296 (Parsels et al. 2011) and phosphorylation of a number of downstream targets involved in DNA repair and cell cycle arrest. CHK1 controls entry into mitosis via the G2/M checkpoint, and S-phase progression via the intra S-phase checkpoint. Following RS, ATR mediated activation of CHK1 leads to the phosphorylation of the CDC25 phosphatase proteins CDC25A and B. This results in the inhibition of phosphatase activity, which in turn leads to the persistence of an inhibitory phosphorylation event on CDK1. In addition, CHK1 phosphorylates and activates the Wee1 kinase, which directly induces the inhibitory phosphorylation on CDK1 (Fig. 4.1) (Sorensen and Syljuasen 2012; Chen et al. 2003; Dai and Grant 2010; Lee et al. 2001). The outcome of this cascade is to block CDK1-mediated mitotic progression. In doing so the ATR-CHK1 response prevents cells with damaged chromosomes from entering mitosis, which could otherwise lead to gross genetic deformations or mitotic catastrophe. In addition to a role in preventing entry into mitosis, recent evidence suggests that ATR, via CHK1 activation, can also impact the progression of cells with damaged DNA through mitosis. ATR-CHK1 activation leads to phosphorylation of Aurora-B, a kinase that is involved in the mitotic spindle checkpoint. This checkpoint serves to ensure that duplicated chromosomes are correctly segregated to opposing cell poles. Accordingly, defective chromosomes that arise from persistent DNA damage or aberrant repair are not segregated and progressed through to cytokinesis as a result of CHK1 mediated Aurora-B activation (Mackay and Ullman 2015).

ATR-mediated phosphorylation of CHK1 and its downstream effects on CDC25 protein stability are also a key event in the regulation of the intra-S-phase checkpoint. Cdc25A removes an inactivating phosphorylation on the CDK2/Cyclin A or E complexes, which promotes S-phase. Following exposure to a variety of DNA damaging agents, including IR (Sorensen et al. 2003), UV and hydroxurea (HU)

(Mailand et al. 2000; Xiao et al. 2003), CHK1 promotes the rapid degradation of Cdc25A, preventing S-phase entry (Dai and Grant 2010). Accordingly, ATR knockdown has been shown to stabilise Cdc25A (Sorensen et al. 2004). In addition to a role in regulating cell cycle checkpoints, ATR-mediated phosphorylation of CHK1 can also suppress global firing of new replication origins, via the CDC25-mediated suppression of CDK activity. This acts to stop DNA replication, avoiding the potential to form multiple unstable forks and catastrophic DNA damage. Interestingly, recent studies have shown that ATR activity can also suppress replication origin firing via a CHK1 independent route that involves the helicase SMARCAL1 (Couch et al. 2013). The effect of ATR-mediated CHK1 activation on DNA replication and cell cycle progression is therefore fourfold: phosphorylation of CDC25 is inhibitory, thereby preventing S phase entry and preventing G2/M transition; Wee1 is phosphorylated and stabilised resulting in inactivation of CDK1, Aurora-B is activated blocking G2/M transition; and CDC25 mediated suppression of origin firing.

The impact of ATR on DNA replication and S and G2/M cell cycle progression following DNA damage is important when considering the potential benefit from inhibiting ATR. Specifically, impairment of G1 control in cancer is almost ubiquitous (Massague 2004), caused by multiple mechanisms such as loss of function of key G1 control proteins including p53 or Rb. For example, the *TP53* gene is the most commonly mutated gene in cancer with >50% of all solid tumours harboring mutations largely in the DNA binding domain of the *TP53* gene (Olivier et al. 2010). This sets up an hypothesis that cancer cells defective in the G1 checkpoint may be reliant on the ATR mediated S and G2/M checkpoints for survival from DNA damage. In contrast, non-cancer cells with their full complement of cell cycle checkpoints may better tolerate ATR inhibition. The most convincing data regarding G1 dependence comes from experiments using paired isogenic cell lines that differ only in their p53 status (discussed in more detail below). For example, ATR depletion sensitised human colorectal cells with inactive p53 to cisplatin but when wt p53 was knocked in survival was increased (Sangster-Guity et al. 2011). However, it is important to acknowledge that other studies have shown p53 competent cancer cells can also be sensitive to ATR inhibitors. This may be associated with other defects in the G1 checkpoint. For example, ATR silencing sensitized p53 wild-type U2OS cells, which have G1 dysfunction by virtue of p16 deletion, to topoisomerase I poisons (Flatten et al. 2005). Moreover, U2OS sensitivity to dominant negative inactivation of ATR was further enhanced by inducing additional defects in G1 control (Nghiem et al. 2001).

4.1.2 ATR Signaling to DNA Repair

Once DNA damage is detected, the cell can employ a series of distinct repair processes. This is determined by a number of factors most notable of which is the nature of the damage lesion e.g., small vs. bulky adducts, single strand vs. double strand breaks; and the phase of cell cycle in which the damage is detected. During the S- and G2 phases of cell cycle the cell can use the sister chromatid DNA as a template for repair, enabling high fidelity repair by HRR. In contrast, outside of these cell cycle phases, multiple repair pathways are available. Lesions affecting one strand of DNA can be repaired with high fidelity using the complementary strand as a template but for lesions affecting both strands there is a considerable risk of incorrect repair, resulting in genome instability. HRR involves three major steps; end-resection (as described above) of a DSB to reveal a region of ssDNA (redundant in the case of a stalled fork), invasion of the DNA into the sister chromatid and then finally damage resolution, a process which includes extension of the DNA chain by DNA polymerase activity and reannealing of the DNA ends. Although it is far from clear exactly how ATR affects DNA damage repair, multiple strands of evidence implicate ATR in the regulation of HRR. Firstly, a number of studies have shown that depletion of ATR leads to a decrease in the efficiency or frequency of HRR (Wang et al. 2004; Brown et al. 2014). Secondly, ATR expression is cell cycle dependent peaking at S and G2, coincident with HRR: ATR is associated with chromatin throughout the cell cycle in the absence of genotoxic stress, however this degree of association appears to be much higher in S phase when the threat to genomic integrity is the greatest (Dart et al. 2004). Thirdly, inhibition of ATR has been shown to decrease a number of HRR markers most notable amongst which is the RAD51 filament protein that is involved in the homology search. Fourthly, ATR is associated with, or phosphorylates a number of proteins that are involved in HRR. These include the RecQ helicases BLM and WRN (Blm suppresses inapproprtiate sister chromatid exchange and WRN prevents the collapse of stalled forks); the breast cancer type 1 susceptibility protein (BRCA, which is involved with the recruitment of HRR essential repair proteins); and a minor variant of histone H2A (H2AX, which colocalises with a series of HRR proteins including BRCA1 and RAD51). Finally, TopBP1, an important regulator of the ATR protein complex, has been shown to interact with NBS1. This protein forms part of the MRN complex that plays an important role in activating HRR (Morishima et al. 2007).

At sites of RS, in the event that ATR fails to stabilize the replication fork and repair the causative lesion, the replication fork can rapidly collapse to form a potentially lethal DSB. Once a DSB is formed a surveillance pathway, mediated by the ATR homolog ATM, determines the fate of the cell. ATM signals to cell cycle arrest via phosphorylation of critical downstream substrates such as p53 and CHK2, and also triggers repair of the DSB by HRR. Notably, it has been widely reported that components of the ATM DSB pathway are very commonly dysfunctional in cancer. Most notable examples include loss of the ATM activating complex MRN, which has been observed in breast cancer (Bartkova et al. 2008; Jiang et al. 2009); loss of function mutations or loss of expression of ATM itself, which has been observed in a number of cancers such as non-small cell lung cancer (Weber et al. 2016); and perhaps most importantly, loss of function mutations in the key ATM substrate, p53. This defect is highly prevalent in some aggressive diseases such as serous ovarian cancer (>95%) (The Cancer Genome Atlas Research Network 2011; Cole et al. 2016), basal-like breast cancer (80%) (Cancer Genome Atlas Network 2012a) and squamous cell lung cancers (>80%) (Cancer Genome Atlas Network 2012b).

Defective DSB repair associated with defects in ATM signaling has been suggested to be an early event in tumourgenesis and provides the nascent tumour with an environment that supports genomic instability, as a result of persistent unrepaired DNA damage. Although a defective ATM-p53 response may provide a growth advantage to the tumour it increases the reliance on the ATR RS response to survive DNA damage during replication (Halazonetis et al. 2008).

In addition to a role in HRR, ATR has also been implicated in the regulation of the interstrand crosslink (ICL) repair pathway. This complex pathway acts to resolve adducts formed between two complementary DNA strands, and utilizes numerous repair processes. Typically, such adducts arise from treatment with anti-cancer drugs such as the bifunctional N-mustards, platinating agents like cisplatin and carboplatin; and mitomycin C. During replication, at the site of an ICL, a large protein complex is formed—known as the Fanconi Anemia (FA) core. This complex consists of over ten separate proteins and although the full activity of this complex is not yet defined it is clear that one effect is to recruit endonuclease activities (such as the XPF-ERCC1 or FAN1 endonucleases) that cleave either side of the ICL to unhook the adduct from one of the DNA strands. The result is a DSB that is repaired by a combination of translesion synthesis (to fill the gap left by the excised adduct, restoring the growing DNA chain) and HRR. The remaining 'still hooked' strand, which now constitutes a bulky adduct, is resolved by NER. A comprehensive description of ICL has been reviewed elsewhere (Kim and D'Andrea 2012; Haynes et al. 2015; Deans and West 2011). ATR has been associated with ICL through a series of important experimental observations. ATR phosphorylates and regulates many FA proteins. Specifically, ATR has been shown to phosphorylate FANCs A, G, E, I, M and D2. In many cases it has been shown that ATR-mediated phosphorylation directly impacts their function, for example, blocking the ATR site of phosphorylation in FANCM impacts its recruitment to the sites of ICL (Singh et al. 2013). In addition to a role for ATR in the regulation of FA core proteins, the converse has also been shown: FA core proteins can lead to activation of ATR. In response to damage, the FA protein FANCM has been shown to activate ATR and its downstream intra S-phase checkpoint. Additionally, knockdown of *FANCM* or *FAAP24* (a gene that encodes the FA core-complex associated protein 24) reduced ATR-dependent phosphorylation of pCHK1^{Ser317} and p53^{Ser15} following HU and UV, respectively, (Collis et al. 2008); and deletion of *FANCM* reduced levels of the ATR marker pCHK1^{Ser345} following treatment with camptothecin (Schwab et al. 2010). Furthermore, depletion of FANCM in cells leads to a phenotype that is very similar to that seen with loss of ATR: increased DNA damage and cell cycle checkpoint defects in response to RS (Luke-Glaser et al. 2010). Finally, the FA core complex has been reported to increase the binding of ATRIP to chromatin at sites of damage, which in turn leads to activation of ATR (Tomida et al. 2013).

In addition to the potentially beneficial anti-cancer impact inhibiting ATR has on cancer cell cycle control, blocking its impact on DNA damage repair may also provide substantial benefit. This is based on a common finding that many cancer cells have defects in overlapping repair pathways, which in turn may place a burden on remaining repair capacity. The most notable example is a defect in the ATM-p53 mediated DSB response pathway that is described above. In the absence of a functional ATM-p53 response, cells may be especially reliant on ATR to maintain survival in the face of RS. This is discussed in detail later in this chapter. Additionally, defects in other repair pathways may lead to an increase in RS from persistence of unrepaired DNA damage as the cell progresses to S-phase of the cell cycle. In turn this would increase the requirement for ATR activity to maintain cell survival.

The remainder of this chapter is dedicated to reviewing the data that supports the potential for ATR inhibitors to be used in a variety of contexts to provide patient benefit.

4.2 Validation of ATR as a Therapeutic Target

Genomic instability has been identified as an "enabling characteristic" of cancer cells (Hanahan and Weinberg 2011), and commonly arises due to errors in DNA replication and repair machinery. Defects in the DDR are common in cancer, leading to a reduced repair capacity in many cancer cells compared with normal cells. Historically, conventional cytotoxics that act by damaging DNA have relied on exploitation of these defects. Many of the anticancer drugs in routine clinical use act with the intention of inducing lethal levels of DNA damage in the tumour. These drugs can be classified based on the form of DNA damage they induce: single base damage through alkyltation for example by temozolomide or dacarbazine (DTIC); single strand breaks induced by topoisomerase I inhibitors such as irinotecan, topotecan and camptothecin; DSBs induced by topoisomerase II inhibitors such as etoposide, doxorubicin and mitoxantrone; DNA cross-links (inter-or intra strands) induced by bifunctional alkylating agents such as the nitrogen mustards, such as melphalan, and the platinum drugs cisplatin and carboplatin; and finally, the antimetabolite class of drugs typified by the nucleotide analogs gemcitabine, HU and 5-fluoro uracil (5-FU) and antifolates such as methotrexate and pemetrexed that induce DNA damage both by blocking DNA extension via insertion in the extending chain and by inhibiting the synthesis of the deoxynucleotides that are essential for DNA replication (the lack of which will lead to RS). For many patients treatment with these DNA damaging drugs provides limited benefit, and several strands of clinical evidence suggest that functional capacity of the DNA damage response network is an important determinant in response. For example, several studies have been reported where good responses to such drugs are associated with impaired DNA repair processes. Firstly, cisplatin based treatment leads to a remarkable cure rate of >80% in patients with testicular cancer (Masters and Koberle 2003). Cell studies have demonstrated that platinum adducts in testicular cancer cells persist, presumably as a result of failed repair, in contrast to observations with cells from other tumour types. Low levels of key proteins involved in NER, such as ERCC1-XPF and XPA in testicular cancer cells may suggest that defective NER is a driver of the cancer cell sensitivity to cisplatin (Masters and Koberle 2003). Secondly, a recently reported clinical study assessed the response of patients with triple negative breast cancer to carboplatin. The investigators noted that patients with a germline BRCA mutation (a protein that is involved in HR repair) responded better to carboplatin than the BRCA wild type group (68% vs. 28% overall response rate respectively) (Tutt et al. 2015).

Since so many of these agents lead to activation of ATR, it has long been considered a suitable target for anticancer therapy. Importantly, a number of observations in mouse and humans provide confidence that modulation of ATR activity could be tolerated by non-cancer cells. Although ATR knockout mice are not viable (Brown and Baltimore 2000) and significant depletion of ATR in mice and humans leads to developmental issues (Seckel syndrome in humans, which is associated with microcephaly and short stature) (O'Driscoll et al. 2004), conditional knockout in adult mice is well tolerated and no enhanced cancer risk is observed in either Seckel patients or conditional knockout mice (Ruzankina et al. 2007; Schoppy et al. 2012; Murga et al. 2009).

Despite the potential for drugging ATR, the lack of suitable inhibitors meant that initially genetic manipulation was the only means of target validation (Table 4.1). Using a human transformed fibroblast cell line (GM847) or an osteosarcroma line (U2OS) expressing a doxycycline-inducible ATR-kinase dead gene, that acts in a dominant negative fashion (Nghiem et al. 2001, 2002; Cliby et al. 1998, 2002), it was shown that ATR inactivation sensitised cells to the monofunctional alkylating agent, methylmethanosulfonate (MMS), the cross-linking agent cisplatin, the topoisomerase I and II inhibitors topotecan, SN38 (the cell active metabolite of irinotecan), the topoisomerase II poisons, doxorubicin, etoposide and teniposide; IR, and HU but not to taxanes, which exert their antiproliferative effect largely through inhibiting mictotubule dynamics necessary for chromosomal segregation at mitosis (Cliby et al. 1998). A second approach assessed the impact of Seckel mutant ATR expression, which leads to low ATR activity, on the sensitivity of DLD1 cancer cells to a range of drugs and irradiation (Hurley et al. 2007). These cells were six-fold more sensitive to the topoisomerase II poison doxorubicin, 10–20-fold more sensitive to the antimetabolites 5-fluorouracil, gemcitabine, HU and methotrexate and >400-fold more sensitive to cisplatin than DLD1 cells expressing wild-type ATR (Wilsker and Bunz 2007). A third approach, adopted by a number of investigators, used siRNA knockdown of ATR. In a range of cancer cell backgrounds, ATR knockdown led to increased sensitivity, when compared with control siRNA treated cells, to cisplatin, MMS, temozolomide, topotecan, SN38, and the antimetabolite gemcitabine. (Caporali et al. 2004, 2008; Wagner and Karnitz 2009; Huntoon et al. 2013). Taken together these data supported the hypothesis that inhibiting ATR could be an attractive approach to treating cancer, and specifically to improve the benefit from the DNA damaging drugs that are widely used as standard of care across many indications.

Table 4.1 Summary of sensitisation to DNA damaging agents by genetic ATR inactivation

Treatment class	Treatment	Cell line/genetic inactivation	Increased sensitivity?	Reference
X-irradiation	IR	GM847-KD	Yes	Cliby et al. (1998)
		GM637-KD	Yes	Wright et al. (1998)
		U2OS-KD	Yes	Nghiem et al. (2002)
		F02-98 (Seckel patient fibroblasts)	Slight	O'Driscoll et al. (2003)
		DLD1-ATR-Seckel	Yes	Hurley et al. (2007)
UV irradiation	UV	GM847-KD	Slight	Cliby et al. (1998)
		GM637-KD	Yes	Wright et al. (1998)
		U2OS-KD	Yes	Nghiem et al. (2002)
		F02-98 (Seckel patient fibroblasts)	Yes	Yang et al. (2008)
		DLD1-ATR-Seckel	Yes	Hurley et al. (2007)
Alkylating agents	Cisplatin	GM847-KD	Yes	Cliby et al. (1998)
		U2OS-KD	Yes	Nghiem et al. (2002)
		DLD1-ATR-Seckel	Yes	Wilsker and Bunz (2007); Wilsker et al. (2012)
		HeLa siRNA	Yes	Wagner and Karnitz (2009)
		U2OS siRNA	Yes	Wagner and Karnitz (2009)
		HCT116 siRNA	Yes	Wagner and Karnitz (2009)
		OVCAR-8 siRNA	Yes	Wagner and Karnitz (2009)
	Cyclophosphamide	DLD1-ATR-Seckel	Yes	Wilsker and Bunz (2007)
	Mitomycin C (MMC)	F02-98 (Seckel patient fibroblasts)	Yes	Yang et al. (2008)
		DLD1-ATR-Seckel	Yes	Wilsker and Bunz (2007); Wilsker et al. (2012)
	Methyl methanosulfonate	GM847-KD	Yes	Cliby et al. (1998)
		PC3 siRNA	Yes	Collis et al. (2003)
		DU145 siRNA	Yes	Collis et al. (2003)
	Temozolomide	DK0064 (ATR mutant) lymphoblastoid, LN229 glioma and DO3 melanoma siATR	Yes	Eich et al. (2013)

(continued)

Table 4.1 (continued)

Treatment class	Treatment	Cell line/genetic inactivation	Increased sensitivity?	Reference
Topoisomerase I poisons/inhibitors	Topotecan	GM847-KD	Yes	Cliby et al. (2002)
		OVCAR-8 siRNA	Yes	Huntoon et al. (2013)
	SN-38 (irinotecan)	GM847-KD	Yes	Cliby et al. (2002)
		HeLa siRNA	Yes	Flatten et al. (2005)
		U2OS siRNA	Yes	Flatten et al. (2005)
	camptothecin	HeLa siRNA	Yes	Flatten et al. (2005)
Topoisomerase II poisons/inhibitors	Etoposide	GM847-KD	Yes	Cliby et al. (2002)
	Teniposide	DLD1-ATR-Seckel	Yes	Wilsker et al. (2012)
	Doxorubicin	GM847-KD	Yes	Cliby et al. (2002)
		DLD1-ATR-Seckel	Yes	Wilsker and Bunz (2007)
Antimetabolites	5-FU	DLD1-ATR-Seckel	Yes	Wilsker and Bunz (2007)
	Gemcitabine	DLD1-ATR-Seckel	Yes	Wilsker and Bunz (2007)
		HeLa siRNA	Yes	Wagner and Karnitz (2009)
		U2OS siRNA	Yes	Wagner and Karnitz (2009)
		HCT116 siRNA	Yes	Wagner and Karnitz (2009)
		OVCAR-8 siRNA	Yes	Huntoon et al. (2013)
	HU	GM847-KD	Yes	Cliby et al. (1998); Peasland et al. (2011)
		U2OS-KD	Yes	Nghiem et al. (2002)
		DLD1-ATR-Seckel	Yes	Wilsker and Bunz (2007)
	Methotrexate	DLD1-ATR-Seckel	Yes	Wilsker and Bunz (2007)
	Raltitrexed	DLD1-ATR-Seckel	Yes	Wilsker and Bunz (2007)
PARP inhibitor	Rucaparib	GM847-KD	Yes	Peasland et al. (2011)
	Veliparib	OVCAR-8 siRNA	Yes	Huntoon et al. (2013)
Taxanes	Paclitaxel	GM847-KD	No	Cliby et al. (2002)
		DLD1-ATR-Seckel	No	Wilsker and Bunz (2007)

4.3   Development of ATR Inhibitors

For many years the available ATR inhibitors lacked potency and specificity but nev-ertheless were used as tools to support data generated from genetic studies (Table 4.2). One of the earliest ATR inhibitors was caffeine, but it lacked potency (IC_{50} = 1.1 mM) (Cortez 2003) and specificity, as it is a more potent inhibitor of ATM (IC_{50} = 0.2 mM) (Sarkaria et al. 1999). Wortmannin, a fungal metabolite, is a more potent inhibitor of ATR than caffeine (IC_{50} = 1.8 μM) but inhibits multiple PIKKs including ATM (IC_{50} = 150 nM). PI-103, a PI3K inhibitor also inhibits ATR (IC_{50} = 850 nM) but had equivalent potency against ATM (IC_{50} = 920 nM) and greater potency against DNA-PK (IC_{50} = 2 nM) (Knight et al. 2006). The natural product, Schisandrin B is a weak inhibitor of ATR with an in vitro IC_{50} of 7.25 μM, however at concentrations of 30 μM or greater, no inhibition of related kinases was observed (ATM, CHK1, PI3K, DNA-PK and mTOR), indicating potential for ATR selectivity (Nishida et al. 2009). NU6027 (2,6-diamino-4-cyclohexyl-methyloxy-5-nitroso-pyrimidine), originally designed as a Cdk2 inhibitor, was found to be more efficient in inhibiting cellular ATR activity (as determined by CHK1 serine[345] phos-phorylation) than CDK2 activity (IC_{50} = 6.7 μM for ATR and >10 μM for Cdk2), with no effect on ATM and DNA-PK (Peasland et al. 2011). Finally, a high-throughput screen of 623 compounds identified that the PI-3K inhibitor ETP-46464 was a potent ATR inhibitor (IC_{50} = 25 nM) (Toledo et al. 2011; Teng et al. 2015).

The discovery of more potent and specific inhibitors of ATR may have been hampered by challenges in accessing the protein to run high throughput screens and to support medicinal chemistry efforts (ATR is a very large protein (Unsal-Kacmaz and Sancar 2004)). However, in recent years a number of potent and specific ATR inhibitors have been reported (Table 4.1 and reviewed in (Foote et al. 2015)) aided by successful production of recombinant protein, elegant cell screens and optimiza-tion of compounds initially designed to inhibit close analogs of ATR such as mTOR. Of these compounds VE-821 and VE-822 from Vertex Pharmaceuticals (recently licensed to Merck, EMD Serono); and AZ20 and AZD6738 from AstraZeneca, have been most widely used in pre-clinical studies (Foote et al. 2013; Guichard et al. 2013; Jones et al. 2013; Reaper et al. 2011; Charrier et al. 2011). VE-822 (also known as VX-970 and more recently as M6620), an analog VX-803 (M4344) and AZD6738 have all progressed in to clinical development (discussed in detail in Chap. 5 of this volume). These advanced compounds have greatly expanded the tool box available to researchers.

4.4   ATR Inhibition as Combination Therapy with DNA Damaging Chemotherapy

Since the advent of potent and specific ATR inhibitors, more detailed assessments have been possible that have provided insights on the impact ATR inhibition has on non-cancer cells, which cancer cells are most susceptible to ATR inhibition and finally the in vivo profile of ATR inhibition in mouse models of cancer. Early studies

Table 4.2 ATR inhibitors

Compound and structure	Ki or IC$_{50}$ for ATR	Other reported targets
Caffeine	IC$_{50}$ = 1.1 mM	ATM, DNA-PKcs mTOR
Wortmanin	IC$_{50}$ = 1.8 μM	ATM, DNA-PKcs, PI3K
Schisandrin B	IC$_{50}$ = 7.25 μM	
PI-103	IC$_{50}$ = 0.9 μM	PI3K, mTOR, DNA-PKcs
ETP-46464	IC$_{50}$ = 25 nM	

(continued)

Table 4.2 (continued)

Compound and structure	Ki or IC$_{50}$ for ATR	Other reported targets
NU6027	Ki = 100 nM Cellular IC$_{50}$ = 6.7 μM	CDK2
AZ20	IC$_{50}$ = 4.5 nM	
AZD6738	IC$_{50}$ = 1.0 nM	
VE-821	IC$_{50}$ = 13 nM	
VX-970 (M6620)	IC$_{50}$ = 0.2 nM	

with NU6027 revealed that, at concentrations that were not cytotoxic per se, NU6027 sensitised MCF7 breast cancer cells to IR, temozolomide, cisplatin, camptothecin, doxorubicin, and hydroxyurea, but not the anti-tubulin agent paclitaxel (Peasland et al. 2011). Similarly ETP-46464 enhanced the radiation and cisplatin sensitivity of human ovarian, endometrial and cervical cancer cell lines (Teng et al. 2015). Using VE-821 it was shown that ATR inhibition markedly sensitised HCT116 colon cancer cells to gemcitabine, camptothecin, etoposide, carboplatin and cisplatin (addition of VE-821 decreased the IC_{50} value for the DNA damaging drug by up to ten-fold) (Reaper et al. 2011). As expected, no sensitization was observed with taxotere. A number of subsequent experiments have confirmed the strong potentiation of DNA damaging drug induced cell death by ATR inhibition in cancer cells. For example, in a panel of cancer and non-cancer cell lines VE-821 sensitised most of the 14 cancer lines to cisplatin, in stark contrast, potentiation of cisplatin was not observed for any of the six non-cancer cell lines (Reaper et al. 2011). The apparent cancer specific activity of VE-821 was further characterized in H23 cancer cells and HFl1 non-cancer fibroblast cells. In both cell lines at early time points (24 h), VE-821 enhanced the cytostatic activity of cisplatin. By 96 h this had translated to marked potentiation of cell death in the cancer cell line in contrast to the non-cancer cells in which no enhancement of cell death was observed (Reaper et al. 2011). Furthermore, the enhanced growth arrest that was observed in the non-cancer cells was reversed when VE-821 and cisplatin were washed off. Tolerance of the non-cancer cells to treatment of VE-821 with cisplatin was shown by western blot to be associated with a rapid activation of ATM leading to a compensatory DDR involving activation of a number of downstream ATM cell cycle checkpoint proteins such as CHK2 (Reaper et al. 2011). In a complementary experiment using matched or isogenic cell pairs it was shown that loss of p53 by siRNA depletion or expression of the E6 papillomavirus was sufficient to sensitise cells to co-treatment with VE-821 and cisplatin (Reaper et al. 2011). Similarly, loss of expression or inhibition of ATM sensitized cisplatin treated non-cancer cells to ATR inhibition by VE-821 (Reaper et al. 2011). However, a number of studies have shown individual cell lines can respond to ATR inhibition despite being wild type for p53 (Peasland et al. 2011; Hall et al. 2014). This may be due to defects elsewhere in the ATM-p53 pathway or it may suggest that some cells can be reliant on ATR activity under high RS pressure even in the presence of a fully functioning ATM-p53 response. Additional studies to better define markers of response that can be used to identify target patient sub-populations are merited.

In vivo benefit from ATR inhibition in combination with DNA damaging drugs has been demonstrated in a number of separate studies using both human cancer cell line and primary patient derived tumour xenografts. Marked anti-cancer activity associated with substantial synergy has been demonstrated in combination with cisplatin, gemcitabine and irinotecan (Hall et al. 2014; Jossé et al. 2014; Vendetti et al. 2015; Pollard et al. 2016a). As an example, in one study a panel of seven patient derived non-small cell lung cancer xenografts were treated with cisplatin or VX-970

(M6620) alone or with the combination. The ATR inhibitor had no impact on tumour growth alone in any of the models, whereas cisplatin gave a range of responses: three tumours responded well with >70% tumour growth inhibition, one showed a moderate response (50–70% tumour growth inhibition), and three were insensitive (<20% tumour growth inhibition). In six of the seven models the combination was statistically more effective than cisplatin alone. Notably, complete tumour growth inhibition was observed in all three of the cisplatin resistant models and complete tumour regression was observed in one cisplatin responsive model (Hall et al. 2014). This raises the attractive prospect that ATR inhibition may be an approach to resensitise platinum resistant tumours as well as increasing the benefit in cisplatin responsive tumours. In this study, activity was associated with inhibition of CHK1 phosphorylation in tumours and the combination of VX-970 (M6620) and cisplatin was well tolerated. A similarly beneficial profile in combination with cisplatin has been demonstrated with AZD6738 in an H23 lung cancer xenograft model (Vendetti et al. 2015). Robust anti-tumour activity with well-tolerated ATR and DNA damaging drug combinations is consistent with in vitro observations that ATR inhibition leads to cancer cell specific enhancement of cell death. A second important observation was made from a study of irinotecan and VX-970 (M6620), where it was shown that the combination of an ATR inhibitor with a DNA damaging drug was capable of providing greater efficacy than could be obtained with the DNA damaging drug alone at its maximum tolerated dose (MTD) (Jossé et al. 2014).

A key consideration when developing agents with a novel mechanism of action is dose schedule, this is even more relevant when studies involve drug combinations. The first systematic pre-clinical analysis of dose schedule for combinations of ATR inhibitors with DNA damaging drugs was reported at the 2016 Annual AACR meeting (Pollard et al. 2016a). Maximum in vitro and in vivo activity for VX-970 (M6620) in combination with cisplatin or gemcitabine was achieved when the ATR inhibitor was administered after the DNA damaging therapy. Cell studies demonstrated that transient exposure to ATR inhibition for just 2 h was sufficient for response, with optimal activity when addition of the ATR inhibitor was timed to coincide with peak accumulation of cells in S-phase and concomitant activation of ATR (P-CHK1), following treatment with the DNA damaging drug. In mouse models the optimal schedule was VX-970 (M6620) administered 12–24 h after chemotherapy (Pollard et al. 2016a).

Given the marked ability of ATR inhibitors to potentiate the anti-cancer activity of DNA damaging drugs, with minimal impact on non-cancer cell viability, plus the prevalence of these drugs as standard-of-care across most cancer indications, ATR inhibitors represent an exciting novel therapeutic approach. Accordingly, a number of clinical studies are ongoing with AZ6738, VX-970 (M6620) and VX-803 (M4344) in combination with the DNA damaging drugs cisplatin, carboplatin, gemcitabine and topotecan in a range of cancer indications (Reviewed in Chap. 5).

4.5   ATR Inhibition as Combination Therapy with Ionising Radiation (IR)

IR is used to treat about 60% of cancer patients, both as a potentially curative therapy and also to palliate symptoms. Furthermore, IR is one of the most successful curative therapies used in cancer treatment with about 40% of cancer cures involving IR treatment (Ringborg et al. 2003). Cell death from IR is associated with lethal DNA damage arising both from the direct interaction of radiation with the DNA or, more commonly, indirectly via the ionization of water or oxygen molecules to form highly reactive species within the vicinity of the DNA (Lomax et al. 2013). DNA damage from IR treatment includes single stranded breaks, RS and double strand breaks (Lomax et al. 2013). A number of early studies, involving the expression of inactive ATR mutants demonstrated an important role for ATR and downstream HRR in the response to, and repair of, IR mediated DNA damage (Wang et al. 2004; Cliby et al. 1998; Wright et al. 1998). Potentiation of IR by inhibition of ATR was first demonstrated in vitro with the semi-selective inhibitor NU6027 in MCF7 breast cancer cells. In this experiment the ATR inhibitor decreased clonogenic cancer cell survival by >80% in combination with IR, compared with ~50% survival for IR alone (Peasland et al. 2011). A comprehensive assessment of the benefit from ATR inhibition with IR was subsequently reported in a series of in vitro and in vivo studies using VE-821 and VX-970 (M6620). IR alone induced HRR in a number of cancer cell lines, which was blocked by treatment with VE-821. This inhibition of HRR by VE-821 was associated with elevated DNA damage (measured by H2AX and 53BP1 foci) consistent with failed repair and the persistence of unrepaired damage. In clonogenic viability assays VE-821 significantly enhanced IR toxicity in a number of cancer cells, with changes in surviving fractions of about two to sixfold (for the combination vs. IR alone) (Prevo et al. 2012). This observation was confirmed in a second independent study that showed enhanced IR toxicity in a panel of 12 cancer cell lines, with substantial decreases in surviving fraction observed on treatment with VE-821 + IR vs. IR alone (Pires et al. 2012). Consistent with observations from combinations of ATR inhibitors and DNA damaging chemotherapy, it was shown using VX-970 (M6620) that non-cancer cells are able to tolerate the combination of an ATR inhibitor and IR with no enhanced toxicity (Fokas et al. 2012). Notably, it has also been shown that ATR inhibition can substantially radio-sensitise hypoxic cancer cells (Pires et al. 2012). This is an interesting and potentially important observation since tumour hypoxia is a major barrier to successful responses to IR in patients (Pires et al. 2012).

Combinations of ATR inhibition and IR have been studied in a number of mouse xenograft models. Mice bearing either PSN1 or MiaPaCa-2 pancreatic tumours were treated with a single dose of IR ± 6 contiguous daily doses of VX-970 (M6620). In both models remarkable anti-tumour activity was observed for the combination, in contrast to either agent alone. Most impressive was the response in MiaPaCa-2 tumours, where sustained regression was observed in the combination treated group (Fokas et al. 2012). Marked anti-tumour activity was also observed for the combination in a third model when the IR was given using a fractionated regime: IR given as 5 daily doses of 2 Gy each, with VX-970 (M6620) given for 6 contiguous days starting 1 day prior to IR treatment. Anti-tumour activity was associated with a decrease in pCHK1 levels in tumours of IR treated mice, consistent with an ATR mediated mechanism of action (Fokas et al. 2012). In many clinical situations IR treatment is associated with concurrent chemotherapy, and the impact of ATR inhibition with such a treatment was assessed in a PSN-1 mouse xenograft. In this model the combination of VX-970 (M6620) with gemcitabine and IR was markedly more effective than any of the agents alone or gemcitabine plus IR. Notably, in all the models adding VX-970 (M6620) to either IR alone or IR and gemcitabine was well tolerated with no greater body weight loss when compared with control animals treated in the absence of VX-970 (M6620, Fokas et al. 2012). Importantly, the tolerance of normal tissues to VX-970 (M6620) and IR was assessed in tumour bearing mice irradiated ± VX-970 (M6620) treatment through the small bowel and the normal tissue assessed for evidence of intestinal cell death or adverse morphological changes. Treatment with IR alone led to increased TUNEL-positive apoptotic jejunal cells, that was not further increased by VX-970 (M6620). Furthermore, whereas IR alone induced both villus tip loss and villi shortening, neither was enhanced by the addition of VX-970 (M6620, Fokas et al. 2012). These data are consistent with in vitro findings that inhibition of ATR does not increase cell death in non-cancer cells exposed to DNA damaging agents such as IR.

The pre-clinical data demonstrating that ATR inhibition can markedly potentiate the anti-tumour activity of IR in a wide range of cancer models with minimal impact on normal tissue, and furthermore that ATR inhibition can sensitise hypoxic cancer cells to IR (a common mechanism for IR resistance) provides a compelling rationale to test ATR inhibitors with IR in the clinic. A number of clinical studies are ongoing to assess both AZD6738 and VX-970 (M6620) with IR alone or as part of a chemo-radiation therapy (Reviewed in Chap. 5).

4.6 ATR Inhibition as Monotherapy

Tumour DNA is in a more fragile state than in normal cells, leading to elevated background RS, a hallmark of cancer (Macheret and Halazonetis 2015). This can arise for example from dysregulated proliferation and loss of checkpoint control, and elevated levels of oxidative damage (due to mitochondrial dysfunction, altered metabolism and inflammation (Wiseman and Halliwell 1996; Storz 2005; Babior 1999; Berasain et al. 2009)). Accordingly, given the established apical role ATR plays in regulating the cellular responses to RS, there is much interest in the potential for ATR inhibitors to be used as single agents. This could be exacerbated in cells that concurrently carry defects elsewhere in the DNA repair network, placing further reliance on ATR. Both these concepts are discussed below.

Endogenous events that drive RS: Many transforming oncogenes such as K-ras or C-myc act to drive dysregulated S-phase entry and their expression is widespread across cancer. The resulting oncogenic stress has been shown to elevate RS and activate ATR. This can be attributed to a series of events including premature origin firing, exhaustion of the nucleotide pool, oxidative DNA damage and potential clashes between replication and transcription machinery (Davidson et al. 2006; Moiseeva et al. 2009; Dominguez-Sola et al. 2007). The potential for tumours driven by such oncogenes to be dependent on ATR for survival and thus be sensitive to ATR inhibition has been characterised in a number of studies. Transformation of mouse embryonic fibroblast (MEF) cells with either K-ras or H-ras led to marked elevation of ATR activity consistent with elevated RS. Hypomorphic suppression of ATR by shRNA (>80% depletion of ATR protein) led to potent suppression of cell growth and elevated cell death in the transformed cells (Gilad et al. 2010). Similarly, Myc transformation led to elevated RS in MEFs: DNA damage was further enhanced following ATR depletion, which was associated with increased cell death (Murga et al. 2011). Furthermore, shRNA for ATR significantly reduced the viability of Myc upregulated multiple myeloma cells, which was attributed to Myc-induced oncogenic stress and increased reactive oxygen species (ROS). Loss of cell viability was increased by ROS induction using piperlongumine (Cottini et al. 2015) and the sensitivity of Myc transformed cells to ATR depletion was enhanced in p53-deficient cells, consistent with a model in which blockade of compensatory DDR signaling or G1 checkpoint control augments reliance on ATR (Murga et al. 2011). In subsequent studies, oncogene transformation was shown to sensitise cells to inhibition of ATR. Using an analog of VE-821, inhibition of ATR in H-ras or C-myc transformed MEFs increased S-phase DNA damage (γH2AX), the frequency of chromatid breaks, cell growth inhibition and cell death, relative to the impact of the ATR inhibitor in non-oncogene transformed matched cells (Schoppy et al. 2012). Another cell cycle regulator that is commonly amplified in cancer is Cyclin E1: amplification is observed in some cancers such as high-grade serous ovarian cancer. Cyclin E forms a complex with cdk2 to promote S-phase entry (Patch et al. 2015) Inhibition of ATR by ETP-46464 led to substantial elevation of RS in Cyclin E transformed MEFs vs. untransformed cells. The synthetic addiction of Cyclin E1 amplification with ATR inhibition was markedly enhanced in the absence of p53 (Toledo et al. 2011).

In addition to the expression of oncogenes driving dysregulated proliferation and its associated RS, a number of other cancer relevant mechanisms have been shown to elevate RS. Perhaps the most intuitive are defects that impair the DNA replication machinery. The result would be a potential uncoupling of the helicase and the replicase complex, leading to exposed ssDNA. Several synthetic lethal screens using either selective ATR inhibitors or cells expressing the ATR Seckel mutation (associated with substantial reduction of ATR) have shown that silencing of some genes involved in DNA replication is synthetically lethal with ATR inhibition or depletion. Of note, silencing of the RRM1 and 2 genes that form the ribonuclease reductase enzyme (responsible for synthesizing the nucleotide DNA building blocks), PRIM1 that makes the RNA primers required for the lagging strand replication, and POLD1 the DNA polymerase responsible for lagging strand replication, all resulted in marked sensitivity to ATR depletion or inhibition (Hocke et al. 2016; Mohni et al. 2015). In the case of POLD1 more detailed studies showed reducing ATR activity both through transfection of the ATR Seckel gene or inhibition with VX-970 (M6620) increased sensitivity of DLD1 cells to POLD1 silencing by nearly tenfold. In a second experiment, depletion of POLD1 by siRNA in a panel of cell lines increased the growth inhibitory activity of VX-970 (M6620) by up to tenfold. This was associated with increased RS and cell death (Hocke et al. 2016). Missense mutations in the POLD1 gene have recently been identified in colorectal, endometrial, brain and renal cancer (Hocke et al. 2016).

Regions of hypoxia are a hallmark of solid tumours, arising as a result of an inefficient tumour vasculature. Tumour hypoxia leads to a repression of DNA repair pathways and as a consequence an increase in genomic instability. Severe hypoxia also leads to elevated RS, which has been attributed to acute depletion of nucleotide pools, most likely through impairment of oxygen-dependent ribonucleotide reductase activity. Given the elevated RS that accompanies hypoxia it is perhaps unsurprising that ATR activity has been shown to be increased under these conditions (Pires et al. 2012). As such, hypoxia sets up an environment where RS is elevated but where many DNA repair pathways are repressed, a seemingly perfect scenario for dependence on ATR. This was first assessed using siRNA depletion of ATR: hypoxic cells depleted of ATR showed increased cell death compared with control treated cells (Hammond et al. 2004; Hammond and Giaccia 2004). Using VE-821 it was subsequently demonstrated that inhibition of ATR also sensitises cells to hypoxia. Treatment of hypoxic RKO cells with VE-821 led to a substantial decrease in P-CHK1 and a concomitant increase in DNA damage. This was associated with a marked decrease in clonogenic survival in VE-821 treated RKO cells exposed to short periods of hypoxia followed by reoxygenation. Sensitivity to the ATR inhibitor was both dependent on oxygen tension (increased hypoxia leading to greater sensitivity) and the duration cells were left under hypoxic conditions (Pires et al. 2012).

Finally, telomere maintenance is essential for cancer cells to attain immortality and whereas most cancer cells use the telomerase machinery to maintain telomeres, a sub-set of cancer cells use an HRR-dependent process known as Alternative Lengthening of Telomeres (ALT) (Draskovic and Londono-Vallejo 2014). Telomeres also represent hard to replicate, fragile, regions of the genome, which is partly associated with prevalent G-rich hexameric TTAGGG repeats. In ALT positive cells this situation is even worse since ALT telomeres comprise a series of variant hexameres, which disrupt the binding of important telomeric capping proteins. As a consequence, replication of ALT telomeres leads to high levels of RS (Cox et al. 2016). Using VE-821 it has been shown that inhibition of ATR leads to rapid loss of telomeres in ALT positive cancer cells and cell death after just one or two rounds of cell cycle. The IC_{50} values for inhibition of cell viability by VE-821 in ALT positive cell lines were on average over tenfold lower than a similar set of telomerase (ALT negative) cell lines. In addition to compromising the cell response to RS generated during the replication of ALT telomeres, ATR inhibition blocked the process of ALT itself (Flynn et al. 2015). Intriguingly however, in a second independent study, ALT positive cells were not found to be especially more sensitive to the ATR inhibitor VE-821 than cells utilizing a telomerase mechanism (Deeg et al. 2016).

Further studies are clearly required to determine the potential for ATR inhibitors as monotherapy in ALT tumors.

Endogenous events that impair DNA repair driving a reliance on ATR for survival: In addition to events that elevate RS, sensitivity to ATR inhibition as a monotherapy has been shown to be affected by defects elsewhere in the DNA repair network. Interestingly, this sensitivity can arise from defects in proteins associated with the ATR pathway along with defects in alternative surveillance and repair pathways.

In two synthetic lethal screens using VE-821, the strongest hits were with genes on the ATR pathway: ATR itself, ATRIP, RPA, Claspin, Hus1, Rad1 and CHK1 (Mohni et al. 2015, 2014). In subsequent studies, depletion of ATR or CHK1 increased sensitivity of U2OS cells to VE-821 by up to ~5-fold. Interestingly the presence of a heterozygote ATR mutant (on one of the two alleles) was sufficient to sensitise the cells to VE-821. These findings can be interpreted in a number of ways, either partial suppression of the ATR pathway places a greater reliance on the residual capacity and thus increases sensitivity to ATR inhibition; or it could be that the signaling pathway isn't always linear, for example, independent signals may lead to regulation of different ATR pathway proteins or the pathway may comprise regulatory feedback processes (discussed below for CHK1). Regardless of the underlying mechanism, the observation of synthetic lethality between ATR inhibition and depletion of genes on the ATR pathway highlights an interesting opportunity for use of ATR inhibitors as single agents since up to 25% of some cancer types harbor mutations or deletions in ATR pathway genes (Cerami et al. 2012).

RPA (replication protein A) is rapidly recruited to single stranded DNA where it protects it from nuclease cleavage and also recruits ATRIP and ATR. In an elegant in vitro study (Toledo et al. 2013) it was demonstrated that cells express a defined pool of nuclear RPA. When activated at a stressed fork, ATR signals to shut down global origin firing via CHK1, which acts to limit the number of stressed forks and thus depletion of the RPA pool. However, when ATR is inhibited DNA replication continues and RPA is depleted as the number of stalled forks increase. Once the RPA pool is exhausted the exposed, unprotected single stranded DNA at a stalled fork is rapidly converted to a double strand break. Consistent with this model, it was shown that RPA provides a resistance mechanism to ATR inhibition: overexpression of RPA by two to threefold was sufficient to protect cells from ATR inhibition at the time points assessed in the study. Conversely, depletion of the RPA pool markedly enhanced the sensitivity of cells to ATR inhibition (Toledo et al. 2013). This study highlights an attractive potential opportunity for single agent ATR inhibition in tumours with limited RPA pools. Such a situation could arise either from low baseline levels of RPA expression or from a combination of low RPA expression and elevated background RS. Further studies are required to assess and validate this approach and to define the appropriate markers that could support clinical investigation.

Finally, defects in HRR, the repair pathway ATR signals to, have also been shown to confer sensitivity to ATR inhibitors as single agents. In one study, either depletion of the HRR essential protein RAD51 (a recombinase involved in the homology search and strand pairing aspects of HRR) or its inhibition by the compound BO2, rendered cells highly sensitive to ATR inhibition by VE-821. For example, in HeLa cells VE-821 treatment alone led to about 75% clonogenic survival, however following RAD51 depletion by siRNA, viability was reduced to <5% (Krajewska et al. 2015). In a second study, cells defective in the HRR genes BRCA2 (involved in the recruitment of RAD51 to single stranded DNA) or XRCC3 (which complexes with RAD51 to effect homology search and strand pairing) were markedly sensitized to VE-821 compared with parental cells. Specifically, parental Chinese hamster ovary cells tolerated VE-821 with 91% clonogenic survival, in contrast cells defective in XRCC3 showed only 16% survival; and Chinese hamster lung cells with defective BRCA2 were also markedly sensitised compared with parental cells (8% survival compared with 38% survival, respectively) (Middleton et al. 2015).

In addition to defects in ATR pathway genes, loss of function in other DNA repair pathways has been shown to confer sensitivity to ATR inhibitors as single agents. Given that both the ATR and ATM mediated pathways signal to HRR in response to damage during S/G2 phases of cell cycle, and that loss of ATM signaling pathway function appears to sensitise cells to ATR in combination with DNA damaging agents (Cui et al. 2014), it is perhaps unsurprising that a number of studies have provided data that shows defects in ATM pathway signaling can confer sensitivity to single agent ATR inhibition. This was first demonstrated by Wright et al. (Wright et al. 1998) based on the observation that the ATR-kinase dead mutation led to markedly reduced viability of cells with mutant p53 or ATM deficiency. More recently, siRNA of ATM in U2OS cells led to increased sensitivity to the ATR inhibitor AZ20 by almost five-fold (Lee et al. 2011). ATM loss due to deletion of the 11q22-23 locus or promoter methylation has been described in a number of diseases including head and neck squamous cell carcinoma (HNSCC), mantle cell lymphoma (MCL) and chronic lymphocytic leukemia CLL (Lee et al. 2011; Menezes et al. 2015; Boultwood 2001; Schaffner et al. 1999). Treatment of two MCL lines, one with and one without deletion of the 11q22-23 locus, showed a differential sensitivity to AZ20: the ATM wild type line tolerated high concentrations of AZ20 (<20% growth inhibition at 1 μM) in contrast to the ATM null line where substantial growth inhibition was observed (>90% at 1 μM). In a CLL study, ATM defective CLL cells (ATM shRNA depletion) were five-fold more sensitive to treatment with AZD6738 than the ATM wild type parental cells, and similarly, in a panel of 29 primary CLL samples ATM defective (n = 8) or *TP53* defective (n = 6) samples were more sensitive to AZD6738 than ATM/*TP53* wild type cells (EC$_{50}$ 8.7 μM and 8.2 μM vs. 38.3 μM respectively) (Kwok et al. 2016). In mouse patient derived CLL xenograft studies using samples defective in either ATM or *TP53*, treatment with AZD6738 led to marked reduction in the number of CLL cells in the spleen of the mice. In one experiment tumour cell recovery was observed following treatment with AZD6738 and it was noted that the spleens of these mice had a significantly reduced frequency of ATM deficiency compared with the vehicle treated mice, supporting the hypothesis that ATR inhibition can be an effective approach to kill ATM or *TP53* defective tumour cells (Kwok et al. 2016). Interestingly, of the three reported mouse xenograft models based on solid cancer cell lines, where single agent ATR inhibition (AZ20 or AZD6738) has been shown to be effective, two are defective in ATM (Granta519 and LoVo) (Foote et al. 2015; Menezes et al. 2015).

BER and NER act to resolve small and bulky lesions respectively on nucleotides, and defects in BER and NER are widely reported in a variety of cancer types (Wallace et al. 2012; Marteijn et al. 2014). The X-ray repair cross-complimentary gene 1 (XRCC1) protein is a scaffold protein that plays an important role in recruiting key proteins for both BER and NER. (Caldecott 2003; Moser et al. 2007) In three separate studies it has been shown that isogenic cell pairs deficient in XRCC1 are more sensitive to ATR inhibition than their parental counterparts. The semi-selective ATR inhibitor NU6027 reduced clonogenic survival of XRCC1 null CHO derivatives by over 50% in contrast to parental cells, which tolerated the compound well (Peasland et al. 2011). This was associated with a marked increase in apoptosis (Sultana et al. 2013). Similarly, treatment of XRCC1 defective CHO cells with VE-821 led to marked inhibition of clonogenic viability (75%) in stark contrast to parental cells that tolerated VE-821 with minimal impact on survival (<10% loss of viability) (Middleton et al. 2015). Furthermore, inhibition of PARP, a key enzyme in BER, has been shown to dramatically sensitize cells to ATR inhibition (described in detail below).

The ERCC1-XPF nuclease complex functions in a number of repair pathways that act to resolve bulky DNA adducts, double strand breaks and interstrand cross links. Low levels of ERCC1 have been described in some cancers, most notably testicular cancer (Usanova et al. 2010). Depletion of ERCC1 by siRNA in five cell lines increased cell sensitivity to VE-821 in all cases, with IC_{50} shifts for VE-821 of up to 1 order of magnitude. This was associated with elevated DNA damage (by γH2AX) (Mohni et al. 2014). Finally, disruption of proteins in involved in NHEJ was shown to sensitise cells to ATR inhibition. Depletion of Ku80, a protein that binds DSBs and recruits DNA-PK to form the catalytically active enzyme required for NHEJ, sensitised CHO cells to VE-821 with just 20% clonogenic survival compared with >90% for the parental CHO cells. Intriguingly however, loss of DNA-PKcs itself rendered CHO cells marginally *resistant* to VE-821, and overexpression of DNA-PKcs in both human GBM and CHO cells that lacked DNA-PKcs increased their sensitivity to VE-821. Even more intriguingly, the effects of DNA-PKcs expression was not associated with catalytic activity since addition of the DNA-PK inhibitor NU7441 did not rescue the cells. The model proposed to rationalize these data was that elevated levels of DNA-PKcs led to increased loading and persistence of DNA-PKcs on DSBs. Since end resection, revealing regions of ssDNA and recruitment of ATR, is a key step in DSB resolution, persistence of DNA-PKcs may impair this process. The impact of this could be to reduce ATR signaling capacity, placing increased reliance on residual proficient ATR signaling and rendering cells highly sensitive to ATR inhibition (Middleton et al. 2015).

Taken together, the emerging picture is that somatic defects leading to elevated RS, and/or reliance on ATR through impairments in DNA repair processes, have the potential to render cells sensitive to ATR inhibition as a monotherapy. Whilst this provides an exciting opportunity, defining translationally robust markers that support monotherapy activity in the context of the heterogeneity of human cancer remains a very important task.

4.7   ATR Inhibition in Combination with Targeted Drugs

As discussed above, a number of genetic studies have demonstrated that depletion of genes involved in DNA repair can drive a reliance on ATR to survive DNA damage. Accordingly, there is potential for ATR inhibitors to provide benefit when used in combination with agents that block other proteins involved in the surveillance and response to DNA damage. Two examples have been described; ATR inhibition with PARP inhibition and ATR inhibition with CHK1 inhibition.

PARP is a key enzyme involved in the repair of single stranded DNA (ssDNA) breaks, primarily during BER. PARP is recruited to sites of ssDNA damage where it acts to add ADP-ribose moieties to proteins, a process termed PAR-ylation. The result is an increasingly negatively charged region at sites of damage that serves to recruit the BER multi-protein complex including proteins such as DNA ligase III, DNA polymerase beta and the scaffold protein XRCC1 (Curtin 2014). PARP has also been shown to play a role in regulating replication fork dynamics at sites of RS and a direct interaction between PARP and ATR has been demonstrated in response to DNA damage (Bryant et al. 2009; Sugimura et al. 2008; Kedar et al. 2008). PARP inhibition is synthetically lethal with loss of the HRR essential genes BRCA1/2 (Li and Yu 2015). Given these observations it was intriguing to consider whether ATR inhibition could sensitise cells to PARP inhibition. The combination of an ATR and PARP inhibitor was first described in 2011 with NU6027 and the PARP inhibitor rucaparib (Peasland et al. 2011). Rucaparib alone led to elevated DNA damage (γH2AX foci formation) and increased HRR pathway activity (RAD51 foci) in a BRCA wild type cell line. Co-treatment with NU6027 completely blocked RAD51 foci formation consistent with inhibition of HRR. In two different cell lines, both with functional HRR, NU6027 increased the cytotoxic activity of rucaparib: in GM847KD cells, expression of ATR kinase dead or treatment with NU6027 reduced the LC_{50} for rucaparab from >30 μM to about 12 μM, and in MCF7 cells clonogenic survival was reduced from 60% to 70% for rucaparib alone to about 20% on co-treatment with NU6027 (Peasland et al. 2011). ATR depletion and VE-821 also sensitized ovarian cancer cells to the PARP inhibitor, veliparib (Huntoon et al. 2013). In a subsequent study, reported at the AACR annual meeting in 2016, ATR inhibition using VX-970 (M6620) was shown to synergise with all the available clinical PARP inhibitors (veliparib, olaparib, rucaparib, niraparib and talazoparib) across a panel of cancer cell lines. Importantly, synergy was not observed in a non-cancer cell line. Furthermore, in isogeneic cell pairs, loss of either ATM or p53 resulted in marked sensitivity to the combination of VX-970 (M6620) and talazoparib. Consistent with this, across a large panel of over 100 cancer cell lines, greater synergy was observed for the combination of VX-970 (M6620) and talazoparib in cell lines with a mutation of the *TP53* gene (Pollard et al. 2016a, b). A similar profile was reported for AZD6738 and olaparaib, at the EORTC/NCI/AACR triple meeting in 2015 (Lau et al. 2015). These data are comparable with the observations for combinations of ATR inhibitors with cytotoxic chemotherapy and suggest that loss of the compensatory ATM-p53 signaling pathway may be a marker for tumour sensitivity.

Accordingly, activation of the ATM-p53 pathway may provide a mechanism to enable non-cancer cells to tolerate the combination. In vivo benefit for the combination has been reported with AZD6738 and olaparaib in two primary explant mouse xenograft models. In the first model, which was BRCA2 and *TP53* mutant, olparaib alone was active (partial tumour growth inhibition) consistent with the established synthetic lethality of PARP inhibition and BRCA mutation, whereas AZD6738 had no single agent activity. Impressively, the combination led to complete and sustained regression. In the second model, which was ATM and *TP53* mutant but BRCA wild type, the combination led to complete tumour growth inhibition in contrast to either agent alone, which were inactive (Lau et al. 2015). A number of clinical studies are actively assessing the combination of PARP and ATR inhibitors either as doublets or with the addition of chemotherapy (Chap. 5).

CHK1 and ATR function in the same pathway to coordinate cell responses to DNA damage. However, there are circumstances where each appears to function independently. For example, ATR has been reported to control the intra S-phase checkpoint independently of CHK1 activity (Couch et al. 2013; Luciani et al. 2004), and conversely CHK1 has been reported to be activated in response to RS by claspin in an ATR independent manner (Yang et al. 2008). Furthermore, differences in the potential for CHK1 and ATR inhibition to sensitise cells to various DNA damaging drugs was demonstrated from a large panel of lung cancer cell lines. Whereas inhibition of either CHK1 or ATR sensitised many cancer cells to gemcitabine, inhibition of CHK1 had only a moderate impact on cancer cell sensitivity to platinating agents in contrast to ATR inhibition, which induced substantial cell sensitivity (Hall et al. 2014). The potential for ATR and CHK1 inhibitors to provide a beneficial combination therapy was characterized in a series of elegant studies. Against a panel of seven cancer cell lines co-treatment with the CHK1 inhibitor AZD7762 and the ATR inhibitor VE-821 led to synergistic loss of viability in all seven lines. A subsequent experiment in a sub-set of the cell lines showed that AZD7762 reduced the IC_{50} of VE-821 by three to tenfold (Sanjiv et al. 2016). In contrast, the two agents when combined did not impact the viability of a number of non-cancer cell lines. To address a concern that the combination is merely a hypermorphic response i.e., that the combined effect arises through more comprehensive inhibition of the pathway than can be achieved by either agent alone, CHK1 null DLD1 cells were treated with VE-821. Almost complete loss of clonogenic survival was observed (<5% survival), in stark contrast to parental cells that were tolerant to very high concentrations of VE-821 (>70% clonogenic survival). The cytotoxic activity of the combination appeared to be dependent on RS since Myc expressing cells were acutely sensitive to VE-821 plus AZD7762, as opposed to parental non-transformed cells that were resistant to the combined drug treatment. Detailed molecular studies led to the proposal of a model in which CHK1 inhibition leads to a CDK mediated increase in origin firing, which in turn leads to depletion of the dNTP pool, slowed or stalled fork progression, increased levels of RS and a concomitant reliance on ATR. Interestingly, this model suggests that CHK1 could limit the efficacy of ATR inhibition and vice versa. The potential benefit for combined treatment with ATR and CHK1 inhibition was assessed in a mouse H460 cell line xenograft. Treatment with either AZD7762 or VX-970 (M6620) alone had minimal impact on tumour cell growth and survival, however the combination resulted in almost complete tumour growth inhibition and a marked increase in survival. The combination was well tolerated with no body weight loss. This study highlights an interesting intrapathway synthetic lethality that could be exploited to provide a tumour specific anti-cancer therapy (Sanjiv et al. 2016).

4.8 Conclusion

The ATR kinase plays an important role in the cells response to exposed ssDNA, a structure most commonly formed at stalled replication forks (replication stress, RS), but also as an intermediate in a number of repair processes. In the absence of a functional ATR response, unresolved ssDNA can form a lethal DSB. RS and ssDNA can result from many types of DNA damage insult including endogenous events such as oxidative stress and deregulated DNA replication (for example from expression of oncogenes); or from exogenous events such as hypoxia or treatment with DNA damaging chemotherapy or IR. Elevated levels of ssDNA drive an acute reliance on ATR, which can be further exacerbated in cells where alternative DNA damage repair processes are impaired. Both high levels of DNA damage and defective DNA repair are hallmarks of cancer and numerous genetic and pharmacologic studies have demonstrated that many cancer cells are reliant on ATR to survive DNA damage. Inhibition of ATR is frequently lethal to cancer cells either alone or when treated in combination with agents that induce DNA damage. In contrast non-cancer cells can tolerate ATR inhibition through activation of a compensatory DNA damage response. Given the multiple contexts in which RS can be elevated in cancer cells, there are many opportunities where ATR inhibitors have the potential to provide patient benefit. Perhaps the best pre-clinically validated opportunity is as a combination therapy with DNA damaging drugs and IR. This, coupled with the widespread role these agents play in standard of care across multiple cancer types and the emerging role DNA repair has as a clinically relevant mechanism of resistance to such agents, has led to growing interest in the numerous ongoing clinical studies assessing ATR inhibitors with various DNA damaging drugs and IR. A growing body of evidence also supports a potential for ATR inhibitors as monotherapy in cancers with high levels of background DNA damage and/or defects in compensatory repair pathways; and as combination therapies with agents that block other DNA repair processes.

References

Babior BM (1999) NADPH oxidase: an update. Blood 93(5):1464–1476
Bartkova J, Tommiska J, Oplustilova L, Aaltonen K, Tamminen A, Heikkinen T, Mistrik M, Aittomäki K, Blomqvist C, Heikkilä P, Lukas J, Nevanlinna H, Bartek J (2008) Aberrations of the MRE11-RAD50-NBS1 DNA damage sensor complex in human breast cancer: MRE11 as a candidate familial cancer-predisposing gene. Mol Oncol 2:296–316

Berasain C, Castillo J, Perugorria MJ, Latasa MU, Prieto J, Avila MA (2009) Inflammation and liver cancer: new molecular links. Ann N Y Acad Sci 1155:206–221

Boultwood J (2001) Ataxia telangiectasia gene mutations in leukaemia and lymphoma. J Clin Pathol 54(7):512–516

Brown EJ, Baltimore D (2000) ATR disruption leads to chromosomal fragmentation and early embryonic lethality. Genes Dev 14:397–402

Brown AD, Sager BW, Gorthi A, Tonapi SS, Brown EJ, Bishop AJR (2014) ATR suppresses endogenous DNA damage and allows completion of homologous recombination repair. PLoS One 9(3):e91222. https://doi.org/10.1371/journal.pone.0091222

Bryant HE, Petermann E, Schultz N, Jemth AS, Loseva O, Issaeva N, Johansson F, Fernandez S, McGlynn P, Helleday T (2009) PARP is activated at stalled forks to mediate Mre11-dependent replication restart and recombination. EMBO J 28(17):2601–2615

Burdova K, Mihaljevic B, Sturzenegger A, Chappidi N, Janscak P (2015) The mismatch-binding factor MutSbeta can mediate ATR activation in response to DNA double-strand breaks. Mol Cell 59(4):603–614

Caldecott KW (2003) XRCC1 and DNA strand break repair. DNA Repair 2(9):955–969

Cancer Genome Atlas Network (2012a) Comprehensive molecular portraits of human breast tumours. Nature 490:61–80

Cancer Genome Atlas Network (2012b) Comprehensive genomic characterization of squamous cell lung cancers. Nature 489:519–525

Caporali S, Falcinelli S, Starace G, Russo MT, Bonmassar E, Jiricny J, D'Atri S (2004) DNA damage induced by temozolomide signals to both ATM and ATR: role of the mismatch repair system. Mol Pharmacol 66(3):478–491

Caporali S, Levati L, Starace G, Ragone G, Bonmassar E, Alvino E, D'Atri S (2008) AKT is activated in an ataxia-telangiectasia and Rad3-related-dependent manner in response to temozolomide and confers protection against drug-induced cell growth inhibition. Mol Pharmacol 74(1):173–183

Cerami E, Gao J, Dogrusoz U, Gross BE, Sumer SO, Aksoy BA, Jacobsen A, Byrne CJ, Heuer ML, Larsson E, Antipin Y, Reva B, Goldberg AP, Sander C, Schultz N (2012) The cBio cancer genomics portal: an open platform for exploring multidimensional cancer genomics data. Cancer Discov 2(5):401–404

Charrier JD, Durrant SJ, Golec JM, Kay DP, Knegtel RM, MacCormick S Mortimore M, O'Donnell ME, Pinder JL, Reaper PM, Rutherford AP, Wang PS, Young SC, Pollard JR (2011) Discovery of potent and selective inhibitors of ataxia telangiectasia mutated and Rad3 related (ATR) protein kinase as potential anticancer agents. J Med Chem **54**:2320–2330

Chen MS, Ryan CE, Piwnica-Worms H (2003) CHK1 kinase negatively regulates mitotic function of Cdc25A phosphatase through 14-3-3 binding. Mol Cell Biol 23(21):7488–7497

Choi JH, Lindsey-Boltz LA, Kemp M, Mason AC, Wold MS, Sancar A (2010) Reconstitution of RPA-covered single-stranded DNA-activated ATR-CHK1 signaling. Proc Natl Acad Sci U S A 107(31):13660–13665

Cleaver JE (2016) Profile of Thomas Lindahl, Paul Modrich ans Aziz Sancar, 2015 Noel Laureates in chemistry. Proc Natl Acad Sci U S A 113(2):242–245

Cliby WA, Roberts CJ, Cimprich KA, Stringer CM, Lamb JR, Schreiber SL, Friend SH (1998) Overexpression of a kinase-inactive ATR protein causes sensitivity to DNA-damaging agents and defects in cell cycle checkpoints. EMBO J 17(1):159–169

Cliby WA, Lewis KA, Lilly KK, Kaufmann SH (2002) S phase and G2 arrests induced by topoisomerase I poisons are dependent on ATR kinase function. J Biol Chem 277(2):1599–1606

Cole AJ, Dwight T, Gill AJ, Dickson KA, Zhu Y, Clarkson A, Gard GB, Maidens J, Valmadre S, Clifton-Bligh R, Marsh DJ (2016) Assessing mutant p53 in primary high-grade serous ovarian cancer using immunohistochemistry and massively parallel sequencing. Sci Rep 6:26191

Collis SJ, Swartz MJ, Nelson WG, DeWeese TL (2003) Enhanced radiation and chemotherapy-mediated cell killing of human cancer cells by small inhibitory RNA silencing of DNA repair factors. Cancer Res 63(7):1550–1554

Collis SJ, Ciccia A, Deans AJ, Horejsi Z, Martin JS, Maslen SL, Skehel JM, Elledge SJ, West SC, Boulton SJ (2008) FANCM and FAAP24 function in ATR-mediated checkpoint signaling independently of the Fanconi anemia core complex. Mol Cell 32(3):313–324

Cortez D (2003) Caffeine inhibits checkpoint responses without inhibiting the ataxia-telangiectasia-mutated (ATM) and ATM- and Rad3-related (ATR) protein kinases. J Biol Chem 278(39):37139–37145

Cottini F, Hideshima T, Suzuki R, Tai YT, Bianchini G, Richardson PG, Anderson KC, Tonon G (2015) Synthetic lethal approaches exploiting DNA damage in aggressive myeloma. Cancer Discov 5(9):972–987

Couch FB, Bansbach CE, Driscoll R, Luzwick JW, Glick GG, Bétous R, Carroll CM, Jung SY, Qin J, Cimprich KA, Cortez D (2013) ATR phosphorylates SMARCAL1 to prevent replication fork collapse. Genes Dev 27(14):1610–1623

Cox KE, Marechal A, Flynn RL (2016) SMARCAL1 resolves replication stress at ALT telomeres. Cell Rep 14:1032–1040

Cui Y, Palii SS, Innes CL, Paules RS (2014) Depletion of ATR selectively sensitizes ATM-deficient human mammary epithelial cells to ionizing radiation and DNA-damaging agents. Cell Cycle 13(22):3541–3550

Curtin NJ (2014) PARP inhibitors for anticancer Therapy. Biochem Soc Trans 42:82–88

Dai Y, Grant S (2010) New insights into checkpoint kinase 1 in the DNA damage response signaling network. Clin Cancer Res 16(2):376–383

Dart DA, Adams KE, Akerman I, Lakin ND (2004) Recruitment of the cell cycle checkpoint kinase ATR to chromatin during S-phase. J Biol Chem 269:16433–16440

Davidson IF, Li A, Blow JJ (2006) Deregulated replication licensing causes DNA fragmentation consistent with head-to-tail fork collision. Mol Cell 24:433–443

Deans AJ, West SC (2011) DNA interstrand crosslink repair and cancer. Nat Rev Cancer 24:467–480

Deeg KI, Chung I, Bauer C, Rippe K (2016) Cancer Cells with Alternative Lengthening of Telomeres Do Not Display a General Hypersensitivity to ATR Inhibition. Front Oncol 6:186. https://doi.org/10.3389/fonc.2016.00186

Dominguez-Sola D, Ying CY, Grandori C, Ruggiero L, Chen B, Li M, Galloway DA, Gu W, Gautier J, Dalla-Favera R (2007) Non-transcriptional control of DNA replication by c-Myc. Nature 448:445–451

Draskovic I, Londono-Vallejo A (2014) Telomere recombination and the ALT pathway: a therapeutic perspective for cancer. Curr Pharm Des 20:6466–6471

Durocher D, Jackson SP (2001) DNA-PK, ATM and ATR as sensors of DNA damage: variations on a theme? Curr Opin Cell Biol 13(2):225–231

Eich M, Roos WP, Nikolova T, Kaina B (2013) Contribution of ATM and ATR to the resistance of glioblastoma and malignant melanoma cells to the methylating anticancer drug temozolomide. Mol Cancer Ther 12(11):2529–2540

Fang WH, Li GM, Longley M, Holmes J, Thilly W, Modrich P (1993) Mismatch repair and genetic stability in human cells. Cold Spring Harb Symp Quant Biol 58:597–603

Flatten K, Dai NT, Vroman BT, Loegering D, Erlichman C, Karnitz LM, Kaufmann SH (2005) The role of checkpoint kinase 1 in sensitivity to topoisomerase I poisons. J Biol Chem 280(14):14349–14355

Flynn RL, Cox KE, Jeitany M, Wakimoto H, Bryll AR, Ganem NJ, Bersani F, Pineda JR, Suva ML, Benes CH et al (2015) Alternative lengthening of telomeres renders cancer cells hypersensitive to ATR inhibitors. Science 347:273–277

Fokas E, Prevo R, Pollard JR, Reaper PM, Charlton PA, Cornelissen B, Vallis KA, Hammond EM, Olcina MM, Gillies McKenna W, Muschel RJ, Brunner TB (2012) Targeting ATR in vivo using the novel inhibitor VE-822 results in selective sensitization of pancreatic tumors to radiation. Cell Death Dis 3:e441

Foote KM, Blades K, Cronin A, Fillery S, Guichard SS, Hassall L, Hickson I, Jacq X, Jewsbury PJ, McGuire TM, Nissink JW, Odedra R, Page K, Perkins P, Suleman A, Tam K, Thommes P, Broadhurst R, Wood C (2013) Discovery of 4-{4-[(3R)-3-Methylmorpholin-4-yl]-6-[1-

(methylsulfonyl)cyclopropyl]pyrimidin-2-yl}-1H-indole (AZ20): a potent and selective inhibitor of ATR protein kinase with monotherapy in vivo antitumor activity. J Med Chem 56(5):2125–2138

Foote KM, Lau A, Nissink JW (2015) Drugging ATR: progress in the development of specific inhibitors for the treatment of cancer. Future Med Chem 7:873–891

Gaillard H, García-Muse T, Aguilera A (2015) Replication stress and cancer. Nat Rev Cancer 15:276–289

Genschel J, Modrich P (2009) Functions of MutLalpha, replication protein A (RPA), and HMGB1 in 5′-directed mismatch repair. J Biol Chem 284(32):21536–21544

Gilad O, Nabet BY, Ragland RL, Schoppy DW, Smith KD, Durham AC, Brown EJ (2010) Combining ATR suppression with oncogenic Ras synergistically increases genomic instability, causing synthetic lethality or tumorigenesis in a dosage-dependent manner. Cancer Res 70(23):9693–9702

Guichard SM, Brown E, Odedra R, Hughes A, Heathcote D, Barnes J, Lau A, Powell S, Jones CD, Nissink JW, Foote KM, Jewsbury PJ, Pass M (2013) The pre-clinical *in vitro* and *in vivo* activity of AZD6738: a potent and selective inhibitor of ATR kinase. Cancer Res 73(8 Suppl):Abstract nr 3343

Halazonetis TD, Gorgoulis VG, Bartek J (2008) An oncogene-induced DNA damage model for cancer development. Science 319:1352–1355

Hall AB, Newsome D, Wang Y, Boucher DM, Eustace B, Gu Y, Hare B, Johnson MA, Milton S, Murphy CE, Takemoto D, Tolman C, Wood M, Charlton P, Charrier JD, Furey B, Golec J, Reaper PM, Pollard JR (2014) Potentiation of tumor responses to DNA damaging therapy by the selective ATR inhibitor VX-970. Oncotarget 5:5674–5685

Hammond EM, Giaccia AJ (2004) The role of ATM and ATR in the cellular response to hypoxia and re-oxygenation. DNA Repair (Amst). 3(8-9):1117–1122

Hammond EM, Dorie MJ, Giaccia AJ (2004) Inhibition of ATR leads to increased sensitivity to hypoxia/reoxygenation. Cancer Res 64(18):6556–6562

Hanahan D, Weinberg RA (2011) Hallmarks of cancer: the next generation. Cell 144(5):646–674

Haynes B, Saadat N, Myung B, Shekhar MP (2015) Crosstalk between translesion synthesis, Fanconi anemia network, and homologous recombination repair pathways in interstrand DNA crosslink repair and development of chemoresistance. Mutat Res 763:258–266

Hocke S, Guo Y, Job A, Orth M, Ziesch A, Lauber K, De Toni EN, Gress TM, Herbst A, Göke B, Gallmeier EA (2016) synthetic lethal screen identifies ATR-inhibition as a novel therapeutic approach for POLD1-deficient cancers. Oncotarget 7(6):7080–7095

Huntoon CJ, Flatten KS, Wahner Hendrickson AE, Huehls AM, Sutor SL, Kaufmann SH, Karnitz LM (2013) ATR inhibition broadly sensitizes ovarian cancer cells to chemotherapy independent of BRCA status. Cancer Res 73(12):3683–3691

Hurley PJ, Wilsker D, Bunz F (2007) Human cancer cells require ATR for cell cycle progression following exposure to ionizing radiation. Oncogene 26(18):2535–2542

Itakura E, Umeda K, Sekoguchi E, Takata H, Ohsumi M, Matsuura A (2004) ATR-dependent phosphorylation of ATRIP in response to genotoxic stress. Biochem Biophys Res Commun 323(4):1197–1202

Jiang H, Reinhardt HC, Bartkova J, Tommiska J, Blomqvist C, Nevanlinna H, Bartek J, Yaffe MB, Hemann MT (2009) The combined status of ATM and p53 link tumor development with therapeutic response. Genes Dev 23:1895–1909

Jones CD, Blades K, Foote KM, Guichard SM, Jewsbury PJ, McGuire T, Nissink JW, Odedra R, Tam K, Thommes P, Turner P, Wilkinson G, Wood C, Yates JW (2013) Discovery of AZD6738, a potent and selective inhibitor with the potential to test the clinical efficacy of ATR kinase inhibition in cancer patients. [abstract]. Cancer Res 73(8 Suppl):Abstract nr 2348

Jossé R, Martin SE, Guha R, Ormanoglu P, Pfister TD, Reaper PM, Barnes CS, Jones J, Charlton P, Pollard JR, Morris J, Doroshow JH, Pommier Y (2014) ATR inhibitors VE-821 and VX-970 sensitize cancer cells to topoisomerase i inhibitors by disabling DNA replication initiation and fork elongation responses. Cancer Res 74(23):6968–6979

Kedar PS, Stefanick DF, Horton JK, Wilson SH (2008) Interaction between PARP-1 and ATR in mouse fibroblasts is blocked by PARP inhibition. DNA Repair (Amst) 7(11):1787–1798

Kim H, D'Andrea AD (2012) Regulation of DNA cross-link repair by the Fanconi anemia/BRCA pathway. Genes Dev 26:1393–1408

Knight ZA, Gonzalez B, Feldman ME, Zunder ER, Goldenberg DD, Williams O, Loewith R, Stokoe D, Balla A, Toth B, Balla T, Weiss WA, Williams RL, Shokat KM (2006) A pharmacological map of the PI3-K family defines a role for p110alpha in insulin signaling. Cell 125(4):733–747

Krajewska M, Fehrmann RS, Schoonen PM, Labib S, de Vries EG, Franke L, van Vugt MA (2015) ATR inhibition preferentially targets homologous recombination-deficient tumor cells. Oncogene 34(26):3474–3481

Kwok M, Davies N, Agathanggelou A, Smith E, Oldreive C, Petermann E, Stewart G, Brown J, Lau A, Pratt G, Parry H, Taylor M, Moss P, Hillmen P, Stankovic T (2016) ATR inhibition induces synthetic lethality and overcomes chemoresistance in TP53- or ATM-defective chronic lymphocytic leukemia cells. Blood 127(5):582–595

Lau A, Brown E, Thomason A, Odedra R, Sheridan V, Cadogan E, Xu S, Cui A, Gavine PR, O'Connor M (2015) Pre-clinical efficacy of the ATR inhibitor AZD6738 in combination with the PARP inhibitor olaparib. Mol Cancer Ther 14(12 Suppl 2):Abstract nr C60

Lee J, Kumagai A, Dunphy WG (2001) Positive regulation of Wee1 by CHK1 and 14-3-3 proteins. Mol Biol Cell 12(3):551–563

Lee KW, Tsai YS, Chiang FY, Huang JL, Ho KY, Yang YH, Kuo WR, Chen MK, Lin CS (2011) Lower ataxia telangiectasia mutated (ATM) mRNA expression is correlated with poor outcome of laryngeal and pharyngeal cancer patients. Ann Oncol 22:1088–1093

Li M, Yu X (2015) The role of poly(ADP-ribosyl)ation in DNA damage response and cancer chemotherapy. Oncogene 34(26):3349–3356

Lindahl T (1993) Instability and decay of the primary structure of DNA. Nature 362(6422):709–715

Lindsey-Boltz LA, Sancar A (2011) Tethering DNA damage checkpoint mediator proteins topoisomerase IIbeta-binding protein 1 (TopBP1) and Claspin to DNA activates ataxia-telangiectasia mutated and RAD3-related (ATR) phosphorylation of checkpoint kinase 1 (CHK1). J Biol Chem 286(22):19229–19236

Liu Q, Guntuku S, Cui XS, Matsuoka S, Cortez D, Tamai K, Luo G, Carattini-Rivera S, DeMayo F, Bradley A, Donehower LA, Elledge SJ (2000) CHK1 is an essential kinase that is regulated by Atr and required for the G(2)/M DNA damage checkpoint. Genes Dev 14(12):1448–1459

Liu Y, Fang Y, Shao H, Lindsey-Boltz L, Sancar A, Modrich P (2010) Interactions of human mismatch repair proteins MutSalpha and MutLalpha with proteins of the ATR-CHK1 pathway. J Biol Chem 285(8):5974–5982

Lomax ME, Folkes LK, O'Neill P (2013) Biological consequences of radiation-induced DNA damage: relevance to radiotherapy. Clin Oncol 25:578–585

Luciani MG, Oehlmann M, Blow JJ (2004) Characterization of a novel ATR-dependent, Chk1-independent, intra-S-phase checkpoint that suppresses initiation of replication in Xenopus. J Cell Sci 117(Pt 25):6019–6030

Luke-Glaser S, Luke B, Grossi S, Constantinou A (2010) FANCM regulates DNA chain elongation and is stabilized by S-phase checkpoint signalling. EMBO J 29(4):795

Macheret M, Halazonetis TD (2015) DNA replication stress as a hallmark of cancer. Annu Rev Pathol 10:425–448

Mackay DR, Ullman KS (2015) ATR and a CHK1-Aurora B pathway coordinate postmitotic genome surveillance with cytokinetic abscission. Mol Biol Cell 26(12):2217–2226

Mailand N, Falck J, Lukas C, Syljuasen RG, Welcker M, Bartek J, Lukas J (2000) Rapid destruction of human Cdc25A in response to DNA damage. Science 288(5470):1425–1429

Marteijn JA, Lans H, Vermeulen W, Hoeijmakers JH (2014) Understanding nucleotide excision repair and its roles in cancer and ageing. Nat Rev Mol Cell Biol 15(7):465–481

Massague J (2004) G1 cell-cycle control and cancer. Nature 432(7015):298–306

Masters JRW, Koberle B (2003) Curing metastatic cancer: lessons from testicular germ-cell tumours. Nat Rev Cancer 3:517–525

Matsuoka S, Ballif BA, Smogorzewska A, ER MD III, Hurov KE, Luo J, Bakalarski CE, Zhao Z, Solimini N, Lerenthal Y, Shiloh Y, Gygi SP, Elledge SJ (2007) ATM and ATR substrate analysis reveals extensive protein networks responsive to DNA damage. Science 316(5828):1160–1166

Menezes DL, Holt J, Tang Y, Feng J, Barsanti P, Pan Y, Ghoddusi M, Zhang W, Thomas G, Holash J, Lees E, Taricani L (2015) A synthetic lethal screen reveals enhanced sensitivity to ATR inhibitor treatment in mantle cell lymphoma with ATM loss-of-function. Mol Cancer Res 13(1):120–129

Middleton FK, Patterson MJ, Elstob CJ, Fordham S, Herriott A, Wade MA, McCormick A, Edmondson R, May FE, Allan JM, Pollard JR, Common CNJ (2015) cancer-associated imbalances in the DNA damage response confer sensitivity to single agent ATR inhibition. Oncotarget 6(32):32396–32409

Mlasenov E, Mahin S, Soni A, Illiakis G (2016) DNA double-strand-break repair in higher eukaryotes and its role in genomic instability and cancer: cell cycle and proliferation-dependent regulation. Semin Cancer Biol 37-38:51–64

Mohni KN, Kavanaugh GM, Cortez D (2014) ATR pathway inhibition is synthetically lethal in cancer cells with ERCC1 deficiency. Cancer Res 74(10):2835–2845. https://doi.org/10.1158/0008-5472.CAN-13-3229

Mohni KN, Thompson PS, Luzwick JW, Glick GG, Pendleton CS, Lehmann BD, Pietenpol JA, Cortez DA (2015) Synthetic lethal screen identifies DNA repair pathways that sensitize cancer cells to combined ATR inhibition and cisplatin treatments. PLoS One 10(5):e0125482

Moiseeva O, Bourdeau V, Roux A, Deschenes-Simard X, Ferbeyre G (2009) Mitochondrial dysfunction contributes to oncogene-induced senescence. Mol Cell Biol 29:4495–4507

Morishima K, Sakamoto S, Kobayashi J, Izumi H, Suda T, Matsumoto Y, Tauchi H, Ide H, Komatsu K, Matsuura S (2007) TopBP1 associates with NBS1 and is involved in homologous recombination repair. Biochem Biophys Res Commun 362(4):872–879

Moser J, Kool H, Giakzidis I, Caldecott K, Mullenders LH, Fousteri MI (2007) Sealing of chromosomal DNA nicks during nucleotide excision repair requires XRCC1 and DNA ligase III alpha in a cell-cycle-specific manner. Mol Cell 27(2):311–323

Murga M, Bunting S, Montaña MF, Soria R, Mulero F, Cañamero M, Lee Y, McKinnon PJ, Nussenzweig A, Fernandez-Capetillo O (2009) A mouse model of ATRSeckel shows embryonic replicative stress and accelerated aging. Nat Genet 41:891–899

Murga M, Campaner S, Lopez-Contreras AJ, Toledo LI, Soria R, Montaña MF, D'Artista L, Schleker T, Guerra C, Garcia E, Barbacid M, Hidalgo M, Amati B, Fernandez-Capetillo O (2011) Exploiting oncogene-induced replicative stress for the selective killing of Myc-driven tumors. Nat Struct Mol Biol 18(12):1331–1335

Myers K, Gagou ME, Zuazua-Villar P, Rodriguez R, Meuth M (2009) ATR and Chk1 suppress a caspase-3–dependent apoptotic response following DNA replication stress. PLoS Genet 5(1):e1000324. https://doi.org/10.1371/journal.pgen.1000324

Nghiem P, Park PK, Kim YS, Vaziri C, Schreiber SL (2001) ATR inhibition selectively sensitizes G1 checkpoint-deficient cells to lethal premature chromatin condensation. Proc Natl Acad Sci U S A 98(16):9092–9097

Nghiem P, Park PK, Kim Ys YS, Desai BN, Schreiber SL (2002) ATR is not required for p53 activation but synergizes with p53 in the replication checkpoint. J Biol Chem 277(6):4428–4434

Nishida H, Tatewaki N, Nakajima Y, Magara T, Ko KM, Hamamori Y, Konishi T (2009) Inhibition of ATR protein kinase activity by schisandrin B in DNA damage response. Nucleic Acids Res 37(17):5678–5689

O'Driscoll M, Ruiz-Perez VL, Woods CG, Jeggo PA, Goodship JA (2003) A splicing mutation affecting expression of ataxia-telangiectasia and Rad3-related protein (ATR) results in Seckel syndrome. Nat Genet 33(4):497–501

O'Driscoll M, Gennery AR, Seidel J, Concannon P, Jeggo PA (2004) An overview of three new disorders associated with genetic instability: LIG4 syndrome, RS-SCID and ATR-Seckel syndrome. DNA Repair (Amst) 3(8-9):1227–1235

Olivier M, Hollstein M, Hainaut P (2010) TP53 mutations in human cancers: origins, consequences, and clinical use. Cold Spring Harb Perspect Biol 2(1):a001008

Parsels LA, Qian Y, Tanska DM, Gross M, Zhao L, Hassan MC, Arumugarajah S, Parsels JD, Hylander-Gans L, Simeone DM, Morosini D, Brown JL, Zabludoff SD, Maybaum J, Lawrence TS, Morgan MA (2011) Assessment of CHK1 phosphorylation as a pharmacodynamic biomarker of CHK1 inhibition. Clin Cancer Res 17(11):3706–3715

Patch AM, Christie EL, Etemadmoghadam D, Garsed DW, George J, Fereday S, Nones K, Cowin P, Alsop K, Bailey PJ, Kassahn KS, Newell F, Quinn MC, Kazakoff S, Quek K, Wilhelm-Benartzi C, Curry E, Leong HS (2015) Australian Ovarian Cancer Study Group, et al. Whole-genome characterization of chemoresistant ovarian cancer. Nature 521:489–494

Peasland A, Wang LZ, Rowling E, Kyle S, Chen T, Hopkins A, Cliby WA, Sarkaria J, Beale G, Edmondson RJ, Curtin NJ (2011) Identification and evaluation of a potent novel ATR inhibitor, NU6027, in breast and ovarian cancer cell lines. Br J Cancer 105(3):372–381

Pires IM, Olcina MM, Anbalagan S, Pollard JR, Reaper PM, Charlton PA, McKenna WG, Hammond EM (2012) Targeting radiation-resistant hypoxic tumour cells through ATR inhibition. Br J Cancer 107(2):291–299

Pollard J, Reaper P, Peek A, Hughes S, Gladwell S, Jones J, Chiu P, Wood M, Tolman C, Johnson M, Littlewood P, Penney M, McDermott K, Hare B, Fields SZ, Asmal M, O'Carrigan B, Yap TA (2016a) Defining optimal dose schedules for ATR inhibitors in combination with DNA damaging drugs: informing clinical studies of VX-970, the first-in-class ATR inhibitor. Cancer Res 76(14 Suppl):Abstract nr 3717

Pollard J, Reaper P, Peek A, Hughes S, Dheja H, Cummings S, Larbi K, Penney M, Sullivan J, Takemoto D, Defranco C (2016b) Pre-clinical combinations of ATR and PARP inhibitors: defining target patient populations and dose schedule. Cancer Res 76(14 Suppl):Abstract nr 3711

Prevo R, Fokas E, Reaper PM, Charlton PA, Pollard JR, McKenna WG, Muschel RJ, Brunner TB (2012) The novel ATR inhibitor VE-821 increases sensitivity of pancreatic cancer cells to radiation and chemotherapy. Cancer Biol Ther 13(11):1072–1081

Reaper PM, Griffiths MR, Long JM, Charrier JD, Maccormick S, Charlton PA, Golec JM, Pollard JR (2011) Selective killing of ATM- or p53-deficient cancer cells through inhibition of ATR. Nat Chem Biol 7(7):428–430

Ringborg U, Bergqvist D, Brorsson B, Cavallin-Ståhl E, Ceberg J, Einhorn N, Frödin JE, Järhult J, Lamnevik G, Lindholm C, Littbrand B, Norlund A, Nylén U, Rosén M, Svensson H, Möller TR (2003) The Swedish Council on Technology Assessment in Health Care (SBU) systematic overview of radiotherapy for cancer including a prospective survey of radiotherapy practice in Sweden 2001 — summary and conclusions. Acta Oncol 42:357–365

Ruzankina Y, Pinzon-Guzman C, Asare A, Ong T, Pontano L, Cotsarelis G, Zediak VP, Velez M, Bhandoola A, Deletion BEJ (2007) of the developmentally essential gene ATR in adult mice leads to age-related phenotypes and stem cell loss. Cell Stem Cell 1:113–126

Sangster-Guity N, Conrad BH, Papadopoulos N, Bunz F (2011) ATR mediates cisplatin resistance in a p53 genotype-specific manner. Oncogene 30(22):2526–2533

Sanjiv K, Hagenkort A, Calderón-Montaño JM, Koolmeister T, Reaper PM, Mortusewicz O, Jacques SA, Kuiper RV, Schultz N, Scobie M, Charlton PA, Pollard JR, Berglund UW, Altun M, Helleday T (2016) Cancer-specific synthetic lethality between ATR and CHK1 kinase activities. Cell Rep 14(2):298–309

Sarkaria JN, Busby EC, Tibbetts RS, Roos P, Taya Y, Karnitz LM, Abraham RT (1999) Inhibition of ATM and ATR kinase activities by the radiosensitizing agent, caffeine. Cancer Res 59(17):4375–4382

Schaffner C, Stilgenbauer S, Rappold GA, Döhner H, Lichter P, Somatic ATM (1999) mutations indicate a pathogenic role of ATM in B-cell chronic lymphocytic leukemia. Blood 94(2):748–753

Schoppy DW, Ragland RL, Gilad O, Shastri N, Peters AA, Murga M et al (2012) Oncogenic stress sensitizes murine cancers to hypomorphic suppression of ATR. J Clin Invest 122:241–252

Schwab RA, Blackford AN, Niedzwiedz W (2010) ATR activation and replication fork restart are defective in FANCM-deficient cells. EMBO J 29(4):806–818

Shiotani B, Zou L (2009) Single-stranded DNA orchestrates an ATM-to-ATR switch at DNA breaks. Mol Cell 33(5):547–558

Sibghatullah HI, Carlton W, Sancar A (1989) Human nucleotide excision repair in vitro: repair of pyrimidine dimers, psoralen and cisplatin adducts by HeLa cell-free extract. Nucleic Acids Res 17(12):4471–4484

Singh TR, Ali AM, Paramasivam M, Pradhan A, Wahengbam K, Seidman MM, Meetei AR (2013) ATR-dependent phosphorylation of FANCM at serine 1045 is essential for FANCM functions. Cancer Res 73(14):4300–4310

Sorensen CS, Syljuasen RG (2012) Safeguarding genome integrity: the checkpoint kinases ATR, CHK1 and WEE1 restrain CDK activity during normal DNA replication. Nucleic Acids Res 40(2):477–486

Sorensen CS, Syljuasen RG, Falck J, Schroeder T, Ronnstrand L, Khanna KK, Zhou BB, Bartek J, Lukas J (2003) CHK1 regulates the S phase checkpoint by coupling the physiological turnover and ionizing radiation-induced accelerated proteolysis of Cdc25A. Cancer Cell 3(3):247–258

Sorensen CS, Syljuasen RG, Lukas J, Bartek J (2004) ATR, Claspin and the Rad9-Rad1-Hus1 complex regulate CHK1 and Cdc25A in the absence of DNA damage. Cell Cycle 3(7):941–945

Storz P (2005) Reactive oxygen species in tumor progression. Front Biosci 10:1881–1896

Sugimura K, Takebayashi S, Taguchi H, Takeda S, Okumura K (2008) PARP-1 ensures regulation of replication fork progression by homologous recombination on damaged DNA. J Cell Biol 183(7):1203–1212

Sultana R, Abdel-Fatah T, Perry C, Moseley P, Albarakti N, Mohan V, Seedhouse C, Chan S, Madhusudan S (2013) Ataxia telangiectasia mutated and Rad3 related (ATR) protein kinase inhibition is synthetically lethal in XRCC1 deficient ovarian cancer cells. PLoS One 8(2):e57098

Symington LS, Gautier J (2011) Double-strand break end resection and repair pathway choice. Annu Rev Genet 45:247–271

Taylor EM, Lindsay HD (2016) DNA replication stress and cancer: cause or cure? Future Oncol 12:221–237

Teng PN, Bateman NW, Darcy KM, Hamilton CA, Maxwell GL, Bakkenist CJ, Conrads TP (2015) Pharmacologic inhibition of ATR and ATM offers clinically important distinctions to enhancing platinum or radiation response in ovarian, endometrial, and cervical cancer cells. Gynecol Oncol 136(3):554–561

The Cancer Genome Atlas Research Network (2011) Integrated genomic analyses of ovarian carcinoma. Nature 474:609–615

Toledo LI, Murga M, Zur R, Soria R, Rodriguez A, Martinez S, Oyarzabal J, Pastor J, Bischoff JR, Fernandez-Capetillo O (2011) A cell-based screen identifies ATR inhibitors with synthetic lethal properties for cancer-associated mutations. Nat Struct Mol Biol 18(6):721–727

Toledo LI, Altmeyer M, Rask MB, Lukas C, Larsen DH, Povlsen LK, Bekker-Jensen S, Mailand N, Bartek J, Lukas J (2013) ATR prohibits replication catastrophe by preventing global exhaustion of RPA. Cell 155(5):1088–1103

Tomida J, Itaya A, Shigechi T, Unno J, Uchida E, Ikura M, Masuda Y, Matsuda S, Adachi J, Kobayashi M, Meetei AR, Maehara Y, Yamamoto K, Kamiya K, Matsuura A, Matsuda T, Ikura T, Ishiai M, Takata M (2013) A novel interplay between the Fanconi anemia core complex and ATR-ATRIP kinase during DNA cross-link repair. Nucleic Acids Res 41(14):6930–6941

Tutt A, Ellis P, Kilburn L, Gilett C, Pinder S, Abraham J, Barrett S, Barrett-Lee P, Chan S, Cheang M, Fox L, Grigoriadis A, Harper-Wynne C, Hatton M, Kernaghan S, Owen J, Parker P, Rahman N, Roylance R, Smith I, Thompson R, Tovey H, Wardley A, Wilson G, Harries M, Bliss J (2015) The TNT trial: a randomized phase III trial of carboplatin (C) compared with docetaxel (D) for patients with metastatic or recurrent locally advanced triple negative or BRCA1/2 breast cancer (CRUK/07/012). Cancer Res 75(9 Suppl):Abstract nr S3-01

Unsal-Kacmaz K, Sancar A (2004) Quaternary structure of ATR and effects of ATRIP and replication protein A on its DNA binding and kinase activities. Mol Cell Biol 24(3):1292–1300

Usanova S, Piée-Staffa A, Sied U, Thomale J, Schneider A, Kaina B, Köberle B (2010) Cisplatin sensitivity of testis tumour cells is due to deficiency in interstrand-crosslink repair and low ERCC1-XPF expression. Mol Cancer 9:248

Vendetti FP, Lau A, Schamus S, Conrads TP, O'Connor MJ, Bakkenist CJ (2015) The orally active and bioavailable ATR kinase inhibitor AZD6738 potentiates the anti-tumor effects of cisplatin to resolve ATM-deficient non-small cell lung cancer in vivo. Oncotarget 6(42):44289–44305

Wagner JM, Karnitz LM (2009) Cisplatin-induced DNA damage activates replication checkpoint signaling components that differentially affect tumour cell survival. Mol Pharmacol 76(1):208–214

Wallace SS, Murphy DL, Sweasy JB (2012) Base excision repair and cancer. Cancer Lett 327(1-2):73–89

Wang Y, Qin J (2003) MSH2 and ATR form a signaling module and regulate two branches of the damage response to DNA methylation. Proc Natl Acad Sci U S A 100(26):15387–15392

Wang H, Wang H, Powell SN, Iliakis G, Wang Y (2004) ATR affecting cell radiosensitivity is dependent on homologous recombination repair but independent of nonhomologous end joining. Cancer Res 64(19):7139–7143

Weber AM, Drobnitzky N, Devery AM, Bokobza SM, Adams RA, Maughan TS, Ryan AJ (2016) Phenotypic consequences of somatic mutations in the ataxia-telangiectasia mutated gene in non-small cell lung cancer. Oncotarget 7(38):60807. https://doi.org/10.18632/oncotarget.11845

Wilsker D, Bunz F (2007) Loss of ataxia telangiectasia mutated- and Rad3-related function potentiates the effects of chemotherapeutic drugs on cancer cell survival. Mol Cancer Ther 6(4):1406–1413

Wilsker D, Chung JH, Pradilla I, Petermann E, Helleday T, Bunz F (2012) Targeted mutations in the ATR pathway define agent-specific requirements for cancer cell growth and survival. Mol Cancer Ther 11(1):98–107

Wiseman H, Halliwell B (1996) Damage to DNA by reactive oxygen and nitrogen species: role in inflammatory disease and progression to cancer. Biochem J 313(Pt 1):17–29

Wright JA, Keegan KS, Herendeen DR, Bentley NJ, Carr AM, Hoekstra MF, Concannon P (1998) Protein kinase mutants of human ATR increase sensitivity to UV and ionizing radiation and abrogate cell cycle checkpoint control. Proc Natl Acad Sci U S A 95(13):7445–7450

Xiao Z, Chen Z, Gunasekera AH, Sowin TJ, Rosenberg SH, Fesik S, Zhang H (2003) CHK1 mediates S and G2 arrests through Cdc25A degradation in response to DNA-damaging agents. J Biol Chem 278(24):21767–21773

Yamane K, Taylor K, Kinsella TJ (2004) Mismatch repair-mediated G2/M arrest by 6-thioguanine involves the ATR-CHK1 pathway. Biochem Biophys Res Commun 318(1):297–302

Yang XH, Shiotani B, Classon M, Zou L (2008) Chk1 and Claspin potentiate PCNA ubiquitination. Genes Dev 22(9):1147–1152

Zhao H, Piwnica-Worms H (2001) ATR-mediated checkpoint pathways regulate phosphorylation and activation of human CHK1. Mol Cell Biol 21(13):4129–4139

Zou L, Elledge SJ (2003) Sensing DNA damage through ATRIP recognition of RPA-ssDNA complexes. Science 300(5625):1542–1548

Chapter 5
Targeting ATR for Cancer Therapy: ATR-Targeted Drug Candidates

Magnus T. Dillon and Kevin J. Harrington

Abstract ATR inhibitors are a new class of anti-cancer compounds reaching early phase clinical trials. They are predicted to have anti-cancer activity as monotherapy, and in combination with DNA damaging chemotherapies and ionizing radiation. We outline the clinical trials in progress using the current clinical candidates VX-970 (M6620) and AZD6738, discuss potential biomarkers for this class of drug and consider future avenues for development of ATR inhibitors.

Keywords Cell cycle checkpoint · ATR inhibitor · Radiosensitization · Chemosensitization

5.1 Background

Targeting cell cycle checkpoints has been considered to be an attractive approach for cancer therapy for some time (Dillon et al. 2014). The knowledge that most tumour cells lack a functional G1 checkpoint led to the hypothesis that they are more heavily reliant on the remaining S and G2/M checkpoints for appropriate cell cycle arrest and DNA repair. Following on from this observation, it is reasonable to suppose that, in combination with DNA damaging chemotherapy or ionizing radiation, pharmacological inhibition of the remaining S and G2/M checkpoints will result in uncontrolled cell division without time for DNA repair. As a result, cells will subsequently suffer cell death by mitotic catastrophe or other mechanisms. Inhibition of the ATR-CHK1 axis may also prevent the critical actions of these kinases in cell division and DNA repair: stabilizing stalled replication forks, regulating the firing of replication origins, and directly promoting the repair of DNA breaks by homologous recombination which may result in lethality in cancer cells

M. T. Dillon · K. J. Harrington (✉)
The Institute of Cancer Research, London, UK

The Royal Marsden NHS Foundation Trust, London, UK

© Springer International Publishing AG, part of Springer Nature 2018
J. Pollard, N. Curtin (eds.), *Targeting the DNA Damage Response for Anti-Cancer Therapy*, Cancer Drug Discovery and Development, https://doi.org/10.1007/978-3-319-75836-7_5

with high levels of replication stress (either in the context of single-agent therapy or in combination with DNA-damaging agents), or in combination with other small molecule inhibitors of DNA repair. Hence, targeting S and G2/M checkpoint kinases can be viewed as an extremely promising anti-cancer strategy and one that carries with it a high degree of tumour selectivity.

CHK1 was the first clinically targeted element of this pathway; the first generation of CHK1 inhibitors were not developed further due to toxicity, but showed evidence of target inhibition (Perez et al. 2006; Fracasso et al. 2011). The development of ATR inhibitors has been slower, but a number of agents have been developed (Table 5.1) and there are currently two compounds in early phase clinical

Table 5.1 ATR inhibitors and their current status

Compound	Pre-clinical evidence	Current clinical status
Caffeine (Powell et al. 1995; Sarkaria et al. 1999)	Radiosensitization via ATM and ATR inhibition	None—non-specific inhibitor
Schisandrin B (Nishida et al. 2009)	Sensitization to UV and abrogation of G2 checkpoint	None
VE-821 (Reaper et al. 2011; Pires et al. 2012; Prevo et al. 2012)	Growth inhibition, radiosensitization and chemosensitization, overcoming hypoxic radioresistance	None
NU6027 (Peasland et al. 2011)	Sensitization to hydroxyurea and genotoxic chemotherapy, but not mitotic poisons. Synthetic lethal with impaired SSB repair. Also inhibits CDK1/2, DNA-PK	None
VE-822/VX-970 (M6620) (Fokas et al. 2012; Hall et al. 2014; Josse et al. 2014)	Radiosensitization, chemosensitization in vivo	Phase 1 study [NCT02157792]: monotherapy and combination with cytotoxic chemotherapy: gemcitabine, gemcitabine-cisplatin, cisplatin, cisplatin-etoposide
VX-803 (M4344)	None published	Phase 1 study [NCT02278250]: monotherapy and combination with cytotoxic chemotherapy: carboplatin, gemcitabine, cisplatin
AZ20 (Jacq et al. 2012; Foote et al. 2013)	Growth inhibition in vivo, increased gamma-H2AX foci; synergy in combination with ATM inhibitor	None
AZD6738 (Guichard et al. 2013; Jones et al. 2013a)	Monotherapy growth inhibition in vivo in ATM deficient xenografts; chemosensitization and radiosensitization	Phase 1 monotherapy study [NCT01955668] (terminated) Phase 1 monotherapy and combination with radiation [NCT02223923] Phase 1 Combination with cytotoxic chemotherapy and olaparib [NCT02264678]

trials. ATR inhibitors have promise as anticancer agents as monotherapy and in combination with DNA-damaging agents. In this chapter, we will explore ATR inhibitors that are currently clinical candidates and will discuss active clinical trials. We will also consider future directions for ATR inhibition, including the importance of combination studies and the role of predictive and pharmacodynamic biomarkers.

A wealth of pre-clinical data shows that ATR inhibition and CHK1 inhibition have different effects. Although CHK1 is the best studied downstream target of ATR (Dai and Grant 2010), many other targets are also phosphorylated by this kinase. Hence, it is reasonable to expect a different spectrum of activities between ATR inhibition and CHK1 inhibition. ATM and ATR share similar substrate specificities, and it has been difficult definitively to identify substrates which rely more heavily on ATR modulation. However, there is also evidence that points towards differing specificities of ATM and ATR (Kim et al. 1999; Stokes et al. 2007). As well as protein site specificity, the differential phosphorylation of targets by ATR and ATM may depend upon spatial and contextual factors.

ATR and CHK1 also share some substrates. ATR inhibition may, therefore, result in a broader activity, due to more proximal pathway inhibition. Preclinical data have confirmed some differences between ATR and CHK1 inhibition for radiosensitization (Gamper et al. 2013), and sensitization to DNA damaging chemotherapy (Huntoon et al. 2013): where ATRi may sensitize more effectively than CHK1i to platinum (Wagner and Karnitz 2009; Huntoon et al. 2013), and CHK1i may be more effective than ATRi in sensitizing to microtubule inhibition (Zhang et al. 2009; Reaper et al. 2011). This is not, however, a consistent finding (Huntoon et al. 2013).

5.2 Current Clinical Candidates

5.2.1 VX-970 (M6620)

VX-970 (M6620 Merck KGaA) (Hall et al. 2014; Josse et al. 2014), also known as VE-822, is an aminopyrazine closely related to the ATR inhibitor VE-821(Charrier et al. 2011). VE-821 has an extensive pre-clinical data package showing sensitization to DNA-damaging chemotherapy (Reaper et al. 2011) and radiotherapy (Prevo et al. 2012), and radiosensitization under hypoxic conditions (Pires et al. 2012). VX-970 (M6620) has improved pharmacokinetic properties and potency compared with VE-821, and preclinical data with this compound have also demonstrated chemosensitzation and radiosensitization of tumour cell lines and xenograft models, sparing normal cell lines (Fokas et al. 2012; Hall et al. 2014).

Lung tumour cell lines were sensitized to cisplatin, oxaliplatin, gemcitabine, etoposide and SN38. In addition, patient-derived xenografts demonstrated effective growth inhibition in combination with cisplatin, compared with either single-agent therapy (Hall et al. 2014). The authors felt that lung cancer was an attractive target for this combination because there are high levels of p53 loss and frequent oncogene activation, resulting in increased levels of replication stress.

5.2.1.1 NCT02157792: First-in-Human Study of VX-970 (M6620) in Combination with Cytotoxic Chemotherapy

This phase 1 study tested VX-970 (M6620) monotherapy and in combination with cytotoxic chemotherapy in advanced cancers. In the monotherapy part of the study, 11 patients were treated in dose-escalation, with weekly administration; no dose-limiting toxicity was encountered and one patient with colorectal cancer with ATM loss had a durable complete response, with four further patients experiencing stable disease. The recommended phase 2 dose of VX-970 (M6620) monotherapy is 240 mg/m^2 weekly. Combination with carboplatin at this dose (given as carboplatin at an area under the plasma concentration-time curve of 5 (AUC5) day 1, VX-970 (M6620) day 2 and 9 of a 21-day cycle), required carboplatin dose delay or reduction in 3/3 patients due to haematological toxicity; dose-limiting toxicities were febrile neutropenia and hypersensitivity. The recommended phase 2 dose in combination with carboplatin is 90 mg/m^2. This combination yielded one durable partial response in a patient with germline BRCA1 mutation and ovarian cancer resistant to platinum and PARP inhibition. VX-970 (M6620) pharmacokinetics were dose-proportional with no interaction with carboplatin and drug-on-target activity was demonstrated by reduction of phospho-CHK1 on paired tumour biopsies (O'Carrigan et al. 2016). A separate part of the study treated 50 patients with gemcitabine (M6620) (day 1 and 8 of a 21-day cycle) in combination with VX-970 (M6620) (day 2, 9, 16). Dose-limiting toxicities were elevated liver transaminases (n = 4) and thrombocytopenia (n = 1). Four patients had partial responses and a further two had prolonged stable disease. The recommended phase 2 dose is VX-970 (M6620) 210 mg/m^2 with gemcitabine 1000 mg/m^2 (Plummer et al. 2016).

5.2.2 AZD6738

The morpholino-pyrimidine, AZD6738 (AstraZeneca) (Guichard et al. 2013; Jones et al. 2013a), is an orally bioavailable ATR inhibitor and is currently under evaluation in a number of early phase clinical trials. Data using the predecessor compound AZ20 showed monotherapy activity in xenograft models (Jacq et al. 2012; Foote et al. 2013). Published data that report on AZD6738 have shown single-agent activity across a variety of cell lines, which appears to be enhanced in cells with ATM pathway deficiencies (Vendetti et al. 2015; Kwok et al. 2016; Min et al. 2017). In addition, synergy has been reported with combinations of AZD6738 and gemcitabine, cisplatin (Vendetti et al. 2015) or radiation (Dillon et al. 2017a) in cell lines and in xenograft models (Guichard et al. 2013). Preclinical studies have shown evidence of gamma-H2AX focus formation in normal bone marrow and gut epithelium, which is transient compared with the persistent increase in foci that is seen in tumour tissue. This observation suggests the possibility of on-target normal tissue toxicities in these organs, but also provides hope that a therapeutic window will exist that will allow this agent to be used safely and effectively in the clinic. Published abstracts and clinical trial information have tended to focus on ATM-deficient tumours (see below) in the monotherapy context, since these have proven to be more sensitive to ATR inhibition in preclinical models.

5.2.2.1 NCT01955668: AZD6738 in 11q-Deleted Chronic Lymphocytic Leukaemia

The first-in-man study of AZD6738 focused on ATM-deficient chronic lymphocytic leukaemia (CLL). Loss of the 11q.23 locus (containing the ATM gene) is a relatively common chromosomal aberration in a number of haematological malignancies, including CLL. Therefore, enrichment for 11q deletion (by FISH) enriches for a population that is deficient in at least one allele of ATM. In CLL, 10–20% of patients have 11q deletion at diagnosis (Byrd et al. 2006) and an estimated 25% have ATM alteration, including deletion and mutation (Guarini et al. 2012). This is associated with poorer survival (Dohner et al. 2000) and more rapid disease progression (Dohner et al. 1997). Mutation of the remaining allele of ATM (Schaffner et al. 1999) is a frequent event at relapse and is associated with worse survival and resistance to therapy (Austen et al. 2007; Rossi and Gaidano 2012; Skowronska et al. 2012). In vitro, ATM mutations in CLL cells resulted in an impaired DNA-damage response (DDR). Interestingly, however, those 11q-deleted CLL cells with a remaining wild-type allele had a preserved DDR (Stankovic et al. 2002; Austen et al. 2005).

Unfortunately, despite the excellent preclinical and clinical rationale for this study, it was terminated early due to the changing treatment landscape in B cell malignancies. Given the preclinical evidence of increased sensitivity to ATR inhibitors in tumours deficient in ATM, it will be interesting to see if loss of 11q can be used as a predictive biomarker for ATR inhibition in other tumour types. This matter is discussed further below.

5.2.2.2 PATRIOT (NCT02223923): AZD6738 Monotherapy and in Combination with Palliative Radiotherapy in Advanced Solid Tumours

The PATRIOT study is a phase 1 trial of AZD6738 in advanced solid tumours (Fig. 5.1). It is a complex three-part study (Dillon et al. 2016) that will allow investigators to assess single-agent AZD6738 and also to combine it with palliative radiotherapy. In the initial part of the trial (part A), single-agent AZD6738 was dose-escalated in a standard phase 1 3 + 3 design with safety as the primary endpoint. In addition, a number of exploratory investigations were performed, including analysis of tumour and surrogate normal tissues for drug-on-target effects (loss of CHK1 phosphorylation, gamma-H2AX and Rad51 foci, see below). The maximum tolerated dose (MTD) was 160 mg BID, dose-limiting toxicities were haematological (thrombocytopenia, n = 3; pancytopenia, n = 1) and one episode of elevated amylase, pharmacokinetics were dose-proportional and there was preliminary

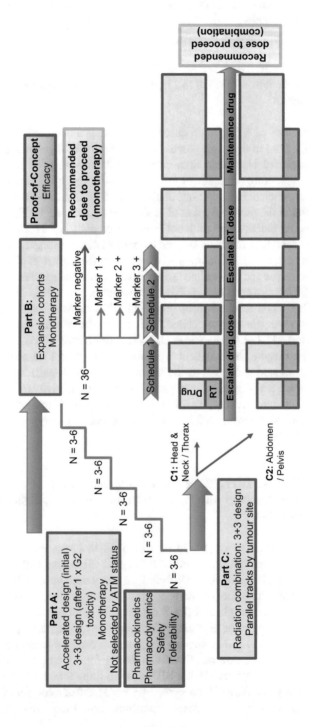

Fig. 5.1 Design of the PATRIOT study

evidence of target engagement (Dillon et al. 2017b). There was one partial response and a number of durable cases of stabilization of disease. Subsequently, in part B, expansion cohorts are being recruited at MTD that has been defined in part A, in an effort to study the value of different schedules of the drug and the possibility of using biomarkers to predict response to ATR inhibition. The final part C of the study is combining AZD6738 with palliative radiation therapy.

Overall, the objectives of this study are to define a suitable monotherapy dose and schedule, and to find a dose and schedule which is tolerable in combination with radiotherapy as a prelude to later-phase studies in each of these contexts.

During the radiation combination part of this study (part C), participants in whom a palliative course of radiotherapy is appropriate will also be treated with AZD6738. The course of radiation will be delivered using the 2 Gy fraction size that is typically used in radical radiotherapy, as opposed to 3, 4 or 5 Gy per fraction as typically used in short-course palliative treatment. In the initial stages of part C, a radiation dose of 20 Gy in 10 fractions will be used, giving a slightly lower biologically-effective dose than the 20 Gy in 5 fractions typically prescribed in this situation. The dose of AZD6738 will be escalated and, if this is tolerated, the radiation dose will be escalated to 30 Gy in 15 fractions, giving a biologically-effective dose comparable to, or slightly greater than, the standard palliative radiation dose. In addition, in order to take account of the fact that radiation-drug toxicities may vary depending on the site in the body which is being treated, parallel tracks in part C will evaluate patients with tumour sites above and below the diaphragm. If possible, accessible tumours and skin within the radiation field will be biopsied at baseline, prior to fraction 1 and prior to fraction 2. These will be analysed for gamma-H2AX (Olive 2011) and Rad51 foci to compare DNA damage and repair dynamics in normal and tumour tissues after radiation and ATR inhibition.

Combining novel agents with radiation presents a specific set of challenges due to the nature of clinical radiotherapy (Harrington et al. 2011). First, toxicity may be acute or chronic, and levels of acute toxicity do not necessarily predict long-term toxicities. Hence, any study of a novel radiosensitizer must include some element of long-term follow-up where possible. Second, the long-term aim for radiosensitization must be to develop drugs that can be used in the radical setting in order to improve tumour control rates as part of a radical therapeutic regimen. However, most tumours which are treated with radiation as a primary therapy are better controlled with concomitant platin-based chemoradiation (e.g. head and neck, lung and cervical cancers), and total radiation doses are usually of the order of 60–70 Gy over 5–7 weeks.

This presents a number of specific challenges when attempting to combine with novel agents (such as modifiers of DDR). The prolonged course of treatment may require the new agent to be administered for up to 7 weeks. Accurate knowledge of pharmacokinetics is required in order to decide when the agent should be started and stopped in relation to radiotherapy, and, in the case of continuously dosed drugs, whether weekend breaks or other intermittent schedules are possible. The combination of radiation with concomitant chemotherapy will often mean treatment is already at the limit of toxicity for many patients. Therefore, adding in a novel agent with potentially overlapping toxicities may mean that the new combination regimen becomes intolerable. In the context of a radical treatment, any fractions of radiation that are missed or any prolonged delays in treatment delivery due to toxicity will have a real effect in reducing cure rates. So, trials must be designed to avoid this at all costs. This may be achieved by cautious dose escalation of the novel agent, by exploiting window-of-opportunity trial designs, or by reducing the dose of concomitant therapies. An alternative method is that used in the PATRIOT study, where palliative radiation is used as a starting point for the combination therapy. Palliative radiotherapy is delivered at lower doses than radical therapy and the consequences of missed doses are less grave. A next step could also be using these agents in situations where either high-dose palliative radiotherapy is used alone, or where radical-dose radiotherapy is used without concomitant chemotherapy, due to patient comorbidities. However, in the context of an early phase study, it is unlikely that participants who are excluded from standard treatment on the basis of comorbidity will be well enough to enter these studies. Hence, it is likely that there will always be some inevitable risk when translating these new agents to combination with radical radiotherapy regimens.

5.2.2.3   NCT02264678: AZD6738 in Combination with Carboplatin or Olaparib

Combination with platinum is another attractive approach for combination studies with ATR inhibition, given the preclinical data indicating sensitization to these agents. The first part of this study is dose-escalating AZD6738 in combination with carboplatin AUC5, in order to establish the MTD and optimal schedule of the ATR inhibitor/carboplatin combination. This will then be tested in patients with platinum-resistant disease (ovarian cancer) or ATM-deficient disease (lung adenocarcinoma).

A second module of this study is investigating combination of AZD6738 and the PARP inhibitor olaparib. Again, this combination has demonstrated efficacy in preclinical studies (Peasland et al. 2011). Initially, there will be a dose-optimisation phase in combination with olaparib, followed by expansion to treat patients with advanced gastric and gastro-oesophageal cancers with low ATM expression. Patients will be divided into those who have had no previous PARP inhibitor treatment and those who have previously received a PARP inhibitor.

The modular design of this study enables the investigators to add further novel anti-cancer agents (such as immunotherapies) in combination with AZD6738 on the basis of emerging pre-clinical and clinical data.

5.3   Biomarkers

5.3.1   Pharmacodynamic Biomarkers for ATRi

ATR phosphorylates CHK1. While an autophosphorylation site (T1989) on ATR has been found to be a marker of activated ATR (Nam et al. 2011), inhibition of CHK1 phosphorylation at the ATR-specific serine 345 has been established as a pharmacodynamic biomarker for ATR inhibition in cell line and in vivo studies. Other serine residues on CHK1 have been investigated (Zhao and Piwnica-Worms 2001), including S317, but there may be greater specificity of the effect of ATR on S345 (Peasland et al. 2011). This direct marker of ATR function is useful in tissues where the ATR-CHK1 axis is activated at baseline (tumours with activated pathway) or when chemotherapy- or radiation-induced DNA damage causes activation of ATR-CHK1—since abrogation of this effect can be demonstrated with ATR inhibition. However, in the monotherapy setting, it is entirely possible that a signal may not be found in the absence of (i) exogenous DNA damage or (ii) high basal levels of replication stress. Such considerations may lead to problems detecting monotherapy drug-on-target effects, particularly in normal tissues (where high basal levels of replication are very unlikely).

For example, peripheral blood mononuclear cells (PBMC) are frequently used for pharmacodynamic (PD) sampling, but ATR inhibition may not result in any signal unless the PBMC are treated *ex vivo* with ultraviolet light (UV), hydroxyurea or the UV-mimetic 4-nitroquinoline 1-oxide (4NQO) (Chen et al. 2015). This is also likely to be the case in other normal tissues commonly used for PD analyses, such as hair follicles and skin biopsies. In tumour samples, it is more likely that there will be basal activation of the ATR-CHK1 axis, but repeated tumour sampling for PD is not always safe or practicable.

Because of these limitations, other PD biomarkers may be useful, even though they are likely to be less specific. Increased gamma-H2AX foci (Bonner et al. 2008) may be seen in tumour tissue as a result of increased double-strand breaks subsequent to ATR inhibition. One would expect that there would be less modulation in gamma-H2AX in normal tissues, especially if the agent is tumour-selective. In combination with DNA damaging agents, one may expect persistence and delayed resolution of gamma-H2AX foci after administration of the DNA-damaging agent. It is also likely that such changes would be accompanied by reduced homologous recombination, as shown by decreased formation of Rad51 foci.

The evaluation of circulating tumour cells (CTCs) as a biomarker is an area of growing interest (Yap et al. 2014). Enumeration of CTCs has proven useful in a number of tumour types, and there is also the possibility of characterizing CTCs in terms of their protein expression. Measurement of pCHK1 in CTCs has not been described, but it may be possible to use gamma-H2AX as an indirect biomarker in clinical studies of ATR inhibition. However, the utility of this potential biomarker is likely to be limited by a number of factors specific to CTCs: the possibility of differences between CTCs that are represented in the circulation and the tumour cells that comprise solid tumour masses; significant heterogeneity between individual CTCs; and the possibility that CTCs will be exposed to higher drug concentrations than solid tumour masses. All of these considerations may limit the relevance of CTCs for use in PD studies. Additionally, CTCs may not be abundant in all malignancies.

5.3.2   Predictive Biomarkers for ATR Inhibitors

There is considerable uncertainty regarding the selection of predictive markers for response to ATR inhibition. Preclinical studies have attempted to find a somatic tumour defect which would prove 'synthetically lethal' in combination with ATR inhibition, and a number of candidates have been identified which seem to sensitise to ATR inhibition in vitro (Fig. 5.2). However, there does not seem to be an overarching rule for sensitization, potentially due to the pleiotropic effect ATR has on

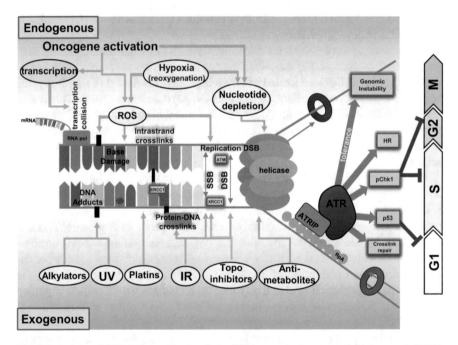

Fig. 5.2 Actions of ATR at the replication fork. ATR is recruited to sites of single-stranded DNA (ssDNA) coated in RpA (replication protein A). These are exposed during replication stress that can occur due to DNA lesions which slow the DNA replication apparatus, such as DNA adducts, base damage, intrastrand crosslinks, protein-DNA complexes and crosslinks, single-strand (SSB) and double-strand breaks (DSB). Endogenous lesions, increased by oncogene activation, include increased protein transcription causing replication-transcription collisions and reduced pools of nucleotides that can slow down DNA replication. Hypoxia slows replication forks due to depletion of cellular deoxyribonucleotides (Scanlon and Glazer 2015) and reoxygenation results in production of reactive oxygen species (ROS), causing base damage and single-strand lesions, which can degenerate into DSB during replication. Cancer cells have a pro-oxidant state resulting in endogenous ROS production (Manda et al. 2015). Exogenous DNA damage due to chemotherapy or radiotherapy will also cause replication stress. Activated ATR serves to stabilise the replication fork, control the firing of DNA replication origins, activate cell cycle checkpoints and DNA repair pathways (including homologous recombination, HR; and crosslink repair). An activated DNA repair pathway is important for cellular tolerance to genomic instability. Processes and proteins outlined in red represent potential biomarkers for sensitivity to ATR inhibitors. *UV* Ultraviolet, *IR* ionizing radiation, *ATM* ataxia-telangiectasia mutated, *ERCC1* excision repair cross-complementation group 1, *XRCC1* X-ray repair cross-complementing protein 1, *ATRIP* ATR interacting protein

cellular processes. As noted above, some of these strategies are being prospectively explored in ongoing clinical trials. It will also be important to bear in mind that there may be differences between markers of sensitivity to monotherapy ATR inhibition and its combination with DNA-damaging agents.

5.3.2.1 ATM Loss

Apart from ATR, ATM is the other proximal DDR kinase. It is activated by DSBs and signals to a wide variety of cellular components, including CHK2 and p53, to facilitate G1/S arrest, and, depending upon the level of DNA damage, activation of apoptotic, senescence or alternate cell death pathways.

ATM loss is a relatively frequent occurrence in a number of malignancies, including haematological (Stankovic et al. 1999), breast (Angele et al. 2000), head and neck (Bolt et al. 2005) and lung cancers (Ding et al. 2008). This occurs through a variety of mechanisms, including 11q23 deletion, promoter hypermethylation (Bai et al. 2004), loss-of-function mutation of which 80% are truncations that cause loss of protein expression (Lavin et al. 2004) and micro-RNA (miRNA)-mediated gene silencing (Hu et al. 2010). ATM loss has also been associated with poorer prognosis in some tumour types (Ai et al. 2004; Ding et al. 2008; Bueno et al. 2014; Lee et al. 2014).

ATM is lost in a variety of malignancies at varying rates. Exact rates depend upon the cohort being studied, but levels have been quoted above 25% in head and neck squamous cell cancers (Ai et al. 2004; Lim et al. 2012). Because of the multiple potential mechanisms of ATM loss, a biomarker needs to take all these into account. Expression of total protein as measured by immunohistochemistry (IHC) would take most mechanisms into account, but may miss expression of mutant protein which still contains the epitope that allows antibody recognition. Therefore, ultimately, a combination of methods may be better.

The potential use of ATM loss as a biomarker for response to ATR inhibition is predicated on the hypothesis that there is functional overlap and redundancy between these two kinases: in response to DNA damage, cells lacking ATM will rely more heavily on the function of ATR. In fact, direct evidential support for this notion is sparse, and the hypothesis will be tested by ongoing clinical trials. Nonetheless, given the current importance of this potential biomarker, the basis for its selection will be considered using existing lines of evidence.

(i) ATR as a 'back-up' DSB repair initiator. Typically, ATM is felt to be crucial for the response of cells to DSB. ATR has been shown to be activated following DSB, especially at ssDNA-dsDNA junctions, and this may rely on the ATM-dependent end-resection of DSBs by exonucleases, resulting in stretches of ATR-activating ssDNA coated with RPA (Jazayeri et al. 2006; Cimprich and Cortez 2008). However, there is also some evidence for ATM-independent activation of ATR by DSB. For example, ATR becomes activated (albeit slowly) in ataxia telangiectasia cells (which lack functional ATM), after ATM-independent end-resection (Shiloh 2003). Likewise, overexpression of ATR in ataxia telangiectasia cells (which lack ATM) restores their ability to stop DNA synthesis after ionizing radiation (Cliby et al. 1998).

(ii) Replication-associated DSBs will occur in the context of ATR inhibition and at least some of these will require the ATM pathway for stabilization and repair (Chanoux et al. 2009). Absence of this pathway will be likely to result in persistent DNA breaks which cannot be repaired.

(iii) ATM null cells are able to undergo G1/S arrest on ectopic expression of ATR (Toledo et al. 2008).

(iv) Genetic assessment of an outlier response to CHK1 inhibition revealed mutation in Rad50 (part of the ATM-activating MRN complex), and suggested that inhibition of signaling through both the ATM (via the Rad50 mutation) and ATR (via CHK1 inhibition by AZD7762) axes resulted in extreme sensitivity to irinotecan (Al-Ahmadie et al. 2014). This mutation appeared to be clonal, having occurred early in tumour development and, hence, this may have improved the response at all sites of disease.

(v) Preclinical data suggest that ATM-deficient cell lines and xenografts are more sensitive to ATR inhibition in combination with DNA damaging therapies: in combination with cisplatin, ATR inhibitors were synergistic in ATM knockdown, but not isogenic ATM wild-type, cells (Reaper et al. 2011). ATR inhibition increased cell death if there was combined ATM and p53 loss (Weber et al. 2013). In CLL cells, ATR inhibition resulted in ATM activation and ATM- or p53-deficient CLL cells were more sensitive to AZD6738 than their proficient counterparts. *In vivo*, patient-derived CLL xenografts had significantly lower tumour load after AZD6738 in cases with p53 deletion or mutation, or ATM deletion (Kwok et al. 2016). ATM-deficient non-small cell lung cancer (NSCLC) cell lines were sensitive to the combination of AZD6738 and cisplatin *in vitro* and *in vivo*, and knock-down of ATM sensitized a NSCLC cell line to ATR inhibition (Vendetti et al. 2015), this effect has also been noted in cell lines originating from other tumour types (Middleton et al. 2015; Min et al. 2017).

(vi) ATM is thought to be involved in homologous recombination (Morrison et al. 2000; Bolderson et al. 2004), so ATM-deficient cells have defective homologous recombination, which has been shown to sensitise to ATRi (see below).

A further issue with the use of ATM loss as a biomarker is the degree of ATM loss that is required. It is unclear whether heterozygosity of ATM has a significant effect on cellular function. It has been observed that ATM heterozygotes have a modest increase in breast cancer risk and that heterozygous cells have a modest increase in radiosensitivity. Likewise, ATM haploinsufficient mouse models have increased levels of carcinogen-induced tumours. As mentioned above, a subset of poorer-prognosis CLL have 11q deletion and even losing one allele has an effect on prognosis—it seems that this may be due to compound loss of one allele of a number of genes involved in the DDR at the same locus, since 11q deletion carries a poorer prognosis than monoallelic ATM mutation (Ouillette et al. 2010).

Hence, it seems likely that, in the absence of a dominant-negative effect inhibiting ATM dimerization, that complete ATM loss would be necessary to have a significant effect on cellular ATM functions during DSB signaling.

5.3.2.2 Replication Stress

Replication stress (RS) (Toledo et al. 2011a; Lecona and Fernandez-Capetillo 2014; Zeman and Cimprich 2014; Gaillard et al. 2015) can be defined as accumulation of ssDNA at the replication fork, for example due to uncoupling of the leading and lagging strands of the DNA replication machinery. The cell will encounter RS under normal circumstances, and the ATR-CHK1 pathway is one of the mechanisms that is used to circumvent this. As well as that generated by DNA-damaging therapy, cancer cells have increased levels of endogenous RS for a number of reasons:

(i) Oncogene activation (López-Contreras et al. 2012): This occurs through unclear mechanisms, possibly as a result of increased origin firing stimulated by activated oncogenes, depletion of nucleotides (Bester et al. 2011) or replication-transcription collisions (Ciccia and Elledge 2010).

(ii) Replication-transcription collisions: Cancer cells have higher levels of protein transcription and active replication. This results in an increased chance of the replication machinery colliding with the enzymes responsible for transcription of mRNA (Jones et al. 2013b).

(iii) DNA lesions: These can arise from products of cellular metabolism (including ROS) (Tanaka et al. 2006).

ATR or CHK1 loss is very rare in cancers, and upregulation is frequent, most likely because cells need to upregulate the RS response in order to tolerate the high levels of RS after oncogene activation (Lecona and Fernandez-Capetillo 2014). Upregulation of this axis in breast cancer is associated with a more aggressive phenotype (Abdel-Fatah et al. 2015), and increased levels of CHK1 protect against oncogene-induced RS (López-Contreras et al. 2012). Inhibition of this signaling pathway may, therefore, target a cancer-specific 'addiction' and represent a route to synthetic lethality of tumour cells.

In vitro, RS can be identified by direct examination of 5-bromo-2'-deoxyuridine (BrDU) incorporation into DNA, or by DNA fibre assays. However, there is no accepted test for RS in clinical samples. Possibilities would include examination for RPA foci, indicating exposed expanses of ssDNA, or to look for downstream phosphorylations by ATR, for example on CHK1 S345, or RPA S33. Gamma-H2AX may also increase under RS and at collapsed replication forks, which has been demonstrated in clinical trials of PARP inhibitors (Camidge et al. 2005; Fong et al. 2009). However, the levels of this can increase in multiple circumstances, with numerous types of DNA damage and during the process of apoptosis. Markers of proliferation or examination for oncogene activation (such as *RAS* (Gilad et al. 2010), *MYC* (Murga et al. 2011), cyclin E amplification +/− p53 inactivation (Toledo et al. 2011a, b)) may be useful as proxy measures for RS.

In the combination setting, RS is increased by conventional DNA-damaging therapies that can have activity in both tumour and normal tissues (see below). Successful clinical exploitation of ATR inhibition will rely on a therapeutic window due to DDR being more effective in the normal cells.

5.3.2.3 p53

Most cancer cells have a defective G1 cell cycle checkpoint. The most common reason for this is inactivation of p53. Loss of p53 allows promiscuous entry into S phase and, hence, one may expect cells with loss of functional p53 to have higher levels of RS and increased sensitivity to ATR inhibition. Additionally, in combination with DNA damage, they will rely more heavily on their remaining intra-S and G2/M checkpoints to arrest the cell cycle and allow DNA repair prior to ongoing division. The effect of p53 status on sensitivity to ATR inhibition is not clear. Some groups have noted increased sensitivity to ATRi in p53 mutant cells (Reaper et al. 2011). In mice, knockout of both ATR and p53 led to high levels of DNA damage in cells and this combination appeared to by synthetically lethal (Murga et al. 2009; Ruzankina et al. 2009). Prior to the development of selective ATR inhibitors, studies using caffeine as an ATR inhibitor showed synergy with loss of p53 function; however, it was clear that this sensitization also occurred with a number of other common mechanisms of G1 checkpoint loss including expression of human papillomavirus (HPV) E6 protein, cyclin D1, cyclin-dependent kinase 2 (CDK2), mouse double minute 2 homolog (mdm2), or cyclin E overexpression (Nghiem et al. 2001). Transforming cells with overexpression of cell cycle promoting oncogenes resulted in RS, addition of ATR inhibitors caused DNA damage and cell death, and this was enhanced in the presence of p53 dysfunction (Toledo et al. 2011a, b). Other studies have found that ATR inhibition seemed to radiosensitise cell lines regardless of p53 status (Pires et al. 2012), and that chemosensitization with cisplatin appeared to be greater in p53 functional cells, but sensitization to temozolomide was greater in p53 dysfunctional cells (Peasland et al. 2011). Furthermore, when using VX-970 (M6620) in an isogenic model with p53 short-hairpin RNA silencing, there was more effective sensitization to DNA damage in the p53 knockdown cells. On examining a panel of cell lines, no significant correlation was found between p53 mutational status and sensitization to DNA-damaging chemotherapy, although there was a trend towards sensitization of p53 defective cells to cisplatin (Hall et al. 2014). Taken together, these data indicate that loss of p53 may not be a reliable marker of sensitivity to ATR inhibition.

5.3.2.4 DNA Damage Response Defects

DSB Repair

Some evidence suggests loss of ATM pathway function may sensitise to ATR inhibition; this has been described above.

The effect of loss of components of the non-homologous end-joining pathway is more complex. Loss of Ku-80, the DNA-binding component, sensitized cells to ATRi, but cells expressing high levels of the catalytic subunit DNA-PKcs were hypersensitive to ATR inhibition, and correcting a DNA-PKcs defect in a cell line restored sensitivity to ATRi. This effect was thought to be due to increased inhibition of homologous recombination by ATRi in DNA-PKcs proficient cells—high levels of this protein may influence repair pathway choice towards NHEJ and effectively create a homologous recombination defect (Middleton et al. 2015).

SSB Repair

ATR inhibition has been shown to have a synthetic lethal interaction with inactivation of two components involved in SSB repair, PARP or XRCC1 (Peasland et al. 2011; Sultana et al. 2013; Middleton et al. 2015). Inhibition of SSB repair leads to these lesions degenerating into replication-associated DSBs at replication forks. This process activates ATR, which would normally activate replication fork stabilization and repair by HR. Loss of XRCC1 has also been shown to result in sensitivity to a variety of genotoxic agents (Caldecott 2003).

HR Deficiency

HR-deficient tumours are highly genomically unstable, with mechanisms to tolerate this to allow ongoing proliferation. These include loss of p53 and amplification of ATR or CHK1, which induce tolerance of chromosomal instability. Combining reduced HR capacity with inhibition of ATR or CHK1 has resulted in decreased clonogenic survival in vitro (Krajewska et al. 2015; Middleton et al. 2015).

Although germline mutation of BRCA1 and BRCA2 are commonly described sources of HR deficiency, tumours may have HR deficiency through a variety of mechanisms: numerous genes can be inactivated in various ways (Walsh 2015). There are a number of approaches to detection of HR deficiency regardless of mechanism and these are based on detecting the genomic aberrations resulting from loss of HR and reliance on alternative DNA repair pathways (Watkins et al. 2014).

Other DNA Repair Enzymes

ERCC1 (excision repair cross-complementation group 1) forms a complex with XPF (xeroderma pigmentosum, complementation group F) and functions in nucleotide-excision repair (NER), where it repairs bulky DNA adducts and inter-strand crosslinks. Silencing of ERCC1 and XPF (by small interfering RNA (siRNA)) sensitized to both ATR and CHK1 inhibition, creating S-phase arrest and increasing both focal and pan-nuclear gamma-H2AX staining, indicating RS and DNA damage (Mohni et al. 2014). Silencing other NER genes did not replicate this, indicating that the other functions of ERCC1-XPF may be responsible—including replication of fragile sites and repair of intra-strand crosslinks (Kirschner and Melton 2010). A further screen identified the loss of translesion DNA polymerase ζ as synergising with ATR inhibition when combined with cisplatin (Mohni et al. 2015). This polymerase also has functions in repair of intra-strand crosslinks, and may be important for the RS response (Bhat et al. 2013; Kotov et al. 2014).

ATR Pathway Defects

In the same synthetic lethality siRNA screen that identified the synergy between ATR inhibition and ERCC1-XPF deficiency, it was found that pre-existing deficiency in the ATR pathway sensitizes to further ATR inhibition (Mohni et al. 2014). Defects that were identified included RPA, ATRIP, CHK1 and ATR heterozygosity, amongst others.

5.3.2.5 Alternative Lengthening of Telomeres (ALT)

Overcoming replicative senescence is a hallmark of cancer (Hanahan and Weinberg 2011). Cancer cells generally achieve this by activating telomerase to maintain telomere length. More rarely, an alternative mechanism (alternative lengthening of telomeres, ALT) uses recombination to lengthen telomeres. Links between ATR and telomere function are becoming increasingly apparent in the literature (d'Adda di Fagagna et al. 2003; Bi et al. 2005; McNees et al. 2010; Pennarun et al. 2010; Thanasoula et al. 2012). In cells that use ALT as their principal mechanism of avoiding replicative senescence, RpA accumulates on telomeres, recruiting ATR-ATRIP. Frequently, ALT cells have lost function of ATRX (α-thalassaemia/mental retardation syndrome X-linked), which usually allows the release of RpA from telomeres. Hence, loss of ATRX may imply the use of ALT, although loss of ATRX is not sufficient to recapitulate reliance on ALT (Heaphy et al. 2011; Lovejoy et al. 2012). Cells using the ALT mechanism are selectively killed by ATR inhibition (Flynn et al. 2015). This raises the possibility that identification of cells that rely on ALT, through testing for loss of ATRX or other markers such as absence of telomerase upregulation, may select tumours sensitive to ATR inhibition.

5.3.2.6 Hypoxia

Interactions between the response to hypoxia-reoxygenation and the DNA damage response has led to interest in hypoxia as a predictor of response to ATR inhibition. Hypoxic conditions cause replication arrest, which activates ATR which, in turn, results in p53 phosphorylation (Hammond et al. 2002; Pires et al. 2010). Additionally, hypoxia-reoxygenation results in DNA damage through the formation of ROS and activation of ATM and ATR (Hammond et al. 2003). A number of DDR processes have been shown to be suppressed under hypoxic conditions (Hammond et al. 2007; Bristow and Hill 2008), including HR DNA repair. Reduction in the HR protein, Rad51, in hypoxic tumour areas can result in a 'conditional synthetic lethality' which has been demonstrated with PARP inhibitors: hypoxia results in replication fork stalling (Olcina et al. 2010), the role of PARP in stabilization of replication forks is demonstrated by the S-phase toxicity of PARP inhibition under hypoxic conditions (Chan et al. 2010). The fact that ATR is also crucial in maintaining replication fork stability may also indicate an effect under hypoxia. Hypoxia-activated

ATR and CHK1 phosphorylation is reduced by using the ATRi VE-821 (Pires et al. 2012). This leads to a corresponding decrease in replication speed and increase in markers of DNA damage, consistent with the hypothesis that ATR inhibition under hypoxic conditions would result in replication fork collapse and DNA break accumulation (Hammond et al. 2004). Hypoxia is a major determinant of radiation resistance (Bristow and Hill 2008), sensitizing the hypoxic fraction of cells to radiation may enable increased tumour control rates. There is some evidence that ATR inhibitors may achieve this: VE-821 sensitized hypoxic, radioresistant cells to radiation (Pires et al. 2012), as well as sensitizing pancreatic cancer cell lines to both radiation and gemcitabine under oxic and hypoxic conditions, with corresponding evidence of persistent DNA damage and reduced homologous recombination after irradiation (Prevo et al. 2012).

5.3.2.7 Upregulation of DDR Components

It has been established that increased therapy resistance in certain tumour cells is related to upregulation of components of the DNA damage response. For example, glioblastoma cancer stem cells demonstrate radioresistance and this is associated with both increased basal activation of DDR proteins and their increased phosphorylation and activation after radiation. This was associated with enhanced recovery from DNA damage, a phenomenon that could be reversed by inhibition of CHK1 and CHK2 (Bao et al. 2006). Additionally, ATR and CHK1 are frequently upregulated in tumours, particularly those with high levels of genomic instability (Krajewska et al. 2015) or RS (López-Contreras et al. 2012). This allows tumour cells to tolerate these conditions and continue proliferation without catastrophic effects.

5.4 Future Directions

5.4.1 Hazards of ATR Inhibtion

Concerns regarding off-target effects and tolerability of ATR inhibitors will be addressed by the ongoing phase 1 clinical trials. Previous clinical studies of earlier generations of CHK1 inhibitors were limited by the toxicities of these agents (Chen et al. 2012). Preclinical data have indicated that the current clinical candidate ATR inhibitors have high specificity for ATR with potencies against similar kinases (mTOR, PI3-kinase, DNA-PK and ATM) that are not significant at relevant doses (Foote et al. 2015).

One additional concern which will not be addressed by early phase studies in advanced cancer patients is the possibility of an effect of ATR in suppression of tumours at early stages in their development. It is known that the DDR (Halazonetis et al. 2008), and specifically ATR (Lopez-Contreras and Fernandez-Capetillo 2010), plays a role in tumour suppression. Engagement of the DDR after oncogene activation allows oncogene-induced senescence and, therefore, inactivation of the DDR promotes malignant transformation (Di Micco et al. 2006). Hence, 'pre-cancers' or neoplasia in early stages of development may be held in check and prevented from acquiring a malignant phenotype by an effective DDR (Bartek et al. 2007). Whether specific ATR inhibition will increase progression of these lesions or whether other redundant mechanisms may be capable of transcomplementing this function remains to be seen. Additionally, inhibition of ATR may increase genomic instability in normal proliferating cells (Park et al. 2015), with a risk of subsequent tumorigenesis. However, it is likely that normal cells will be able to overcome this effect through activation of their intact DNA repair mechanisms.

Investigation of these concerns in animal models has not been conclusive. Mice expressing hypomorphic ATR did not develop tumours (Murga et al. 2009), but ATR heterozygotes did have an increased propensity to tumour development (Brown and Baltimore 2000). Combination of ATR heterozygosity and mismatch repair defects (MLH1 homozygous loss) led to increased chromosomal instability and development of tumours in mice (Fang et al. 2004). K-ras activation led to stimulation of the ATR pathway, presumably as a normal protective response. However, ATR heterozygous mice developed increased neoplasia compared with ATR +/+ mice; further reduction of ATR levels resulted in synthetic lethality in the context of oncogene activation, suggesting that there may be a dose-related effect (Gilad et al. 2010). Importantly, humans with Seckel syndrome (hypomorphic ATR) have an increased risk of myelodysplasia, hypoplastic bone marrow (Chanan-Khan et al. 2003) and possibly myeloid leukaemia (Hayani et al. 1994), although propensity to solid tumour development has not been described (O'Driscoll et al. 2004).

5.4.2 Monotherapy

Using ATR inhibition as monotherapy depends upon the identification of predictive biomarkers. As outlined above, there are a number of possibilities for this. The presence of monotherapy responses in ongoing phase 1 clinical trials is encouraging (O'Carrigan et al. 2016; Dillon et al. 2017b), and these studies may provide further information regarding predictive markers of single-agent responses. However, in the absence of any accepted method to assess RS levels within tumours prior to starting treatment, this may prove difficult.

Notably, in the small amount of published data using the clinical candidate compounds, single agent responses in xenografts have been reported in abstracts using AZD6738 (Guichard et al. 2013). In vivo studies using VE-821 and VE-822 have been carried out in combination with radiation (Fokas et al. 2012) or chemotherapy (Hall et al. 2014; Josse et al. 2014), and the monotherapy arms of the study have not shown significant difference from controls. However, drug dosing in these cases was short-term during the course of DNA-damaging therapy, and no continuous-dosing in vivo experiments have been reported.

5.4.3 Combination with Genotoxic Chemotherapy

Most preclinical studies of ATRi have shown sensitization to DNA-damaging chemotherapy (Wilsker and Bunz 2007), such as antimetabolite therapy, topoisomerase inhibitors, platinum and alkylating agents, but not with antimicrotubule agents (Peasland et al. 2011). Clinical trials of these agents with ATRi have already started. In the absence of toxicity data from monotherapy studies of ATRi, it is difficult to make informed decisions regarding rational combination regimens in terms of their likely toxicities, but there are ample preclinical data suggesting that these combinations will be efficacious.

- Antimetabolites: gemcitabine, cytarabine, 5-fluorouracil (5-FU). These nucleoside analogues cause premature termination of replication and stalling of replication forks. They have been shown to activate the ATR-CHK1 axis and to synergise with ATR inhibition or loss (Prevo et al. 2012; Huntoon et al. 2013).
- Topoisomerase inhibitors have been combined with VX-970 (M6620) in vivo and shown synergy without additional toxicity (Josse et al. 2014). ATR was shown to be required for the G2 and S phase arrests after topoisomerase inhibitors (Cliby et al. 2002). Colony formation after exposure to SN-38 or camptothecin was reduced when ATR or CHK1 was downregulated, with minimal effect of downregulation of ATM or CHK2 (Flatten et al. 2005).
- Platinum induces DNA crosslinks which block replication. ATR seems to sensitize more to cisplatin than to oxaliplatin (Lewis et al. 2009; Hall et al. 2014). This sensitization is most likely due to the role of ATR in activation of the Fanconi anaemia pathway, which is critical for the repair of platinum-induced crosslinks (Wang 2007; Singh et al. 2013).
- Alkylating agents, such as temozolomide, cause cell death after the damaged DNA undergoes attempted repair by the mismatch repair system. This misrepair activates the ATR pathway (Caporali et al. 2004) and induces G2 arrest with subsequent apoptosis, mitotic catastrophe or senescence. Temozolomide has been shown to synergise with ATR inhibition (Peasland et al. 2011).

5.4.4 Combination with Other Targeted Agents

Combination of ATR and PARP inhibition has been shown to be synergistic in vitro in a number of studies (Peasland et al. 2011; Huntoon et al. 2013; Mohni et al. 2015). This may be due to single-strand breaks (caused by DNA replication in the presence of PARP inhibition) degenerating in to replicative lesions which would normally activate ATR for HR repair. Combining ATR and PARP inhibition results in persistent replication-induced double-strand breaks and cell death. Ongoing phase 1 studies of this combination will inform us further of the tumour selectivity of this combination.

Combination with ATR and CHK1 inhibitors has also been shown to be synergistic in preclinical models (Sanjiv et al. 2016), with an increase in DNA breaks, S-phase arrest and apoptosis with the combination therapy. CHK1 inhibition causes an increased firing of replication origins, causing replication stress and ATR activation which protects the stalled replication forks. Inhibition of ATR leads to collapse of these replication forks. This effect appeared to be specific to cancer cells and underscores the distinct roles that these two kinases have, as well as pointing to potential mechanisms of resistance to ATRi or CHK1i monotherapy.

5.4.5 Combination with Radical Radiation

The combination of ATRi and radiotherapy is being investigated in a phase 1 study. This study investigates the combination in the context of low-dose palliative radiation, in order to accurately assess the normal tissue toxicity in this first-in-man combination. Pre-clinical data support the sensitizing effect of ATRi on radiation (Dillon et al. 2017a) and the combination has resulted in significant xenograft tumour growth retardation (Fokas et al. 2012; Guichard et al. 2013). The difficulties in making the step between a low-dose phase 1 study and combination with radical doses of radiation or chemoradiation in the curative setting are certainly complex and have been outlined above. However, this has been achieved successfully with a variety of novel agents in combination with radical radiation and chemoradiation and there is reason for optimism that the same will be true with ATRi (Dillon and Harrington 2015).

5.4.6 Combination with Immune Oncology Agents

The advent of effective immunotherapies with the promise of durable responses in metastatic disease has revolutionised oncology research. Efforts to increase response rates using combination therapies have been extensive and, although there are sparse preclinical data to support such a strategy as yet, combination studies of ATR inhibitors with anti-programmed death ligand-1 (PDL-1) antibodies have been initiated (NCT02264678). A further window-of-opportunity study has been initiated to examine the effect of pre-operative treatment with inhibitors of the DDR, including AZD6738, on the immune environment of the tumour—specifically investigating the effect of these agents on tumour-infiltrating lymphocytes (CD3- and CD8-positive) and modulation of gene expression, examining T_h1/interferon gamma responses to DDR agents (NCT03022409).

5.5 Summary

Three ATR inhibitors have reached clinical trials and these are currently ongoing. The current portfolio of ATR trials, all of which are being conducted in patients with advanced solid cancers, covers monotherapy, combination with genotoxic chemotherapy, combination with ionising radiation and combination with PARP inhibitors. There is a compelling pre-clinical rationale for each of these combinations and, as the data accrue, we can be confident that we will learn how to refine patient selection and optimise rational approaches to the development of this novel class of agents.

References

Abdel-Fatah TM, Middleton FK, Arora A, Agarwal D, Chen T, Moseley PM, Perry C, Doherty R, Chan S, Green AR, Rakha E, Ball G, Ellis IO, Curtin NJ, Madhusudan S (2015) Untangling the ATR-CHEK1 network for prognostication, prediction and therapeutic target validation in breast cancer. Mol Oncol 9(3):569–585

Ai L, Vo QN, Zuo C, Li L, Ling W, Suen JY, Hanna E, Brown KD, Fan CY (2004) Ataxia-telangiectasia-mutated (ATM) gene in head and neck squamous cell carcinoma: promoter hypermethylation with clinical correlation in 100 cases. Cancer Epidemiol Biomarkers Prev 13(1):150–156

Al-Ahmadie H, Iyer G, Hohl M, Asthana S, Inagaki A, Schultz N, Hanrahan AJ, Scott SN, Brannon AR, McDermott GC, Pirun M, Ostrovnaya I, Kim P, Socci ND, Viale A, Schwartz GK, Reuter V, Bochner BH, Rosenberg JE, Bajorin DF, Berger MF, Petrini JH, Solit DB, Taylor BS (2014) Synthetic lethality in ATM-deficient RAD50-mutant tumors underlies outlier response to cancer therapy. Cancer Discov 4(9):1014–1021

Angele S, Treilleux I, Taniere P, Martel-Planche G, Vuillaume M, Bailly C, Bremond A, Montesano R, Hall J (2000) Abnormal expression of the ATM and TP53 genes in sporadic breast carcinomas. Clin Cancer Res 6(9):3536–3544

Austen B, Powell JE, Alvi A, Edwards I, Hooper L, Starczynski J, Taylor AMR, Fegan C, Moss P, Stankovic T (2005) Mutations in the ATM gene lead to impaired overall and treatment-free survival that is independent of IGVH mutation status in patients with B-CLL. Blood 106(9):3175–3182

Austen B, Skowronska A, Baker C, Powell JE, Gardiner A, Oscier D, Majid A, Dyer M, Siebert R, Taylor AM, Moss PA, Stankovic T (2007) Mutation status of the residual ATM allele is an important determinant of the cellular response to chemotherapy and survival in patients with chronic lymphocytic leukemia containing an 11q deletion. J Clin Oncol 25(34):5448–5457

Bai AH, Tong JH, To KF, Chan MW, Man EP, Lo KW, Lee JF, Sung JJ, Leung WK (2004) Promoter hypermethylation of tumor-related genes in the progression of colorectal neoplasia. Int J Cancer 112(5):846–853

Bao S, Wu Q, McLendon RE, Hao Y, Shi Q, Hjelmeland AB, Dewhirst MW, Bigner DD, Rich JN (2006) Glioma stem cells promote radioresistance by preferential activation of the DNA damage response. Nature 444(7120):756–760

Bartek J, Bartkova J, Lukas J (2007) DNA damage signalling guards against activated oncogenes and tumour progression. Oncogene 26(56):7773–7779

Bester AC, Roniger M, Oren YS, Im MM, Sarni D, Chaoat M, Bensimon A, Zamir G, Shewach DS, Kerem B (2011) Nucleotide deficiency promotes genomic instability in early stages of cancer development. Cell 145(3):435–446

Bhat A, Andersen PL, Qin Z, Xiao W (2013) Rev3, the catalytic subunit of Polzeta, is required for maintaining fragile site stability in human cells. Nucleic Acids Res 41(4):2328–2339

Bi X, Srikanta D, Fanti L, Pimpinelli S, Badugu R, Kellum R, Rong YS (2005) Drosophila ATM and ATR checkpoint kinases control partially redundant pathways for telomere maintenance. Proc Natl Acad Sci U S A 102(42):15167–15172

Bolderson E, Scorah J, Helleday T, Smythe C, Meuth M (2004) ATM is required for the cellular response to thymidine induced replication fork stress. Hum Mol Genet 13(23):2937–2945

Bolt J, Vo QN, Kim WJ, McWhorter AJ, Thomson J, Hagensee ME, Friedlander P, Brown KD, Gilbert J (2005) The ATM/p53 pathway is commonly targeted for inactivation in squamous cell carcinoma of the head and neck (SCCHN) by multiple molecular mechanisms. Oral Oncol 41(10):1013–1020

Bonner WM, Redon CE, Dickey JS, Nakamura AJ, Sedelnikova OA, Solier S, Pommier Y (2008) GammaH2AX and cancer. Nat Rev Cancer 8(12):957–967

Bristow RG, Hill RP (2008) Hypoxia and metabolism. Hypoxia, DNA repair and genetic instability. Nat Rev Cancer 8(3):180–192

Brown EJ, Baltimore D (2000) ATR disruption leads to chromosomal fragmentation and early embryonic lethality. Genes Dev 14(4):397–402

Bueno RC, Canevari RA, Villacis RA, Domingues MA, Caldeira JR, Rocha RM, Drigo SA, Rogatto SR (2014) ATM down-regulation is associated with poor prognosis in sporadic breast carcinomas. Ann Oncol 25(1):69–75

Byrd JC, Gribben JG, Peterson BL, Grever MR, Lozanski G, Lucas DM, Lampson B, Larson RA, Caligiuri MA, Heerema NA (2006) Select high-risk genetic features predict earlier progression following chemoimmunotherapy with fludarabine and rituximab in chronic lymphocytic leukemia: justification for risk-adapted therapy. J Clin Oncol 24(3):437–443

Caldecott KW (2003) XRCC1 and DNA strand break repair. DNA Repair 2(9):955–969

Camidge DR, Randall KR, Foster JR, Sadler CJ, Wright JA, Soames AR, Laud PJ, Smith PD, Hughes AM (2005) Plucked human hair as a tissue in which to assess pharmacodynamic end points during drug development studies. Br J Cancer 92(10):1837–1841

Caporali S, Falcinelli S, Starace G, Russo MT, Bonmassar E, Jiricny J, D'Atri S (2004) DNA damage induced by temozolomide signals to both ATM and ATR: role of the mismatch repair system. Mol Pharmacol 66(3):478–491

Chan N, Pires IM, Bencokova Z, Coackley C, Luoto KR, Bhogal N, Lakshman M, Gottipati P, Oliver FJ, Helleday T, Hammond EM, Bristow RG (2010) Contextual synthetic lethality of cancer cell kill based on the tumor microenvironment. Cancer Res 70(20):8045–8054

Chanan-Khan A, Holkova B, Perle M, Reich E, Wu C, Inghirami G, Takeshita K (2003) T-cell clonality and myelodysplasia without chromosomal fragility in a patient with features of Seckel syndrome. Haematologica 88(5):ECR14

Chanoux RA, Yin B, Urtishak KA, Asare A, Bassing CH, Brown EJ (2009) ATR and H2AX cooperate in maintaining genome stability under replication stress. J Biol Chem 284(9):5994–6003

Charrier JD, Durrant SJ, Golec JM, Kay DP, Knegtel RM, MacCormick S, Mortimore M, O'Donnell ME, Pinder JL, Reaper PM, Rutherford AP, Wang PS, Young SC, Pollard JR (2011) Discovery of potent and selective inhibitors of ataxia telangiectasia mutated and Rad3 related (ATR) protein kinase as potential anticancer agents. J Med Chem 54(7):2320–2330

Chen T, Middleton FK, Falcon S, Reaper PM, Pollard JR, Curtin NJ (2015) Development of pharmacodynamic biomarkers for ATR inhibitors. Mol Oncol 9(2):463–472

Chen T, Stephens PA, Middleton FK, Curtin NJ (2012) Targeting the S and G2 checkpoint to treat cancer. Drug Discov Today 17(5-6):194–202

Ciccia A, Elledge SJ (2010) The DNA damage response: making it safe to play with knives. Mol Cell 40(2):179–204

Cimprich KA, Cortez D (2008) ATR: an essential regulator of genome integrity. Nat Rev Mol Cell Biol 9(8):616–627

Cliby WA, Lewis KA, Lilly KK, Kaufmann SH (2002) S phase and G2 arrests induced by topoisomerase I poisons are dependent on ATR kinase function. J Biol Chem 277(2):1599–1606

Cliby WA, Roberts CJ, Cimprich KA, Stringer CM, Lamb JR, Schreiber SL, Friend SH (1998) Overexpression of a kinase-inactive ATR protein causes sensitivity to DNA-damaging agents and defects in cell cycle checkpoints. EMBO J 17(1):159–169

d'Adda di Fagagna F, Reaper PM, Clay-Farrace L, Fiegler H, Carr P, Von Zglinicki T, Saretzki G, Carter NP, Jackson SP (2003) A DNA damage checkpoint response in telomere-initiated senescence. Nature 426(6963):194–198

Dai Y, Grant S (2010) New insights into checkpoint kinase 1 in the DNA damage response signaling network. Clin Cancer Res 16(2):376–383

Di Micco R, Fumagalli M, Cicalese A, Piccinin S, Gasparini P, Luise C, Schurra C, Garre M, Nuciforo PG, Bensimon A, Maestro R, Pelicci PG, d'Adda di Fagagna F (2006) Oncogene-induced senescence is a DNA damage response triggered by DNA hyper-replication. Nature 444(7119):638–642

Dillon M, Ellis S, Grove L, McLellan L, Clack G, Smith DS, Laude J, Viney Z, Adeleke S, Lazaridis G, Spicer JF, Forster MD, Harrington KJ (2016) PATRIOT: a phase I study to assess the tolerability, safety and biological effects of a specific ataxia telangiectasia and Rad3-related (ATR) inhibitor (AZD6738) as a single agent and in combination with palliative radiation therapy in patients with solid tumours. ASCO Meet Abstr 34(15_suppl):TPS2603

Dillon MT, Barker HE, Pedersen M, Hafsi H, Bhide SA, Newbold KL, Nutting CM, McLaughlin M, Harrington KJ (2017a) Radiosensitization by the ATR Inhibitor AZD6738 through Generation of Acentric Micronuclei. Mol Cancer Ther 16(1):25–34

Dillon MT, Espinasse A, Ellis S, Mohammed K, Grove L, McLellan L, Smith SA, Ross G, Woo K, Adeleke S, Josephides E, Spicer J, Forster MD, Harrington KJ (2017b) A phase I multicenter dose-escalation study of AZD6738 ATR inhibitor monotherapy in advanced solid tumors (PATRIOT Part A): preliminary results. AACR Annual Meeting, Washington, DC

Dillon MT, Good JS, Harrington KJ (2014) Selective targeting of the G2/M cell cycle checkpoint to improve the therapeutic index of radiotherapy. Clin Oncol (R Coll Radiol) 26(5):257–265

Dillon MT, Harrington KJ (2015) Human Papillomavirus-Negative Pharyngeal Cancer. J Clin Oncol 33(29):3251–3261

Ding L, Getz G, Wheeler DA, Mardis ER, McLellan MD, Cibulskis K, Sougnez C, Greulich H, Muzny DM, Morgan MB, Fulton L, Fulton RS, Zhang Q, Wendl MC, Lawrence MS, Larson DE, Chen K, Dooling DJ, Sabo A, Hawes AC, Shen H, Jhangiani SN, Lewis LR, Hall O, Zhu Y, Mathew T, Ren Y, Yao J, Scherer SE, Clerc K, Metcalf GA, Ng B, Milosavljevic A, Gonzalez-Garay ML, Osborne JR, Meyer R, Shi X, Tang Y, Koboldt DC, Lin L, Abbott R, Miner TL, Pohl C, Fewell G, Haipek C, Schmidt H, Dunford-Shore BH, Kraja A, Crosby SD, Sawyer CS, Vickery T, Sander S, Robinson J, Winckler W, Baldwin J, Chirieac LR, Dutt A, Fennell T, Hanna M, Johnson BE, Onofrio RC, Thomas RK, Tonon G, Weir BA, Zhao X, Ziaugra L, Zody MC, Giordano T, Orringer MB, Roth JA, Spitz MR, Wistuba II, Ozenberger B, Good PJ, Chang AC, Beer DG, Watson MA, Ladanyi M, Broderick S, Yoshizawa A, Travis WD, Pao W, Province MA, Weinstock GM, Varmus HE, Gabriel SB, Lander ES, Gibbs RA, Meyerson M, Wilson RK (2008) Somatic mutations affect key pathways in lung adenocarcinoma. Nature 455(7216):1069–1075

Dohner H, Stilgenbauer S, Benner A, Leupolt E, Krober A, Bullinger L, Dohner K, Bentz M, Lichter P (2000) Genomic aberrations and survival in chronic lymphocytic leukemia. N Engl J Med 343(26):1910–1916

Dohner H, Stilgenbauer S, James MR, Benner A, Weilguni T, Bentz M, Fischer K, Hunstein W, Lichter P (1997) 11q deletions identify a new subset of B-cell chronic lymphocytic leukemia characterized by extensive nodal involvement and inferior prognosis. Blood 89(7):2516–2522

Fang Y, Tsao CC, Goodman BK, Furumai R, Tirado CA, Abraham RT, Wang XF (2004) ATR functions as a gene dosage-dependent tumor suppressor on a mismatch repair-deficient background. EMBO J 23(15):3164–3174

Flatten K, Dai NT, Vroman BT, Loegering D, Erlichman C, Karnitz LM, Kaufmann SH (2005) The role of checkpoint kinase 1 in sensitivity to topoisomerase I poisons. J Biol Chem 280(14):14349–14355

Flynn RL, Cox KE, Jeitany M, Wakimoto H, Bryll AR, Ganem NJ, Bersani F, Pineda JR, Suva ML, Benes CH, Haber DA, Boussin FD, Zou L (2015) Alternative lengthening of telomeres renders cancer cells hypersensitive to ATR inhibitors. Science 347(6219):273–277

Fokas E, Prevo R, Pollard JR, Reaper PM, Charlton PA, Cornelissen B, Vallis KA, Hammond EM, Olcina MM, Gillies W, McKenna RJM, Brunner TB (2012) Targeting ATR in vivo using the novel inhibitor VE-822 results in selective sensitization of pancreatic tumors to radiation. Cell Death Dis 3:e441

Fong PC, Boss DS, Yap TA, Tutt A, Wu P, Mergui-Roelvink M, Mortimer P, Swaisland H, Lau A, O'Connor MJ, Ashworth A, Carmichael J, Kaye SB, Schellens JH, de Bono JS (2009) Inhibition of poly(ADP-ribose) polymerase in tumors from BRCA mutation carriers. N Engl J Med 361(2):123–134

Foote KM, Blades K, Cronin A, Fillery S, Guichard SS, Hassall L, Hickson I, Jacq X, Jewsbury PJ, McGuire TM, Nissink JW, Odedra R, Page K, Perkins P, Suleman A, Tam K, Thommes P, Broadhurst R, Wood C (2013) Discovery of 4-{4-[(3R)-3-methylmorpholin-4-yl]-6-[1-(methylsulfonyl)cyclopropyl]pyrimidin-2-y 1}-1H-indole (AZ20): a potent and selective inhibitor of ATR protein kinase with monotherapy in vivo antitumor activity. J Med Chem 56(5):2125–2138

Foote KM, Lau A, JW MN (2015) Drugging ATR: progress in the development of specific inhibitors for the treatment of cancer. Future Med Chem 7(7):873–891

Fracasso PM, Williams KJ, Chen RC, Picus J, Ma CX, Ellis MJ, Tan BR, Pluard TJ, Adkins DR, Naughton MJ, Rader JS, Arquette MA, Fleshman JW, Creekmore AN, Goodner SA, Wright LP, Guo Z, Ryan CE, Tao Y, Soares EM, Cai S-r, Lin L, Dancey J, Rudek MA, McLeod HL, Piwnica-Worms H (2011) A Phase 1 study of UCN-01 in combination with irinotecan in patients with resistant solid tumor malignancies. Cancer Chemother Pharmacol 67(6):1225–1237

Gaillard H, Garcia-Muse T, Aguilera A (2015) Replication stress and cancer. Nat Rev Cancer 15(5):276–289

Gamper AM, Rofougaran R, Watkins SC, Greenberger JS, Beumer JH, Bakkenist CJ (2013) ATR kinase activation in G1 phase facilitates the repair of ionizing radiation-induced DNA damage. Nucleic Acids Res 41(22):10334–10344

Gilad O, Nabet BY, Ragland RL, Schoppy DW, Smith KD, Durham AC, Brown EJ (2010) Combining ATR suppression with oncogenic Ras synergistically increases genomic instability, causing synthetic lethality or tumorigenesis in a dosage-dependent manner. Cancer Res 70(23):9693–9702

Guarini A, Marinelli M, Tavolaro S, Bellacchio E, Magliozzi M, Chiaretti S, De Propris MS, Peragine N, Santangelo S, Paoloni F, Nanni M, Del Giudice I, Mauro FR, Torrente I, Foà R (2012) ATM gene alterations in chronic lymphocytic leukemia patients induce a distinct gene expression profile and predict disease progression. Haematologica 97(1):47–55

Guichard SM, Brown E, Odedra R, Hughes A, Heathcote D, Barnes J, Lau A, Powell S, Jones CD, Nissink W, Foote KM, Jewsbury PJ, Pass M (2013) Abstract 3343: the pre-clinical in vitro and in vivo activity of AZD6738: a potent and selective inhibitor of ATR kinase. Cancer Res 73(8 Supplement):3343

Halazonetis TD, Gorgoulis VG, Bartek J (2008) An oncogene-induced DNA damage model for cancer development. Science 319(5868):1352–1355

Hall AB, Newsome D, Wang Y, Boucher DM, Eustace B, Gu Y, Hare B, Johnson MA, Milton S, Murphy CE, Takemoto D, Tolman C, Wood M, Charlton P, Charrier J-D, Furey B, Golec J, Reaper PM, Pollard JR (2014) Potentiation of tumor responses to DNA damaging therapy by the selective ATR inhibitor VX-970. Oncotarget 5(14):5674–5685

Hammond EM, Denko NC, Dorie MJ, Abraham RT, Giaccia AJ (2002) Hypoxia links ATR and p53 through replication arrest. Mol Cell Biol 22(6):1834–1843

Hammond EM, Dorie MJ, Giaccia AJ (2003) ATR/ATM targets are phosphorylated by ATR in response to hypoxia and ATM in response to reoxygenation. J Biol Chem 278(14):12207–12213

Hammond EM, Dorie MJ, Giaccia AJ (2004) Inhibition of ATR leads to increased sensitivity to hypoxia/reoxygenation. Cancer Res 64(18):6556–6562

Hammond EM, Kaufmann MR, Giaccia AJ (2007) Oxygen sensing and the DNA-damage response. Curr Opin Cell Biol 19(6):680–684

Hanahan D, Weinberg RA (2011) Hallmarks of cancer: the next generation. Cell 144(5):646–674

Harrington KJ, Billingham LJ, Brunner TB, Burnet NG, Chan CS, Hoskin P, Mackay RI, Maughan TS, Macdougall J, McKenna WG, Nutting CM, Oliver A, Plummer R, Stratford IJ, Illidge T (2011) Guidelines for preclinical and early phase clinical assessment of novel radiosensitisers. Br J Cancer 105(5):628–639

Hayani A, Suarez CR, Molnar Z, LeBeau M, Godwin J (1994) Acute myeloid leukaemia in a patient with Seckel syndrome. J Med Genet 31(2):148–149

Heaphy CM, de Wilde RF, Jiao Y, Klein AP, Edil BH, Shi C, Bettegowda C, Rodriguez FJ, Eberhart CG, Hebbar S, Offerhaus GJ, McLendon R, Rasheed BA, He Y, Yan H, Bigner DD, Oba-Shinjo SM, Marie SKN, Riggins GJ, Kinzler KW, Vogelstein B, Hruban RH, Maitra A, Papadopoulos N, Meeker AK (2011) Altered telomeres in tumors with ATRX and DAXX mutations. Science 333(6041):425

Hu H, Du L, Nagabayashi G, Seeger RC, Gatti RA (2010) ATM is down-regulated by N-Myc-regulated microRNA-421. Proc Natl Acad Sci U S A 107(4):1506–1511

Huntoon CJ, Flatten KS, Wahner Hendrickson AE, Huehls AM, Sutor SL, Kaufmann SH, Karnitz LM (2013) ATR inhibition broadly sensitizes ovarian cancer cells to chemotherapy independent of BRCA status. Cancer Res 73(12):3683–3691

Jacq X, Smith L, Brown E, Hughes A, Odedra R, Heathcote D, Barnes J, Powell S, Maguire S, Pearson V, Boros J, Caie P, Thommes PA, Nissink W, Foote K, Jewsbury PJ, Guichard SM (2012) Abstract 1823: AZ20, a novel potent and selective inhibitor of ATR kinase with in vivo antitumour activity. Cancer Res 72(8 Supplement):1823

Jazayeri A, Falck J, Lukas C, Bartek J, Smith GC, Lukas J, Jackson SP (2006) ATM- and cell cycle-dependent regulation of ATR in response to DNA double-strand breaks. Nat Cell Biol 8(1):37–45

Jones CD, Blades K, Foote KM, Guichard SM, Jewsbury PJ, McGuire T, Nissink JW, Odedra R, Tam K, Thommes P, Turner P, Wilkinson G, Wood C, Yates JW (2013a) Abstract 2348: discovery of AZD6738, a potent and selective inhibitor with the potential to test the clinical efficacy of ATR kinase inhibition in cancer patients. Cancer Res 73(8 Supplement):2348

Jones RM, Mortusewicz O, Afzal I, Lorvellec M, Garcia P, Helleday T, Petermann E (2013b) Increased replication initiation and conflicts with transcription underlie Cyclin E-induced replication stress. Oncogene 32(32):3744–3753

Josse R, Martin SE, Guha R, Ormanoglu P, Pfister TD, Reaper PM, Barnes CS, Jones J, Charlton P, Pollard JR, Morris J, Doroshow JH, Pommier Y (2014) ATR inhibitors VE-821 and VX-970 sensitize cancer cells to topoisomerase I inhibitors by disabling DNA replication initiation and fork elongation responses. Cancer Res 74(23):6968–6979

Kim ST, Lim DS, Canman CE, Kastan MB (1999) Substrate specificities and identification of putative substrates of ATM kinase family members. J Biol Chem 274(53):37538–37543

Kirschner K, Melton DW (2010) Multiple roles of the ERCC1-XPF endonuclease in DNA repair and resistance to anticancer drugs. Anticancer Res 30(9):3223–3232

Kotov IN, Siebring-van Olst E, Knobel PA, van der Meulen-Muileman IH, Felley-Bosco E, van Beusechem VW, Smit EF, Stahel RA, Marti TM (2014) Whole genome RNAi screens reveal a critical role of REV3 in coping with replication stress. Mol Oncol 8(8):1747–1759

Krajewska M, Fehrmann RS, Schoonen PM, Labib S, de Vries EG, Franke L, van Vugt MA (2015) ATR inhibition preferentially targets homologous recombination-deficient tumor cells. Oncogene 34(26):3474

Kwok M, Davies N, Agathanggelou A, Smith E, Oldreive C, Petermann E, Stewart G, Brown J, Lau A, Pratt G, Parry H, Taylor M, Moss P, Hillmen P, Stankovic T (2016) ATR inhibition induces synthetic lethality and overcomes chemoresistance in TP53- or ATM-defective chronic lymphocytic leukemia cells. Blood 127(5):582–595

Lavin MF, Scott S, Gueven N, Kozlov S, Peng C, Chen P (2004) Functional consequences of sequence alterations in the ATM gene. DNA Repair 3(8–9):1197–1205

Lecona E, Fernandez-Capetillo O (2014) Replication stress and cancer: it takes two to tango. Exp Cell Res 329(1):26–34

Lee HE, Han N, Kim MA, Lee HS, Yang HK, Lee BL, Kim WH (2014) DNA damage response-related proteins in gastric cancer: ATM, Chk2 and p53 expression and their prognostic value. Pathobiology 81(1):25–35

Lewis KA, Lilly KK, Reynolds EA, Sullivan WP, Kaufmann SH, Cliby WA (2009) Ataxia telangiectasia and rad3-related kinase contributes to cell cycle arrest and survival after cisplatin but not oxaliplatin. Mol Cancer Ther 8(4):855–863

Lim AM, Young RJ, Collins M, Fox SB, McArthur GA, Corry J, Peters L, Rischin D, Solomon B (2012) Correlation of Ataxia-Telangiectasia-Mutated (ATM) gene loss with outcome in head and neck squamous cell carcinoma. Oral Oncol 48(8):698–702

Lopez-Contreras AJ, Fernandez-Capetillo O (2010) The ATR barrier to replication-born DNA damage. DNA Repair (Amst) 9(12):1249–1255

López-Contreras AJ, Gutierrez-Martinez P, Specks J, Rodrigo-Perez S, Fernandez-Capetillo O (2012) An extra allele of Chk1 limits oncogene-induced replicative stress and promotes transformation. J Exp Med 209(3):455–461

Lovejoy CA, Li W, Reisenweber S, Thongthip S, Bruno J, de Lange T, De S, Petrini JHJ, Sung PA, Jasin M, Rosenbluh J, Zwang Y, Weir BA, Hatton C, Ivanova E, Macconaill L, Hanna M, Hahn WC, Lue NF, Reddel RR, Jiao Y, Kinzler K, Vogelstein B, Papadopoulos N, Meeker AK, ALT Starr Cancer Consortium (2012) Loss of ATRX, genome instability, and an altered DNA damage response are hallmarks of the alternative lengthening of telomeres pathway. PLoS Genet 8(7):e1002772

Manda G, Isvoranu G, Comanescu MV, Manea A, Debelec Butuner B, Korkmaz KS (2015) The redox biology network in cancer pathophysiology and therapeutics. Redox Biol 5:347–357

McNees CJ, Tejera AM, Martínez P, Murga M, Mulero F, Fernandez-Capetillo O, Blasco MA (2010) ATR suppresses telomere fragility and recombination but is dispensable for elongation of short telomeres by telomerase. J Cell Biol 188(5):639–652

Middleton FK, Patterson MJ, Elstob CJ, Fordham S, Herriott A, Wade MA, McCormick A, Edmondson R, May FE, Allan JM, Pollard JR, Curtin NJ (2015) Common cancer-associated imbalances in the DNA damage response confer sensitivity to single agent ATR inhibition. Oncotarget 6(32):32396–32409

Min A, Im SA, Jang H, Kim S, Lee M, Kim DK, Yang Y, Kim HJ, Lee KH, Kim JW, Kim TY, Oh DY, Brown J, Lau A, O'Connor MJ, Bang YJ (2017) AZD6738, a novel oral inhibitor of ATR, induces synthetic lethality with ATM deficiency in gastric cancer cells. Mol Cancer Ther 16(4):566–577

Mohni KN, Kavanaugh GM, Cortez D (2014) ATR pathway inhibition is synthetically lethal in cancer cells with ERCC1 deficiency. Cancer Res 74(10):2835–2845

Mohni KN, Thompson PS, Luzwick JW, Glick GG, Pendleton CS, Lehmann BD, Pietenpol JA, Cortez D (2015) A synthetic lethal screen identifies DNA repair pathways that sensitize cancer cells to combined ATR inhibition and cisplatin treatments. PLoS One 10(5):e0125482

Morrison C, Sonoda E, Takao N, Shinohara A, Yamamoto K, Takeda S (2000) The controlling role of ATM in homologous recombinational repair of DNA damage. EMBO J 19(3):463–471

Murga M, Bunting S, Montana MF, Soria R, Mulero F, Canamero M, Lee Y, McKinnon PJ, Nussenzweig A, Fernandez-Capetillo O (2009) A mouse model of ATR-Seckel shows embryonic replicative stress and accelerated aging. Nat Genet 41(8):891–898

Murga M, Campaner S, Lopez-Contreras AJ, Toledo LI, Soria R, Montana MF, D'Artista L, Schleker T, Guerra C, Garcia E, Barbacid M, Hidalgo M, Amati B, Fernandez-Capetillo O (2011) Exploiting oncogene-induced replicative stress for the selective killing of Myc-driven tumors. Nat Struct Mol Biol 18(12):1331–1335

Nam EA, Zhao R, Glick GG, Bansbach CE, Friedman DB, Cortez D (2011) Thr-1989 phosphorylation is a marker of active ataxia telangiectasia-mutated and Rad3-related (ATR) kinase. J Biol Chem 286(33):28707–28714

Nghiem P, Park PK, Kim Y, Vaziri C, Schreiber SL (2001) ATR inhibition selectively sensitizes G1 checkpoint-deficient cells to lethal premature chromatin condensation. Proc Natl Acad Sci U S A 98(16):9092–9097

Nishida H, Tatewaki N, Nakajima Y, Magara T, Ko KM, Hamamori Y, Konishi T (2009) Inhibition of ATR protein kinase activity by schisandrin B in DNA damage response. Nucleic Acids Res 37(17):5678–5689

O'Carrigan B, de Miguel Luken MJ, Papadatos-Pastos D, Brown J, Tunariu N, Perez Lopez R, Ganegoda M, Riisnaes R, Figueiredo I, Carreira S, Hare B, Yang F, McDermott K, Penney MS, Pollard J, Lopez JS, Banerji U, De Bono JS, Fields SZ, Yap TA (2016) Phase I trial of a first-in-class ATR inhibitor VX-970 as monotherapy (mono) or in combination (combo) with carboplatin (CP) incorporating pharmacodynamics (PD) studies. ASCO Meet Abstr 34(15_suppl):2504

O'Driscoll M, Gennery AR, Seidel J, Concannon P, Jeggo PA (2004) An overview of three new disorders associated with genetic instability: LIG4 syndrome, RS-SCID and ATR-Seckel syndrome. DNA Repair (Amst) 3(8-9):1227–1235

Olcina M, Lecane PS, Hammond EM (2010) Targeting hypoxic cells through the DNA damage response. Clin Cancer Res 16(23):5624–5629

Olive PL (2011) Retention of gammaH2AX foci as an indication of lethal DNA damage. Radiother Oncol 101(1):18–23

Ouillette P, Fossum S, Parkin B, Ding L, Bockenstedt P, Al-Zoubi A, Shedden K, Malek SN (2010) Aggressive chronic lymphocytic leukemia with elevated genomic complexity is associated with multiple gene defects in the response to DNA double-strand breaks. Clin Cancer Res 16(3):835–847

Park JS, Na HJ, Pyo JH, Jeon HJ, Kim YS, Yoo MA (2015) Requirement of ATR for maintenance of intestinal stem cells in aging Drosophila. Aging (Albany N Y) 7(5):307–318

Peasland A, Wang LZ, Rowling E, Kyle S, Chen T, Hopkins A, Cliby WA, Sarkaria J, Beale G, Edmondson RJ, Curtin NJ (2011) Identification and evaluation of a potent novel ATR inhibitor, NU6027, in breast and ovarian cancer cell lines. Br J Cancer 105(3):372–381

Pennarun G, Hoffschir F, Revaud D, Granotier C, Gauthier LR, Mailliet P, Biard DS, Boussin FD (2010) ATR contributes to telomere maintenance in human cells. Nucleic Acids Res 38(9):2955–2963

Perez RP, Lewis LD, Beelen AP, Olszanski AJ, Johnston N, Rhodes CH, Beaulieu B, Ernstoff MS, Eastman A (2006) Modulation of cell cycle progression in human tumors: a pharmacokinetic and tumor molecular pharmacodynamic study of cisplatin plus the Chk1 inhibitor UCN-01 (NSC 638850). Clin Cancer Res 12(23):7079–7085

Pires IM, Bencokova Z, Milani M, Folkes LK, Li JL, Stratford MR, Harris AL, Hammond EM (2010) Effects of acute versus chronic hypoxia on DNA damage responses and genomic instability. Cancer Res 70(3):925–935

Pires IM, Olcina MM, Anbalagan S, Pollard JR, Reaper PM, Charlton PA, McKenna WG, Hammond EM (2012) Targeting radiation-resistant hypoxic tumour cells through ATR inhibition. Br J Cancer 107(2):291–299

Plummer ER, Dean EJ, Evans TRJ, Greystoke A, Herbschleb K, Ranson M, Brown J, Zhang Y, Karan S, Pollard J, Penney MS, Asmal M, Fields SZ, Middleton MR (2016) Phase I trial of first-in-class ATR inhibitor VX-970 in combination with gemcitabine (Gem) in advanced solid tumors (NCT02157792). J Clin Oncol 34(suppl):abstr 2513

Powell SN, DeFrank JS, Connell P, Eogan M, Preffer F, Dombkowski D, Tang W, Friend S (1995) Differential sensitivity of p53(-) and p53(+) cells to caffeine-induced radiosensitization and override of G2 delay. Cancer Res 55(8):1643–1648

Prevo R, Fokas E, Reaper PM, Charlton PA, Pollard JR, McKenna WG, Muschel RJ, Brunner TB (2012) The novel ATR inhibitor VE-821 increases sensitivity of pancreatic cancer cells to radiation and chemotherapy. Cancer Biol Ther 13(11):1072–1081

Reaper PM, Griffiths MR, Long JM, Charrier JD, Maccormick S, Charlton PA, Golec JM, Pollard JR (2011) Selective killing of ATM- or p53-deficient cancer cells through inhibition of ATR. Nat Chem Biol 7(7):428–430

Rossi D, Gaidano G (2012) ATM and chronic lymphocytic leukemia: mutations, and not only deletions, matter. Haematologica 97(1):5

Ruzankina Y, Schoppy DW, Asare A, Clark CE, Vonderheide RH, Brown EJ (2009) Tissue regenerative delays and synthetic lethality in adult mice after combined deletion of Atr and Trp53. Nat Genet 41(10):1144–1149

Sanjiv K, Hagenkort A, José M, Calderón-Montaño TK, Philip M, Reaper OM, Sylvain A, Jacques RV, Kuiper NS, Scobie M, Peter A, Charlton JR, Pollard UW, Berglund MA, Helleday T (2016) Cancer-specific synthetic lethality between ATR and CHK1 kinase activities. Cell Rep 14(2):298–309

Sarkaria JN, Busby EC, Tibbetts RS, Roos P, Taya Y, Karnitz LM, Abraham RT (1999) Inhibition of ATM and ATR kinase activities by the radiosensitizing agent, caffeine. Cancer Res 59(17):4375–4382

Scanlon SE, Glazer PM (2015) Multifaceted control of DNA repair pathways by the hypoxic tumor microenvironment. DNA Repair (Amst) 32:180

Schaffner C, Stilgenbauer S, Rappold GA, Döhner H, Lichter P (1999) Somatic ATM mutations indicate a pathogenic role of ATM in B-cell chronic lymphocytic leukemia. Blood 94:748

Shiloh Y (2003) ATM and related protein kinases: safeguarding genome integrity. Nat Rev Cancer 3(3):155–168

Singh TR, Ali AM, Paramasivam M, Pradhan A, Wahengbam K, Seidman MM, Meetei AR (2013) ATR-dependent phosphorylation of FANCM at serine 1045 is essential for FANCM functions. Cancer Res 73(14):4300–4310

Skowronska A, Parker A, Ahmed G, Oldreive C, Davis Z, Richards S, Dyer M, Matutes E, Gonzalez D, Taylor AM, Moss P, Thomas P, Oscier D, Stankovic T (2012) Biallelic ATM inactivation significantly reduces survival in patients treated on the United Kingdom Leukemia Research Fund Chronic Lymphocytic Leukemia 4 trial. J Clin Oncol 30(36):4524–4532

Stankovic T, Stewart GS, Fegan C, Biggs P, Last J, Byrd PJ, Keenan RD, Moss PAH, Taylor AMR (2002) Ataxia telangiectasia mutated–deficient B-cell chronic lymphocytic leukemia occurs in pregerminal center cells and results in defective damage response and unrepaired chromosome damage. Blood 99(1):300

Stankovic T, Weber P, Stewart G, Bedenham T, Murray J, Byrd PJ, Moss PA, Taylor AM (1999) Inactivation of ataxia telangiectasia mutated gene in B-cell chronic lymphocytic leukaemia. Lancet 353(9146):26–29

Stokes MP, Rush J, Macneill J, Ren JM, Sprott K, Nardone J, Yang V, Beausoleil SA, Gygi SP, Livingstone M, Zhang H, Polakiewicz RD, Comb MJ (2007) Profiling of UV-induced ATM/ATR signaling pathways. Proc Natl Acad Sci U S A 104(50):19855–19860

Sultana R, Abdel-Fatah T, Perry C, Moseley P, Albarakti N, Mohan V, Seedhouse C, Chan S, Madhusudan S (2013) Ataxia telangiectasia mutated and Rad3 related (ATR) protein kinase inhibition is synthetically lethal in XRCC1 deficient ovarian cancer cells. PLoS One 8(2):e57098

Tanaka T, Halicka HD, Huang X, Traganos F, Darzynkiewicz Z (2006) Constitutive histone H2AX phosphorylation and ATM activation, the reporters of DNA damage by endogenous oxidants. Cell Cycle 5(17):1940–1945

Thanasoula M, Escandell JM, Suwaki N, Tarsounas M (2012) ATM/ATR checkpoint activation downregulates CDC25C to prevent mitotic entry with uncapped telomeres. EMBO J 31(16):3398–3410

Toledo LI, Murga M, Fernandez-Capetillo O (2011a) Targeting ATR and Chk1 kinases for cancer treatment: a new model for new (and old) drugs. Mol Oncol 5(4):368–373

Toledo LI, Murga M, Gutierrez-Martinez P, Soria R, Fernandez-Capetillo O (2008) ATR signaling can drive cells into senescence in the absence of DNA breaks. Genes Dev 22(3):297–302

Toledo LI, Murga M, Zur R, Soria R, Rodriguez A, Martinez S, Oyarzabal J, Pastor J, Bischoff JR, Fernandez-Capetillo O (2011b) A cell-based screen identifies ATR inhibitors with synthetic lethal properties for cancer-associated mutations. Nat Struct Mol Biol 18(6):721–727

Vendetti FP, Lau A, Schamus S, Conrads TP, O'Connor MJ, Bakkenist CJ (2015) The orally active and bioavailable ATR kinase inhibitor AZD6738 potentiates the anti-tumor effects of cisplatin to resolve ATM-deficient non-small cell lung cancer in vivo. Oncotarget 6(42):44289–44305

Wagner JM, Karnitz LM (2009) Cisplatin-induced DNA damage activates replication checkpoint signaling components that differentially affect tumor cell survival. Mol Pharmacol 76(1):208–214

Walsh CS (2015) Two decades beyond BRCA1/2: homologous recombination, hereditary cancer risk and a target for ovarian cancer therapy. Gynecol Oncol 137(2):343–350

Wang W (2007) Emergence of a DNA-damage response network consisting of Fanconi anaemia and BRCA proteins. Nat Rev Genet 8(10):735–748

Watkins JA, Irshad S, Grigoriadis A, Tutt AN (2014) Genomic scars as biomarkers of homologous recombination deficiency and drug response in breast and ovarian cancers. Breast Cancer Res 16(3):211

Weber AM, Bokobza SM, Devery AM, Ryan AJ (2013) Abstract B91: combined ATM and ATR kinase inhibition selectively kills p53-mutated non-small cell lung cancer (NSCLC) cells. Mol Cancer Ther 12(11 Supplement):B91

Wilsker D, Bunz F (2007) Loss of ataxia telangiectasia mutated- and Rad3-related function potentiates the effects of chemotherapeutic drugs on cancer cell survival. Mol Cancer Ther 6(4):1406–1413

Yap TA, Lorente D, Omlin A, Olmos D, de Bono JS (2014) Circulating tumor cells: a multifunctional biomarker. Clin Cancer Res 20(10):2553–2568

Zeman MK, Cimprich KA (2014) Causes and consequences of replication stress. Nat Cell Biol 16(1):2–9

Zhang C, Yan Z, Painter CL, Zhang Q, Chen E, Arango ME, Kuszpit K, Zasadny K, Hallin M, Hallin J, Wong A, Buckman D, Sun G, Qiu M, Anderes K, Christensen JG (2009) PF-00477736 mediates checkpoint kinase 1 signaling pathway and potentiates docetaxel-induced efficacy in xenografts. Clin Cancer Res 15(14):4630–4640

Zhao H, Piwnica-Worms H (2001) ATR-mediated checkpoint pathways regulate phosphorylation and activation of human Chk1. Mol Cell Biol 21(13):4129–4139

Chapter 6
ATM: Its Recruitment, Activation, Signalling and Contribution to Tumour Suppression

Atsushi Shibata and Penny Jeggo

Abstract DNA double strand breaks (DSBs) are a critical lesion for cancer etiology. Most cancer cells incur increased DNA breakage to enhance genomic instability. The DSB damage response encompasses pathways of repair and a signal transduction pathway. The ataxia telangiectasia mutated (ATM) kinase lies at the centre of the signalling response. ATM is not essential for the major DSB repair process in mammalian cells but influences DSB repair, including its accuracy, in multiple ways. ATM is activated by DSBs to promote cell cycle checkpoint arrest and apoptosis. There is mounting evidence that ATM is active endogenously and/or that it can be activated by non-DSB routes, including oxidative damage. It plays an important role in regulating cellular redox status. The tumour suppressor functions of ATM are discussed. Paradoxically, since elevated DSBs arise in cancer cells, despite being a tumour suppressor, pharmacological inhibition of ATM is a promising route for cancer therapy.

Keywords DNA damage signalling · Radiosensitivity · DNA double-strand break repair · Cell cycle checkpoints · Apoptosis · Ataxia telangiectasia

6.1 Introduction

Ataxia telangiectasia mutated (*ATM*) was identified as the gene mutated in the autosomal recessive disorder, ataxia telangiectasia (A-T), in 1995 via a stirling, collaborative effort headed by Yossi Shiloh (Savitsky et al. 1995). The marked

A. Shibata
Eduction and Research Support Centre, Graduate School of Medicine, Gunma University, Maebashi, Gunma, Japan
e-mail: shibata.at@gunma-u.ac.jp

P. Jeggo (✉)
Genome Damage and Stability Centre, Life Sciences, University of Sussex, Brighton, UK
e-mail: P.a.jeggo@sussex.ac.uk

© Springer International Publishing AG, part of Springer Nature 2018
J. Pollard, N. Curtin (eds.), *Targeting the DNA Damage Response for Anti-Cancer Therapy*, Cancer Drug Discovery and Development,
https://doi.org/10.1007/978-3-319-75836-7_6

radiosensitivity and chromosomal instability of cell lines derived from ataxia telangiectasia (A-T) patients had already provided clues to ATM function. The dramatic clinical manifestation of A-T, which includes progressive ataxia, immunodeficiency, clinical radiosensitivity and cancer predisposition, demonstrated the broad impact of ATM's function, although the underlying basis for some of these features has remained unclear for the 20 intervening years since *ATM's* identification. The enormous size of the protein (370 kDa) and transcript created limitations for analysis but sequencing revealed the gene to be a member of the phosphatidyl inositol 3-kinase-like kinase (PIKK) superfamily, similar to the DNA dependent protein kinase catalytic subunit (DNA-PKcs), which had been identified several years earlier. For many years, the enigma of A-T cell lines was that, despite their dramatic radiosensitivity, they were largely proficient in the repair of DNA double strand breaks (DSBs) but showed a phenotype called radioresistant DNA synthesis (RDS), representing a failure to shut down replication following exposure to ionising radiation (IR) (Painter 1981). Subsequently, a key concept in understanding ATM's function was the demonstration that ATM activates a mammalian cell cycle checkpoint pathway involving p53 (Kastan et al. 1992). The identification of ATM as a kinase and the evidence that, like DNA-PKcs, it is a protein kinase rather than a lipid kinase, provided fuel to consolidate the notion that ATM regulates a signal transduction pathway. Substantial intervening studies have shown that ATM signalling is activated by DSBs, explaining the marked sensitivity of A-T cells to agents, including IR, that induce DSBs. However, this simple notion is now being challenged with current models proposing that other lesions or stresses can also activate ATM. In the 20 intervening years since *ATM's* identification, we have gained enormous insight into its function. Yet fundamental questions remain and we have little understanding of the basis underlying A-T's most dramatic feature, progressive ataxia. In this chapter, a summary of the progress made in understanding ATM function, particularly of relevance to its role in tumour suppression, will be presented. In ensuing chapters, discussion will be made as to how this insight can be exploited for translational benefit for cancer therapy.

6.2   Domains and Structure of the ATM Kinase

As a PIKK family member, ATM has a conserved PI3K domain at its C-terminus (Fig. 6.1). However, unlike PI3K lipid kinases, PIKK family members additionally have a conserved FRAP-ATM-TRAPP (FAT) and a FAT carboxy-terminus (FATC) domain, which confers protein kinase activity (Lovejoy and Cortez 2009). The FAT domain, which lies adjacent and N-terminal to the kinase domain, consists of HEAT (**H**untintin, **E**longation factor 3, **A** subunit of protein phosphatase 2A and **TOR**1) repeats. There are further HEAT repeats throughout the N-terminal part of all PIKK proteins, which occur in linear arrays and can consist of more than 50 repeat units (Perry and Kleckner 2003). There is also a PIKK-regulatory domain (PRD) between

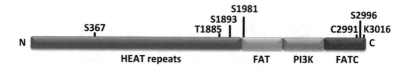

Fig. 6.1 Domain structure of ATM. The figure highlights domains and sites important for ATM function. S367, T1885, S1893, S1981 and S2996 are autophosphorylation sites; phosphorylation of S1981 is required to activate ATM via dimer dissociation. C2991 undergoes disulphide bridge formation and is required for activation following oxidative stress. K3016 undergoes TIP60-dependent acetylation, which enhances ATM activation

the kinase and FATC domain. The HEAT repeats form superhelical scaffolding structures which promote protein interactions (Perry and Kleckner 2003). They also provide an elastic, flexible structure, rendering the protein responsive to mechanical signalling by linking force with catalysis (Grinthal et al. 2010). However, despite these insights into ATM structure based on the sequence, additional structural information is still limited.

6.3   Hierarchical Regulation of ATM Signalling and Protein Assembly at DSBs

Although ATM recruitment and retention at DSBs represent the first steps in ATM-dependent signalling, the complexity of proteins associating at DSBs needs to be understood to comprehend these early steps. Therefore, we will commence with an overview of the choreography of protein recruitment at DSBs and how it leads to irradiation-induced foci (IRIF) formation (Fig. 6.2).

H2AX represents one of the earliest ATM substrates following ATM's recruitment and activation. H2AX is phosphorylated at Serine 139 and the spreading of phosphorylation at H2AX away for the DSB site creates the renowned γH2AX foci, which are often used as a marker for DSB formation and repair (Lobrich et al. 2010). pS139-H2AX (H2AX phosphorylated at the ATM-dependent site; γH2AX represents pS139-H2AX), serves to recruit the mediator of damage-checkpoint 1 (MDC1/NFBD1, hereafter called MDC1), the first of the mediator proteins that assemble at DSBs (Stucki et al. 2005). MDC1 recruitment occurs via its BRCT repeat domain, a characterised phosphorylation binding motif. ATM then phosphorylates MDC1 on its TQXF motifs, promoting binding of the E3 ubiquitin ligase, RNF8, via its FHA domain (Huen et al. 2007; Mailand et al. 2007). RNF8, together with another E3 ligase, RNF168, which is recruited downstream of RNF8, ubiquitylate H2A in the flanking chromatin, facilitating assembly of BRCA1 and 53BP1, two additional mediator proteins. 53BP1 is a reader of mononucleosomes containing histone H4 dimethylated at lysine20 (H4K20 Me^2), which it binds via its Tudor domain. H4K20 Me^2 residues become exposed at DSBs following proteasome-dependent degradation of the H4K20Me^2 binding protein, KDM4A/JMJD2A in an RNF8/RNF168-dependent

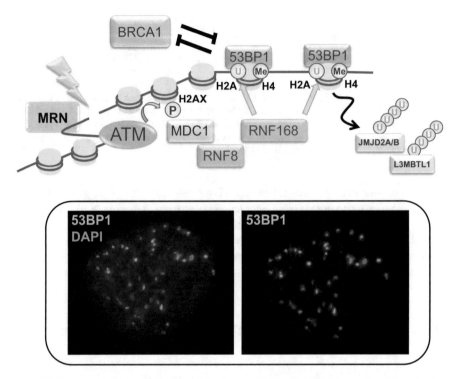

Fig. 6.2 Steps in radiation induced foci formation. Following DSB formation after IR, the MRE11/RAD50/NBS1 (MRN) complex rapidly senses and binds DSB ends, promoting ATM activation. ATM phosphorylates S139 H2AX. Phosphorylated H2AX recruits MDC1, a mediator protein, promoting the recruitment of two ubiquitin ligases, RNF8 and RNF168. RNF8/168 ubiquitylates histone H2A as well as JMJD2A/B and L3MBTL1. Ubiquitylated JMJD2A/B and L3MBTL1 is degraded and released from chromatin, promoting the exposure of dimethylated H4 K20 (H4K20 Me^2). 53BP1 binds to nucleosomes via RNF168-dependent ubiquitylation of H2A (H2AK15ub) and H4K20Me^2. The presence of 53BP1 suppresses the recruitment of BRCA1, with its final recruitment to chromatin being influenced by additional factors (not shown). 53BP1 inhibits resection and BRCA1 counteracts this inhibitory effect. Thus, the balance between NHEJ and HR seems to be regulated by the competition between 53BP1 and BRCA1

manner (Mallette et al. 2012). 53BP1 recruitment is also promoted by interaction with H2AK15ub via its ubiquitination-dependent recruitment (UDR) motif (Fradet-Turcotte et al. 2013). H2AK15ub is also effected by RNF8. RNF8-dependent ubiquitylation of MDC1 also recruits RAP80-BRCA1 to DSBs, which occurs most robustly in S and G2 phase (Watanabe et al. 2013). Interestingly, mice and cells expressing S139A-H2AX, which fail to undergo phosphorylation show radiosensitivity and genomic instability although they are less sensitive than mice and cell lines lacking ATM, demonstrating that the ability to form γH2AX foci is important but that ATM has additional functions (Celeste et al. 2002).

6.4   ATM Recruitment, Activation and Retention at DSBs

ATM does not have strong DNA binding capacity but is recruited and tethered at DSBs by several factors, which act independently and in concert. For DSBs induced by agents such as IR, the most significant DSB sensor that recruits ATM is the MRE11/RAD50/NBS1 (MRN) complex (Fig. 6.3) (Uziel et al. 2003). Patients with hypomorphic mutations in MRE11 display ataxia telangiectasia like disorder (ATLD), a disorder with features milder than, but overlapping with, A-T (Stewart et al. 1999). Whilst this demonstrates that MRE11 is intimately involved in ATM-dependent signalling, its precise role is unclear, in part due to the fact that the syndrome caused by mutations in NBS1, Nijmegen Breakage Syndrome (NBS), has a somewhat distinct clinical presentation (International Nijmegen Breakage Syndrome Study Group 2000). In 2003, ATLD cell lines were shown to have reduced ATM-dependent substrate phosphorylation, suggesting that MRN activates ATM

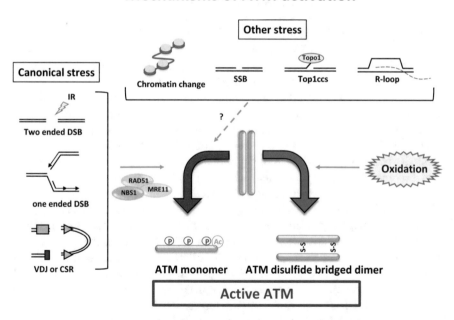

Fig. 6.3 Mechanisms of ATM activation. The mechanism of ATM activation at DSBs (called canonical stress) has been well described and involves the MRN complex, dimer to monomer formation and p1981-ATM autophosphorylation. At two ended DSBs, spreading of the ATM signal away from the DSB end occurs via γH2AX, MDC1, RNF8, RNF168 and 53BP1. ATM has also been shown to be activated by disulphide bond formation from oxidative damage to ATM protein. Although several disulphide bonds form after treatment of ATM with H_2O_2, Cys2991 is essential for ATM activation, and the process is MRN-independent. Finally, there is provocative evidence that ATM can be activated without DSB formation following transcription arrest, Top1cc formation, impeded SSB repair or chromatin changes

(Uziel et al. 2003). Subsequently, the Paull laboratory substantiated this model demonstrating that MRN binds DSB ends, recruits inactive ATM dimers which drives ATM monomerization and activation (Lee and Paull 2005). The recruitment of ATM by MRN involves an interaction between ATM and a conserved motif in the NBS1 C-terminus. This motif also regulates KU80-DNA-PKcs and ATR-ATRIP interactions, two other protein complexes that can influence DNA repair (Falck et al. 2005; You et al. 2005). One model for this process postulates the generation of single stranded DNA (ssDNA) by MRN-dependent unwinding of DNA ends although such a model is difficult to reconcile with the rapidity of Ku recruitment to DSB ends and its function in end-protection, since Ku recruitment and ATM activation appear to occur in unison at all DSBs. The lack of, or less demanding, requirement for NBS1 could be due to the presence of ATM-interacting protein (ATMIN), a protein, which, in some situations, has an overlapping function with NBS1 (Zhang et al. 2012; Kanu and Behrens 2007). As mentioned above, ATM is predominantly held as an inactive dimer in undamaged cells via binding of the kinase domain of one molecule to the FAT domain of another (Bakkenist and Kastan 2003; Du et al. 2014). Following IR, there is rapid intermolecular autophosphorylation on S1981, promoting dimer dissociation. Additional ATM autophosphorylation sites have been reported and some residues (S367 and S1893) also contribute to ATM activation (Kozlov et al. 2006). However, serine to alanine mutation of the equivalent sites in mice do not influence ATM activation (Daniel et al. 2008). In addition to this well characterised route of ATM activation, there is increasing evidence that ATM can be activated via routes that do not involve DSBs (see below).

Whilst MRN initiates ATM activation, there is also a cascade process that enhances MRN retention at DSBs, thereby increasing retention of active ATM at DSBs, leading to ATM foci formation. This process promotes the spreading of histone modifications at increasing distances from the DSB, giving rise to defined pH2AX foci (γH2AX foci). Following initial ATM activation, MDC1 is recruited and becomes hyperphosphorylated, which, in addition to promoting interaction with RNF8, also facilitates interaction with MRE11 via MDC1's forkhead associated (FHA) and BRCT domains (Goldberg et al. 2003). Additionally, NBS1 binds to MDC1 in a damage dependent manner via NBS1's FHA domain (Lukas et al. 2004). Whilst these interactions are not essential for ATM activation, they increase its retention at DSBs and are required for efficient cell cycle checkpoint arrest. The retention of active ATM around the DSB allows the phosphorylation of more distal H2AX, the recruitment of MDC1 at more distal sites, and hence the stepwise enlargement of IRIF (Lukas et al. 2004). A further and distinct step in MRN recruitment involves an interaction between the RAD50 component of MRN and the BRCT domains of the downstream mediator protein, 53BP1, in a phosphorylation-independent manner, thereby further promoting the recruitment of MRN complexes at DSBs (Lee et al. 2010). This distinct step is critical for the formation of detectable p1981-ATM foci and is required for specific ATM substrate phosphorylation events, such as discrete pKAP-1 foci (see further discussion below) (Noon et al. 2010). Consistent with this model, a genetic analysis of factors involved in interactions with MRN reveal distinct steps influencing the level of NBS1 at DSBs; a basal level detectable in cells lacking H2AX, a further layer which is MDC1/RNF8 dependent and a final layer which is 53BP1 dependent (Noon et al. 2010).

A discussion of factors regulating ATM recruitment and activation would not be completed without mention of TIP60-dependent acetylation. TIP60, an acetyltransferase, acetylates ATM at K3016, a residue within ATM's conserved FATC domain (Sun et al. 2007). Mutation of K3016 reduces ATM monomerisation and substrate phosphorylation. In undamaged cells, TIP60 is complexed with the transcription factor, ATF2 and the E3 ubiquitin ligase, Cul3, and Cul3-dependent ubiquitylation of TIP60 promotes its proteasome mediated degradation (Bhoumik et al. 2008). Following DNA damage, TIP60 degradation is disturbed allowing ATM acetylation. Further, at DSBs TIP60 interacts with H3K9me3 via its chromodomain, which promotes TIP60 acetylation activity, thereby further stimulating ATM acetylation and activation (Sun et al. 2010). The regulation of ATM via acetylation, however, appears to modulate activation rather than being an essential factor.

6.5 ATM Activation in the Absence of DSB Formation

6.5.1 ATM Activation by Oxidative Stress

For many years, ATM was thought to be solely activated by DSBs. However, this simplistic view was challenged initially by the demonstration that ATM can be activated and phosphorylate specific substrates in a pan-nuclear manner by agents that perturb chromatin structure, such as hypotonic buffer or chloroquine, without DSB formation, γH2AX phosphorylation or pS1981-ATM foci formation (Bakkenist and Kastan 2015). There is now an emerging consensus that ATM can be endogenously activated at a low level compared to its hyperactivation at DSBs. Such a model is consistent with some clinical features of A-T patients, which suggest developmental roles for ATM that do not correlate with DSB formation.

A range of findings have provided evidence that A-T cells and patients are oxidatively stressed and that ATM has a central role in regulating the cellular redox status (Fig. 6.3) (Barzilai et al. 2002; Kamsler et al. 2001; Takao et al. 2000). One underlying mechanism is that ATM regulates the expression of several antioxidants. Other studies have shown that ATM localises with the anti-oxidant, catalase, in the cytoplasm in peroxisomes, raising the possibility that ATM can sense and respond to oxidative stress (Watters et al. 1999). This raises the question whether ATM is activated by stress induced DNA damage or directly senses the cellular redox status in a DNA-damage independent manner. A significant finding in this context was the observation that ATM can be directly activated by reactive oxygen species (ROS) damage (Guo et al. 2010). The underlying mechanism is genetically and structurally distinct to the DSB-dependent process, requiring a Cysteine-2991 residue in the C-terminus of ATM rather than S-1981. Furthermore, MRE11 is dispensable for ROS-induced ATM activation. At the structural level, the process involves the formation of covalent homodimers of ATM via intermolecular disulphide bond formation, a mechanism distinct to the disruption of constitutive dimers into monomers as occurs following DSB-induced activation. Interestingly, a recent report described how ATM in mice can be activated in immature vessels due to ROS accumulation (Okuno et al. 2012). Failure to activate this process by global or endothelial-specific ATM inactivation prevented pathological neoangiogenesis in the retina, via a process that correlated with ROS levels and mitogen activated kinase p38α. Such a model confers a critical role for ATM in oxidative defence distinct from a response to DSBs.

A somewhat distinct DSB-independent role for ATM is its regulation of carbon metabolism. Recent studies have shown that ATM can modulate the metabolic flux from glycolysis to the pentose phosphate pathway (PPP) by phosphorylation of Hsp27, which binds to glucose-6-phosphate dehydrogenase (G6PD) (Cosentino et al. 2011; Kruger and Ralser 2011). The PPP pathway regulates the production of NADPH, an essential anti-oxidant. This process insinuates ATM as a regulator of glucose metabolism with a direct link to oxidative stress. It was proposed that this role for ATM may directly influence its role in DNA repair, both by stimulating NADPH production and promoting the synthesis of nucleotides required for DSB repair (Cosentino et al. 2011). Whilst there is indirect evidence for links between these alternative roles of ATM and its function during the DDR, it remains unclear whether they involve DSB-induced ATM activation and are a component of a master strategy to deal with DSBs, or whether there is a distinct role for ATM in regulating metabolism (involving DSB-independent ATM activation). A role for ATM in metabolism is consistent with the A-T clinical presentation, where there is evidence for metabolic abnormalities, including an enhanced frequency of type-II diabetes in A-T patients, and a mechanistic link between ATM and insulin regulation (Schalch et al. 1970; Yang and Kastan 2000). Further, A-T patients have constitutively reduced expression of Insulin like Growth Factor-1 receptor (IGF1-R), which has a strong association with metabolic syndrome. Finally, a further aspect which may correlate with ATM's role in stress response signalling and ATM's metabolic function is mitochondria dysfunction, a feature consistently reported in A-T cells (Eaton et al. 2007). However, it remains unclear whether the mitochondria abnormalities arise as a consequence of an abnormal redox balance or cause it. Clearly there is a complex relationship which requires further defining. Furthermore, the contribution of these factors in the response to DNA damage needs to be clarified. The impact of ATM inhibitors on mitochondrial function is also an important aspect to consider when using such inhibitors for cancer therapy.

6.5.2   ATM Activation by Other DNA Lesions

Intriguingly, a recent study reported ATM activation by transcription blocking lesions following UV treatment (Tresini et al. 2015). The proposed model is that R-loop formation, which arises following RNA polymerase pausing at DNA lesions, activates ATM, which affects spliceosome organisation and alternative splicing at a genome wide level. This important finding could be significant if promoted by a wider range of DNA lesions, since the neuronal cells most affected in A-T patients are highly transcriptionally active. It will also be important to define the mechanism by which ATM is activated by R-loops.

There is also recent provocative evidence that ATM can be activated by single strand breaks (SSBs) or another non-DSB lesion or that ATM is endogenously activated and influences SSB repair. Such a role for ATM could be clinically relevant since progressive ataxia, a profound feature of A-T patients, arises in patients defective in components of the SSB repair machinery and is not a general consequence of impeded DSB repair (McKinnon 2012). In one study, ATM was shown to regulate the stability of Topoisomerase I (Top1) cleavable complexes (Top1cc), trapped Top1-DNA complexes, which arise during normal cell growth, by precluding Top1 SUMO/ubiquitin mediated turnover (Katyal et al. 2014). Intriguingly, this role was not dependent on ATM kinase activity. However, the same study demonstrated that ATM was activated by camptothecin-induced Top1ccs in quiescent cells, when DSBs do not form, and in an MRN-independent manner, suggesting a route for ATM activation distinct to canonical DSB-induced activation. Another study provided evidence that ATM can be activated by SSBs persisting in SSB repair deficient cells and promote checkpoint arrest (Khoronenkova and Dianov 2015). This provocative study provides evidence that ATM has a critical role in regulating SSB repair capacity, although to date ATM cells have not been observed to have an SSB repair defect. It is possible that these findings can be explained by the activation of ATM at R-loops, which could arise if transcription is impeded by SSBs.

Finally, a recent study suggested that ATM can be activated at a one-ended DSB generated by fork regression following replication fork stalling (Fugger et al. 2015). FBH1 is a helicase that promotes stalled fork regression, generating a chicken foot structure. FBH1 activity at stalled forks activated ATM signalling and subsequent CHK2 phosphorylation, an ATM-specific substrate, and downstream checkpoint signalling. Although such fork regression generates a structure that represents a one-ended DSB, which is not conceptually distinct from an IR-induced DSB, such a process is significant in demonstrating ATM activation without DNA breakage *per se*, and widens the role of ATM to encompass replication fork recovery.

Collectively, these findings are provocative in suggesting that ATM can be activated by more diverse lesions or mechanisms than the canonical process at DSBs (summarised in Fig. 6.2). Such a response could contribute to the unexplained mechanism underlying the progressive ataxia of A-T patients.

6.6 Consequences of ATM Dependent Signalling at DSBs

6.6.1 Chromatin Changes at the DSB

Chromatin is organised in states that range from highly compacted (e.g. heterochromatic DNA) through to decompacted or open states (e.g. transcribed sequences). Highly compacted chromatin is normally transcriptionally repressed. ATM promotes substantial modification to histones (phosphorylation, methylation, ubiquitylation, sumoylation and neddylation) in the DSB vicinity, with some of these modifications, such as ubiquitylation, directly affecting histone compaction. Further, such modifications can promote protein recruitment at DSBs, including chromatin modelling complexes, which modify the chromatin structure around the DSB. The role of chromatin remodelling complexes at DSBs is complex and still poorly understood at a mechanistic level. Since several reviews are available, the role of chromatin remodellers will only be discussed here where a functional role has been defined (Jeggo and Downs 2014; Seeber et al. 2013).

A range of studies have demonstrated that both compaction and decompaction of chromatin occur in the DSB vicinity. It is likely that this arises in a temporal and proximity-dependent manner, although details remain unclear. Localised chromatin relaxation and histone eviction has been well described (Berkovich et al. 2007; Kruhlak et al. 2006; Ziv et al. 2006). More recent studies have also provided evidence for chromatin compaction at DSBs. One approach using procedures to monitor compaction/expansion at site specific DSBs concluded that there was initial chromatin relaxation followed by condensation, with repression being necessary for DDR signalling (Burgess et al. 2014). Other studies, however, have provided evidence for the early recruitment of repressive factors to DSBs including KAP-1, HP1, SUV39-1 (Ziv et al. 2006; Baldeyron et al. 2011; Ayrapetov et al. 2014). Together these factors enhance the level of H3K9me3 in the DSB vicinity and promote localised repressive chromatin (Fig. 6.4). These factors also activate

Impact of ATM on the fidelity of DNA repair

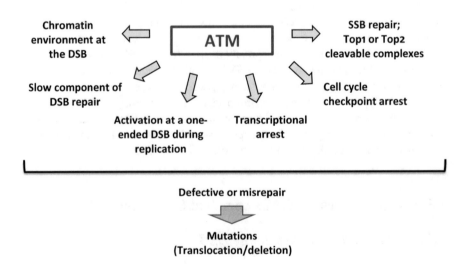

Fig. 6.4 Ways in which ATM can influence the fidelity of DNA repair. ATM influences a range of processes that can directly or indirectly affect the fidelity of DNA repair. The role of ATM in the slow component of DSB repair results in a DSB repair defect but this could result in the formation of translocations, deletions or rearrangements following replication. Similarly ATM's role in the other processes highlighted may enhance the opportunity for mis-repair events or, as in the case of checkpoint arrest, compromise the opportunity for accurate repair

TIP60 acetyl transferase activity, enhancing ATM activation as discussed above (Ayrapetov et al. 2014). However, the models from these two approaches, though overlapping in arguing for chromatin compaction at DSBs, differ in the timing of when repression occurs. The former study argues for initial relaxation followed by compression; the later finds the recruitment of repressive factors occurs at an early stage with subsequent localised dismantling of the compacted state to promote relaxation, which is required for DSB repair.

6.6.2 Influence of ATM and DDR Signalling on DNA Repair

6.6.2.1 Role for ATM in the Slow Process of DSB Repair

The two major DSB repair mechanisms are canonical DNA non-homologous end-joining (c-NHEJ) and homologous recombination (HR), with c-NHEJ occurring in all cell cycle phases and HR functioning solely in S/G2 phase, where a sister chromatid is available. These processes have been described previously and will not be detailed here (Jasin and Rothstein 2013; Lieber 2010). Of relevance here is that c-NHEJ represents a compact process that does not require extensive homology, and most likely little chromatin decompaction. Indeed, the process involves simply the binding of DNA-PK to the DSB ends, followed by the recruitment of a ligation complex (XRCC4/XLF/DNA ligase IV and potentially PAXX). Depending on the nature of the DSB end, some end processing is likely required. c-NHEJ proceeds via two overlapping but distinct processes, which differ in kinetics and genetic requirements. Following IR, ~80% of DSBs are repaired with fast kinetics via an ATM-independent process that requires the c-NHEJ proteins (Ku, DNA-PKcs, XRCC4, XLF, DNA ligase IV and PAXX). However, a sub-fraction of DSBs (15–20%) are rejoined via a slower process that, in addition to c-NHEJ proteins, requires ATM, the mediator proteins (H2AX, MDC1, RNF8, RNF168 and 53BP1) and the nuclease, Artemis. This finding of a subtle repair defect in A-T cells was consistent with earlier chromosomal studies examining chromosome breakage and rejoining of prematurely condensed chromosomes in G1 phase A-T cells, where the rate of DSB rejoining was similar to that in control cells whilst the fraction of unrejoined DSBs was greater (Cornforth and Bedford 1985). The DSBs repaired with slow kinetics have been argued to represent those located at regions of heterochromatin (HC) with the role of ATM correlating with its phosphorylation of KAP-1 at S824. Further, relaxation of the HC superstructure by siRNA-mediated depletion of compacting factors, including KAP-1, bypasses the need for ATM for DSB repair. A model proposed is that HC acts as a barrier to c-NHEJ and ATM-dependent HC relaxation is required for HC-DSB repair to ensue but it is also possible that chromatin compaction could take place during the repair process. These possible models, however, do not explain the requirement for Artemis in the slow rejoining process, particularly since depletion of compacting factors does not relieve the need for Artemis for HC-DSB repair. It has, therefore, been argued that DSBs which are not rapidly rejoined by c-NHEJ, due, for example, to a barrier created by chromatin compaction, undergo limited end resection prior to rejoining by c-NHEJ. Indeed, the slow process of DSB rejoining in G1 phase cells has recently been shown to involve resection factors (as well as the nuclease, Artemis) and has been called resection-dependent c-NHEJ (Biehs et al. 2017). This process may utilise small regions of microhomology and thus represent a form of microhomology mediated end-joining (MMEJ) but it should not be confused with Alt-NHEJ, which also uses microhomology, but involves DNA ligase I/III as opposed to DNA ligase IV, which functions during c-NHEJ. Another factor influencing both the kinetics of repair and genetic factor requirement is the complexity of the DNA end. Indeed, the repair of DSBs induced by high linear energy transfer (LET) radiation, such as carbon ions, which are known to occur with slow kinetics, has a greater requirement for Artemis, consistent with the notion that there is a switch to a resection-dependent process if c-NHEJ does not rapidly occur. It should also be noted that nearly all assays that monitor NHEJ involve some form of mis-rejoining (e.g. small deletions) since accurate rejoining merely reconstitutes the original restriction site. It is possible that this type of assay monitors the slow DSB rejoining process rather than the fast process that does not involve any defined resection factors. Of relevance in the context of chromatin changes is the likelihood that the slow DSB repair process involving Artemis may require a greater level of chromatin opening than the compact process of core NHEJ.

As mentioned above, the slow process of DSB repair in G1 phase also requires ATM dependent signalling proteins, including MRN, H2AX, MDC1, RNF8/RNF168 and 53BP1. 53BP1 is essential for the visualisation of p1981-ATM foci at DSBs suggesting that it is a critical late step in promoting ATM retention at DSBs. The requirement for the mediator proteins for the slow component of DSB repair, therefore, may reflect their role in recruiting and retaining 53BP1. This has led to the model that 53BP1-dependent ATM retention at DSBs is required for localised, concentrated p824 KAP-1 foci formation and subsequent HC relaxation. Consistent with this model, p824 KAP-1 foci are ATM and 53BP1-dependent although pan nuclear KAP-1 phosphorylation at S824 requires only ATM.

In summary, ATM is dispensable for the core process of NHEJ and, *vice versa*, ATM-dependent signalling occurs in cells lacking NHEJ proteins. However, cells lacking ATM activity have a repair defect due to a failure to carry out the slow DSB repair process (Fig. 6.3). The available data suggest that this role for ATM represents its ability to modify the chromatin structure at a subset of DSBs, most likely at those DSBs that are in pre-existing HC regions or at regions that become repressed and HC-like during the DDR. This role of ATM requires its sustained tethering at DSBs; hence ATM has a role in promoting 53BP1 foci formation as well as in p824 KAP-1 foci formation.

6.6.2.2 Impact of ATM in the Repair of DSBs in the Vicinity of Active Transcription

There is mounting recognition that DNA transactions such as transcription and replication can hinder DSB repair and that, *vice versa*, unrepaired DSBs can impede such metabolic processes. RNA polymerase I (Pol1)-dependent transcription is transiently repressed in a genome wide manner following exposure to genotoxic stress, via a process dependent upon ATM, NBS1 and MDC1 (Kruhlak et al. 2007). Further, although genome wide Pol II transcription is not inhibited, there is evidence for localised repression. Greenberg et al. established an elegant system to examine transcription in the vicinity of DSBs and revealed an ATM-dependent process that uniquely silences Pol II-dependent transcription flanking DSBs (Fig. 6.3) (Shanbhag et al. 2010). Subsequent analysis showed that failure to arrest transcription enhances DSB levels in a transcription dependent manner, suggesting impeded DSB repair (Kakarougkas et al. 2014). Significantly, this process additionally requires the BAF180 and BRG1 components of the remodelling complex, PBAF, as well as the PRC1 and PRC2 subunits of the polycomb group complex, and H2A K119 ubiqui-tylation. ATM phosphorylates a unique site on BAF180. Additionally, the transcrip-tional elongation factor, ENL is phosphorylated by ATM at conserved SQ sites, which promotes an interaction between ENL and PRC1 and subsequent H2A K119 ubiquitylation (Ui et al. 2015). Loss of these steps ablates transcriptional silencing in the proximity of DSBs. Thus, ATM appears to exert two distinct functions in Pol II DSB-dependent transcriptional repression. It is noteworthy that the role of ATM in Pol II transcriptional silencing does not require factors downstream of RNF8 but rather a specific set of proteins (PBAF, PRC1 and PRC2), which, although inducing H2A K119 ubiquitylation at all DSBs, only exerts a function at DSBs in transcrip-tionally active regions. Thus, the repair of specific DSBs (e.g. those close to tran-scriptionally active regions or in HC regions) require specific ATM-dependent chromatin modifications. It is noteworthy that these experiments were undertaken in G1 cells, arguing that DSBs in the vicinity of transcriptionally active genes can be repaired by NHEJ (the only repair process in G1 phase). A distinct study has reported that DSBs induced in active genes enriched in H3K36me3 are specifically repaired by HR in a manner dependent upon the trimethyltransferase, SETD2, suggesting that repair pathway usage can be regulated by transcriptional status (Clouaire and Legube 2015).

6.6.2.3 Role for ATM in HR at a Two-Ended DSB

NHEJ is a compact process. HR, in contrast, demands that DNA end-processing extends a substantial distance from the DSB, which most likely involves histone eviction or sliding and/or histone modifications over a substantial distance. In brief, HR involves the initiation and elongation of resection, engagement of the ssDNA with the sister homologue, replacement of RPA, which coats the ssDNA, with RAD51 and generation of a heteroduplex. Fill in of the resected DNA, including regenerating any sequence information lost at the DSB, occurs using the undam-aged strand as a template. HR is completed following branch migration and resolu-tion of the Holliday junction formed when the strands cross over. As stated above, in mammalian cells, HR only functions in the presence of a sister homologue restricting the process to S/G2 phase. HR has its major role in S phase cells to pro-mote replication fork restart following fork stalling/collapse, where the lesion pro-moting HR may be a one-ended DSB or ssDNA (Petermann and Helleday 2010).

In contrast, HR has only a minor function in the repair of direct IR-induced DSBs. Thus, in G2 phase fibroblasts from normal individuals, where both HR and NHEJ can function, the majority of DSBs are repaired by NHEJ with only a subset of 10–15% DSBs undergoing repair by HR (Beucher et al. 2009). Similar to the slow component of DSB repair in G1 phase (which requires NHEJ proteins), the DSBs that undergo repair by HR in G2 phase appear to be HC-DSBs (Shibata et al. 2011). Given these findings, it has been proposed that NHEJ represents the first choice of pathway for DSB repair in G1 and G2 phase but, if NHEJ is transiently stalled or slowed, then repair proceeds by a resection mediated NHEJ pathway in G1 phase and by HR in G2 phase (following more robust resection than in G1 phase) (Shibata et al. 2014; Jeggo and Lobrich 2015). Whilst ATM appears to be dispensable for HR in S phase, it is required for the initiating step of resection at DSBs in G2 phase (Fig. 6.3). CtIP is essential for the initiation of 5′ to 3′ resection and ATM phosphorylates CtIP at S664/745 (Shibata et al. 2011; Li et al. 2000). Since HR occurs at HC-DSBs in G2 phase, ATM has an additional role in phosphorylating S824 KAP-1 to relax the HC similar to its role in the slow repair component in G1 phase (Noon et al. 2010; Shibata et al. 2011). Expression of S664A/S745A CtIP does not prevent ATM dependent pKAP-1 formation but DSB repair in G2 proceeds by NHEJ rather than HR due to a failure to initiate resection (Shibata et al. 2011).

Interestingly, as resection ensues, ATR becomes activated at ssDNA regions, promoting a switch from ATM to ATR signalling (Shiotani and Zou 2009). Thus, ATM is required for the initiation of resection at two-ended DSBs but may be dispensable for later steps due to ATR activation. Moreover, resection or ssDNA can arise in a distinct manner at lesions arising following replication fork stalling/collapse, explaining the lack of an essential role for ATM for HR in S phase (Petermann and Helleday 2010).

6.6.2.4 Requirement for Chromatin Compaction During HR

As mentioned above, IRIF promote ATM retention at DSBs, a prerequisite for pKAP-1 foci formation and HC-DSB repair by NHEJ in G1 and HR in G2 phase (Shibata et al. 2011). IRIF also promotes localised chromatin relaxation. However, as also discussed above, compacting factors, including KAP-1, SUV39H1/H2, SETDB1 and HP1 are also recruited to DSBs (Baldeyron et al. 2011; Ayrapetov et al. 2014; Alagoz et al. 2015). The recruitment of these factors appears to be dispensable for NHEJ but obligatory for HR. Since siRNA-mediated depletion of these factors results in enhanced sister chromatid separation assessed using a centromeric marker in undamaged cells, a model has been presented whereby the recruitment of repressive factors promotes engagement of the damaged strand with the undamaged sister chromatid (Alagoz et al. 2015). Consistent with this proposal, siRNA mediated depletion of repressive factors allows the initiation but reduces the extension of resection, impairs RAD51 loading and abolishes the completion of HR at two-ended DSBs in G2 phase (Alagoz et al. 2015). Verification that engagement with the sister homologue is impaired, however, awaits the development of novel technology. Notwithstanding the precise role of chromatin compaction during HR, the evidence that repressive factors are recruited to DSBs is compelling.

Another step that appears to be critical for HR is the appropriate regulation of H2A.Z, another variant form of histone H2A. In undamaged cells, nucleosomes containing H2A.Z are located at some transcriptional start sites but H2A.Z also functions during the DNA damage response in a process involving the INO80 family of chromatin remodelling enzymes. Significantly, H2A.Z is recruited to DSBs in a TIP60 dependent manner, promoting the recruitment of NHEJ factors and restricting resection (Xu et al. 2012). However, the recruitment of H2A.Z at chromatin flanking DSBs is transient, with H2A.Z being rapidly removed via a process dependent upon INO80 and the histone chaperone ANP32E, which is known to function in removal of H2A.Z from chromatin. Significantly, the failure to remove H2A.Z by siRNA of INO80 or ANP32E partially diminishes RAD51 foci formation and confers a marked HR defect assessed by sister chromatid exchange (SCE) formation. Both these steps were rescued by H2A.Z co-depletion i.e. a situation where H2A.Z is not deposited at DSBs. This model is consistent with the notion that H2A.Z is initially recruited to DSBs to help promote NHEJ, the first choice DSB repair pathway, by inhibiting resection. However, to switch to HR, H2AZ must be removed by INO80 and ANP32E (Alatwi and Downs 2015). Significantly, other chromatin remodelling complexes have been reported to be required for HR (Jeggo and Downs 2014; Seeber et al. 2013) consistent with the notion that HR requires a greater level of chromatin remodelling than NHEJ. However, mechanistic details of the role played by these remodelling complexes remains unclear.

6.6.3 ATM-Dependent Cell Cycle Checkpoint Arrest After DNA Damage

The concept of cell cycle checkpoint arrest, whereby DNA damage promotes arrest of cell cycle progression from one phase to the next, or, indeed, progression through a cell cycle phase, has been appreciated for many years. Significantly, the RDS phenotype of A-T was described in the early 1980s, although its significance was obscure (Painter 1981). In late 1980/early 1990, work progressed apace on the role of p53 in the response to DNA damage and in 1992, the seminal observation was made that A-T cells fail to appropriately activate a p53-dependent cell cycle checkpoint arrest after IR, although such arrest was proficient after other forms of DNA damage (Kastan et al. 1992). This was significant in identifying p53 as a determinant of the DNA damage checkpoint response as well as defining A-T as a checkpoint disorder. Since A-T cells are dramatically radiosensitive but failed to show any marked DSB repair deficiency, the finding argued that the checkpoint response was critical in determining radioresistance. Although we now appreciate that ATM regulates an extensive signalling response, and that the checkpoint defect plays only

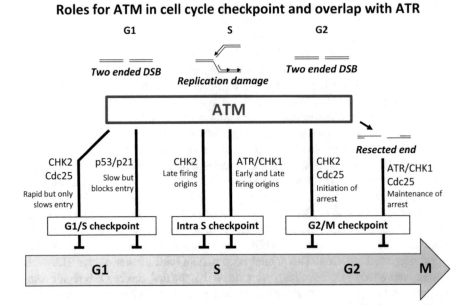

Fig. 6.5 Role of ATM in cell cycle checkpoint arrest and overlap with ATR. Processes shown are in response to ionising radiation. ATM regulates a fast process that slows entry into S phase, which is CHK2 and CDC25-dependent, and a slower p53/p21 dependent process which blocks S phase entry. ATM functions during S phase to arrest late firing origins, whilst ATR affects early and late firing origins. In G2 phase, ATM is activated at non-resected DSBs inducing CHK2/CDC25 checkpoint arrest. Following resection, ATR/CHK1 is activated, functioning with ATM to activate and maintain checkpoint arrest

a modest role in radiosensitivity, in the context of cancer onset and maintenance of genome stability the checkpoint response is important (Fig. 6.5).

Three major checkpoints have been described; G1-S, G2-M and intra-S phase arrest, with evidence for additional regulatory processes including, for example, a spindle checkpoint, which can halt progression through mitosis. These processes have been described previously and the discussion here will focus on the relevance to maintaining genomic stability.

6.6.3.1 G1/S Checkpoint Arrest

The IR-induced G1/S checkpoint is p53 dependent, with ATM phosphorylating both p53 and MDM2, the ubiquitin ligase that regulates p53 proteasome mediated degradation. Since p53 is frequently mutated in cancer, many cancer cells fail to activate G1/S checkpoint arrest. In brief, this process involves upregulation of the p53 substrate, p21, a cyclin-dependent kinase (CDK) inhibitor. For G1/S arrest, p21 inhibits CDK2, thereby preventing phosphorylation of retinoblastoma protein (Rb), which is required for release of the transcription factor, E2F (Wahl et al. 1997). The process is now known to activate arrest of progression through G1, rather than specifically arresting cells at the G1/S boundary (Deckbar et al. 2010, 2011). However, since there is a restriction point which commits to S phase entry once a threshold level of Rb phosphorylation has been reached, and since the activation of p21 requires transcription, a slow process, p53-dependent G1/S checkpoint arrest is not fully activated until 4–6 h post IR even after high doses (Deckbar et al. 2007). Additionally, arrest is not always efficiently maintained. These two factors provide limitations in the ability of the G1/S checkpoint to maintain genomic stability although this should not undermine the high efficiency of the process in preventing genomic instability. Importantly, activation of the checkpoint is highly sensitive being detectable after 100 mGy (Deckbar et al. 2010).

In addition to the well described p53-dependent process, the Bartek laboratory uncovered another process which arises at early times post IR, that delays rather than completely abolishes S phase entry (Bartek and Lukas 2001; Mailand et al. 2000). This process is ATM and CHK1/2 dependent but p53 independent. Akin to the activation of G2/M checkpoint arrest (see below), the process involves phosphorylation of the phosphatase CDC25A by the CHK1/2 kinases with subsequent inhibition of cyclin E-CDK2. Thus, a dual wave of responses leading to diminished S phase entry occurs in G1; an initial transient response dependent on CHK2 that is activated within 20–30 min and lasts several hours followed by a more slowly activated but sustained process involving p53/p21. Both processes are ATM dependent.

6.6.3.2 G2/M Arrest

The Lavin laboratory was pivotal in identifying a role for ATM in G2/M checkpoint arrest (Beamish and Lavin 1994; Lavin et al. 1994). Early studies demonstrated the failure of A-T cells to arrest mitotic entry at 1–2 h post IR, in contrast to control cells, via a process that involves ATM-dependent phosphorylation of the CDC25A, B and C phosphatases, which counterbalance the inhibitory tyrosine phosphorylation of CDK1. The CDC25 phosphatases are not direct ATM substrates but are phosphorylated by the transducer kinases, CHK1 or CHK2. At early times after IR, CHK2, a specific ATM substrate, is the most significant. Phosphorylation of the CDC25 phosphatases exerts several impacts including inhibition of their activity and degradation (Bartek and Lukas 2007). However, this early checkpoint response does not appear to be highly sensitive and is, in most cell types, only efficiently activated following exposure to doses of IR greater than 0.5 Gy (Deckbar et al. 2007). Nonetheless, this process has a significant impact on restricting genomic instability by preventing the progression of cells with DSBs into mitosis, where DSB repair is less efficient due to chromatin compaction. However, it does not have a major impact on radiation sensitivity, since it only affects the subset of cells in G2 phase at the time of IR. Interestingly, however, failure to undergo G2/M checkpoint arrest at low doses underlies the low dose radiation hypersensitivity phenotype, which reflects the hypersensitivity of a small subset of cells (those in G2 phase) at low doses (Krueger et al. 2010).

Finally, following the description of ATM-dependent G2/M checkpoint arrest, which can be detected 1–3 h post IR, it was recognised that at later times, A-T cells actually accumulate in G2. Such findings led to the description of two molecularly distinct processes effecting G2/M checkpoint arrest; an early ATM-dependent process activated by DSBs in G2 phase cells followed by a process detectable at later times post IR, when cells in S phase at the time of IR have progressed into G2 phase (Xu et al. 2002). This later process is ATR and CHK1-dependent. DSBs which fail to be appropriately repaired or replication-induced DSBs activate the ATR-dependent process. Thus, A-T cells show enhanced G2 accumulation at later times post IR.

6.6.3.3   Intra S Phase Arrest

As mentioned above, the concept of RDS, described in early 1980 was effectively the first description of a checkpoint defect in A-T cells (Painter 1981). Although the notion of a "checkpoint" was not well defined at that time, the finding revealed that A-T cells fail to shut down replication in the face of DNA damage. Two parallel ATM-dependent pathways contribute to RDS; one is NBS1-MRE11 dependent and the other CHK2-CDC25A-CDK2 dependent (Falck et al. 2002; Bartek et al. 2004). The latter process involves ATM-dependent phosphorylation of CHK2 and CHK2-dependent phosphorylation of CDC25A on S123, which prevents dephosphorylation of CDK2 (Falck et al. 2001). This prevents CDK2-dependent loading of CDC45 onto replication origins. ATM appears to predominantly regulate late firing origins (Bartek et al. 2004). ATR, which is activated following replication fork stalling, regulates a similar process during replication, with the two responses acting in concert to fully inhibit replication after IR (Bartek et al. 2004).

6.6.3.4   The Spindle Assembly Checkpoint

Recent studies have provided evidence for abnormalities in mitosis in A-T cells, with evidence of a defective spindle checkpoint (Takagi et al. 1998; Shigeta et al. 1999; Yang et al. 2011). Defects in metaphase to anaphase transition in A-T cells has also been reported to cause aneuploidy. Intriguingly, and consistent with the notion that ATM has roles outside of the DDR, a recent study showed that Aurora-B can phosphorylate and activate ATM during normal mitosis, and that this response is essential for the spindle assembly checkpoint (SAC) (Yang et al. 2011). This important finding adds to roles of ATM in undamaged cells, and provides a mechanism of ATM activation involving Aurora-B kinase.

6.6.4   Role of ATM in Activating Apoptosis

The identification of p53 as an ATM substrate implicated ATM in the regulation of damage induced apoptosis. As the number of ATM substrates has increased, ATM's role in regulating apoptosis broadened to encompass other direct substrates as well as pro-apoptotic genes transcriptionally regulated by p53.

Significantly, IR does not activate apoptosis in most normal, differentiated cells or tissues. Human fibroblasts, for example, do not undergo apoptosis even after high X-ray doses but rather succumb to prolonged G1-S arrest leading to senescence. Since fibroblasts readily activate p53, the fate of cell death after IR must be determined downstream of ATM and p53 activation. Certain tissues exploit apoptosis during development (e.g. cells with non-productive V(D)J rearrangements can be removed by apoptosis) (Lam et al. 2007). Specific stem cells also appear able to sensitively activate apoptosis both endogenously and after IR (e.g. stem or early progenitor cells in the crypt, embryonic neural and haematopoietic stem cells sensitively activate apoptosis endogenously and after IR) (Barazzuol et al. 2015; Ijiri and Potten 1986; Insinga et al. 2013). In these cases, such apoptosis is ATM dependent and can arise after exposure to low doses, conferring high radiosensitivity of these tissues.

ATM directly and indirectly (via p53) regulates pro-apoptotic proteins, including those belonging to the intrinsic, mitochondrial pathway and extrinsic, receptor-mediated apoptosis (Matt and Hofmann 2016). Such regulation will not be covered in depth here. Intriguingly, and of relevance here, is the observation that in certain situations ATM can regulate pro-survival pathways in contrast to apoptosis (Grosjean-Raillard et al. 2009). One such example is the ATM-dependent activation of NF-kB, which can occur in myelodysplastic syndromes and acute myeloid leukemia (AML). NF-kB activation can be stimulated by several ATM-dependent pathways, such as the activation of PIDD, a p53 inducible gene. Although NF-kB activation can have diverse consequences, when activated by ATM it can function as a pro-survival, anti-apoptotic transcription factor. Consequently, pharmacological inhibition of ATM can result in apoptosis in malignant myeloblasts, a feature which lies at the centre of a translational strategy for treating AML (Box 6.1) (Grosjean-Raillard et al. 2009). Such a role for ATM in malignant myeloblasts may arise due to its constitutive activation by oxidative or replicative stress in such cells.

Box 6.1 Potential exploitation of ATM inhibitors for cancer therapy

- Radiotherapy—targeted delivery of ATMi to tumours to enhance radiosensitisation.
- Enhancing the efficacy of agents such as etoposide by treating/preventing resistance to etoposide.
- Preventing NFKβ activation for AML treatment (see text and Grosjean-Raillard et al. 2009).
- Tumours with increased DSB levels particularly if arising separately from replication fork arrest (i.e. non ATR dependent).
- Synthetic lethality for tumours with mutations/expression changes in ATR.
- Synthetic lethality for tumours with mutations/expression changes in FA proteins (Kennedy et al. 2007).
- Synthetic lethality for tumours with mutations in XRCC1 (early breast and ovarian cancers) (Sultana et al. 2013).
- Synthetic lethality with BRCA1-BER deficient breast cancer (Albarakati et al. 2015).
- Other synthetic lethality for tumours with DDR defects.

6.7 Tumour Suppressor Function of ATM and Its Dysregulation in Cancer

The pronounced cancer predisposition of A-T patients provided the first evidence that ATM functions as a tumour suppressor gene. This notion was substantiated by the downregulation of ATM and identification of ATM mutations in tumours, especially breast cancer and chronic lymphoid leukaemia (Lin et al. 2016; Nadeu et al. 2016; Tavtigian et al. 2009). Finally, our understanding of the role played by ATM in the DDR, and its possible role in oxidative stress, has consolidated the significance of ATM's tumour suppressor function. Perhaps paradoxically such studies have also provided routes for exploitation of ATM-inhibiting drugs in cancer therapy (Box 6.1).

In earlier sections of this chapter, we reviewed the multifarious roles of ATM which contribute to its tumour suppressor function. Below, we summarise these roles in the specific context of tumour suppression and radioresistance. Firstly, although ATM is dispensable for NHEJ, it contributes to DSB repair via its requirement for the slow DSB repair process, its role in activating HR at two-ended DSBs, and in transcriptional arrest in the vicinity of DSBs (Fig. 6.2). As importantly, ATM can influence the fidelity of repair by regulating appropriate modifications to the chromatin structure around a DSB or by activating checkpoint arrest. ATM deficient cells incur increased translocations, attesting to ATM's role in promoting accurate DSB repair or precluding aberrant repair (Stumm et al. 2001). These roles are also important in promoting radioresistance. Cell cycle checkpoint arrest also contributes to the fidelity of DSB repair by providing time for accurate repair prior to progression through critical phases, such as mitosis or replication. Additionally, the activation of pathways that eliminate (e.g. apoptosis) or prevent the proliferation of (e.g. permanent checkpoint arrest and senescence) damaged cells, represent important steps that both restrict initiating steps in carcinogenesis as well as restrict tumour cell proliferation. Finally, a role for ATM in regulating ROS production, represents a further, but somewhat distinct, contribution to the maintenance of genomic stability. Collectively ATM's contribution to maintaining genomic stability is extensive.

Given that cancer cells evolve to gain genomic instability, it is not unsurprising that down regulation of ATM is observed in cancer cells, a feature which should be evaluated when using ATM inhibitors for anti-cancer therapy. However, many cancer cells endure enhanced levels of DSB formation as a consequence of replicative or oxidative stress as well as via the downregulation or loss of other factors or pathways that contribute to the maintenance of genomic stability. Indeed, enhancing DSB formation is a critical step in generating the genomic instability desired by cancer cells. Paradoxically, such changes can place a greater reliance on ATM to allow survival coupled with genomic instability. This raises the possibility that loss of or diminished ATM function could confer synthetic lethality in cancer cells. As discussed above, there are also situations where ATM signalling can promote pro-survival responses, providing a further possibility for a synthetic lethal relationship by inhibiting ATM function (Box 6.1). Additionally, ATM inhibition in the vicinity of tumours could provide a route to enhance tumour radiosensitivity following radiotherapy. For these reasons, ATM inhibiting drugs have the potential to be exploited for cancer therapy, which will be the subject of further chapters in this book.

6.8 Summary

The history of our understanding of A-T and ATM has progressed from early findings that A-T is a devastating disorder displaying dramatic radiosensitivity yet proficiency to repair DSBs, the main IR-induced lethal lesion. We now know that there is a subtle DSB repair defect but, more significantly, that ATM lies at the heart of an extensive response to DSBs with a myriad of consequences, some of which are common to all cell types but many of which are tissue or cell type specific. This demonstrates that ATM signalling interfaces with other signalling responses including growth factor and tumour suppressor signalling. Although enhanced sensitivity to the lethal effects of radiation is characteristic of ATM deficiency, the dramatically increased genomic instability is of equal significance. Thus, ATM serves to protect us from DSB-induced cell lethality or trigger lethality/senescence to maintain genomic stability. Paradoxically, whilst this underlies the tumour suppressor function of ATM, it also provides us with the ability to exploit ATM inhibitors for therapeutic benefit. Optimally exploiting this route to cancer therapy, however, requires a more in depth understanding of ATM cellular functions, the interface between DDR and growth factor signalling pathways and the close interplay between ATM's ability to promote cell survival or cell death under different condition.

References

Alagoz M, Katsuki Y, Ogiwara H, Ogi T, Shibata A, Kakarougkas A, Jeggo P (2015) SETDB1, HP1 and SUV39 promote repositioning of 53BP1 to extend resection during homologous recombination in G2 cells. Nucleic Acids Res 43:7931–7944

Alatwi HE, Downs JA (2015) Removal of H2A.Z by INO80 promotes homologous recombination. EMBO Rep 16:986–994

Albarakati N, Abdel-Fatah TM, Doherty R, Russell R, Agarwal D, Moseley P, Perry C, Arora A, Alsubhi N, Seedhouse C et al (2015) Targeting BRCA1-BER deficient breast cancer by ATM or DNA-PKcs blockade either alone or in combination with cisplatin for personalized therapy. Mol Oncol 9:204–217

Ayrapetov MK, Gursoy-Yuzugullu O, Xu C, Xu Y, Price BD (2014) DNA double-strand breaks promote methylation of histone H3 on lysine 9 and transient formation of repressive chromatin. Proc Natl Acad Sci U S A 111:9169–9174

Bakkenist CJ, Kastan MB (2003) DNA damage activates ATM through intermolecular autophosphorylation and dimer dissociation. Nature 421:499–506

Bakkenist CJ, Kastan MB (2015) Chromatin perturbations during the DNA damage response in higher eukaryotes. DNA Repair 36:8–12

Baldeyron C, Soria G, Roche D, Cook AJ, Almouzni G (2011) HP1alpha recruitment to DNA damage by p150CAF-1 promotes homologous recombination repair. J Cell Biol 193:81–95

Barazzuol L, Rickett N, Ju L, Jeggo PA (2015) Low levels of endogenous or X-ray-induced DNA double-strand breaks activate apoptosis in adult neural stem cells. J Cell Sci 128:3597–3606

Bartek J, Lukas J (2001) Pathways governing G1/S transition and their response to DNA damage. FEBS Lett 490:117–122

Bartek J, Lukas J (2007) DNA damage checkpoints: from initiation to recovery or adaptation. Curr Opin Cell Biol 19:238–245

Bartek J, Lukas C, Lukas J (2004) Checking on DNA damage in S phase. Nat Rev Mol Cell Biol 5:792–804

Barzilai A, Rotman G, Shiloh Y (2002) ATM deficiency and oxidative stress: a new dimension of defective response to DNA damage. DNA Repair 1:3–25

Beamish H, Lavin MF (1994) Radiosensitivity in ataxia-telangiectasia: anomalies in radiation-induced cell cycle delay. Int J Radiat Biol 65:175–184

Berkovich E, Monnat RJ Jr, Kastan MB (2007) Roles of ATM and NBS1 in chromatin structure modulation and DNA double-strand break repair. Nat Cell Biol 9:683–690

Beucher A, Birraux J, Tchouandong L, Barton O, Shibata A, Conrad S, Goodarzi AA, Krempler A, Jeggo PA, Lobrich M (2009) ATM and Artemis promote homologous recombination of radiation-induced DNA double-strand breaks in G2. EMBO J 28:3413–3427

Bhoumik A, Singha N, O'Connell MJ, Ronai ZA (2008) Regulation of TIP60 by ATF2 modulates ATM activation. J Biol Chem 283:17605–17614

Biehs R, Steinlage M, Barton O, Juhasz S, Kunzel J, Spies J, Shibata A, Jeggo PA, Lobrich M (2017) DNA double-strand break resection occurs during non-homologous end joining in G1 but is distinct from resection during homologous recombination. Mol Cell 65:671–684.e5

Burgess RC, Burman B, Kruhlak MJ, Misteli T (2014) Activation of DNA damage response signaling by condensed chromatin. Cell Rep 9:1703–1717

Celeste A, Petersen S, Romanienko PJ, Fernandez-Capetillo O, Chen HT, Sedelnikova OA, Reina-San-Martin B, Coppola V, Meffre E, Difilippantonio MJ et al (2002) Genomic instability in mice lacking histone H2AX. Science 296:922–927

Clouaire T, Legube G (2015) DNA double strand break repair pathway choice: a chromatin based decision? Nucleus 6:107–113

Cornforth MN, Bedford JS (1985) On the nature of a defect in cells from individuals with ataxia-telangiectasia. Science 227:1589–1591

Cosentino C, Grieco D, Costanzo V (2011) ATM activates the pentose phosphate pathway promoting anti-oxidant defence and DNA repair. EMBO J 30:546–555

Daniel JA, Pellegrini M, Lee JH, Paull TT, Feigenbaum L, Nussenzweig A (2008) Multiple autophosphorylation sites are dispensable for murine ATM activation in vivo. J Cell Biol 183:777–783

Deckbar D, Birraux J, Krempler A, Tchouandong L, Beucher A, Walker S, Stiff T, Jeggo P, Lobrich M (2007) Chromosome breakage after G2 checkpoint release. J Cell Biol 176:749–755

Deckbar D, Stiff T, Koch B, Reis C, Lobrich M, Jeggo PA (2010) The limitations of the G1-S checkpoint. Cancer Res 70:4412–4421

Deckbar D, Jeggo PA, Lobrich M (2011) Understanding the limitations of radiation-induced cell cycle checkpoints. Crit Rev Biochem Mol Biol 46:271–283

Du F, Zhang M, Li X, Yang C, Meng H, Wang D, Chang S, Xu Y, Price B, Sun Y (2014) Dimer monomer transition and dimer re-formation play important role for ATM cellular function during DNA repair. Biochem Biophys Res Commun 452:1034–1039

Eaton JS, Lin ZP, Sartorelli AC, Bonawitz ND, Shadel GS (2007) Ataxia-telangiectasia mutated kinase regulates ribonucleotide reductase and mitochondrial homeostasis. J Clin Invest 117:2723–2734

Falck J, Mailand N, Syljuasen RG, Bartek J, Lukas J (2001) The ATM-Chk2-Cdc25A checkpoint pathway guards against radioresistant DNA synthesis. Nature 410:842–847

Falck J, Petrini JH, Williams BR, Lukas J, Bartek J (2002) The DNA damage-dependent intra-S phase checkpoint is regulated by parallel pathways. Nat Genet 30:290–294

Falck J, Coates J, Jackson SP (2005) Conserved modes of recruitment of ATM, ATR and DNA-PKcs to sites of DNA damage. Nature 434:605–611

Fradet-Turcotte A, Canny MD, Escribano-Diaz C, Orthwein A, Leung CC, Huang H, Landry MC, Kitevski-LeBlanc J, Noordermeer SM, Sicheri F et al (2013) 53BP1 is a reader of the DNA-damage-induced H2A Lys 15 ubiquitin mark. Nature 499:50–54

Fugger K, Mistrik M, Neelsen KJ, Yao Q, Zellweger R, Kousholt AN, Haahr P, Chu WK, Bartek J, Lopes M et al (2015) FBH1 catalyzes regression of stalled replication forks. Cell Rep. https://doi.org/10.1016/j.celrep.2015.02.028

Goldberg M, Stucki M, Falck J, D'Amours D, Rahman D, Pappin D, Bartek J, Jackson SP (2003) MDC1 is required for the intra-S-phase DNA damage checkpoint. Nature 421:952–956

Grinthal A, Adamovic I, Weiner B, Karplus M, Kleckner N (2010) PR65, the HEAT-repeat scaffold of phosphatase PP2A, is an elastic connector that links force and catalysis. Proc Natl Acad Sci U S A 107:2467–2472

Grosjean-Raillard J, Tailler M, Ades L, Perfettini JL, Fabre C, Braun T, De Botton S, Fenaux P, Kroemer G (2009) ATM mediates constitutive NF-kappaB activation in high-risk myelodysplastic syndrome and acute myeloid leukemia. Oncogene 28:1099–1109

Guo Z, Kozlov S, Lavin MF, Person MD, Paull TT (2010) ATM activation by oxidative stress. Science 330:517–521

Huen MS, Grant R, Manke I, Minn K, Yu X, Yaffe MB, Chen J (2007) RNF8 transduces the DNA-damage signal via histone ubiquitylation and checkpoint protein assembly. Cell 131:901–914

Ijiri K, Potten CS (1986) Radiation-hypersensitive cells in small intestinal crypts; their relationships to clonogenic cells. Br J Cancer Suppl 7:20–22

Insinga A, Cicalese A, Faretta M, Gallo B, Albano L, Ronzoni S, Furia L, Viale A, Pelicci PG (2013) DNA damage in stem cells activates p21, inhibits p53, and induces symmetric self-renewing divisions. Proc Natl Acad Sci U S A 110:3931–3936

International Nijmegen Breakage Syndrome Study Group (2000) Nijmegen breakage syndrome. The International Nijmegen Breakage Syndrome Study Group. Arch Dis Child 82:400–406

Jasin M, Rothstein R (2013) Repair of strand breaks by homologous recombination. Cold Spring Harb Perspect Biol 5:a012740

Jeggo PA, Downs JA (2014) Roles of chromatin remodellers in DNA double strand break repair. Exp Cell Res 329:69–77

Jeggo PA, Lobrich M (2015) How cancer cells hijack DNA double-strand break repair pathways to gain genomic instability. Biochem J 471:1–11

Kakarougkas A, Ismail A, Chambers AL, Riballo E, Herbert AD, Kunzel J, Lobrich M, Jeggo PA, Downs JA (2014) Requirement for PBAF in transcriptional repression and repair at DNA breaks in actively transcribed regions of chromatin. Mol Cell 55:723–732

Kamsler A, Daily D, Hochman A, Stern N, Shiloh Y, Rotman G, Barzilai A (2001) Increased oxidative stress in ataxia telangiectasia evidenced by alterations in redox state of brains from Atm-deficient mice. Cancer Res 61:1849–1854

Kanu N, Behrens A (2007) ATMIN defines an NBS1-independent pathway of ATM signalling. EMBO J 26:2933–2941

Kastan MB, Zhan Q, el-Deiry WS, Carrier F, Jacks T, Walsh WV, Plunkett BS, Vogelstein B, Fornace AJ Jr (1992) A mammalian cell cycle checkpoint pathway utilizing p53 and GADD45 is defective in ataxia-telangiectasia. Cell 71:587–597

Katyal S, Lee Y, Nitiss KC, Downing SM, Li Y, Shimada M, Zhao J, Russell HR, Petrini JH, Nitiss JL et al (2014) Aberrant topoisomerase-1 DNA lesions are pathogenic in neurodegenerative genome instability syndromes. Nat Neurosci 17:813–821

Kennedy RD, Chen CC, Stuckert P, Archila EM, De la Vega MA, Moreau LA, Shimamura A, D'Andrea AD (2007) Fanconi anemia pathway-deficient tumor cells are hypersensitive to inhibition of ataxia telangiectasia mutated. J Clin Invest 117:1440–1449

Khoronenkova SV, Dianov GL (2015) ATM prevents DSB formation by coordinating SSB repair and cell cycle progression. Proc Natl Acad Sci U S A 112:3997–4002

Kozlov SV, Graham ME, Peng C, Chen P, Robinson PJ, Lavin MF (2006) Involvement of novel autophosphorylation sites in ATM activation. EMBO J 25:3504–3514

Krueger SA, Wilson GD, Piasentin E, Joiner MC, Marples B (2010) The effects of G2-phase enrichment and checkpoint abrogation on low-dose hyper-radiosensitivity. Int J Radiat Oncol Biol Phys 77:1509–1517

Kruger A, Ralser M (2011) ATM is a redox sensor linking genome stability and carbon metabolism. Sci Signal 4:pe17. https://doi.org/10.1126/scisignal.2001959

Kruhlak MJ, Celeste A, Nussenzweig A (2006) Spatio-temporal dynamics of chromatin containing DNA breaks. Cell Cycle 5:1910–1912

Kruhlak M, Crouch EE, Orlov M, Montano C, Gorski SA, Nussenzweig A, Misteli T, Phair RD, Casellas R (2007) The ATM repair pathway inhibits RNA polymerase I transcription in response to chromosome breaks. Nature 447:730–734

Lam QL, Lo CK, Zheng BJ, Ko KH, Osmond DG, Wu GE, Rottapel R, Lu L (2007) Impaired V(D) J recombination and increased apoptosis among B cell precursors in the bone marrow of c-Abl-deficient mice. Int Immunol 19:267–276

Lavin MF, Khanna KK, Beamish H, Teale B, Hobson K, Watters D (1994) Defect in radiation signal transduction in ataxia-telangiectasia. Int J Radiat Biol 66:S151–S156

Lee JH, Paull TT (2005) ATM activation by DNA double-strand breaks through the Mre11-Rad50-Nbs1 complex. Science 308:551–554

Lee JH, Goodarzi AA, Jeggo PA, Paull TT (2010) 53BP1 promotes ATM activity through direct interactions with the MRN complex. EMBO J 29:574–585

Li S, Ting NS, Zheng L, Chen PL, Ziv Y, Shiloh Y, Lee EY, Lee WH (2000) Functional link of BRCA1 and ataxia telangiectasia gene product in DNA damage response. Nature 406:210–215

Lieber MR (2010) The mechanism of double-strand DNA break repair by the nonhomologous DNA end-joining pathway. Annu Rev Biochem 79:181–211

Lin PH, Kuo WH, Huang AC, Lu YS, Lin CH, Kuo SH, Wang MY, Liu CY, Cheng FT, Yeh MH et al (2016) Multiple gene sequencing for risk assessment in patients with early-onset or familial breast cancer. Oncotarget. https://doi.org/10.18632/oncotarget.7027

Lobrich M, Shibata A, Beucher A, Fisher A, Ensminger M, Goodarzi AA, Barton O, Jeggo PA (2010) Gamma H2AX foci analysis for monitoring DNA double-strand break repair: strengths, limitations and optimization. Cell Cycle 9:662–669

Lovejoy CA, Cortez D (2009) Common mechanisms of PIKK regulation. DNA Repair 8:1004–1008

Lukas C, Melander F, Stucki M, Falck J, Bekker-Jensen S, Goldberg M, Lerenthal Y, Jackson SP, Bartek J, Lukas J (2004) Mdc1 couples DNA double-strand break recognition by Nbs1 with its H2AX-dependent chromatin retention. EMBO J 23:2674–2683

Mailand N, Falck J, Lukas C, Syljuasen RG, Welcker M, Bartek J, Lukas J (2000) Rapid destruction of human Cdc25A in response to DNA damage. Science 288:1425–1429

Mailand N, Bekker-Jensen S, Faustrup H, Melander F, Bartek J, Lukas C, Lukas J (2007) RNF8 ubiquitylates histones at DNA double-strand breaks and promotes assembly of repair proteins. Cell 131:887–900

Mallette FA, Mattiroli F, Cui G, Young LC, Hendzel MJ, Mer G, Sixma TK, Richard S (2012) RNF8- and RNF168-dependent degradation of KDM4A/JMJD2A triggers 53BP1 recruitment to DNA damage sites. EMBO J 31:1865–1878

Matt S, Hofmann TG (2016) The DNA damage-induced cell death response: a roadmap to kill cancer cells. Cell Mol Life Sci 73(15):2829–2850

McKinnon PJ (2012) ATM and the molecular pathogenesis of ataxia telangiectasia. Annu Rev Pathol 7:303–321

Nadeu F, Delgado J, Royo C, Baumann T, Stankovic T, Pinyol M, Jares P, Navarro A, Martin-Garcia D, Bea S et al (2016) Clinical impact of clonal and subclonal TP53, SF3B1, BIRC3, NOTCH1 and ATM mutations in chronic lymphocytic leukemia. Blood 127(17):2122–2130

Noon AT, Shibata A, Rief N, Lobrich M, Stewart GS, Jeggo PA, Goodarzi AA (2010) 53BP1-dependent robust localized KAP-1 phosphorylation is essential for heterochromatic DNA double-strand break repair. Nat Cell Biol 12:177–184

Okuno Y, Nakamura-Ishizu A, Otsu K, Suda T, Kubota Y (2012) Pathological neoangiogenesis depends on oxidative stress regulation by ATM. Nat Med 18:1208–1216

Painter RB (1981) Radioresistant DNA synthesis: an intrinsic feature of ataxia telangiectasia. Mutat Res 84:183–190

Perry J, Kleckner N (2003) The ATRs, ATMs, and TORs are giant HEAT repeat proteins. Cell 112:151–155

Petermann E, Helleday T (2010) Pathways of mammalian replication fork restart. Nat Rev Mol Cell Biol 11:683–687

Savitsky K, Bar-Shira A, Gilad S, Rotman G, Ziv Y, Vanagaite L, Tagle DA, Smith S, Uziel T, Sfez S et al (1995) A single ataxia telangiectasia gene with a product similar to PI-3 kinase. Science 268:1749–1753

Schalch DS, McFarlin DE, Barlow MH (1970) An unusual form of diabetes mellitus in ataxia telangiectasia. N Engl J Med 282:1396–1402

Seeber A, Hauer M, Gasser SM (2013) Nucleosome remodelers in double-strand break repair. Curr Opin Genet Dev 23:174–184

Shanbhag NM, Rafalska-Metcalf IU, Balane-Bolivar C, Janicki SM, Greenberg RA (2010) ATM-dependent chromatin changes silence transcription in cis to DNA double-strand breaks. Cell 141:970–981

Shibata A, Conrad S, Birraux J, Geuting V, Barton O, Ismail A, Kakarougkas A, Meek K, Taucher-Scholz G, Lobrich M et al (2011) Factors determining DNA double-strand break repair pathway choice in G2 phase. EMBO J 30:1079–1092

Shibata A, Moiani D, Arvai AS, Perry J, Harding SM, Genois MM, Maity R, van Rossum-Fikkert S, Kertokalio A, Romoli F et al (2014) DNA double-strand break repair pathway choice is directed by distinct MRE11 nuclease activities. Mol Cell 53:7–18

Shigeta T, Takagi M, Delia D, Chessa L, Iwata S, Kanke Y, Asada M, Eguchi M, Mizutani S (1999) Defective control of apoptosis and mitotic spindle checkpoint in heterozygous carriers of ATM mutations. Cancer Res 59:2602–2607

Shiotani B, Zou L (2009) Single-stranded DNA orchestrates an ATM-to-ATR switch at DNA breaks. Mol Cell 33:547–558

Stewart GS, Maser RS, Stankovic T, Bressan DA, Kaplan MI, Jaspers NG, Raams A, Byrd PJ, Petrini JH, Taylor AM (1999) The DNA double-strand break repair gene hMRE11 is mutated in individuals with an ataxia-telangiectasia-like disorder. Cell 99:577–587

Stucki M, Clapperton JA, Mohammad D, Yaffe MB, Smerdon SJ, Jackson SP (2005) MDC1 directly binds phosphorylated histone H2AX to regulate cellular responses to DNA double-strand breaks. Cell 123:1213–1226

Stumm M, Neubauer S, Keindorff S, Wegner RD, Wieacker P, Sauer R (2001) High frequency of spontaneous translocations revealed by FISH in cells from patients with the cancer-prone syndromes ataxia telangiectasia and Nijmegen breakage syndrome. Cytogenet Cell Genet 92:186–191

Sultana R, Abdel-Fatah T, Abbotts R, Hawkes C, Albarakati N, Seedhouse C, Ball G, Chan S, Rakha EA, Ellis IO et al (2013) Targeting XRCC1 deficiency in breast cancer for personalized therapy. Cancer Res 73:1621–1634

Sun Y, Xu Y, Roy K, Price BD (2007) DNA damage-induced acetylation of lysine 3016 of ATM activates ATM kinase activity. Mol Cell Biol 27:8502–8509

Sun Y, Jiang X, Price BD (2010) Tip60: connecting chromatin to DNA damage signaling. Cell Cycle 9:930–936

Takagi M, Delia D, Chessa L, Iwata S, Shigeta T, Kanke Y, Goi K, Asada M, Eguchi M, Kodama C et al (1998) Defective control of apoptosis, radiosensitivity, and spindle checkpoint in ataxia telangiectasia. Cancer Res 58:4923–4929

Takao N, Li Y, Yamamoto K (2000) Protective roles for ATM in cellular response to oxidative stress. FEBS Lett 472:133–136

Tavtigian SV, Oefner PJ, Babikyan D, Hartmann A, Healey S, Le Calvez-Kelm F, Lesueur F, Byrnes GB, Chuang SC, Forey N et al (2009) Rare, evolutionarily unlikely missense substitutions in ATM confer increased risk of breast cancer. Am J Hum Genet 85:427–446

Tresini M, Warmerdam DO, Kolovos P, Snijder L, Vrouwe MG, Demmers JA, van IJcken WF, Grosveld FG, Medema RH, Hoeijmakers JH et al (2015) The core spliceosome as target and effector of non-canonical ATM signalling. Nature 523:53–58

Ui A, Nagaura Y, Yasui A (2015) Transcriptional elongation factor ENL phosphorylated by ATM recruits polycomb and switches off transcription for DSB repair. Mol Cell 58:468–482

Uziel T, Lerenthal Y, Moyal L, Andegeko Y, Mittelman L, Shiloh Y (2003) Requirement of the MRN complex for ATM activation by DNA damage. EMBO J 22:5612–5621

Wahl GM, Linke SP, Paulson TG, Huang LC (1997) Maintaining genetic stability through TP53 mediated checkpoint control. Cancer Surv 29:183–219

Watanabe S, Watanabe K, Akimov V, Bartkova J, Blagoev B, Lukas J, Bartek J (2013) JMJD1C demethylates MDC1 to regulate the RNF8 and BRCA1-mediated chromatin response to DNA breaks. Nat Struct Mol Biol 20:1425–1433

Watters D, Kedar P, Spring K, Bjorkman J, Chen P, Gatei M, Birrell G, Garrone B, Srinivasa P, Crane DI et al (1999) Localization of a portion of extranuclear ATM to peroxisomes. J Biol Chem 274:34277–34282

Xu B, Kim ST, Lim DS, Kastan MB (2002) Two molecularly distinct G(2)/M checkpoints are induced by ionizing irradiation. Mol Cell Biol 22:1049–1059

Xu Y, Ayrapetov MK, Xu C, Gursoy-Yuzugullu O, Hu Y, Price BD (2012) Histone H2A.Z controls a critical chromatin remodeling step required for DNA double-strand break repair. Mol Cell 48:723–733

Yang DQ, Kastan MB (2000) Participation of ATM in insulin signalling through phosphorylation of eIF-4E-binding protein 1. Nat Cell Biol 2:893–898

Yang C, Tang X, Guo X, Niikura Y, Kitagawa K, Cui K, Wong ST, Fu L, Xu B (2011) Aurora-B mediated ATM serine 1403 phosphorylation is required for mitotic ATM activation and the spindle checkpoint. Mol Cell 44:597–608

You Z, Chahwan C, Bailis J, Hunter T, Russell P (2005) ATM activation and its recruitment to damaged DNA require binding to the C terminus of Nbs1. Mol Cell Biol 25:5363–5379

Zhang T, Penicud K, Bruhn C, Loizou JI, Kanu N, Wang ZQ, Behrens A (2012) Competition between NBS1 and ATMIN controls ATM signaling pathway choice. Cell Rep 2:1498–1504

Ziv Y, Bielopolski D, Galanty Y, Lukas C, Taya Y, Schultz DC, Lukas J, Bekker-Jensen S, Bartek J, Shiloh Y (2006) Chromatin relaxation in response to DNA double-strand breaks is modulated by a novel ATM- and KAP-1 dependent pathway. Nat Cell Biol 8:870–876

Chapter 7
Pre-clinical Profile and Expectations for Pharmacological ATM Inhibition

Anika M. Weber and Anderson J. Ryan

Abstract The central DNA damage response (DDR) kinase Ataxia-telangiectasia mutated (ATM) has become an attractive target for cancer therapy. Pre-clinical studies have encouraged the further clinical development of ATM inhibitors, both in combination with chemo- or radiotherapy and as a single agent for the treatment of tumours harbouring deficiencies in certain DDR pathways. The challenges for the successful future development of ATM inhibitors for the clinic will be to translate the knowledge of the cellular phenotypes caused by inhibition of ATM function into the identification of the most beneficial combination strategies and treatment schedules, and to identify robust biomarkers for patient selection and assessment of target inhibition. In this chapter we will review the current knowledge of the cellular defects caused by ATM kinase inhibition and the differences from the known defects observed in ATM-deficient cells. We will also discuss some of the pre-clinical data from in vitro studies with pharmacological ATM inhibitors, the (thus far) most promising combinations of ATM inhibitors with genotoxic modalities, potential synthetic lethal approaches and potential biomarkers for patient selection and assessment of target inhibition.

Keywords DDR · Ataxia-telangiectasia mutated · ATM · ATM inhibitor · KU-55933 · KU-60019 · Radiosensitisation · Chemosensitisation · Synthetic lethality

7.1 Introduction

Ataxia-telangiectasia mutated (ATM) plays crucial roles in the detection and repair of DNA double-strand breaks (DSBs) and in the enforcement of DNA damage-induced cell cycle checkpoints. It lies at the heart of the cellular response that

A. M. Weber · A. J. Ryan (✉)
Cancer Research UK and Medical Research Council Oxford Institute for Radiation Oncology,
The Department of Oncology, University of Oxford, Oxford, UK
e-mail: anika.weber@oncology.ox.ac.uk; anderson.ryan@oncology.ox.ac.uk

© Springer International Publishing AG, part of Springer Nature 2018
J. Pollard, N. Curtin (eds.), *Targeting the DNA Damage Response for Anti-Cancer Therapy*, Cancer Drug Discovery and Development,
https://doi.org/10.1007/978-3-319-75836-7_7

allows cells, including cancer cells, to evade the lethal effects of various genotoxic modalities, such as radio- and chemotherapy. ATM has therefore sparked considerable scientific interest as a potential target for cancer therapy. ATM inhibitors with increasing potency and specificity have been developed in recent years and pre-clinical studies support the clinical development of ATM kinase inhibitors in two therapeutic approaches: as a monotherapy, aiming for synthetic lethal responses in tumours with DDR defects, and in combination with chemo- or radiotherapy. However, in order to identify potential combination approaches and to promote the identification of biomarkers and the future clinical development of a compound, it will be important to better understand the physiological functions of the target and the cellular phenotypes that its inhibition or depletion produces.

7.2   The Cellular Phenotypes of ATM-Deficiency

Germline mutations in the ATM gene are responsible for the autosomal recessive human hereditary disorder Ataxia-telangiectasia (A-T). This disease, caused by a loss of ATM function, is characterised by progressive cerebellar degeneration, oculocutaneous telangiectasia, immunodeficiency, growth retardation, genomic instability, cancer susceptibility and profound sensitivity to ionising radiation (IR) (Taylor et al. 1975; Lavin 2008; Lavin and Shiloh 1997; Rotman and Shiloh 1998). Studies focussing on the characterisation of the cellular defects of A-T cells provided important insight into the cellular functions of ATM, even before the ATM gene was identified in 1995 (Savitsky et al. 1995). A link between ATM and activation of DNA damage-induced cell cycle checkpoints was predicted on the basis of early studies, which demonstrated that A–T cells are unable to arrest cell cycle progression at the G1/S boundary following exposure to ionising radiation and have a characteristic inability to reduce DNA synthesis rates following the induction of DNA DSBs, a phenotype referred to as radiation-resistant DNA synthesis (Fig. 7.1) (Houldsworth and Lavin 1980; Painter and Young 1980; Kastan et al. 1992). In addition, A–T cells that are in the G2-phase of the cell cycle at the time of irradiation fail to delay mitotic entry (Beamish and Lavin 1994) (Fig. 7.1).

   As well as cell-cycle checkpoint defects, one of the most prominent phenotypes of ATM-deficient cells is a hypersensitivity to ionising radiation and radiomimetic drugs (Taylor et al. 1975; Lavin and Shiloh 1997). Despite many advances in our understanding of ATM activation and function, the underlying cause of this increased radiosensitivity is not yet fully resolved. While some studies suggested that the radiation sensitivity of A–T cells results from cell cycle checkpoint defects (Painter and Young 1980; Beamish and Lavin 1994), others implied that a DNA repair defect is primarily responsible for this phenotype.

   The idea that a DNA repair defect may, at least in part, underlie the increased radiation sensitivity of A-T cells gained acceptance in the mid-1980's. It was demonstrated that even though both A-T cells and normal human fibroblasts show the same initial levels of induced DNA DSBs and the same initial rate for re-joining of the

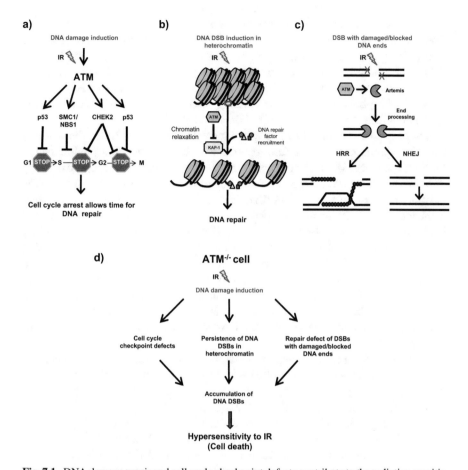

Fig. 7.1 DNA damage repair and cell cycle checkpoint defects contribute to the radiation sensitivity of ATM-defective cells. (**a**) Exposure of cells to IR induces DNA damage, which leads to activation of ATM and, depending on the cell cycle stage at the time of irradiation, to the enforcement of G1/S, intra-S or G2/M cell cycle checkpoints via the downstream targets of ATM. (**b**) ATM plays an important role in the repair of IR-induced DNA DSBs localised in heterochromatic regions of the genome. It causes local chromatin relaxation through phosphorylation of the heterochromatin-building factor KAP-1 (TRIM28), which allows DNA repair factors to gain access to the breakage site. (**c**) ATM plays an important role in the repair of DNA DSBs with damaged/blocked DNA termini, at least in part via regulation of Artemis activity, which mediates the end processing to generate ligatable DNA ends that can then be further processed through either NHEJ or HRR in order to repair the break. (**d**) Cells lacking functional ATM have defects in the activation and maintenance of cell cycle checkpoints and the repair of DNA DSBs located in heterochromatin or with blocked/damaged DNA termini. Together, these defects are the likely cause underlying the hypersensitivity of ATM-deficient cells to ionising radiation

DSBs following exposure to IR, the fraction of residual breaks that remain unrepaired was five to six times greater for the A-T cells (Cornforth and Bedford 1985). This increased level of residual DNA damage in A-T cells after IR-exposure was observed even under non-proliferating conditions, suggesting that progression of cells into

S-phase is not a prerequisite for the increased frequency of chromosome breaks observed in mitosis after irradiation of A-T cells in G1, thus arguing that cell cycle checkpoint defects are not responsible for this phenotype (Cornforth and Bedford 1985). This observation was confirmed by subsequent studies, which demonstrated that A-T cells have the same, or perhaps even higher, initial rates of DSB repair, but a lower final capacity of DNA DSB re-joining, leading to increased levels of residual DNA DSBs following exposure to IR (Foray et al. 1997).

It has since been established that following exposure of cells to IR, the majority of DSBs (approximately 85%) are repaired with fast kinetics in a predominantly ATM-independent manner. The remaining radiation-induced DSBs (approximately 15%) are repaired with markedly slower kinetics via a process that requires ATM and other DNA repair factors (Goodarzi et al. 2010). Recent studies have shed light on the reasons underlying this two-phased repair response. It has been demonstrated that DSBs repaired with slow kinetics in an ATM-dependent manner predominantly localise to heterochromatic (HC) areas of the genome. Indeed, there is increasing evidence that ATM facilitates the repair of heterochromatic DNA DSBs, at least in part via phosphorylation and inactivation of the heterochromatin-building factor KAP-1 (TRIM28), which leads to local chromatin relaxation (Ziv et al. 2006; Goodarzi et al. 2008, 2010; Woodbine et al. 2011). The local modification of chromatin structure in turn allows access of DNA repair factors to the breakage site, thus promoting DNA repair (Fig. 7.1).

The role of ATM in chromatin remodelling might, at least in part, explain the different cellular phenotypes of A-T cells and cells with defects in non-homologous end-joining (NHEJ), the repair process primarily responsible for the fast component of DNA DSB repair (Kakarougkas and Jeggo 2014; Goodarzi et al. 2010). While A-T cells show normal initial DNA repair kinetics following IR-exposure, cells defective in NHEJ (for example due to depletion of DNA-PKcs or DNA Ligase IV) initially fail to repair a large fraction of the IR-induced DNA DSBs. However, NHEJ-defective cells continue the repair of DSBs for many days and thus finally reach a level of unrepaired DSBs similar to that of wild-type cells, whereas A-T cells show increased levels of residual unrepaired DNA DSBs (Kühne et al. 2004; Jeggo 1998).

Chromatin remodelling and phosphorylation of KAP-1 are, however, not the only functions of ATM in the detection and repair of DNA DSBs. Early studies suggested that a recombination-based mechanism involved in the repair of DNA DSBs might be defective in A-T cells and thus, at least in part, be responsible for the radiation sensitivity, immune defects, and karyotypic abnormalities observed in A-T (Luo et al. 1996; Powell et al. 1993; Dar et al. 1997; Meyn 1993; Oxford et al. 1975; Lipkowitz et al. 1990). Following the induction of DNA DSBs and their recognition by the MRN complex, ATM is recruited to the sites of DSBs and activated (Lee and Paull 2005; You et al. 2005). Through phosphorylation of numerous downstream targets, activated ATM then initiates a signalling cascade which mediates both the recruitment of DNA repair factors and cell cycle checkpoint activation (Weber and Ryan 2015; Shiloh 2003; Shiloh and Ziv 2013; Sancar et al. 2004; Jeggo and Löbrich 2006). Amongst its many downstream targets are several proteins crucially involved in homologous recombination repair (HRR) of DNA DSBs, including CtIP (RBBP8) and BRCA1 (Cortez et al. 1999; Wang et al. 2013; Li et al. 2000; Gatei et al. 2001). Numerous studies have investigated a potential role of ATM in HRR, however, the precise function of ATM in the resection process and subsequent recombination steps during homologous recombination has not been determined.

A recent study pointed towards a role for ATM in the initial steps of HRR, as it was found to stimulate the nucleolytic activity of CtIP through phosphorylation (Wang et al. 2013). CtIP is a core HRR factor, which is essential for DNA end resection to generate 3'-ssDNA overhangs. This is followed by RPA loading and RAD51 nucleofilament formation, each of which are central processes required for HRR (You and Bailis 2010; Sartori et al. 2007; Huertas and Jackson 2009; Chen et al. 2008; Krejci et al. 2012; Helleday et al. 2007). This finding is in support of a previous study, which demonstrated altered kinetics of RAD51 foci formation in ATM-depleted cells (Morrison et al. 2000). A-T cells show significantly delayed recruitment of RAD51 to sites of DNA DSBs and it was suggested that this phenotype might be the result of both insufficient DNA end resection and/or delayed H2AX phosphorylation, a prerequisite for timely RAD51 recruitment to sites of DNA damage (Yuan et al. 2003; Paull et al. 2000; Köcher et al. 2012). In contrast, another study demonstrated that inhibition of ATM kinase activity with KU-55933 did not reduce or delay RAD51 foci formation following IR (Cornell et al. 2015) perhaps suggesting that ATM kinase inhibition and ATM loss of function produce distinct phenotypes. When studying the role of ATM in HRR during S-phase, Köcher et al. found that following delayed RAD51 recruitment to sites of DNA DSBs in A-T cells, a persistence of RAD51 foci becomes evident. The authors concluded that the recombination process is initiated in A-T cells, but remains incomplete (Köcher et al. 2012). An HRR defect in ATM-depleted cells has also been described in the G2-phase of the cell cycle, characterised by inefficient formation of replication protein A (RPA) and RAD51 foci following IR-induced DNA DSB formation (Beucher et al. 2009). This ATM-dependent DSB-repair defect was, however, relieved following depletion of KAP-1, suggesting that the role of ATM in HRR during G2 may be related to its role in the repair of DNA DSBs localised in heterochromatin and thus may not reflect a defect in the HRR process per se.

Of note, ATM-deficient and HRR-mutant cells show clear phenotypic differences, particularly with regard to their sensitivity to genotoxic modalities. Mammalian cells that are defective in homologous recombination repair, for example due to mutation or depletion of BRCA1/2 or RAD51, show only mild sensitivity to IR, but are hypersensitive to DNA cross-linking agents (Helleday 2010; Yun et al. 2005; Moynahan et al. 2001; Bhattacharyya et al. 2000). A-T cells, on the other hand, are hypersensitive to IR, but do not manifest an increased sensitivity to cross-linking agents (Fedier et al. 2003; Jaspers et al. 1982; Taylor et al. 1975). These differences in cellular phenotypes suggest that functional impairment of ATM does not cause a gross defect in the general process of HRR. It seems likely that the contribution of ATM to HRR of DNA DSBs might be dependent on the cell cycle stage and the chromatin context, and could also be confined to the recognition or repair of a subclass of DSBs.

Importantly, the role of ATM in the repair of DNA DSBs is not limited to cells in the S- or G2-phase of the cell cycle or to HRR, but it is also required in non-cycling G0 cells for the repair of a subset of radiation-induced DSBs by NHEJ (Riballo et al. 2004; Wang et al. 2005; Darroudi et al. 2007). It has been suggested that in this context, ATM is required for Artemis-dependent processing of DNA DSBs with damaged termini (blocked/non-ligatable DNA ends), indicating that ATM might be important for the repair of complex/blocked DNA DSBs ((Riballo et al. 2004); Fig. 7.1). Artemis (DCLRE1C) is a nuclease that is implicated in the DNA end-processing steps of NHEJ repair of DNA DSBs where it is believed to remove chemically modified and unligatable end groups to generate ligatable ends, and in the opening of hairpin end structures during V(D)J-recombination (Pannicke et al. 2004; Ma et al. 2002, 2005; Yannone et al. 2008; Kurosawa and Adachi 2010).

ATM and Artemis were also shown to be required for the promotion of homologous recombination repair of a subset of IR-induced DNA DSBs during G2, which are re-joined with slow kinetics (Beucher et al. 2009). As Artemis endonuclease activity was found to be crucial for this process, it was suggested that Artemis mediates the removal of lesions or secondary structures at the sites of a subset of DNA DSBs, followed by promotion of end-resection and initiation of HRR. The contribution of ATM was attributed to its role in heterochromatin-remodelling (Beucher et al. 2009). It should be noted, however, that in response to IR, Artemis is hyperphosphorylated in an ATM-dependent manner, identifying it as a downstream component of ATM-dependent signalling (Riballo et al. 2004). Therefore, it seems plausible that the role of ATM may extend to the regulation of Artemis activity. Considering the important role of Artemis in V(D)J-recombination (Pannicke et al. 2004; Ma et al. 2002), regulation of Artemis activity by ATM might be partly responsible for the immunodeficiency and immunoglobulin class switch deficiency observed in ATM knockout mice and some A-T patients (Reina-San-Martin et al. 2004; Lumsden et al. 2004; Mohammadinejad et al. 2015).

Interestingly, cells derived from patients with Artemis-deficiency show comparable IR sensitivity to A-T cells (Riballo et al. 2004). Furthermore, the DNA repair defect observed in Artemis-defective cells differs from that observed in NHEJ-defective cells, but is similar to the DSB repair defect observed in A-T cells (Riballo et al. 2004; Nicolas et al. 1998; Moshous et al. 2001). Of particular importance is the observation that the fraction of unrepaired DNA DSBs observed in ATM- or Artemis-deficient cells is dependent on the nature of the DNA DSB and is much greater following exposure to modalities that induce more complex lesions, such as α-particles (Riballo et al. 2004). These observations further support the concept that ATM plays an important role in the repair of damaged/blocked DNA termini, likely at least in part via regulation of Artemis activity.

Additional support for this concept comes from a study which demonstrated that ATM functions specifically in the re-joining of blocked DSBs, in a manner that is independent of the chromatin status of the lesions (Álvarez-Quilón et al. 2014). This requirement for ATM in the repair of blocked DNA DSBs might underlie the increased sensitivity of ATM-defective cells to topoisomerase inhibitors, which inhibit the re-ligation step of topoisomerases and thus cause the formation of DSBs with peptidic blockages at the 5'-ends of the DNA—either directly (topoisomerase II inhibitors) or in association with DNA replication, following the collision of topoisomerase I-DNA complexes with ongoing replication forks (Smith et al. 1989; Fedier et al. 2003; Álvarez-Quilón et al. 2014; Köcher et al. 2013; Ryan et al. 1991; Strumberg et al. 2000). ATM deficiency might thus cause a defect in the repair of DNA DSBs with non-ligatable ends, independently of the chromatin context (Fig. 7.1). Such a repair defect is likely to contribute to the observed IR-hypersensitivity of ATM-defective cells.

In conclusion, the hypersensitivity of A-T cells to IR is likely to be the result of several defects, which lead to incomplete repair of DNA DSBs, particularly in heterochromatic regions of the genome and at sites of blocked DNA termini (Fig. 7.1). The inability of ATM-deficient cells to activate and maintain DNA damage-induced cell cycle checkpoints is also most probably a contributing factor, as mitotic onset or DNA replication in the presence of DNA damage is likely to cause the induction of further DNA damage, chromosomal aberrations and mis-segregation of genetic material during cell division, eventually leading to cell death.

7.3 The Cellular Phenotype of ATM Inhibition Differs from that Observed After Loss of ATM Protein Expression

It has become clear in recent years that the loss of ATM protein expression results in a different cellular phenotype than expression of a kinase-dead (kd) ATM protein.

While ATM knockout mice are viable and recapitulate many of the symptoms characteristic of A-T (Elson et al. 1996; Barlow et al. 1996), expression of physiological levels of kinase inactive ATM was found to be lethal during early mouse embryogenesis, without displaying dominant-negative interfering activity, suggesting that the expression of kd ATM protein is more detrimental to cells than its loss (Daniel et al. 2012; Yamamoto et al. 2012). Both these studies demonstrated that cells expressing kd ATM showed a higher degree of genomic instability compared with ATM null cells, in particular an increase in chromatid breaks. Chromatid breaks suggest DNA DSB repair defects during the S- and G2-phases of the cell cycle, as unrepaired DSBs generated during G1 generally cause whole chromosome breaks (Yamamoto et al. 2012). This finding could indicate a more severe HRR defect in ATM kd cells compared with ATM null cells as HRR is only active during the S- and G2-phases of the cell cycle. Furthermore, it was demonstrated that kinase-dead ATM protein retains the ability to bind to sites of DNA DSBs, suggesting that its presence may block access of DNA repair factors to the DSB site in a manner that does not occur in the absence of ATM protein, thereby disturbing DDR signalling and causing persistence of DNA damage (Daniel et al. 2012; Yamamoto et al. 2012). The observation that expression of kd ATM protein is not well tolerated by cells may explain why loss of ATM function in A-T is generally associated with loss of protein expression (Gilad et al. 1996; Lavin 2008).

These findings are of particular importance for the pre-clinical evaluation of ATM inhibitors, as ATP-competitive ATM inhibitors (like KU-55933 or KU-60019) may act in a way more similar to kinase-dead ATM protein, rather than loss of ATM protein expression. Following exposure to IR, repair of damaged DNA replication forks was found to be normal in A-T cells, but defective in wild-type cells when ATM was inhibited by KU-55933 or KU-60019 (White et al. 2010). The authors hypothesised that kinase-inhibited ATM presents a physical impediment to homologous recombination repair of DSBs at damaged replication forks (White et al. 2010; Choi et al. 2010), reminiscent of the findings reported for cells expressing kd ATM protein. This finding is supported by a more recent study, which demonstrated that inhibition of ATM following exposure of cells to IR results in persistence of RAD51 foci and a reduced sister chromatid exchange (SCE) rate, suggesting a HRR deficiency (Bakr et al. 2015). However, pharmacological ATM inhibition failed to enhance the sensitivity of ovarian, endometrial, and cervical cancer cells to the DNA cross-linking agent cisplatin (Teng et al. 2015). As HRR-mutants are generally hypersensitive to cross-linking agents (Helleday 2010; Yun et al. 2005; Moynahan et al. 2001; Bhattacharyya et al. 2000), this finding suggests that even though ATM kinase inhibition may cause a greater HRR defect than ATM loss, the defect is still mild compared to, for example, deficiency in BRCA1/2.

Nonetheless, these findings impact on the further clinical development of ATM inhibitors for two reasons: First, considering the increased genomic instability and the exacerbated DNA repair defects observed in ATM-inhibited versus ATM-depleted cells, ATM inhibitors may, upon prolonged exposure, cause greater side effects in vivo than a loss of ATM protein expression would. This possibility may need to be carefully considered when planning treatment schedules and combination approaches for ATM inhibitors in the clinic.

Secondly, the differences in the cellular phenotype between ATM-depleted and ATM-kinase inhibited cells need to be considered when interpreting the results of pre-clinical studies. To confirm the specificity of a compound for a target and/or to validate the specificity of biomarkers of cellular response, results obtained from experiments using inhibitors are often compared to results obtained using isogenic cell lines (with/without functional ATM), or following transient siRNA-mediated depletion of ATM protein. However, in the case of ATM kinase inhibitors such a comparison might have the potential to produce conflicting conclusions.

7.4 Utility of ATM Inhibitors for Chemo- and Radiosensitisation

Many established cancer treatments, such as radio- and chemotherapy, rely on the induction of DNA damage, which is particularly cytotoxic for proliferating cells and hence effective in targeting highly proliferative cancer cells. Since genotoxic therapies generally lack selectivity towards cancer cells, the toxicity induced in non-tumour tissues and the resulting side effects are limiting factors for both the dose and duration of therapy. The hypersensitivity of ATM-defective cells to IR and the increased sensitivity of A-T cells to topoisomerase inhibitors and radiomimetic drugs identified ATM as an attractive target for chemo- or radiosensitisation. Small molecule ATM kinase inhibitors have been developed with the aim of increasing the cytotoxicity of genotoxic modalities in highly proliferative tumour cells, while only minimally affecting less proliferative normal tissues, thus improving the therapeutic window of radio- and chemotherapy.

Support for this concept came from early studies, which demonstrated that inhibition of ATM sensitises cells to genotoxic modalities, particularly ionising radiation (Sarkaria et al. 1999, 1998; Blasina et al. 1999; Price and Youmell 1996). Several studies indicated that the observed radiosensitisation was more pronounced in cells with deficiency in p53 (*TP53*) (Powell et al. 1995; Yao et al. 1996; Bracey et al. 1997) mostly likely due to reduced G2 cell cycle delay/arrest in p53 deficient cells when treated with ATM inhibitors. This is of particular interest, as p53 is one of the most commonly mutated tumour suppressor genes in many different types of cancer (Goh et al. 2011), indicating that ATM inhibition could show increased efficacy in p53-mutated tumours and thus selectivity towards tumour vs. non-tumour tissue. However, the drugs used in those early studies (caffeine and wortmannin) are rather non-specific and also inhibit other phosphatidylinositol 3-kinase-related kinase (PIKK) family members, including ATR and DNA-PKcs (PRKDC) (Sarkaria et al. 1998, 1999). Therefore, it is uncertain how much of the observed effects were due to inhibition of ATM activity. The development of more potent and selective ATM inhibitors allowed for the validation of the radiosensitising effect mediated by pharmacological ATM inhibition in vitro (Rainey et al. 2008; Hickson et al. 2004; Golding et al. 2009, 2012; Biddlestone-Thorpe et al. 2013). With one exception, most of the specific ATM inhibitors developed thus far do not possess sufficient bioavailability to study the effects of pharmacological inhibition in animal models. Yet, despite this limitation, it was demonstrated that ATM inhibition markedly radiosensitises cancer cells in vivo (Biddlestone-Thorpe et al. 2013). The authors bypassed the limitation of poor bioavailability of the compound (KU-60019) by directly injecting the inhibitor into orthotopically grown gliomas in mice (Biddlestone-Thorpe et al. 2013). Importantly, the observed radiosensitising effect was even greater in p53-mutant glioma xenografts, resulting in significantly extended survival and, in some cases, even apparent cure of the treated mice (Biddlestone-Thorpe et al. 2013). It should be noted that this increased sensitivity of p53-deficient glioma cells to the combination of ATM inhibition and ionising radiation was only evident in vivo and not in vitro. This might explain why other studies did not observe an improved radiosensitisation of p53-deficient cells, as those studies only investigated the response in vitro (Batey et al. 2013; Teng et al. 2015). Taken together, this proof-of-principle study provided evidence that pharmacological ATM inhibition has the potential to confer potent radiosensitisation of cancer cells in vivo.

As ATM plays a vital role in the cellular response to DNA DSB formation in normal as well as cancer cells, there are concerns that the radiosensitising properties of pharmacological ATM inhibition will also increase normal tissue toxicity. These concerns are supported by the finding that—at least in vitro—normal human fibroblasts are radiosensitised by ATM inhibition to a similar extent as glioma cells (Golding et al. 2009). Thus, the tumour specificity of ATM kinase inhibition in vivo would likely have to depend on the precision of radiation administration. However, in vitro studies demonstrated that short-term exposure to pharmacological ATM inhibition did not affect the viability of cultured human astrocytes, which are terminally differentiated and not actively dividing, thus indicating that transient ATM inhibition alone is not toxic for less proliferative tissue and normal tissues outside the radiation field (Golding et al. 2012). Furthermore, a recent study has demonstrated that the radiosensitisation conferred by depletion of ATM may be significantly greater in proliferating cells (Moding et al. 2014). As normal tissue is generally less proliferative than tumour tissue, this suggests the possibility of greater radiosensitisation in tumour versus non-tumour tissues, although the potential differential benefit in highly proliferative normal tissues such as in the bone marrow and gastrointestinal tract may be less. Another important observation was that transient inhibition of ATM is sufficient to confer a marked increase in the radiation-induced cytotoxicity (Rainey et al. 2008), suggesting that long-term exposure to ATM inhibitors may not be necessary to achieve clinically relevant radiosensitisation. This may help to reduce the toxicity induced in non-tumour tissue and thus the side effects, indicating that a favourable therapeutic index might be achievable with appropriate scheduling.

In addition to the utility of ATM inhibitors to act as radiosensitisers, several studies have demonstrated that, similar to the observations made in A-T cells, pharmacological ATM inhibition confers marked sensitisation to topoisomerase inhibitors (etoposide, doxorubicin and irinotecan) in vitro (Hickson et al. 2004). Using the first selective ATM inhibitor with sufficient solubility and bio-availability to allow for the study of effects of pharmacological ATM inhibition in animal models (KU-59403), this effect was also confirmed in vivo (Batey et al. 2013). Importantly, the authors demonstrated that ATM had to be inhibited at the time of treatment with the topoisomerase inhibitor etoposide to observe chemosensitisation, and that delaying administration of the ATM inhibitor by only 4 h completely abolished this effect (Batey et al. 2013). This observation is in agreement with the findings from combination studies of ATM inhibitors with IR and further supports the concept that short-term treatment with ATM inhibitors might be sufficient to achieve clinically relevant chemo- or radiosensitisation.

The aim of ATM kinase inhibition in this setting is primarily to increase the effectiveness of established genotoxic treatments and to improve the clinical benefit of chemotherapy (e.g. response rate, duration of response, overall survival) or radiotherapy (e.g. complete response rate, local control rate, overall survival) without increasing toxicity. Therefore, identifying the combinations and treatment schedules that have the greatest potential for tumour selective effects will be important. Future pre-clinical studies will need to determine the drug levels and duration of treatment required to achieve chemo- and radiosensitisation in relevant in vivo models and to determine whether scheduling plays a significant role in optimising the therapeutic window of ATM inhibitor combinations. The duration of treatment with an ATM inhibitor would likely be determined by the established therapy, with chemotherapy given typically every 1–4 weeks and radiotherapy 5 days per week for 5–7 weeks. Although oral formulations are likely to be more convenient where daily dosing is required (e.g. combinations with radiotherapy) and would help to reduce treatment costs, oral administration can be affected by variable intestinal absorption and drug interactions. An intravenous formulation might be suitable for combinations with certain chemotherapies and could help to reduce the differences in bioavailability between patients, which could be important in maximising therapeutic effect and margins.

Many radiotherapy regimens are currently given in combination with DNA-damaging and radiosensitising chemotherapy (e.g. cisplatin, 5-FU, or gemcitabine) at the maximum tolerated dose for patients, and therefore careful pre-clinical evaluation of ATM inhibitors will be required to understand the potential risk/benefit in this complex therapeutic setting. Furthermore, the level of selectivity of ATM inhibitors is likely to be of particular importance as inhibiting other PIKK family members (such as ATR or DNA-PK) will potentially contribute to chemo- and radiosensitisation of both tumour cells and normal tissues, rendering the role of ATM inhibition difficult to assess and increasing the risk of severe side effects (Table 7.1).

Table 7.1 Potential attributes of small molecule ATM kinase inhibitors for cancer therapy

ATM inhibitor attribute	Proposed therapeutic setting	
	Exploiting synthetic lethal interactions in tumour cells	Combination with established DNA damaging therapies
Selectivity	High vs. other PIKK family members	Very high vs other PIKK family members
Route of administration	Oral	Oral or intravenous
Duration or treatment	Chronic (until disease progression)	Acute or prolonged; for the duration of RTX or CTX treatment
In vivo preclinical efficacy benchmarks	Single-agent activity in genetically defined models (DDR-deficient). Delayed tumour growth, tumour shrinkage	Combination activity in models of CTX and RTX resistant disease. Increased tumour shrinkage, evidence of tumour eradication
Normal tissue toxicity	Genome instability, immunosuppression	Increase in RTX- and CTX-related toxicity
Therapeutic margin	High	Moderate
Biomarkers of target inhibition	pATM (S1981), pKAP-1 (S824), pCHEK2 (Thr68)	pATM (S1981), pKAP-1 (S824), pCHEK2 (Thr68)
Biomarkers for patient selection	Genetic mutation/loss of function in certain DDR genes (e.g. *TP53*, FANCD2, XRCC1)	Increased DNA repair or DDR signalling prior to, or following, RTX or CTX (e.g. ATM S1981), *TP53* mutation status for RTX combination or combination with topoisomerase inhibitors
Therapeutic outcomes	Increased tumour shrinkage (objective response rate), delayed tumour growth (progression-free survival), increased overall survival	Increased tumour shrinkage, delayed tumour growth, increased local control rate (radiotherapy), increased complete response rate, increased overall survival
Resistance mechanisms	Unknown	Unknown

7.5   Synthetic Lethal Approaches

In addition to the potential utility of ATM inhibitors as chemo- or radiosensitisers, recent studies suggest that such compounds may have single-agent activity in certain subsets of patients through induction of pharmacological "synthetic lethality". According to the concept of synthetic lethality, two genes or gene products are considered to have a synthetic lethal relationship, if inactivation of either gene product alone does not impair cellular viability, whereas simultaneous defects in both gene products induces cell death (Kaelin 2005).

To date, several potential targets for such a synthetic lethal approach in ATM-deficient or ATM-inhibited cells have been suggested (Fig. 7.2). For instance, it was demonstrated that inhibitors of poly(ADP-ribose) polymerase (PARP), a protein centrally involved in the detection and repair of DNA single-strand breaks (SSBs) and base excision repair (BER), possess single-agent activity in ATM-deficient tumour cells in vitro and in vivo (Weston et al. 2010; Williamson et al. 2010; Aguilar-Quesada et al. 2007). Further enhancement of the cytotoxicity of PARP inhibitors was observed when the function of both ATM and p53 was lost (Williamson et al. 2012; Kubota et al. 2014), suggesting that functional p53 may ameliorate

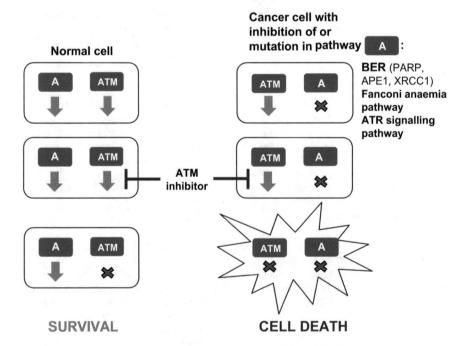

Fig. 7.2 Pharmacological synthetic lethality through ATM kinase inhibition. Cancer cells harbouring somatic mutations in a certain signalling pathway (pathway A; e.g. BER, FA or ATR pathway) may become reliant on ATM signalling for survival. Pharmacological inhibition of ATM would thus induce cell death selectively in those cancer cells, while non-tumour cells with retained function of pathway A would be spared

the otherwise detrimental effects of PARP inhibitors following functional loss of ATM. Deficiency or inhibition of two additional components of the BER pathway, namely APE1 (APEX1) and XRCC1, has been demonstrated to be synthetically lethal in combination with ATM inhibition or deficiency (Sultana et al. 2012, 2013), suggesting that a general synthetic lethal interaction between ATM and the BER pathway might exist. Defects in BER pathways lead to the accumulation of AP (apurinic/apyrimidinic) sites and ssDNA breaks which in turn can lead to replication fork associated DNA DSBs. Since ATM, at least in part, has a role in the resolution of replication-associated DNA DSBs (Köcher et al. 2012) this may underlie the synthetic lethal relationship between loss of BER capacity and loss/inhibition of ATM activity. A phase I clinical trial of an ATM inhibitor (AZD0156) alone and in combination with cytotoxic chemotherapies or novel anti-cancer agents, including a PARP inhibitor (olaparib) is ongoing (ClinicalTrials.gov: NCT02588105). As XRCC1 is frequently deregulated in breast and ovarian cancers (Sultana et al. 2013; Abdel-Fatah et al. 2013), ATM inhibitors may have particular utility for the treatment of these cancer types. Another DDR pathway that is commonly mutated or deregulated in cancer is the Fanconi anaemia (FA) pathway (Kennedy et al. 2007; Kennedy and D'Andrea 2006), which is particularly important for the repair of DNA inter-strand crosslinks (ICLs). Inhibition of ATM kinase activity or knockdown of ATM protein expression has been shown to be particularly cytotoxic for cells with defects in components of this pathway, suggesting a synthetic lethal interaction (Kennedy et al. 2007). Reciprocally, depletion or inhibition of FA pathway components was found to be particularly cytotoxic for ATM-deficient cells (Landais et al. 2009; Jenkins et al. 2012). DNA ICLs present a major barrier to DNA replication and, in the absence of FA activity, stalled DNA replication forks due to ICLs are thought to be primarily repaired in an ATM-dependent manner which may be the basis of the synthetic lethal interaction between these two pathways (Kennedy et al. 2007).

Also of particular interest is a synthetic lethal interaction between the ATM and the ATR (Ataxia-telangiectasia and Rad3-related) signalling pathways. ATR, like ATM, is one of the apical mediators of the cellular response to genotoxic stress and an inducer of cell cycle checkpoints in response to DNA damage. Together, ATM and ATR ensure the maintenance of genomic stability by coordinating cell cycle progression with DNA repair (Cimprich and Cortez 2008; Shiloh 2003; Abraham 2001). Although ATM and ATR are activated by different types of DNA damage and act in distinct pathways, their downstream targets and the responses they mediate are partially overlapping and dependent on the type of genotoxic stress (Helt et al. 2005; Matsuoka et al. 2007). One example is the enforcement of the intra-S-phase checkpoint, where both ATM and ATR can target the CDC25A phosphatase for ubiquitin-dependent degradation thereby regulating the timing of replication origin firing in response to DNA damage (Xiao et al. 2003; Bartek et al. 2004; Falck et al. 2001). Furthermore, both ATM and ATR have been shown to mediate G2/M cell cycle checkpoint activation through phosphorylation of CDC25C via their downstream effectors CHK1 and CHK2 (Shiloh 2003, 2001; Matsuoka et al. 1998; Peng et al. 1997; Sanchez et al. 1997). This overlap in substrates and the partial convergence of the two signalling pathways in their downstream effectors suggests that deficits in one pathway might be, at least to some extent, compensated for by the activity of the respective other pathway.

The first report that ATM and ATR may share a synthetic lethal interaction in cells exposed to genotoxic stress was published in 2011 and was based on in vitro studies using the selective ATR inhibitor VE-821 (Reaper et al. 2011). Interestingly, the authors reported that this synthetic lethality was not only effective in ATM- but also in p53-deficient cells, pointing to a possible G1 cell cycle checkpoint defect as of particular importance for the underlying mechanism. In our own studies we were able to show that non-small cell lung cancer (NSCLC) cells deficient in both ATM and p53 are particularly sensitive to ATR inhibition in vitro, suggesting that the functional status of both ATM and p53 may be important in this setting (Weber et al. 2013). Subsequently, in vivo studies have demonstrated that the ATR inhibitor AZD6738 shows single-agent anti-tumour activity in ATM-deficient but not ATM-proficient xenograft models (Jones et al. 2013; Guichard et al. 2013). Two phase I clinical trials involving AZD6738 are currently recruiting, and one of them in combination with radiation (ClinicalTrials.gov: NCT02223923), and the other assessing AZD6738 alone and in combination with carboplatin or olaparib in ATM-deficient NSCLC, ATM-deficient gastric cancer and advanced solid malignancies (ClinicalTrials.gov: NCT02264678). The progress of this trial will be of great interest as it may give the first clinical proof of a synthetic lethal interaction involving ATM and the emerging results may help to better guide future synthetic lethal approaches.

While several pre-clinical studies suggest that short-term treatment with ATM inhibitors may be sufficient to confer chemo- or radiosensitisation (Rainey et al. 2008; Batey et al. 2013), synthetic lethal approaches may require prolonged target inhibition. The duration of treatment with an ATM inhibitor would likely be determined by the duration of ongoing clinical benefit, until there was evidence of tumour regrowth or unmanageable toxicity. In this setting, daily oral dosing would be most convenient, but may need to achieve sustained target inhibition during the inter-dosing period. Although toxicology studies of ATM inhibitors have not been reported, extrapolation from patients with Ataxia-telangiectasia, and from basic scientific studies in cellular systems and in knockout mice, would suggest that there is the potential for increased genomic instability and thus induction of secondary cancers, immunodeficiency, sensitisation to genotoxic stress and potentially neurological toxicity from sustained inhibition of ATM, which would need careful investigation pre-clinically (Barlow et al. 1996; Elson et al. 1996; Lavin 2008; Lavin and Shiloh 1997; Shiloh and Ziv 2013). The anticipated clinical benefits of ATM inhibition as a synthetic lethal approach are difficult to predict, but previous experience with PARP inhibitors in BRCA-mutated ovarian and breast cancer suggests that prolonged tumour regressions might be achieved in selected patients. Since the selectivity of this approach relies on genetic or epigenetic changes leading to loss of gene function in the tumour cells, developing robust patient selection biomarkers (e.g. impairment of BER, FA or other DDR pathways) in addition to biomarkers of target inhibition will be required ahead of clinical development.

Pre-clinical studies to identify potential mechanisms of resistance to ATM kinase inhibition have not yet been reported, but evidence from other classes of kinase inhibitors in clinical development suggest that resistance to treatment is a likely consequence of chronic target inhibition (Niederst and Engelman 2013; Sullivan and Flaherty 2013; Lovly and Shaw 2014).

7.6 Exploiting Tumor Loss of ATM-Function as Intrinsic Chemo- or Radiosensitiser

In addition to the clinical potential of ATM inhibitors as chemo- or radiosensitisers, it should be noted that ATM deficiency in tumours, caused by epigenetic silencing of the ATM gene or somatic mutations, might be exploitable as an intrinsic radio- or chemosensitiser. However, identifying patients with tumoral loss of ATM function is not without challenges.

ATM is frequently mutated in a broad range of human cancers including lung (Cancer Genome Atlas Research Network 2014, 2012b), colorectal (Cancer Genome Atlas Research Network 2012a), breast (Cancer Genome Atlas Research Network 2012c) and haematopoietic cancers (Landau and Wu 2013; Beà et al. 2013). Amongst the ATM mutations identified in cancer thus far are frame-shift mutations, splice site mutations and nonsense mutations resulting in a truncation of the protein due to introduction of a premature stop codon (Fig. 7.3).When homozygous or occurring coincidentally with heterozygous loss of the ATM gene locus, these mutations are likely to affect ATM protein expression and function (Mitui et al. 2009). However, a substantial proportion of the cancer-associated ATM mutations reported

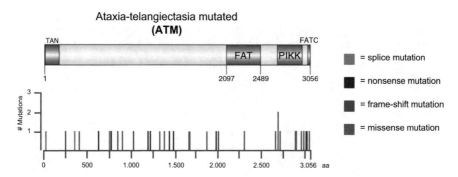

Fig. 7.3 Distribution and types of ATM mutations in NSCLC. A schematic of the ATM protein with the positions of somatic ATM mutations reported in NSCLC (Cancer Genome Atlas Research Network 2012b, 2014). The scale represents the amino acid positions and lines indicate the positions of the reported splice site, frame-shift, missense or nonsense mutations (see legend for colour coding). The length of the lines specifies the number of samples in which the respective mutation occurred (scale on the left). FAT (FRAP-ATM-TRRAP domain), FATC (FAT C-terminal domain), PIKK (phosphatidylinositol 3-kinase-related kinase domain), TAN (Tel1/ATM N-terminal motif)

to date are missense variants, which occur scattered across the entire length of the ATM protein with no apparent hotspots (Fig. 7.3). This is in contrast to the mutation spectrum observed in Ataxia-telangiectasia, where approximately 85% of the mutations are predicted to lead to a truncation of the ATM protein and only 15% of mutations are missense variants (Lavin et al. 2004). Considering the large size of the ATM gene, which spans over 150 kb of genomic DNA, and the characteristic genomic instability of cancer cells, it is likely that a large proportion of the missense changes occurring in cancer cells are neutral passenger mutations rather than deleterious or driver mutations. Currently, distinguishing deleterious missense mutations from benign nonsynonymous polymorphisms or passenger mutations is not possible without functional studies (Gnad et al. 2013).

However, studies in cells derived from A-T patients have shown that the vast majority of missense mutations which lead to functional impairment of ATM do so by destabilising the protein, leading to reduced or absent protein levels (Sandoval et al. 1999; Mitui et al. 2009; Jacquemin et al. 2012; Lavin et al. 2004; Gilad et al. 1996). This is likely due to the aforementioned deleterious effects of expression of kinase dead ATM protein.

When studying the functional consequences of ATM mutations in NSCLC cell lines, we found that the presence of a somatic ATM missense substitution, particularly when heterozygous, indeed does not necessarily imply a functional impairment of ATM signalling. However, in line with observations from missense mutations occurring in A-T, we found that cancer-associated ATM mutations do in some cases lead to a reduction or loss of ATM protein expression and consequently impairment of the ATM signalling pathway. Based on this observation we were able to develop an immunohistochemistry-based assay, which may allow for the identification of tumoral loss of ATM protein expression and thus function in a clinical setting (Weber et al. 2016) (Fig. 7.4). As ATM is constitutively expressed

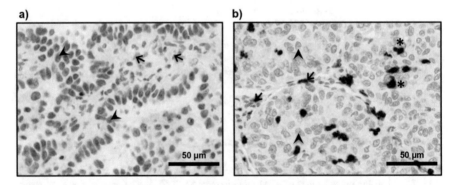

Fig. 7.4 Immunohistochemical analysis of ATM protein expression in NSCLC samples performed to identify tumours with ATM-deficiency due to loss of ATM protein expression. (**a**) Representative image of a NSCLC adenocarcinoma specimen in which the nuclear staining for ATM in tumour cells (arrowheads) is similar to that seen in stromal cells (arrows). (**b**) Representative image of a NSCLC adenocarcinoma specimen with loss of ATM protein expression. Tumour cells (arrowheads), stromal cells (arrows). Intratumour lymphocytes (asterisk) show strong staining for ATM. Images were taken at a 200× magnification

(Brown et al. 1997), we found that the tumour stroma offers a suitable positive control within each sample (Fig. 7.4) and thus helps to correct for variations in the staining intensity between samples and to avoid potential false negative results caused by poor staining or tissue quality.

In addition to somatic point mutations, loss or rearrangement of the ATM gene could also contribute to the loss of ATM protein expression in tumours, as could epigenetic silencing of gene expression. Indeed, hypermethylation of the ATM promoter resulting in decreased protein levels and increased radiosensitivity has been described for colorectal and glioma cell lines (Kim et al. 2002; Roy et al. 2006). Furthermore, studies in locally advanced breast cancer have shown that the ATM gene is a target for epigenetic silencing (Vo et al. 2004).

A recent study demonstrated a potential link between somatic ATM mutations in tumours and exceptional responses to radiotherapy (Ma et al. 2017). Therefore, it seems likely that tumoral loss of ATM expression would confer many of the cellular phenotypes characteristic of A-T cells, including hypersensitivity to ionising radiation and increased sensitivity to topoisomerase inhibitors. Identifying loss of ATM function in tumours might therefore allow for the identification of a patient subset that could receive increased benefit from radiation therapy or certain chemotherapeutic drugs such as topoisomerase inhibitors. Several of the synthetic lethal interactions that have been described for ATM were also identified in studies of cells with loss of ATM expression rather than ATM inhibition. Thus, targeted therapies may have single agent anti-tumour activity in cases with tumoral loss of ATM function and, at least in the cases of ATR or PARP inhibitors, this has already been demonstrated in in vivo studies (Williamson et al. 2010, 2012; Weston et al. 2010; Menezes et al. 2014; Jones et al. 2013; Guichard et al. 2013). Thus, results obtained from studies on ATM-deficient tumours, particularly regarding the responses to standard chemo- or radiotherapy or novel targeted therapies, could be helpful to guide the future clinical development of ATM inhibitors.

7.7   Biomarkers and Patient Selection

DNA replication stress and the induction of DNA damage is characteristic of aberrant oncogene activation during cancer development (Bartkova et al. 2006; Di Micco et al. 2006). Several studies have demonstrated activation of various DDR pathways and cell cycle checkpoint mediators during early stages of tumorigenesis in response to the occurrence of such genotoxic stresses (Bartkova et al. 2005; Gorgoulis et al. 2005). Activation of DDR pathways may act as a barrier to cancer development through inhibition of the proliferation of aberrant cells (Bartkova et al. 2005; Gorgoulis et al. 2005). The tumour suppressor protein p53, which acts as an important cell cycle checkpoint mediator, may be of particular importance for this mechanism, providing a potential explanation for the high frequency of inactivating p53 mutations observed in certain human cancers (Halazonetis et al. 2008). Many human tumours also show functional loss or deregulation of other key proteins involved in the DDR and cell cycle regulation that may allow pre-cancerous cells to overcome the proliferation barrier posed by the DDR and thereby allow pre-malignant lesions to progress to malignant carcinomas (Kandoth et al. 2013; Negrini et al. 2010). These DDR defects offer the potential to employ ATM inhibitors in synthetic lethal approaches, analogous to the use of PARP inhibitors in BRCA1/2 defective tumours (Fong et al. 2009; Tutt et al. 2010; Audeh et al. 2010; Bryant et al. 2005; Farmer et al. 2005). However, for synthetic lethal approaches to be successful, it will be critical to identify the right patient subsets with DDR defects that confer sensitivity towards ATM inhibitors. Current sequencing techniques can identify mutations in DDR genes that may impact on the response of cancer cells to ATM inhibitor treatments, for example XRCC1, *TP53* or components of the FA pathway. However, without functional studies, the consequences of these mutations are generally difficult to predict. Developing biomarkers that can robustly determine the functional status of DDR pathways in tumours and help differentiate between deleterious and benign mutations will therefore be essential. We found that immunohistochemical (IHC) analysis of ATM protein expression might be a promising approach to identify patients with tumoral loss of ATM function (Weber et al. 2016). Similar approaches have been developed to assess tumoral activity of DDR components such as the MRN complex component MRE11 (MRE11A). A study evaluating the protein expression of MRE11 by immunohistochemistry has demonstrated low expression in bladder cancer, which was associated with worse survival following radiotherapy, but not surgery (Choudhury et al. 2010). Furthermore, IHC analysis of the protein expression levels of the BER protein XRCC1 in breast and ovarian cancer specimen revealed frequent tumoral loss or downregulation of XRCC1 (Abdel-Fatah et al. 2013; Sultana et al. 2013). As pre-clinical in vitro data suggests that XRCC1-deficiency may confer sensitivity to ATM inhibitors through a synthetic lethal interaction (Sultana et al. 2013), such an approach may allow for the identification of potential cases for single-agent activity of ATM inhibitors.

In the early stages of clinical development, particularly for the optimisation of dosing and treatment schedules, it is crucial to identify biomarkers that allow for the assessment of target inhibition. For ATM inhibitors, a number of potential measures of ATM activity have been identified in vitro, including ATM autophosphorylation at serine 1981 (S1981). Current models of ATM activation suggest that ATM forms homodimers or higher order multimers in its inactive state. Upon ATM activation, intermolecular autophosphorylation at S1981 then allows for the dissociation into active monomers (Bakkenist and Kastan 2003). Therefore, S1981 autophosphorylation is considered a potential hallmark of activated human ATM (Shiloh and Ziv 2013) and several studies have demonstrated that mutation of this site to alanine (S1981A) leads to defects in the monomerisation of ATM, the stabilisation of ATM at sites of DNA DSBs and the efficient phosphorylation of its downstream targets after DNA damage induction (Berkovich et al. 2007; So et al. 2009; Kozlov et al. 2006). Interestingly, a recent study suggested that elevated ATM S1981 levels prior to radiotherapy is associated with radioresistance and poor prognosis in cervical cancer (Roossink et al. 2012). This suggests that the response of tumours to radiotherapy might be associated with the levels of ATM activity, and that reduced ATM expression or activity might confer radiosensitivity in a clinical setting. Furthermore, elevated levels of ATM protein expression or ATM activity in tumour tissues may identify radioresistant tumours, and therefore this could serve as a potential bio-marker to identify patients that might get the greatest benefit from a combination of ATM inhibitor treatment and radiotherapy.

It should be noted however, that the physiological significance of ATM S1981 autophosphorylation is still controversial, as mutation of mouse ATM at S1987 (the mouse homologue of human S1981) to alanine did not affect the localisation of ATM to DNA DSBs or the phosphorylation of its downstream targets when expressed in an ATM knockout background (Pellegrini et al. 2006). Several other ATM autophosphorylation sites have also been shown to be dispensable for the function and activity of murine ATM in vivo (Daniel et al. 2008). Further studies will need to address the question whether these differential observations are due to species-specific differences in ATM activation, or whether S1981 autophosphorylation is a consequence of, rather than a requirement for, ATM activation.

Additional potential biomarkers for the assessment of ATM activity, and conse-quently its inhibition, include phosphorylation levels of several ATM downstream targets such as KAP-1 (S824), CHK2 (Thr68), p53 (S15) or H2AX (γH2AX) (Shiloh and Ziv 2013; Guo et al. 2014). The most likely challenges for the use of these bio-markers are first, that the background levels of these protein modifications in cells are likely to be very low, unless the cells are challenged by genotoxic treatments, such as IR, and thus they may not perform very well in single-agent studies. Secondly, several of these markers, including p53 and γH2AX are not specific measures of ATM kinase activity as they may also be targets of other DDR kinases, including DNA-PKcs and ATR, which have been shown to be activated in response to ATM inhibition, most likely in an attempt to compensate for the functional loss of ATM (Hammond et al. 2003; Mukherjee et al. 2006). Therefore, it may be necessary to use a panel of these markers to evaluate the activity of ATM inhibitors in the clinic (Bartkova et al. 2005; Kozlov et al. 2011).

7.8   Conclusion

The DDR kinase ATM is emerging as a promising new target for cancer therapy, both as a monotherapy in synthetic lethal approaches and as a chemo- or radiosen-sitiser. Synthetic lethal approaches have the potential for wide therapeutic margins, as they target cancer cells based on genetic or epigenetic changes that are confined to the cancer cells. Considering the high specificity only for cancer cells with defects in certain signalling pathways, the development of robust biomarkers for patient selection will be critical for the successful future development of synthetic lethal approaches in the clinic. The somatic mutations and epigenetic changes that allow for these approaches to be successful also constitute a potential limitation, as they generally occur relatively infrequently and thus limit the number of eligible patients to test such an approach. Conversely, the combination of ATM kinase inhibitors with chemo- or radiotherapy allows for a broader treatment approach that may be suitable for a higher proportion of patients. The limitation of this approach will likely be normal tissue toxicity as the selectivity towards cancer cells is likely to be considerably less than with synthetic lethal approaches. Due to the potential for increased normal tissue effects, ATM inhibitors will need careful preclinical evaluation, particularly in combination with cytotoxic therapies. Several studies have indicated that the functional status of *TP53* may be important for the extent of radiosensitisation achieved by ATM inhibitors in vivo. As mutations in the *TP53* gene are very common in human cancers this finding suggests, that the combination of ATM inhibitors and radiotherapy may have broad utility for cancer treatment. Optimisation of treatment schedules will also be important to achieve the best possible anti-tumour effect while minimising normal tissue effects. In vitro studies carried out thus far are very encouraging, as they suggest that short-term exposure to ATM inhibitors is sufficient to achieve chemo- and radiosensitisation, which suggests that a favourable therapeutic window may be achievable. As a potent and selective ATM inhibitor (AZD0156) with good pharmacological properties has now entered clinical development, we await the results of first clinical studies with great interest.

References

Abdel-Fatah T, Sultana R, Abbotts R, Hawkes C, Seedhouse C, Chan S, Madhusudan S (2013) Clinicopathological and functional significance of XRCC1 expression in ovarian cancer. Int J Cancer 132:2778–2786

Abraham RT (2001) Cell cycle checkpoint signaling through the ATM and ATR kinases. Genes Dev 15:2177–2196

Aguilar-Quesada R, Muñoz-Gámez JA, Martín-Oliva D, Peralta A, Valenzuela MT, Matínez-Romero R, Quiles-Pérez R, Menissier-de Murcia J, de Murcia G, Ruiz de Almodóvar M, Oliver FJ (2007) Interaction between ATM and PARP-1 in response to DNA damage and sensitization of ATM deficient cells through PARP inhibition. BMC Mol Biol 8:29

Álvarez-Quilón A, Serrano-Benítez A, Lieberman JA, Quintero C, Sánchez-Gutiérrez D, Escudero LM, Cortés-Ledesma F (2014) ATM specifically mediates repair of double-strand breaks with blocked DNA ends. Nat Commun 5:3347

Audeh MW, Carmichael J, Penson RT, Friedlander M, Powell B, Bell-McGuinn KM, Scott C, Weitzel JN, Oaknin A, Loman N, Lu K, Schmutzler RK, Matulonis U, Wickens M, Tutt A (2010) Oral poly(ADP-ribose) polymerase inhibitor olaparib in patients with BRCA1 or BRCA2 mutations and recurrent ovarian cancer: a proof-of-concept trial. Lancet 376:245–251

Bakkenist CJ, Kastan MB (2003) DNA damage activates ATM through intermolecular autophosphorylation and dimer dissociation. Nature 421:499–506

Bakr A, Oing C, Kocher S, Borgmann K, Dornreiter I, Petersen C, Dikomey E, Mansour WY (2015) Involvement of ATM in homologous recombination after end resection and RAD51 nucleofilament formation. Nucleic Acids Res 43:3154–3166

Barlow C, Hirotsune S, Paylor R, Liyanage M, Eckhaus M, Collins F, Shiloh Y, Crawley JN, Ried T, Tagle D, Wynshaw-Boris A (1996) Atm-deficient mice: a paradigm of ataxia telangiectasia. Cell 86:159–171

Bartek J, Lukas C, Lukas J (2004) Checking on DNA damage in S phase. Nat Rev Mol Cell Biol 5:792–804

Bartkova J, Horejsi Z, Koed K, Krämer A, Tort F, Zieger K, Guldberg P, Sehested M, Nesland JM, Lukas C, Ørntoft T, Lukas J, Bartek J (2005) DNA damage response as a candidate anti-cancer barrier in early human tumorigenesis. Nature 434:864–870

Bartkova J, Rezaei N, Liontos M, Karakaidos P, Kletsas D, Issaeva N, Vassiliou L-VF, Kolettas E, Niforou K, Zoumpourlis VC, Takaoka M, Nakagawa H, Tort F, Fugger K, Johansson F, Sehested M, Andersen CL, Dyrskjot L, Ørntoft T, Lukas J et al (2006) Oncogene-induced senescence is part of the tumorigenesis barrier imposed by DNA damage checkpoints. Nature 444:633–637

Batey MA, Zhao Y, Kyle S, Richardson C, Slade A, Martin NMB, Lau A, Newell DR, Curtin NJ (2013) Preclinical evaluation of a novel ATM inhibitor, KU59403, in vitro and in vivo in p53 functional and dysfunctional models of human cancer. Mol Cancer Ther 12:959–967

Beà S, Valdés-Mas R, Navarro A, Salaverria I, Martín-Garcia D, Jares P, Giné E, Pinyol M, Royo C, Nadeu F, Conde L, Juan M, Clot G, Vizán P, Di Croce L, Puente DA, López-Guerra M, Moros A, Roue G, Aymerich M et al (2013) Landscape of somatic mutations and clonal evolution in mantle cell lymphoma. Proc Natl Acad Sci U S A 110:18250–18255

Beamish H, Lavin MF (1994) Radiosensitivity in ataxia-telangiectasia: anomalies in radiation-induced cell cycle delay. Int J Radiat Biol 65:175–184

Berkovich E, Monnat RJ, Kastan MB (2007) Roles of ATM and NBS1 in chromatin structure modulation and DNA double-strand break repair. Nat Cell Biol 9:683–690

Beucher A, Birraux J, Tchouandong L, Barton O, Shibata A, Conrad S, Goodarzi AA, Krempler A, Jeggo PA, Löbrich M (2009) ATM and Artemis promote homologous recombination of radiation-induced DNA double-strand breaks in G2. EMBO J 28:3413–3427

Bhattacharyya A, Ear US, Koller BH, Weichselbaum RR, Bishop DK (2000) The breast cancer susceptibility gene BRCA1 is required for subnuclear assembly of Rad51 and survival following treatment with the DNA cross-linking agent cisplatin. J Biol Chem 275:23899–23903

Biddlestone-Thorpe L, Sajjad M, Rosenberg E, Beckta JM, Valerie NCK, Tokarz M, Adams BR, Wagner AF, Khalil A, Gilfor D, Golding SE, Deb S, Temesi DG, Lau A, O'Connor MJ, Choe KS, Parada LF, Lim SK, Mukhopadhyay ND, Valerie K (2013) ATM kinase inhibition preferentially sensitizes p53-mutant glioma to ionizing radiation. Clin Cancer Res 19:3189–3200

Blasina A, Price BD, Turenne GA, McGowan CH (1999) Caffeine inhibits the checkpoint kinase ATM. Curr Biol 9:1135–1138

Bracey TS, Williams AC, Paraskeva C (1997) Inhibition of radiation-induced G2 delay potentiates cell death by apoptosis and/or the induction of giant cells in colorectal tumor cells with disrupted p53 function. Clin Cancer Res 3:1371–1381

Brown KD, Ziv Y, Sadanandan SN, Chessa L, Collins FS, Shiloh Y, Tagle DA (1997) The ataxia-telangiectasia gene product, a constitutively expressed nuclear protein that is not up-regulated following genome damage. Proc Natl Acad Sci U S A 94:1840–1845

Bryant HE, Schultz N, Thomas HD, Parker KM, Flower D, Lopez E, Kyle S, Meuth M, Curtin NJ, Helleday T (2005) Specific killing of BRCA2-deficient tumours with inhibitors of poly(ADP-ribose) polymerase. Nature 434:913–917

Cancer Genome Atlas Research Network (2012a) Comprehensive molecular characterization of human colon and rectal cancer. Nature 487:330–337

Cancer Genome Atlas Research Network (2012b) Comprehensive genomic characterization of squamous cell lung cancers. Nature 489:519–525

Cancer Genome Atlas Research Network (2012c) Comprehensive molecular portraits of human breast tumours. Nature 490:61–70

Cancer Genome Atlas Research Network (2014) Comprehensive molecular profiling of lung adenocarcinoma. Nature 511:543–550

Chen L, Nievera CJ, Lee AY-L, Wu X (2008) Cell cycle-dependent complex formation of BRCA1. CtIP.MRN is important for DNA double-strand break repair. J Biol Chem 283:7713–7720

Choi S, Gamper AM, White JS, Bakkenist CJ (2010) Inhibition of ATM kinase activity does not phenocopy ATM protein disruption: implications for the clinical utility of ATM kinase inhibitors. Cell Cycle 9:4052–4057

Choudhury A, Nelson LD, Teo MTW, Chilka S, Bhattarai S, Johnston CF, Elliott F, Lowery J, Taylor CF, Churchman M, Bentley J, Knowles MA, Harnden P, Bristow RG, Bishop DT, Kiltie AE (2010) MRE11 expression is predictive of cause-specific survival following radical radiotherapy for muscle-invasive bladder cancer. Cancer Res 70:7017–7026

Cimprich K, Cortez D (2008) ATR: an essential regulator of genome integrity. Nat Rev Mol Cell Biol 9:616–627

Cornell L, Munck JM, Alsinet C, Villanueva A, Ogle L, Willoughby CE, Televantou D, Thomas HD, Jackson J, Burt AD, Newell D, Rose J, Manas DM, Shapiro GI, Curtin NJ, Reeves HL (2015) DNA-PK-A candidate driver of hepatocarcinogenesis and tissue biomarker that predicts response to treatment and survival. Clin Cancer Res 21:925–933

Cornforth MN, Bedford JS (1985) On the nature of a defect in cells from individuals with ataxia-telangiectasia. Science 227:1589–1591

Cortez D, Wang Y, Qin J, Elledge SJ (1999) Requirement of ATM-dependent phosphorylation of brca1 in the DNA damage response to double-strand breaks. Science 286:1162–1166

Daniel JA, Pellegrini M, Lee JH, Paull TT, Feigenbaum L, Nussenzweig A (2008) Multiple autophosphorylation sites are dispensable for murine ATM activation in vivo. J Cell Biol 183:777–783

Daniel JA, Pellegrini M, Lee BS, Guo Z, Filsuf D, Belkina NV, You Z, Paull TT, Sleckman BP, Feigenbaum L, Nussenzweig A (2012) Loss of ATM kinase activity leads to embryonic lethality in mice. J Cell Biol 198:295–304

Dar ME, Winters TA, Jorgensen TJ (1997) Identification of defective illegitimate recombinational repair of oxidatively-induced DNA double-strand breaks in ataxia-telangiectasia cells. Mutat Res 384:169–179

Darroudi F, Wiegant W, Meijers M, Friedl AA, van der Burg M, Fomina J, van Dongen JJM, van Gent DC, Zdzienicka MZ (2007) Role of Artemis in DSB repair and guarding chromosomal stability following exposure to ionizing radiation at different stages of cell cycle. Mutat Res 615:111–124

Di Micco R, Fumagalli M, Cicalese A, Piccinin S, Gasparini P, Luise C, Schurra C, Garre' M, Nuciforo PG, Bensimon A, Maestro R, Pelicci PG, d'Adda di Fagagna F (2006) Oncogene-induced senescence is a DNA damage response triggered by DNA hyper-replication. Nature 444:638–642

Elson A, Wang Y, Daugherty CJ, Morton CC, Zhou F, Campos-Torres J, Leder P (1996) Pleiotropic defects in ataxia-telangiectasia protein-deficient mice. Proc Natl Acad Sci U S A 93:13084–13089

Falck J, Mailand N, Syljuåsen RG, Bartek J, Lukas J (2001) The ATM-Chk2-Cdc25A checkpoint pathway guards against radioresistant DNA synthesis. Nature 410:842–847

Farmer H, McCabe N, Lord CJ, Tutt ANJ, Johnson DA, Richardson TB, Santarosa M, Dillon KJ, Hickson I, Knights C, Martin NMB, Jackson SP, Smith GCM, Ashworth A (2005) Targeting the DNA repair defect in BRCA mutant cells as a therapeutic strategy. Nature 434:917–921

Fedier A, Schlamminger M, Schwarz VA, Haller U, Howell SB, Fink D (2003) Loss of atm sensitises p53-deficient cells to topoisomerase poisons and antimetabolites. Ann Oncol 14:938–945

Fong PC, Boss DS, Yap TA, Tutt A, Wu P, Marja M-R, Mortimer P, Swaisland H, Lau A, O'Connor MJ, Ashworth A, Carmichael J, Kaye SB, Schellens JHM, de Bono JS (2009) Inhibition of poly(ADP-ribose) polymerase in tumors from BRCA mutation carriers. N Engl J Med 361:123–134

Foray N, Priestley A, Alsbeih G, Badie C, Capulas EP, Arlett CF, Malaise EP (1997) Hypersensitivity of ataxia telangiectasia fibroblasts to ionizing radiation is associated with a repair deficiency of DNA double-strand breaks. Int J Radiat Biol 72:271–283

Gatei M, Zhou BB, Hobson K, Scott S, Young D, Khanna KK (2001) Ataxia telangiectasia mutated (ATM) kinase and ATM and Rad3 related kinase mediate phosphorylation of Brca1 at distinct and overlapping sites. J Biol Chem 276:17276–17280

Gilad S, Khosravi R, Shkedy D, Uziel T, Ziv Y, Savitsky K, Rotman G, Smith S, Chessa L, Jorgensen TJ, Harnik R, Frydman M, Sanal O, Portnoi S, Goldwicz Z, Jaspers NGJ, Gatti RA, Lenoir G, Lavin MF, Tatsumi K et al (1996) Predominance of null mutations in ataxia-telangiectasia. Hum Mol Genet 5:433–439

Gnad F, Baucom A, Mukhyala K, Manning G, Zhang Z (2013) Assessment of computational methods for predicting the effects of missense mutations in human cancers. BMC Genomics 14:S7

Goh AM, Coffill CR, Lane DP (2011) The role of mutant p53 in human cancer. J Pathol 223:116–126

Golding SE, Rosenberg E, Valerie N, Hussaini I, Frigerio M, Cockcroft XF, Chong WY, Hummersone M, Rigoreau L, Menear KA, O'Connor MJ, Povirk LF, van Meter T, Valerie K (2009) Improved ATM kinase inhibitor KU-60019 radiosensitizes glioma cells, compromises insulin, AKT and ERK prosurvival signaling, and inhibits migration and invasion. Mol Cancer Ther 8:2894–2902

Golding S, Rosenberg E, Adams BR, Wignarajah S, Beckta JM, O'Connor MJ, Valerie K (2012) Dynamic inhibition of ATM kinase provides a strategy for glioblastoma multiforme radiosensitization and growth control. Cell Cycle 11:1167–1173

Goodarzi AA, Noon AT, Deckbar D, Ziv Y, Shiloh Y, Löbrich M, Jeggo PA (2008) ATM signaling facilitates repair of DNA double-strand breaks associated with heterochromatin. Mol Cell 31:167–177

Goodarzi AA, Jeggo P, Löbrich M (2010) The influence of heterochromatin on DNA double strand break repair: getting the strong, silent type to relax. DNA Repair (Amst) 9:1273–1282

Gorgoulis VG, Vassiliou LF, Karakaidos P, Zacharatos P, Kotsinas A, Liloglou T, Venere M, Ditullio RA Jr, Kastrinakis NG, Levy B, Kletsas D, Yoneta A, Herlyn M, Kittas C, Halazonetis TD (2005) Activation of the DNA damage checkpoint and genomic instability in human precancerous lesions. Nature 434:907–913

Guichard S, Brown E, Odedra R, Hughes A, Heathcote D, Barnes J, Lau A, Powell S, Jones CD, Nissink W, Foote KM, Jewsbury PJ, Pass M (2013) The pre-clinical in vitro and in vivo activity of AZD6738: a potent and selective inhibitor of ATR kinase [abstract]. In: Proceedings of the 104th annual meeting of the American Association for Cancer Research, Washington, DC, 6–10 Apr 2013. AACR, Philadelphia, PA. Cancer Res 73(8 Suppl):Abstract nr 3343. https://doi.org/10.1158/1538-7445.AM2013-3343

Guo K, Shelat AA, Guy RK, Kastan MB (2014) Development of a cell-based, high-throughput screening assay for ATM kinase inhibitors. J Biomol Screen 19:538–546

Halazonetis TD, Gorgoulis VG, Bartek J (2008) An oncogene-induced DNA damage model for cancer development. Science 319:1352–1355

Hammond EM, Dorie MJ, Giaccia AJ (2003) ATR/ATM targets are phosphorylated by ATR in response to hypoxia and ATM in response to reoxygenation. J Biol Chem 278:12207–12213

Helleday T (2010) Homologous recombination in cancer development, treatment and development of drug resistance. Carcinogenesis 31:955–960

Helleday T, Lo J, van Gent DC, Engelward BP (2007) DNA double-strand break repair: from mechanistic understanding to cancer treatment. DNA Repair 6:923–935

Helt CE, Cliby WA, Keng PC, Bambara RA, O'Reilly MA (2005) Ataxia telangiectasia mutated (ATM) and ATM and Rad3-related protein exhibit selective target specificities in response to different forms of DNA damage. J Biol Chem 280:1186–1192

Hickson I, Zhao Y, Richardson CJ, Green SJ, Martin NMB, Orr AI, Reaper PM, Jackson SP, Curtin NJ, Smith GC (2004) Identification and characterization of a novel and specific inhibitor of the ataxia-telangiectasia mutated kinase ATM. Cancer Res 64:9152–9159

Houldsworth J, Lavin M (1980) Effect of ionizing radiation on DNA synthesis in ataxia teleangiectasia cells. Nucleic Acids Res 8:3709–3720

Huertas P, Jackson SP (2009) Human CtIP mediates cell cycle control of DNA end resection and double strand break repair. J Biol Chem 284:9558–9565

Jacquemin V, Rieunier G, Jacob S, Bellanger D, D'Enghien CD, Laugé A, Stoppa-Lyonnet D, Stern M-H (2012) Underexpression and abnormal localization of ATM products in ataxia telangiectasia patients bearing ATM missense mutations. Eur J Hum Genet 20:305–312

Jaspers NGJ, De Wit J, Regulski MR, Bootsma D (1982) Abnormal regulation of DNA replication and increased lethality in ataxia telangiectasia cells exposed to carcinogenic agents. Cancer Res 42:335–341

Jeggo PA (1998) DNA breakage and repair. Adv Genet 38:185–218

Jeggo PA, Löbrich M (2006) Contribution of DNA repair and cell cycle checkpoint arrest to the maintenance of genomic stability. DNA Repair (Amst) 5:1192–1198

Jenkins C, Kan J, Hoatlin ME (2012) Targeting the fanconi anemia pathway to identify tailored anticancer therapeutics. Anemia 2012:481583

Jones CD, Blades K, Foote KM, Guichard SM, Jewsbury PJ, McGuire T, Nissink JW, Odedra R, Tam K, Thommes P, Turner P, Wilkinson G, Wood C, Yates JW (2013) Discovery of AZD6738, a potent and selective inhibitor with the potential to test the clinical efficacy of ATR kinase inhibition in cancer patients [abstract]. In Proceedings of the 104th annual meeting of the American Association for Cancer Research, Washington, DC, 6–10 Apr 2013. AACR, Philadelphia, PA. Cancer Res 73(8 Suppl):Abstract nr 2348. https://doi.org/10.1158/1538-7445.AM2013-2348

Kaelin WGJ (2005) The concept of synthetic lethality in the context of anticancer therapy. Nat Rev Cancer 5:689–698

Kakarougkas A, Jeggo PA (2014) DNA DSB repair pathway choice: an orchestrated handover mechanism. Br J Radiol 87:20130685

Kandoth C, McLellan MD, Vandin F, Ye K, Niu B, Lu C, Xie M, Zhang Q, McMichael JF, Wyczalkowski MA, Leiserson MDM, Miller CA, Welch JS, Walter MJ, Wendl MC, Ley TJ, Wilson RK, Raphael BJ, Ding L (2013) Mutational landscape and significance across 12 major cancer types. Nature 502:333–339

Kastan MB, Zhan Q, El-Deiry WS, Carrier F, Jacks T, Walsh WV, Plunkett BS, Vogelstein B, Fornace AJJ (1992) A mammalian cell cycle checkpoint pathway utilizing p53 and GADD45 is defective in ataxia-telangiectasia. Cell 71:587–597

Kennedy RD, D'Andrea AD (2006) DNA repair pathways in clinical practice: lessons from pediatric cancer susceptibility syndromes. J Clin Oncol 24:3799–3808

Kennedy RD, Chen CC, Stuckert P, Archila EM, De la Vega MA, Moreau LA, Shimamura A, D'Andrea AD (2007) Fanconi anemia pathway-deficient tumor cells are hypersensitive to inhibition of ataxia telangiectasia mutated. J Clin Invest 117:1140–1149

Kim W-J, Vo QN, Shrivastav M, Lataxes TA, Brown KD (2002) Aberrant methylation of the ATM promoter correlates with increased radiosensitivity in a human colorectal tumor cell line. Oncogene 21:3864–3871

Köcher S, Rieckmann T, Rohaly G, Mansour WY, Dikomey E, Dornreiter I, Dahm-Daphi J (2012) Radiation-induced double-strand breaks require ATM but not Artemis for homologous recombination during S-phase. Nucleic Acids Res 40:8336–8347

Köcher S, Spies-Naumann A, Kriegs M, Dahm-Daphi J, Dornreiter I (2013) ATM is required for the repair of Topotecan-induced replication-associated double-strand breaks. Radiother Oncol 108:409–414

Kozlov SV, Graham ME, Peng C, Chen P, Robinson PJ, Lavin MF (2006) Involvement of novel autophosphorylation sites in ATM activation. EMBO J 25:3504–3514

Kozlov SV, Graham ME, Jakob B, Tobias F, Kijas AW, Tanuji M, Chen P, Robinson PJ, Taucher-Scholz G, Suzuki K, So S, Chen D, Lavin MF (2011) Autophosphorylation and ATM activation: additional sites add to the complexity. J Biol Chem 286:9107–9119

Krejci L, Altmannova V, Spirek M, Zhao X (2012) Homologous recombination and its regulation. Nucleic Acids Res 40:5795–5818

Kubota E, Williamson CT, Ye R, Elegbede A, Peterson L, Lees-Miller SP, Bebb DG (2014) Low ATM protein expression and depletion of p53 correlates with olaparib sensitivity in gastric cancer cell lines. Cell Cycle 13:2129–2137

Kühne M, Riballo E, Rief N, Ku M, Rothkamm K, Jeggo PA, Löbrich M (2004) A double-strand break repair defect in ATM-deficient cells contributes to radiosensitivity. Cancer Res 64:500–508

Kurosawa A, Adachi N (2010) Functions and regulation of Artemis: a goddess in the maintenance of genome integrity. J Radiat Res 51:503–509

Landais I, Hiddingh S, McCarroll M, Yang C, Sun A, Turker MS, Snyder JP, Hoatlin ME (2009) Monoketone analogs of curcumin, a new class of Fanconi anemia pathway inhibitors. Mol Cancer 8:133

Landau DA, Wu CJ (2013) Chronic lymphocytic leukemia: molecular heterogeneity revealed by high-throughput genomics. Genome Med 5:47

Lavin MF (2008) Ataxia-telangiectasia: from a rare disorder to a paradigm for cell signalling and cancer. Nat Rev Mol Cell Biol 9:759–769

Lavin MF, Shiloh Y (1997) The genetic defect in ataxia-telangiectasia. Annu Rev Immunol 15:177–202

Lavin MF, Scott S, Gueven N, Kozlov S, Peng C, Chen P (2004) Functional consequences of sequence alterations in the ATM gene. DNA Repair 3:1197–1205

Lee J-H, Paull TT (2005) ATM activation by DNA double-strand breaks through the Mre11-Rad50-Nbs1 complex. Science 308:551–554

Li S, Ting NS, Zheng L, Chen PL, Ziv Y, Shiloh Y, Lee EY, Lee WH (2000) Functional link of BRCA1 and ataxia telangiectasia gene product in DNA damage response. Nature 406:210–215

Lipkowitz S, Stern M-H, Kirsch IR (1990) Hybrid T cell receptor genes formed by interlocus recombination in normal and ataxia-telangiectasia lymphocytes. J Exp Med 172:409–418

Lovly CM, Shaw AT (2014) Molecular pathways: resistance to kinase inhibitors and implications for therapeutic strategies. Clin Cancer Res 20:2249–2256

Lumsden JM, McCarty T, Petiniot LK, Shen R, Barlow C, Wynn TA, Morse HC, Gearhart PJ, Wynshaw-Boris A, Max EE, Hodes RJ (2004) Immunoglobulin class switch recombination is impaired in Atm-deficient mice. J Exp Med 200:1111–1121

Luo C-M, Tang W, Mekeel KL, DeFrank JS, Rani AP, Powell SN (1996) High frequency and error-prone DNA recombination in ataxia telangiectasia cell lines. J Biol Chem 271:4497–4503

Ma Y, Pannicke U, Schwarz K, Lieber MR (2002) Hairpin opening and overhang processing by an Artemis/DNA-dependent protein kinase complex in nonhomologous end joining and V(D)J recombination. Cell 108:781–794

Ma Y, Schwarz K, Lieber MR (2005) The Artemis:DNA-PKcs endonuclease cleaves DNA loops, flaps, and gaps. DNA Repair 4:845–851

Ma J, Setton J, Morris L, Albornoz PB, Barker C, Lok BH, Sherman E, Katabi N, Beal K, Ganly I, Powell SN, Lee N, Chan TA, Riaz N (2017) Genomic analysis of exceptional responders to radiotherapy reveals somatic mutations in ATM. Oncotarget 8:10312–10323

Matsuoka S, Huang M, Elledge SJ (1998) Linkage of ATM to cell cycle regulation by the Chk2 protein kinase. Science 282:1893–1897

Matsuoka S, Ballif BA, Smogorzewska A, McDonald ER, Hurov KE, Luo J, Bakalarski CE, Zhao Z, Solimini N, Lerenthal Y, Shiloh Y, Gygi SP, Elledge SJ (2007) ATM and ATR substrate analysis reveals extensive protein networks responsive to DNA damage. Science 316:1160–1166

Menezes DL, Holt J, Tang Y, Feng J, Barsanti P, Pan Y, Ghoddusi M, Zhang W, Thomas G, Holash J, Lees E, Taricani L (2014) A synthetic lethal screen reveals enhanced sensitivity to ATR inhibitor treatment in mantle cell lymphoma with ATM loss-of-function. Mol Cancer Res 13(1):120–129

Meyn MS (1993) High spontaneous intrachromosomal recombination rates in ataxia-telangiectasia. Science 260:1327–1330

Mitui M, Nahas SA, Du LT, Yang Z, Lai CH, Nakamura K, Arroyo S, Scott S, Purayidom A, Concannon P, Lavin MF, Gatti RA (2009) Functional and computational assessment of missense variants in the ataxia-telangiectasia mutated (ATM) gene: mutations with increased cancer risk. Hum Mutat 30:12–21

Moding EJ, Lee C-L, Castle KD, Oh P, Mao L, Zha S, Min HD, Ma Y, Das S, Kirsch DG (2014) Atm deletion with dual recombinase technology preferentially radiosensitizes tumor endothelium. J Clin Invest 124:3325–3338

Mohammadinejad P, Abolhassani H, Aghamohammadi A, Pourhamdi S, Ghosh S, Sadeghi B, Nasiri Kalmarzi R, Durandy A, Borkhardt A (2015) Class switch recombination process in ataxia telangiectasia patients with elevated serum levels of IgM. J Immunoass Immunochem 36:16–26

Morrison C, Sonoda E, Takao N, Shinohara A, Yamamoto K, Takeda S (2000) The controlling role of ATM in homologous recombinational repair of DNA damage. EMBO J 19:463–471

Moshous D, Callebaut I, De Chasseval R, Corneo B, Cavazzana-Calvo M, Le Deist F, Tezcan I, Sanal O, Bertrand Y, Philippe N, Fischer A, De Villartay JP (2001) Artemis, a novel DNA double-strand break repair/V(D)J recombination protein, is mutated in human severe combined immune deficiency. Cell 105:177–186

Moynahan ME, Cui TY, Jasin M (2001) Homology-directed DNA repair, mitomycin-C resistance, and chromosome stability is restored with correction of a Brca1 mutation. Cancer Res 61:4842–4850

Mukherjee B, Kessinger C, Kobayashi J, Chen BPC, Chen DJ, Chatterjee A, Burma S (2006) DNA-PK phosphorylates histone H2AX during apoptotic DNA fragmentation in mammalian cells. DNA Repair (Amst) 5:575–590

Negrini S, Gorgoulis VG, Halazonetis TD (2010) Genomic instability—an evolving hallmark of cancer. Nat Rev Mol Cell Biol 11:220–228

Nicolas N, Moshous D, Cavazzana-Calvo M, Papadopoulo D, de Chasseval R, Le Deist F, Fischer A, de Villartay J-P (1998) A human severe combined immunodeficiency (SCID) condition with increased sensitivity to ionizing radiations and impaired V(D)J rearrangements defines a new DNA recombination/repair deficiency. J Exp Med 188:627–634

Niederst MJ, Engelman JA (2013) Bypass mechanisms of resistance to receptor tyrosine kinase inhibition in lung cancer. Sci Signal 6:re6

Oxford JM, Harnden DG, Parrington JM, Delhanty JD (1975) Specific chromosome aberrations in ataxia telangiectasia. J Med Genet 12:251–262

Painter RB, Young BR (1980) Radiosensitivity in ataxia-telangiectasia: a new explanation. Proc Natl Acad Sci U S A 77:7315–7317

Pannicke U, Ma Y, Hopfner K-P, Niewolik D, Lieber MR, Schwarz K (2004) Functional and biochemical dissection of the structure-specific nuclease ARTEMIS. EMBO J 23:1987–1997

Paull TT, Rogakou EP, Yamazaki V, Kirchgessner CU, Gellert M, Bonner WM (2000) A critical role for histone H2AX in recruitment of repair factors to nuclear foci after DNA damage. Curr Biol 10:886–895

Pellegrini M, Celeste A, Difilippantonio S, Guo R, Wang W, Feigenbaum L, Nussenzweig A (2006) Autophosphorylation at serine 1987 is dispensable for murine Atm activation in vivo. Nature 443:222–225

Peng C-Y, Graves PR, Thoma RS, Wu Z, Shaw AS, Piwnica-Worms H (1997) Mitotic and G2 checkpoint control: regulation of 14-3-3 protein binding by phosphorylation of Cdc25C on serine-216. Science 277:1501–1505

Powell S, Whitaker S, Peacock J, McMillan T (1993) Ataxia telangiectasia: an investigation of the repair defect in the cell line AT5BIVA by plasmid reconstitution. Mutat Res 294:9–20

Powell SN, DeFrank JS, Connell P, Eogan M, Preffer F, Dombkowski D, Tang W, Friend S (1995) Differential sensitivity of p53(−) and p53(+) cells to caffeine-induced radiosensitization and override of G2 delay. Cancer Res 55:1643–1648

Price BD, Youmell MB (1996) The phosphatidylinositol 3-kinase inhibitor wortmannin sensitizes murine fibroblasts and human tumor cells to radiation and blocks induction of p53 following DNA damage. Cancer Res 56:246–250

Rainey MD, Charlton ME, Stanton RV, Kastan MB (2008) Transient inhibition of ATM kinase is sufficient to enhance cellular sensitivity to ionizing radiation. Cancer Res 68:7466–7474

Reaper PM, Griffiths MR, Long JM, Charrier J-D, Maccormick S, Charlton PA, Golec JMC, Pollard JR (2011) Selective killing of ATM- or p53-deficient cancer cells through inhibition of ATR. Nat Chem Biol 7:428–430

Reina-San-Martin B, Chen HT, Nussenzweig A, Nussenzweig MC (2004) ATM is required for efficient recombination between immunoglobulin switch regions. J Exp Med 200:1103–1110

Riballo E, Kühne M, Rief N, Doherty A, Smith GCM, Recio MJ, Reis C, Dahm K, Fricke A, Krempler A, Parker AR, Jackson SP, Gennery A, Jeggo PA, Löbrich M (2004) A pathway of double-strand break rejoining dependent upon ATM, Artemis, and proteins locating to γ-H2AX foci. Mol Cell 16:715–724

Roossink F, Wieringa HW, Noordhuis MG, ten Hoor KA, Kok M, Slagter-Menkema L, Hollema H, de Bock GH, Pras E, de Vries EGE, de Jong S, van der Zee AGJ, Schuuring E, Wisman GBA, van Vugt MATM (2012) The role of ATM and 53BP1 as predictive markers in cervical cancer. Int J Cancer 131:2056–2066

Rotman G, Shiloh Y (1998) ATM: from gene to function. Hum Mol Genet 7:1555–1563

Roy K, Wang L, Makrigiorgos GM, Price BD (2006) Methylation of the ATM promoter in glioma cells alters ionizing radiation sensitivity. Biochem Biophys Res Commun 344:821–826

Ryan AJ, Squires S, Strutt HL, Johnson RT (1991) Camptothecin cytotoxicity in mammalian cells is associated with the induction of persistent double strand breaks in replicating DNA. Nucleic Acids Res 19:3295–3300

Sancar A, Lindsey-Boltz LA, Unsal-Kaçmaz K, Linn S (2004) Molecular mechanisms of mammalian DNA repair and the DNA damage checkpoints. Annu Rev Biochem 73:39–85

Sanchez Y, Wong C, Thoma RS, Richman R, Wu Z, Piwnica-Worms H, Elledge SJ (1997) Conservation of the Chk1 checkpoint pathway in mammals: linkage of DNA damage to Cdk regulation through Cdc25. Science 277:1497–1501

Sandoval N, Platzer M, Rosenthal A, Dörk T, Bendix R, Skawran B, Stuhrmann M, Wegner RD, Sperling K, Banin S, Shiloh Y, Baumer A, Bernthaler U, Sennefelder H, Brohm M, Weber BH, Schindler D (1999) Characterization of ATM gene mutations in 66 ataxia telangiectasia families. Hum Mol Genet 8:69–79

Sarkaria JN, Tibbetts RS, Busby EC, Kennedy AP, Hill DE, Abraham RT (1998) Inhibition of phosphoinositide 3-kinase related kinases by the radiosensitizing agent wortmannin. Cancer Res 58:4375–4382

Sarkaria JN, Busby EC, Tibbetts RS, Roos P, Taya Y, Karnitz LM, Abraham RT (1999) Inhibition of ATM and ATR Kinase activities by the radiosensitizing agent, caffeine. Cancer Res 59:4375–4382

Sartori AA, Lukas C, Coates J, Mistrik M, Fu S, Bartek J, Baer R, Lukas J, Jackson SP (2007) Human CtIP promotes DNA end resection. Nature 450:509–514

Savitsky K, Bar-Shira A, Gilad S, Rotman G, Ziv Y, Vanagaite L, Tagle DA, Smith S, Uziel T, Sfez S, Ashkenazi M, Pecker I, Frydman M, Harnik R, Patanjali SR, Simmons A, Clines GA, Sartiel A, Gatti RA, Chessa L et al (1995) A single ataxia telangiectasia gene with a product similar to PI-3 kinase. Science 268:1749–1753

Shiloh Y (2001) ATM and ATR: networking cellular responses to DNA damage. Curr Opin Genet Dev 11:71–77

Shiloh Y (2003) ATM and related protein kinases: safeguarding genome integrity. Nat Rev Cancer 3:155–168

Shiloh Y, Ziv Y (2013) The ATM protein kinase: regulating the cellular response to genotoxic stress, and more. Nat Rev Mol Cell Biol 14:197–210

Smith PJ, Makinson TA, Watson JV (1989) Enhanced sensitivity to camptothecin in ataxia-telangiectasia cells and its relationship with the expression of DNA topoisomerase I. Int J Radiat Biol 55:217–231

So S, Davis AJ, Chen DJ (2009) Autophosphorylation at serine 1981 stabilizes ATM at DNA damage sites. J Cell Biol 187:977–990

Strumberg D, Pilon AA, Smith M, Hickey R, Malkas L, Pommier Y (2000) Conversion of topoisomerase I cleavage complexes on the leading strand of ribosomal DNA into 5'-phosphorylated DNA double-strand breaks by replication runoff. Mol Cell Biol 20:3977–3987

Sullivan RJ, Flaherty KT (2013) Resistance to BRAF-targeted therapy in melanoma. Eur J Cancer 49:1297–1304

Sultana R, McNeill DR, Abbotts R, Mohammed MZ, Zdzienicka MZ, Qutob H, Seedhouse C, Laughton CA, Fischer PM, Patel PM, Wilson DM, Madhusudan S (2012) Synthetic lethal targeting of DNA double-strand break repair deficient cells by human apurinic/apyrimidinic endonuclease inhibitors. Int J Cancer 131:2433–2444

Sultana R, Abdel-Fatah T, Abbotts R, Hawkes C, Albarakati N, Seedhouse C, Ball G, Chan S, Rakha EA, Ellis IO, Madhusudan S (2013) Targeting XRCC1 deficiency in breast cancer for personalized therapy. Cancer Res 73:1621–1634

Taylor AMR, Harnden DG, Arlett CF, Harcourt SA, Lehmann AR, Stevens S, Bridges BA (1975) Ataxia teleangiectasia: a human mutation with abnormal radiation sensitivity. Nature 258:427–429

Teng P, Bateman NW, Darcy KM, Hamilton CA, Larry G, Bakkenist CJ, Conrads TP (2015) Pharmacologic inhibition of ATR and ATM offers clinically important distinctions to enhancing platinumor radiation response in ovarian, endometrial, and cervical cancer cells. Gynecol Oncol 136:554–561

Tutt A, Robson M, Garber JE, Domchek SM, Audeh MW, Weitzel JN, Friedlander M, Arun B, Loman N, Schmutzler RK, Wardley A, Mitchell G, Earl H, Wickens M, Carmichael J (2010) Oral poly(ADP-ribose) polymerase inhibitor olaparib in patients with BRCA1 or BRCA2 mutations and advanced breast cancer: a proof-of-concept trial. Lancet 376:235–244

Vo QN, Kim W-J, Cvitanovic L, Boudreau DA, Ginzinger DG, Brown KD (2004) The ATM gene is a target for epigenetic silencing in locally advanced breast cancer. Oncogene 23:9432–9437

Wang J, Pluth JM, Cooper PK, Cowan MJ, Chen DJ, Yannone SM (2005) Artemis deficiency confers a DNA double-strand break repair defect and Artemis phosphorylation status is altered by DNA damage and cell cycle progression. DNA Repair (Amst) 4:556–570

Wang H, Shi LZ, Wong CCL, Han X, Hwang PYH, Truong LN, Zhu Q, Shao Z, Chen DJ, Berns MW, Yates JR, Chen L, Wu X (2013) The interaction of CtIP and Nbs1 connects CDK and ATM to regulate HR-mediated double-strand break repair. PLoS Genet 9:25–27

Weber AM, Ryan AJ (2015) ATM and ATR as therapeutic targets in cancer. Pharmacol Ther 149:124–138

Weber AM, Bokobza SM, Devery AM, Ryan AJ (2013) Combined ATM and ATR kinase inhibition selectively kills p53-mutated non-small cell lung cancer (NSCLC) cells [abstract]. In Proceedings of the AACR-NCI-EORTC international conference: molecular targets and cancer therapeutics, Boston,MA, 2013 Oct 19–23. AACR, Philadelphia, PA. Mol Cancer Ther 2(11 Suppl):Abstract nr B91. https://doi.org/10.1158/1535-7163.TARG-13-B91

Weber AM, Drobnitzky N, Devery AM, Bokobza SM, Adams RA, Maughan TS, Ryan AJ (2016) Phenotypic consequences of somatic mutations in the ataxia-telangiectasia mutated gene in non-small cell lung cancer. Oncotarget 7:60807–60822

Weston VJ, Oldreive CE, Skowronska A, Oscier DG, Pratt G, Dyer MJS, Smith G, Powell JE, Rudzki Z, Kearns P, Moss PAH, Taylor AMR, Stankovic T (2010) The PARP inhibitor olaparib induces significant killing of ATM-deficient lymphoid tumor cells in vitro and in vivo. Blood 116:4578–4587

White JS, Choi S, Bakkenist CJ (2010) Transient ATM kinase inhibition disrupts DNA damage-induced sister chromatid exchange. Sci Signal 3:ra44

Williamson CT, Muzik H, Turhan AG, Zamò A, O'Connor MJ, Bebb DG, Lees-Miller SP (2010) ATM deficiency sensitizes mantle cell lymphoma cells to poly(ADP-ribose) polymerase-1 inhibitors. Mol Cancer Ther 9:347–357

Williamson CT, Kubota E, Hamill JD, Klimowicz A, Ye R, Muzik H, Dean M, Tu L, Gilley D, Magliocco AM, McKay BC, Bebb DG, Lees-Miller SP (2012) Enhanced cytotoxicity of PARP inhibition in mantle cell lymphoma harbouring mutations in both ATM and p53. EMBO Mol Med 4:515–527

Woodbine L, Brunton H, Goodarzi AA, Shibata A, Jeggo PA (2011) Endogenously induced DNA double strand breaks arise in heterochromatic DNA regions and require ataxia telangiectasia mutated and Artemis for their repair. Nucleic Acids Res 39:6986–6997

Xiao Z, Chen Z, Gunasekera AH, Sowin TJ, Rosenberg SH, Fesik S, Zhang H (2003) Chk1 mediates S and G2 arrests through Cdc25A degradation in response to DNA-damaging agents. J Biol Chem 278:21767–21773

Yamamoto K, Wang Y, Jiang W, Liu X, Dubois RL, Lin C-S, Ludwig T, Bakkenist CJ, Zha S (2012) Kinase-dead ATM protein causes genomic instability and early embryonic lethality in mice. J Cell Biol 198:305–313

Yannone SM, Khan IS, Zhou RZ, Zhou T, Valerie K, Povirk LF (2008) Coordinate 5′ and 3′ endonucleolytic trimming of terminally blocked blunt DNA double-strand break ends by Artemis nuclease and DNA-dependent protein kinase. Nucleic Acids Res 36:3354–3365

Yao S-L, Akhtar AJ, McKenna KA, Bedi GC, David S, Mack M, Rajani R, Collector MI, Jones RJ, Sharkis SJ, Fuchs EJ, Bedi A (1996) Selective radiosensitization of p53-deficient cells by ceffeine-mediated activation of p34cdc2 kinase. Nat Med 2:1140–1143

You Z, Bailis JM (2010) DNA damage and decisions: CtIP coordinates DNA repair and cell cycle checkpoints. Trends Cell Biol 20:402–409

You Z, Chahwan C, Bailis J, Hunter T, Russell P (2005) ATM activation and its recruitment to damaged DNA require binding to the C terminus of Nbs1. Mol Cell Biol 25:5363–5379

Yuan SSF, Chang HL, Lee EYHP (2003) Ionizing radiation-induced Rad51 nuclear focus formation is cell cycle-regulated and defective in both ATM−/− and c-Abl−/− cells. Mutat Res 525:85–92

Yun J, Zhong Q, Kwak J-Y, Lee W-H (2005) Hypersensitivity of Brca1-deficient MEF to the DNA interstrand crosslinking agent mitomycin C is associated with defect in homologous recombination repair and aberrant S-phase arrest. Oncogene 24:4009–4016

Ziv Y, Bielopolski D, Galanty Y, Lukas C, Taya Y, Schultz DC, Lukas J, Bekker-Jensen S, Bartek J, Shiloh Y (2006) Chromatin relaxation in response to DNA double-strand breaks is modulated by a novel ATM- and KAP-1 dependent pathway. Nat Cell Biol 8:870–876

Chapter 8
Targeting ATM for Cancer Therapy: Prospects for Drugging ATM

Ian Hickson, Kurt G. Pike, and Stephen T. Durant

Abstract As discussed in the previous chapter, the rationale for inhibition of ATM as a therapeutic strategy in cancer is both scientifically sound and well explored. The use of experimental models and, thereafter, the availability of tool compounds to inhibit the target, has allowed the role of ATM in cell signalling to be refined and has highlighted the potential utility of ATM inhibition for therapeutic intervention. The role of ATM as the central DNA damage response (DDR) protein, the high sensitivity of cells from A-T patients, who lack functional ATM, to IR and DNA damaging chemotherapy, and the consequences of knocking down ATM in otherwise proficient cells, have been well described and support ATM as a pharmaceutical target of interest. The somewhat atypical nature of ATM (a member of the PIKK family of kinases), combined with the size of the protein, have brought some unique challenges and opportunities to the discovery of inhibitors of ATM. The development of robust, high-throughput biochemical assays for ATM inhibition has proved challenging, thereby requiring the establishment of less conventional assays to facilitate drug discovery efforts. However, the availability of early compounds that were shown to share features of ATM loss (i.e. bringing about sensitisation of cells to IR induced cell damage and death), helped advance the process and over the past decade the research into ATM inhibition has advanced as the quality of available inhibitors has improved. In this chapter, we will explore the evolution of ATM inhibitors from crude but effective tools, through highly selective tool compounds and ultimately to the development of compounds with potential clinical utility as therapeutics for cancer patients.

I. Hickson (✉)
Northern Institute for Cancer Research (NICR), Newcastle University, Newcastle, UK
e-mail: ian.hickson@newcastle.ac.uk

K. G. Pike · S. T. Durant
Oncology IMED Biotech Unit, Innovative Medicines and Early Development, AstraZeneca, Cambridge, UK
e-mail: kurt.pike@astrazeneca.com; stephen.durant@astrazeneca.com

© Springer International Publishing AG, part of Springer Nature 2018
J. Pollard, N. Curtin (eds.), *Targeting the DNA Damage Response for Anti-Cancer Therapy*, Cancer Drug Discovery and Development, https://doi.org/10.1007/978-3-319-75836-7_8

Keywords DDR · Ataxia-telangiectasia mutated · ATM · ATM inhibitor · AZ31 · AZ32 · AZD0156 · AZD1390 · KU-58050 · KU-55933 · KU-59403 · KU-60019 · CP-466722

8.1   Introduction

The biology, rationale and scope of ATM inhibitors has been very well detailed in the previous chapter but it is worth highlighting the key points of the role of ATM in the DNA Damage Response (DDR), as these features relate to the identification of inhibitors of ATM cellular activity. Ataxia telangiectasia (A-T) is a rare autosomal recessive disease, resulting in a syndrome of neurodegenerative disease, causing severe disability. Aside from the associated developmental and immunological effects of germline mutations of the Ataxia-telangiectasia mutated (ATM) gene, A-T patients suffer from genomic instability and cancer susceptibility, which has been linked to profound sensitivity of A-T cells to ionising radiation (IR), and radiomimetic (DNA-damaging) drugs (Lavin 2008; Lavin and Shiloh 1997; Rotman and Shiloh 1998; Taylor et al. 1975; Köcher et al. 2012, 2013). The cell cycle checkpoint defects of A–T cells result in failure to arrest cells at the G1/S boundary following exposure to ionising radiation, radiation-resistant DNA synthesis (Houldsworth and Lavin 1980; Kastan et al. 1992; Painter and Young 1980) and failure to delay mitotic entry (Beamish and Lavin 1994). Thus, inhibitors of ATM administered to ATM proficient cell lines would be expected to result in marked sensitisation to radiation induced DNA damage, disruption of cell cycle and, when combined with either radiation or chemotherapeutics that damage DNA, result in cell death (Weber and Ryan, 2015). It is important to note that the screening, characterisation and development of ATM inhibitors, as described in this chapter, is designed around and dependent upon the observed biology of the cells of A-T patients.

8.2   ATM as a Target

ATM is large protein (350 kDa) comprising 3056 residues and containing a kinase domain with a relatively high degree of similarity to the lipid kinase PI3K, hence its designation as a phosphoinositide 3-kinase (PI3K)-related kinase (PIKK) (Shiloh 2003). These atypical serine/threonine kinases also comprise ATR, DNA-PKcs, mTOR, SMG1 (and non-enzymatic TRRAP) (Fruman et al. 1998). To facilitate drug discovery efforts in identifying ATM inhibitors, assays of biological activity are required. Such assays rely on features of the biological function of ATM. Specifically, the inactive dimeric form of ATM is recruited to the site of a DSB by the DNA-end tethering MRE11-RAD50-NBS1 (MRN) complex that results in the autophosphorylation of ATM on Serine 1981 (Bakkenist and Kastan 2003; Lee and Paull 2005). This auto-phosphorylation event leads to dimer dissociation, activation of ATM and subsequent phosphorylation of nearby histone variant H2AX on Serine 139 (γH2AX), phosphorylation of p53 on serine 15, and of Mdm2 and CHK2 (Banin et al. 1998; Marine and Lozano 2010; Matsuoka et al. 1998). Phosphorylation of p53 results in activation and accumulation in the nucleus, whereupon p53 acts as transcription factor to drive the expression of genes involved in G1/S cell cycle checkpoint activation and apoptosis (Sullivan et al. 2012). Although there are over 700 substrates phosphorylated in an ATM-dependent manner (Bennetzen et al. 2010), these key events have been used to build screening assays for ATM (Guo et al. 2014), that have ultimately led to the discovery of clinical candidate molecules described at the end of this chapter. The importance of the understanding of the biology of ATM in obtaining tractable chemical matter against the target cannot be underestimated. Whilst loss of ATM protein and ATM inhibition are not a phenocopy per se (Choi et al. 2010; Fedier et al. 2003; Foray et al. 1997; Kühne et al. 2004; Yamamoto et al. 2012), small molecule inhibitors of ATM have been shown to largely match A-T signalling events, indicating a specificity and relevant biological function to the molecules developed.

8.3 Early Inhibitors of ATM

During the earliest efforts to find chemical inhibitors of ATM, the fungal metabolite, Wortmannin (1), was identified as an inhibitor of ATM enzyme ($IC_{50} = 0.15$ µM) (Powis et al. 1994). Although the ATM-directed p53 response has been shown to be diminished in these experiments, optimal radiosensitisation and induction of S and G2 cell cycle phase abnormalities occurs at concentrations above those required to inhibit ATM. It is most likely that the increased sensitivity to ionizing radiation observed was manifested through the ability of Wortmannin to inhibit not only ATM but a number of PIKKs, including ATR and DNA-PK, as well as PI3K (DNA-PK $IC_{50} = 0.016$ µM; ATR $IC_{50} = 1.8$ µM; PI3K $IC_{50} = 0.003$ µM). (Izzard et al. 1999; Sarkaria et al. 1998; Ui et al. 1995). This chemical inhibitor approach, however, demonstrated the feasibility of achieving sensitisation to ionising radiation although did not constitute proof that this effect was driven by ATM inhibition alone. Acting as a non-competitive irreversible inhibitor, Wortmannin probably hits too many other targets to be a viable clinical agent and indeed has been demonstrated to have toxicity in in vivo experiments. Attempts to reformulate the compound for nanoparticle delivery and thereby provide some tumour targeting were unable to sufficiently modulate therapeutic index to support clinical use (Karve et al. 2012).

Caffeine (2), is a methyl xanthine that has been shown to sensitise cells to the lethal effects of genotoxic modalities, including IR (Blasina et al. 1999). The molecule is a relatively weak and non-specific ATM inhibitor ($IC_{50} = 200$ µM against enzyme), with similarly weak activity against a number of PIKK enzymes (ATR $IC_{50} = 1100$ µM, DNA-PK $IC_{50} = 10,000$ µM) (Sarkaria et al. 1999). In the case of caffeine and its potential use in vivo, the sensitisation occurs at an effective concentration that is clinically prohibitive; serum concentrations of 1 mM, which are required to achieve radiosensitisation, are associated with fatal tachyarrhythmias (Sarkaria and Eshleman 2001).

The first synthetic specific inhibitor of the PIKKs was the flavonoid quercetin analogue LY294002 (3), developed by Eli Lilly (Vlahos et al. 1994). LY294002 is an ATP competitive inhibitor with modest potency against a variety of PI3K and PIKK enzymes (PI3Kα, β, γ, δ IC$_{50}$ = 0.55, 16, 12 and 1.6 μM respectively; mTOR IC$_{50}$ = 2.5 μM; DNA-PK IC$_{50}$ = 2.5 μM) and has facilitated the improved understanding of the function of PI3K and PIKKs as well as providing a start-point for the subsequent development of more selective PIKK inhibitors. Although the activity of LY294002 against ATM is somewhat limited (IC$_{50}$ > 100 μM) (Knight et al. 2004), the understanding of the binding mode of the inhibitor in PI3Kγ, in particular the importance of the interactions of the morpholine ring (Andrs et al. 2015), was instrumental in the discovery of future potent and selective tools to probe ATM biology. For this reason, LY294002 is rightly placed in a review of ATM chemical matter.

More recently the dual PI3K/mTOR inhibitor NVP-BEZ235 (4), developed by Novartis, has been shown to be a potent inhibitor of ATM. This compound was taken into clinical studies but development ultimately halted due to toxicity and poor efficacy. Although originally described as a dual mTOR/PI3K inhibitor (mTOR IC$_{50}$ = 0.021 μM; PI3Kα, β, γ, δ IC$_{50}$ = 0.004, 0.075, 0.005 and 0.007 μM respectively) (Maira et al. 2008), it has been shown to inhibit ATM and DNA-PK (ATM IC$_{50}$ = 0.007 μM; DNA-PK IC$_{50}$ = 0.005 μM). The subsequent observation of ATR inhibition (IC$_{50}$ = 21 nM, Toledo et al. 2011), and radio-sensitisation of cells overexpressing RAS to the inhibitory effects of NVP-BEZ235 (Konstantinidou et al. 2009), have further highlighted the potential for toxicity as a result of polypharmacology and underscores the requirement for highly selective ATM inhibitors to develop as potential clinical agents.

CGK733 was originally reported as a dual ATM and ATR inhibitor, capable of reversing cellular senescence (Won et al. 2006), and has been used in a number of publications to explore ATM and ATR activity. The data supporting the original publication were called into question along with the validity of the experiments and the original publication was retracted (Won et al. 2008). Subsequent analysis of the ATM inhibitory potential of CGK733 confirmed that the compound was not an ATM inhibitor (Choi et al. 2011), and as such any data generated with this molecule should be treated with caution (Fig. 8.1).

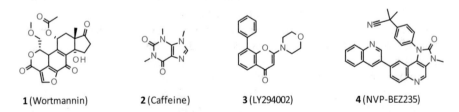

1 (Wortmannin)   **2** (Caffeine)   **3** (LY294002)   **4** (NVP-BEZ235)

Fig. 8.1 Published structures of non-selective ATM inhibitors

8.4 Selective ATM Inhibitors as Probe Molecules

The identification of the pan PI3K/PIKK inhibitors described above has helped advance our understanding of these important targets, but the need to develop selective ATM inhibitors continued.

The compounds used in the above early studies (Caffeine and Wortmannin) are non-specific and also inhibit other phosphatidylinositol 3-kinase-related kinase (PIKK) family members, including ATR and DNA-PKcs (Sarkaria et al. 1998, 1999). Therefore, it is uncertain how much of the observed effects were due to inhibition of ATM activity. The development of more potent and selective ATM inhibitors allowed for the validation of the radio-sensitising effect mediated by pharmacological ATM inhibition in vitro.

As mentioned previously, in addition to increasing the understanding of ATM biology, these non-selective ATM inhibitors also provided important start-points for the development of selective agents. In particular, the morpholine containing scaffold of LY294002, resulted in the development of a number of PIKK targeted inhibitors, a particularly potent and selective example being that of KU-55933 (5). Through screening of a small library of molecules designed around LY294002, the chemistry teams of KuDOS Pharmaceuticals and the Northern Institute for Cancer Research (NICR), described the discovery, synthesis and characterisation of 2-morpholin-4-yl-6-thianthren-1-yl-pyran-4-one, KU-55933 (Hickson et al. 2004; Hollick et al. 2007). KU-55933 potently inhibits ATM in biochemical assays (IC_{50} = 12.9 nM). Counter-screens of KU-55933 against other members of the PIKK family demonstrated at least a 100-fold differential in selectivity (DNA-PK (IC_{50} = 2.5 μM), ATR (IC_{50} > 100 μM), mTOR (IC_{50} = 9.3 μM) and PI3K (IC_{50} = 16.6 μM)). Furthermore, in screening a commercially available panel of 60 kinases at a single concentration of 10 μM, KU-55933 did not significantly inhibit any kinase tested. The evolution of KU-55933 from LY294002 also validates the ability of small molecule ATP-competitive kinase inhibitors to display high levels of selectivity between PIKK family members, a finding further validated by the identification of potent and selective inhibitors of DNA-PK (Hollick et al. 2007).

The role of a hydrogen bond mediated interaction between the morpholine oxygen of LY294002 and the hinge region of PI3K p110γ was highlighted in a crystal structure (Walker et al. 2000). The importance of this moiety for the activity of KU-55933 against ATM was confirmed by the use of the related molecule, 2-piperidin-1-yl-6-thianthren-1-yl-pyran-4-one, KU-58050 (structure not shown), in which the morpholine unit has been replaced by a piperidine unit, thereby removing the possibility of an analogous hydrogen bonding interaction. KU-58050 was found to have significantly reduced ATM activity (IC_{50} = 2.96 μM), indicating the compound to be more than 200 times less effective as an ATM inhibitor when compared to KU-55933. In addition to confirming the importance of the morpholine oxygen for ATM inhibition in this scaffold, KU-58050 also serves as a useful negative control for ATM activity in experiments utilising KU-55933 due to the closely related molecular structure. On the basis of the structural similarity between KU-55933 (compound 5) and LY294002 (compound 3), (Izzard et al. 1999; Vlahos et al. 1994), it was assumed that the inhibition of ATM by KU-55933 would be ATP competitive. Hickson et al. (2004), described the derivation of competitive ATP binding data that was subsequently corroborated by Kevan Shokat's group, who further went on to highlight the extremely selective inhibition of ATM by KU-55933 in an analysis of a broad range of ATP competitive compounds targeting PIKK proteins (Knight et al. 2006). In this publication, the use of the homology models of a number of PIKK proteins and associated inhibitors, in particular for PI3K and ATM binding, supports the earlier model established for KU-55933 binding in the ATM pocket.

KU-55933 was the first potent and selective inhibitor of ATM to be reported and has been adopted by the research community as an effective tool for assessing the cellular role of ATM inhibition. Its use has been broadly reported in the literature in experiments to determine ATM function, basic biology and also the potential therapeutic utility of an ATM inhibitor. Consistent with the previously described biology of ATM loss resulting in sensitivity to genotoxic damage (Blasina et al. 1999; Fedier et al. 2003; Foray et al. 1997; Price and Youmell 1996; Sarkaria et al. 1998, 1999), KU-55933 was shown to sensitize HeLa cells to the cytotoxic effects of topoisomerase I and II inhibitors and to IR. The differentiation of ATM biology is helped by the selective inhibitors that, in the case of KU-55933 for example, are not further sensitising to cells that lack ATM expression (Hickson et al. 2004); data with less selective inhibitors is confounded by activity beyond ATM.

As noted in the previous chapter, the known biology of ATM loss was critical to the development of appropriate tools and ultimately, of course, to the clinical development of an ATM inhibitor. It has been shown that kinase-dead ATM acts in a dominant negative like manner such that expression of physiologically equivalent levels of kinase-dead ATM are lethal in early embryogenesis whereas A-T mice, lacking ATM, are viable (Daniel et al. 2012; Yamamoto et al. 2012). The defect in repair of damaged replication forks observed in KU-55933 treated cells (White et al. 2010), indicated that inhibition of ATM may act in a similar way to kinase-dead ATM protein (Yamamoto et al. 2012) as opposed to that observed for loss of ATM (i.e. kinase inhibited ATM physically blocks homologous recombination repair of DSBs at damaged replication forks) (Choi et al. 2010; White et al. 2010). Parallels could be drawn with the inhibition of PARP, and so-called PARP trapping, that prevents the processing of a lesion in DNA, as distinct from an absence of PARP at the site of damage (Murai et al. 2012).

This observation raises important questions when exploring the biological consequences of ATM inhibition. If 'trapping' of the repair process occurs with ATM inhibitors, could this be more detrimental in vivo than a loss of ATM protein due to the prolonged lesion? It may, therefore, be important to assess if it is possible to achieve exposures that enable sensitisation to chemo- or radiotherapy but that will not cause sustained trapping of ATM on the DNA, which may lead to adverse impacts on normal tissues. The kinetics of binding of the ATM inhibitor are therefore an important factor, which would impact the pharmacokinetic profile for clinical candidates. These key factors are explored further in this chapter wherein the evolution of ATM inhibitors from tools to potential therapeutics is described.

Finally, single agent use, which could exploit potential synthetic lethal interactions, may require different inhibition kinetics and pharmacokinetic profiles for optimal activity. This has been well studied in the case of PARP inhibitors exploiting defects in homologous recombination repair (Bryant et al. 2005; Farmer et al. 2005; Kaelin 2005). It would remain to identify an appropriate patient population (and tumour signature), in whom ATM would cause such synthetic lethality but candidates arising from preclinical work include, APE1 and XRCC1 (Sultana et al. 2012, 2013), and potentially ATR, although it is inhibition of the latter that is reported as synthetic lethal with ATM loss (e.g. Reaper et al. 2011). It is worth noting that PARP inhibition is also synthetically lethal with loss of ATM (Aguilar-Quesada et al. 2007; Weston et al. 2010; Kubota et al. 2014), and this may provide an opportunity to combine two compounds to induce a tumour killing effect, an aspect that may be explored clinically with the appropriate molecules, as addressed at the end of this chapter.

In establishing the potential of ATM as a drug target, KU-55933 laid the foundations for the chemistry to follow, however, the utility of KU-55933 as a tool was limited by its poor physicochemical properties, in particular low aqueous solubility and low oral bioavailability. Whilst the in vitro data generated with the tools described was encouraging, the true nature of the effects on the broader biology may only be apparent when observed in vivo and in pre-clinical evaluation of a potential therapeutic. It was, therefore, apparent additional work was required to improve the physicochemical and pharmacokinetic properties to obtain ATM inhibitors suitable for in vivo assessment.

Optimization of KU-55933 resulted in the discovery of the second generation ATM inhibitors, KU-60019 (6) and KU-59403 (7), in which polar substituents have been appended to the tricyclic core resulting in improved potency and aqueous solubility (Batey et al. 2013; Golding et al. 2009). KU-60019 and KU-59403 are potent inhibitors of ATM enzyme (IC$_{50}$ = 0.006 µM and 0.003 µM respectively), that retain high selectivity over ATR, DNA-PK, mTOR and PI3K (>270 fold and >300 fold respectively). Cellular potency was also improved relative to KU-55933 with KU-60019 and KU-59403 giving effective chemo-sensitisation at a concentrations of 3 µM and 1 µM respectively (concentrations of 10 µM were required in experiments using KU-55933). Cellular potency remains lower than in the biochemical assay, though this is typical of kinase inhibitors due to the target protein affinity for, and high cellular concentration of, ATP; typically a 100-fold drop off is observed for PIKK inhibitors (Knight and Shokat 2005). Although KU-60019 shows improved aqueous solubility when compared to KU-55933, it remains suboptimal for in vivo evaluation. However, by direct intracranial injection of the inhibitor into mice bearing orthotopically grown glioma tumours, in vivo radio-sensitisation was observed (Biddlestone-Thorpe et al. 2013). In this model, it was possible to demonstrate p53 independent inhibition of tumour growth to the point of achieving an apparent cure in some animals. Previous studies into radio-sensitisation of p53-deficient cells were performed in vitro (Teng et al. 2015), and may indicate a limitation of tools used only in vitro. Serendipitously, the use of an in vivo tool was able to unveil another aspect of ATM inhibitor biology.

Whilst the physicochemical and pharmacokinetic properties of KU-59403 were also found to be suboptimal for oral administration, further assessment of ATM inhibition in vivo was conducted with this compound following intraperitoneal (i.p.) injection. When dosed at 50 mg/kg i.p., tumour concentrations of KU-59403 above those required to deliver effective chemo- or radio-sensitisation in vitro were achieved for 4 h. Whilst these exposures may seem modest it has been reported that just transient inhibition of the target is sufficient to yield radio-potentiation (Rainey et al. 2008). Administration of KU-59403 alone did not result in any significant anti-tumour efficacy, consistent with a role as a sensitising agent, but when dosed at either 12.5 or 25 mg/kg i.p. BID for 5 days, sensitisation to cytotoxic therapy was observed. In combination with etoposide, a dose-dependent increase in tumour growth delay was observed in the colorectal tumour models, HCT-116 and SW620 (Batey et al. 2013). A similar dosing schedule combining KU-59403 with irinotecan was also shown to be effective without any obvious unacceptable adverse effects on the animals (as measured by body weight loss). The lack of overt toxicity from KU-59403 was important in establishing that an active ATM inhibitor would not result in inhibition of the target to the detriment of normal tissue, even in combination with cytotoxic therapy and, therefore, that an ATM inhibitor could be developed to enhance the therapeutic effect of chemotherapy (and by inference, radiotherapy). This observation reflected upon the suggestion that too prolonged an inhibition of ATM could be to the detriment of normal cellular processing of DNA damage as the lesion could remain unresolved on the DNA (Choi et al. 2010; White et al. 2010; Yamamoto et al. 2012). Importantly, additional experiments in cells lacking the expression of p53 would explore further the development of ATM inhibitors as clinical candidates. Activity was not compromised by loss of p53, consistent with observed radio-sensitisation that was more pronounced in cells with a p53 deficiency (Bracey et al. 1997; Powell et al. 1995; Yao et al. 1996). In fact, although Batey et al. (2013), reported equivalent activity in p53 deficient and proficient tumours, in another study, ATM inhibition resulted in increased efficacy in p53-mutated tumours (Biddlestone-Thorpe et al. 2013), and thus further selectivity towards tumours might be expected.

AZ32 (8) is a high affinity inhibitor of ATM enzyme ($IC_{50} < 0.006$ μM) discovered in the AstraZeneca laboratories following a focussed screening campaign. This resulted in novel chemistry that lacked the morpholine group that had been present in much of the earlier ATM chemistry, indicating that diversification was possible. AZ32 is a moderately potent inhibitor of ATM in cells ($IC_{50} = 0.31$ μM) but shows good selectivity over ATR in a cell based assay ($IC_{50} > 23$ μM). In addition to being potent and selective (only 4 of 124 kinases found to be inhibited >50% at 10 μM), AZ32 has been shown to be highly permeable in MDCK cell lines overexpressing MDR1 (P_{app} A-B $= 33.7 \times 10^{-6}$ cm/s, efflux ratio $= 0.4$) (Durant et al. 2016) and therefore brain penetrant, and has been shown to be orally bioavailable in rodents. An oral dose of 200 mg/kg in mice was shown to potentiate the effects of irinotecan in a xenograft model, consistent with the data obtained for KU-59403 (Batey et al. 2013). It is interesting to note that the physicochemical properties of AZ32, namely high permeability and low efflux, meant that when dosed at this level, unbound

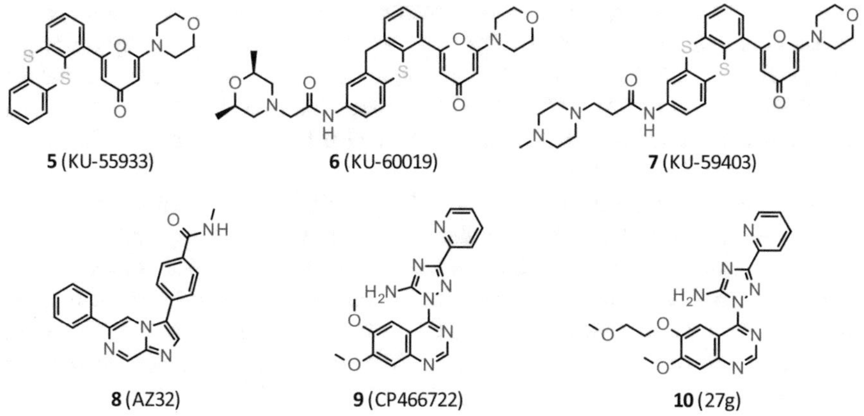

5 (KU-55933)   **6 (KU-60019)**   **7 (KU-59403)**

8 (AZ32)   **9 (CP466722)**   **10 (27g)**

Fig. 8.2 Published structures of selective ATM inhibitors

concentrations in the brain exceeded the cellular IC_{50} for approximately 22 h. This level of ATM engagement in brain tissue would be anticipated to be beyond that required to deliver radiosensitisation. Similar levels of exposure where achieved with a 50 mg/kg oral dose of AZ32 utilising a more optimal formulation and, when combined with IR, this dose resulted in a significant increase in survival of mice bearing orthotopic gliomas (Durant et al. 2016). This result highlights the potential for brain penetrant ATM inhibitors to find therapeutic utility in the treatment of brain cancers (Fig. 8.2).

The quinazoline CP466722 (compound 9) was identified following a screen of 1500 compounds from the Pfizer compound library and shown to be a moderately potent inhibitor of ATM in cells ($IC_{50} = 0.37$ μM). CP466722 selectivity is not optimal and activity against a number of additional kinases was observed, including PIKK enzymes [additional significant activity against 106 out of 451 kinases was observed (tested at 3 μM)]. Importantly for use as a tool to explore the biology of ATM inhibition, little activity was observed against either ATR or DNA-PK in cells (Rainey et al. 2008), thereby allowing the observed radiosensitisation of HeLa cells to be interpreted as ATM dependent. CP466722 has low aqueous solubility (28 μM) and high clearance with a short half-life in mice (CL = 160 mL/h, $t_{1/2} = 1$ h) and was, therefore, unsuited for further in vivo assessment. Optimization of the pharmacokinetic properties resulted in the identification of 27 g (compound 10) which, although being a less potent inhibitor of ATM ($IC_{50} = 1.2$ μM), benefited from an increase in selectivity [active against 41 out of 451 kinases (tested at 3 μM, though it should be noted this is only twofold selective over ATM)] and half-life in C57BL/6 mice ($t_{1/2} = 19$ h) thus facilitating further in vivo evaluation. Despite an approximately fourfold enhancement of radiosensitivity for both CP466722 and 27 g in a clonogenic assay in which MCF7 cells were treated with 10 μM compound and irradiated with increasing doses of IR (0, 2 and 4 Gy), there have only been a small number of other publications reporting data on either compound. Indeed, one of the subsequent publications using CP466722 highlights the need for consideration of the selectivity of the molecule as the potentiation of radiosensitivity observed in breast stem cells at 100 μM of CP466722 could have been caused by off target effects (Kim et al. 2012). An alternative approach using the molecule found that the inhibition of ATM by CP466722 (3 μM), mirrored that of KU-55933 (10 μM) with both molecules sensitising to the effects of temozolomide in a glioblastoma cell model (Nadkarni et al. 2012).

Whilst a range of structurally diverse ATM inhibitors had been identified, the identification of a molecule that combined high levels of potency and selectivity with good oral exposure and other drug like properties, remained elusive. It was appreciated that such a molecule would be required to truly interrogate the biology of ATM inhibition in vivo and to offer the potential for clinical utility. This need encouraged the continued search for novel ATM inhibitors and is described in the next section.

8.5 Evolution of In Vivo Active Probe Molecules

Although BEZ-235 was described earlier in the chapter as an in vivo and indeed clinically active compound, the molecule was classified with the other non-specific inhibitors of ATM and thus is not considered in the evolution of selective ATM inhibitors.

AstraZeneca set about a novel discovery program to identify alternative hit matter that could extend the utility of ATM inhibitors beyond that of the limitations described above. In a directed screen of approximately 15,000 compounds from an internal compound collection, compounds were identified with the ability to inhibit the phosphorylation of ATM on Serine 1981 in HT29 cells following irradiation. Analysis of the data generated identified the quinoline carboxamide hit (compound 11), as a moderately potent inhibitor of ATM in cells ($IC_{50} = 0.82$ μM), but importantly with selectivity for ATM over ATR (as measured by inhibition of pCHK1 in HT29 cells following treatment with 4-nitroquinoline 1-oxide (4NQO), ($IC_{50} = 4.4$ μM)). Compound 11 was shown to be a potent inhibitor of ATM enzyme ($IC_{50} = 0.008$ μM), with selectivity over closely related enzymes (>10-fold selective for ATM over DNA-PK and PI3Kα and >100-fold selective over mTOR, PI3Kβ and PI3Kγ). Compound 11 also showed encouraging selectivity when assessed against a diverse panel of kinases with only eight of the 124 kinases tested showing >50% inhibition when tested at 1 μM. Whilst representing a novel and potentially selective series of ATM inhibitor, it was appreciated that compound 11 shared similar sub-optimal physicochemical properties to many of the early ATM probe molecules. In particular, compound 11 had low aqueous solubility (19 μM), high intrinsic clearance (CL_{int}) in hepatocytes (Rat CL_{int} = 74 μL/min/10^6 cells, Human CL_{int} = 74 μL/min/10^6 cells), and activity against the hERG (human ether-a-go-go related gene) ion channel ($IC_{50} = 2.3$ μM) (Redfern et al. 2003; Waring et al. 2011); however, it was considered that the relatively high lipophilicity of this hit (log $D_{7.4} = 3.5$), may in part, have been responsible for these properties. An optimization campaign was

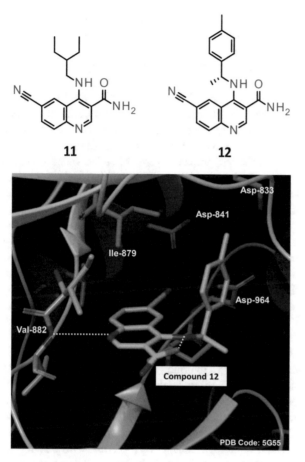

Fig. 8.3 (**a**) Structure of screening hit **11** and closely related PI3K inhibitor **12**. (**b**) X-ray structure of **12** bound into PI3Kγ (PDB code: 5G55)

subsequently initiated with the aim of improving both potency and selectivity whilst simultaneously optimising physicochemical and pharmacokinetic parameters (Degorce et al. 2016) (Fig. 8.3a).

Utilising a strategy similar to that described in the optimisation of KU-55933 the group within AstraZeneca were able to infer key features of the binding interaction between compound 11 and ATM by making an analogy with the interactions observed between a closely related structure, compound 12, and PI3Kγ (Yang et al. 2013) (Fig. 8.3b). Close inspection of the structure [Fig. 8.3b, PDB 5G55, (Degorce et al. 2016)], showed the quinoline nitrogen forming a key interaction with the hinge region of the kinase as well as suggesting the potential to further optimise the 6-cyano and 4-amino substituents. An internal hydrogen bonding interaction between the 4-amino substituent and the 3-carboxamide substituent can also be observed, presumably helping to organise the molecule in a bioactive conformation.

Although compound 12 does not have appreciable activity against ATM in cells ($IC_{50} > 30$ μM), it was hypothesised that a similar binding mode may be adopted by 11 when bound into ATM.

Exploration of the structure-activity relationship, SAR, for the compounds [detailed in (Degorce et al. 2016)], established that significant improvements in both ATM cellular potency and selectivity could be achieved by the introduction of an aromatic group in the 6-position, in particular a 3-pyridine motif. Additional SAR confirmed that small substituents could be introduced to the pyridine ring to further improve potency and selectivity. Parallel with the optimization of the 6-position, high throughput chemistry approaches were utilized to vary the 4-amino substituent with the intent of reducing the lipophilicity and improving physicochemical and pharmacokinetic properties. Opportunities to maintain potency and selectivity whilst improving other properties were identified by incorporating very specific chiral amines in the 4-position. When combined with the optimised substituents in the 6-position, highly potent and selective compounds were identified which showed excellent solubility and good oral bioavailability in rodent and dogs, for example compound 13 (AZ31) and compound 14, Fig. 8.4 [described as compound 74 by (Degorce et al. 2016)].

AZ31 and compound 14, are potent inhibitors of ATM enzyme ($IC_{50} < 0.0012$ μM and <0.0006 μM respectively), with excellent selectivity over closely related enzymes (>500 fold selective over DNA-PK and PI3Kα and >1000 fold selective over mTOR, PI3Kβ and PI3Kγ for both compounds). When tested against a diverse range of kinase targets, AZ31 inhibited 0 out of 126 kinases by >50% when tested at 1 μM, and compound 14 inhibited only 3 out of 386 kinases by >50% when tested at 1 μM. Assessment of permeability using Caco2 cells showed both compounds to be permeable (AZ31: P_{app} A-B $= 5.2 \times 10^{-6}$ cm/s; compound 14: P_{app} A-B $= 14 \times 10^{-6}$ cm/s) and in vivo pharmacokinetic evaluation showed both compounds to orally bioavailable in rat and dog (AZ31: F $= 46\%$ and 31% respectively; compound 14: F $= 29\%$ and 71% respectively). Furthermore, good exposure was observed following oral administration of both compounds to mice with doses of 100 mg/kg QD of AZ31 and 50 mg/kg BID of compound 14 giving unbound plasma exposures in excess of the ATM cell IC_{50} for approximately 24 h. The efficacy of AZ31 was assessed in HT29 tumour-bearing immunocompromised mice following oral administration at 100 mg/kg QD, in combination with IR (2 Gy delivered on

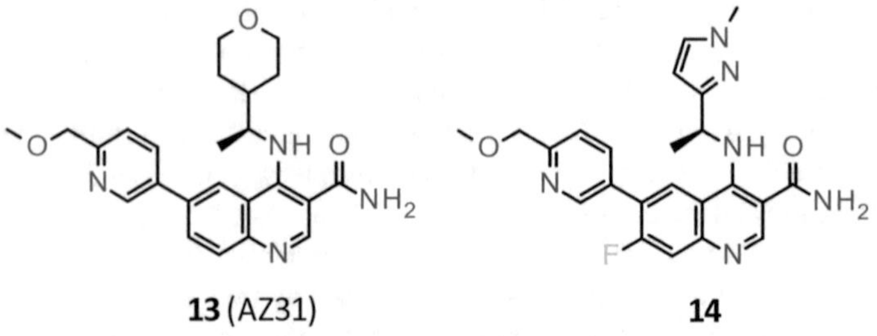

13 (AZ31)   **14**

Fig. 8.4 Structure of AZ31 13 and closely related inhibitor, compound 14

each of days 1–5 of the study). Whilst AZ31 treatment alone did not reduce tumour growth and IR alone gave only a modest benefit, the combination of AZ31 and IR produced a significant reduction of tumour growth highlighting the radio-sensitising effect of ATM inhibition in this in vivo model. The ability for AZ31 to potentiate the effect of DNA BSB inducing chemotherapy was assessed in an SW620 (colorectal cancer cell line) xenograft model. Significant reduction in tumour growth was observed following oral administration of AZ31 at 100 mg/kg QD combined with irinotecan dosed at 50 mg/kg Q7D i.p. Interestingly, in this model tumours started to regrow following the cessation of treatment; however, retreating with the combination again led to tumour regression. No monotherapy effect was seen in this model for AZ31 and monotherapy efficacy for irinotecan was modest. No overt toxicity was observed in these studies and dosing was continued throughout the 21-day dosing period. In a GL261 glioma syngeneic and intracranial model, it was demonstrated that targeted delivery of ionising radiation combined with AZ31, resulted in enhanced therapeutic response compared to radiation alone but without morbidity or overt toxicity (Kahn et al. 2017). In contrast, treatment with ATM inhibitors alone had no therapeutic effect and combination of ATM inhibition with whole head irradiation resulted in mucositis and difficulty eating and drinking, suggestive normal tissue toxicity had occurred. AZ31 was also used in combination experiments with whole body irradiation of mice; combination of irradiation with AZ31 led to a reduced time to the mice becoming moribund and a more marked disruption of crypts leading to gastrointestinal syndrome (Vendetti et al. 2017). Enhancement of radiation induced toxicity in a murine model indicates that ATM inhibition is not restricted to tumour tissue but the data from Kahn et al. (2017), would suggest that targeting of radiation therapy may minimise the risk of toxicity to normal tissues for such combination therapies of ATM inhibitor and irradiation.

The efficacy of compound 14 was explored in SW620 tumour-bearing immuno-compromised mice following oral administration at 50 mg/kg BID (dosed on days 2–4 of a weekly cycle) in combination with irinotecan dosed at 50 mg QD i.p. (dosed on day 1 of a weekly cycle). This combination schedule was tolerated and gave a significant tumour growth reduction following a 3 week regimen which was found to be statistically significant and greater than the reduction observed with irinotecan treatment alone (Degorce et al. 2016).

AZ31 and compound 14 have been demonstrated to be both efficacious and well tolerated and to give unbound exposures of ATM inhibitor in excess of both the enzyme and cell IC_{50}, following oral dosing. As discussed earlier, distinctions between ATM inhibition and kinase dead ATM or ATM loss should also be appreciated. The ability to administer the AZ31 and compound 14 in combination with chemo- and radiotherapy and determine combinatorial effects in the absence of single agent ATM inhibitor activity or toxicity was therefore an important observation and a step forward in the development of ATM inhibitors. However, whilst the potency, selectivity and preclinical pharmacokinetics for AZ31 and compound 14 appear encouraging, more detailed profiling suggested that these compounds were sub-optimal for consideration as a clinical candidate. In particular, AZ31 showed unwanted activity against the human-ether-a-go-go (hERG) potassium ion channel, a known risk for adverse cardiovascular events, and both compounds were predicted to require relatively high doses to drive the desired level and duration of target engagement in the clinic. Detailed modelling of preclinical data suggested that neither AZ31 n or 14 would satisfy stringent criteria for clinical development (Ding et al. 2012; Hilgers et al. 2003; Johnson and Swindell 1996; Page 2016). These observations supported the continued optimisation of the compounds with a particular focus on reducing the predicted clinical dose whilst maintaining the otherwise promising properties. The further evolution of ATM inhibitors and the eventual development of a molecule with the attributes to be considered as a clinical candidate are described in the next section.

8.6   Clinical Candidate ATM Inhibitors

In developing ATM inhibitors to their ultimate clinical utility, it became necessary to substantially expand the medicinal chemistry effort and address critical issues of bioavailability and dosage, beyond the previous explorations of mechanism and feasibility of inhibition as a therapeutic strategy. When considering opportunities for the further optimisation of compounds such as AZ31 and 14, the optimisation of half-life was identified as a promising strategy to reduce the predicted clinical dose. The relatively low metabolic turnover of these compounds directed the strategy towards increasing the volume of distribution (V_{ss}) as a means to increase half-life. The importance of pK_a in determining V_{ss} has been long appreciated with basic compounds often showing considerably higher volumes than neutral and acidic compounds (Smith et al. 2015). Therefore, the opportunity to increase V_{ss}, and thereby half-life, through the incorporation of basic functionality was appreciated and adopted as an optimisation strategy.

Exploration of the 4- and 6-substituents of the quinoline carboxamide scaffold resulted in a wealth of data to aid SAR understanding. Review of these data identified that a basic substituent to support the enhanced V_{ss} strategy could be incorporated in the 6-position, as exemplified by compound 15, Fig. 8.5. Compound 15 is a highly potent and selective inhibitor of ATM in cells ($IC_{50} = 0.0086\ \mu M$), with little or no activity against ATR ($IC_{50} > 30\ \mu M$). Whilst providing evidence that basic functionality could be tolerated with respect to ATM binding, compound 15 was shown to possess a significantly compromised permeability profile (MDCK-MDR1

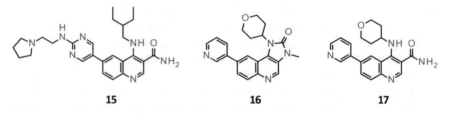

Fig. 8.5 Structures of **15**, **16** and **17**

P_{app} A-B = 0.8×10^{-6} cm/s, efflux ratio = 28). Such a permeability profile was felt to limit the in vivo utility of the molecule and was considered to be driven primarily by a combination of both the basic functionality and the number of hydrogen bond donors present in the molecule. Whilst there remained an opportunity to increase permeability through the continued increase in lipophilicity, this strategy was not adopted due to the likely detrimental impact on many other key properties. Given the important role of both the 3-carboxamide and 4-amino motifs in the pre-organisation of the molecules into a bioactive conformation, the removal of either of these groups as a means to reduce hydrogen bond donor count was considered unlikely to succeed and attention was focussed on the identification of a more permeable scaffold.

The concept of utilising intramolecular hydrogen bonding interactions to constrain molecules in defined conformations is well known and has been used successfully in "scaffold hop" strategies where covalently bonded cyclic systems have been replaced with hydrogen bonded constrained acyclic systems (Furet et al. 2008). In the case of the quinoline carboxamide scaffold there already exists such a hydrogen bonded constrained acyclic system between the 4-amino substituent and the 3-carboxamide substituent suggesting that replacement with a covalently bonded cyclic system may be feasible. Such an approach would result in a significant reduction in hydrogen bond donors. The feasibility of this approach was confirmed by the synthesis of the imidazo[5,4-c]quinolin-2-one containing compound 16 (Fig. 8.5). Indeed, the dual PI3K/mTOR inhibitor NVP-BEZ235 (compound 4), described earlier, contains this same imidazo[5,4-c]quinolin-2-one scaffold, thus providing further evidence of the ability of this scaffold to inhibit ATM, whilst simultaneously highlighting the challenge of achieving the required level of selectivity, not apparent in the earlier example.

Comparison of quinoline carboxamide (17) with the analogous imidazo[5,4-c] quinolin-2-one (16), shows that ATM potency is broadly maintained (17: ATM cell IC_{50} = 0.95 µM, 16: ATM cell IC_{50} = 0.36 µM); however, the selectivity of compound 16 against closely related kinases was significantly reduced and indeed 16 was shown to have greater affinity for ATR than for ATM (16: ATR cell IC_{50} = 0.087 µM). Imidazo[5,4-c]quinolin-2-one,16, did show the anticipated increase in permeability and reduction in efflux compared to quinoline carboxamide analogue 17. This improved permeability was achieved with only a modest increase in lipophilicity (Δ log $D_{7.4}$ = 0.3), supporting the hypothesis that the imidazo[5,4-c] quinolin-2-one is an inherently more permeable scaffold and that this is predominantly driven by reduced number of hydrogen bond donors.

With the identification of a more permeable scaffold attention was once again turned to the incorporation of basic functionality to drive increased V_{ss} and half-life. Significant optimisation of the basic substituent delivered not only improved properties and pharmacokinetics but also delivered a dramatic improvement in ATM affinity and selectivity, as exemplified by compound 18, subsequently known as AZD0156, Fig. 8.6.

AZD0156 is an exceptionally potent inhibitor of ATM, with over 1000-fold improvement on the first generation selective inhibitors such as KU-55933 and

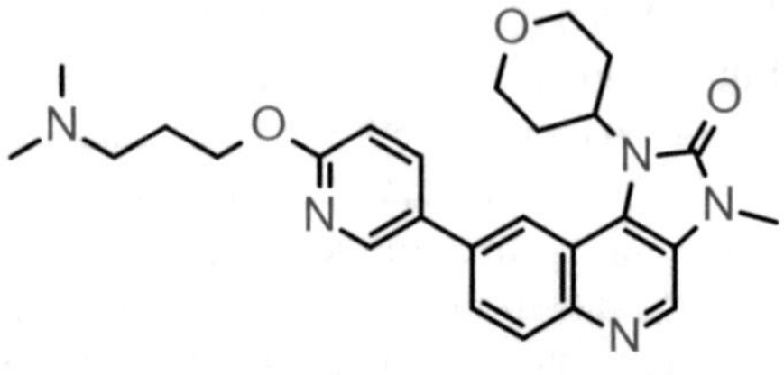

Fig. 8.6 Structure of screening AZD0156 (**18**)

18 (AZD0156)

Table 8.1 Potency and selectivity data for AZD0156

Target	Enzyme IC_{50} (μM)	Cell IC_{50} (μM)
ATM	0.00004[a]	0.00058
ATR	–	6.2
DNA-PK	0.14	–
mTOR	0.20	0.61
PI3Kα	0.32	1.4
PI3Kβ	1.8	–
PI3Kγ	1.1	–
PI3Kδ	0.27	–

[a]IC_{50} value corrected for tight binding

Table 8.2 Physicochemical and pharmacokinetic properties of AZD0156

	AZD0156
Crystalline solubility	>800 μM
% free (rat, dog, human)	11.4%, 40.9%, 29.0%
MDCK P_{app} A–B/efflux ratio	6.6×10^{-6} cm/s/5.1
Caco2 P_{app} A–B/efflux ratio	5.6×10^{-6} cm/s/8.5
Hepatocyte CL_{int} (rat, dog, human)	3.3, 3.3, 5.7 μL/min/10^6 cells
Rat PK (CL, V_{ss}, F)	15.5 mL/min/kg, 4.3 L/kg, 57%
Dog PK (CL, V_{ss}, F)	33.3 mL/min/kg, 17.6 L/kg, 54%
CYP inhibition (3A4, 2D6, 2C9, 1A2, 2C19)	IC_{50} > 30 μM

retaining excellent selectivity over closely related targets in both enzyme and cell based assays, Table 8.1.

When screened at 1 μM against a panel of 397 kinases AZD0156 showed excellent general kinome selectivity with activity above 65% inhibition observed for only 5 kinases (HASPIN: 67%; JAK1 (JH2domain-pseudokinase): 67%; LRRK2: 87%; mTOR: 93%; PIK4CB: 70%). A stable crystalline form of AZD0156 was identified and shown to have good aqueous solubility. AZD0156 has high levels of unbound drug in rat, dog and human plasma, is permeable with good pharmacokinetics in both rat and dog, and does not inhibit any of the five major isoforms of human cytochrome p450 at the concentrations tested (Table 8.2). AZD0156 was predicted to have a low clinically efficacious dose (<10 mg) based on preclinical models and as such was considered suitable for clinical development.

AZD0156 has evolved to become the ultimate tool for ATM inhibition allowing the potential to explore the inhibition of ATM in a clinical setting. In order to support positioning of the compound in the clinic, the ability of AZD0156 to potentiate the efficacy of DNA damage inducing agents was assessed in vitro by combining with either SN-38 (the active agent of the topoisomerase I inhibitor irinotecan) or the PARP inhibitor olaparib. AZD0156 shows good exposure in mice thereby allowing the in vivo assessment of ATM inhibition in mouse xenograft models, at tolerated intermittent schedules with chemotherapy or olaparib. When combined with irinotecan dosed at 50 mg/kg i.p (on day 1 of a weekly cycle), AZD0156 dosed orally at 20 mg/kg QD (on days 2–4 of a weekly cycle) showed clear synergy and caused tumour regression in an SW620 xenograft model. No appreciable efficacy was observed in this model when AZD0156 was dosed as a monotherapy. The addition of AZD0156, dosed orally at 5 mg/kg QD (on days 1–3 of a weekly cycle), to olaparib, dosed orally at 50 mg/kg QD, also resulted in clear synergy and tumour regression when examined in mice bearing an BRCA-2 mutant TNBC patient derived tumour (Pike et al. submitted).

The drug like qualities of AZD0156 has enabled toxicological assessment in both rat and dog and AZD0156 has entered clinical evaluation in a Phase I clinical trial, alone and in combination with olaparib (detailed on clinicaltrials.gov; NCT02588105). The preclinical data support the tolerability of the combination of AZD0156 and olaparib with no interruption of dosing nor overt toxicity observed (no body weight loss) in immune compromised mice harbouring an BRCA2 mutated patient derived xenograft. The clinical studies will establish both the pharmacokinetics of AZD0156 (single agent studies) and tolerated doses for the single agent and combination dosing.

One further opportunity has arisen for the development of ATM inhibitors (Golding et al. 2012). Earlier in the chapter, it was highlighted that brain penetrant nature of AZ32 allows for unbound drug levels in brain tissue to exceed the IC_{50} for ATM inhibition for a sustained period following oral administration. Treatment for Glioblastoma Multiforme (GBM), involves surgery followed by fractionated radiotherapy and temozolomide which provides a median survival of just 12–15 months (Ajaz et al. 2014; Delgado-López and Corrales-García 2016). Poor survival is attributed to an inability to excise all invasive tumour tissue (if operable) and an intrinsic tumour chemo/radioresistance. Equally challenging, is the current poor prognosis of patients with primary malignancies that metastasise to the brain. Single or multiple brain metastases are also refractory to current chemo/radiotherapy regimes and usually signifies end-stage disease (Lin and DeAngelis 2015). One third of GBM tumours contain p53 mutations and ~80% harbour other cell-cycle checkpoint alterations and it has been shown that p53-defective GBM cells are much more radiosensitised that wildtype cells (Roy et al. 2006; Biddlestone-Thorpe et al. 2013; Durant et al. 2016). In addition, reports have shown ATM knock-out mice brains are actually protected from acute adverse effects of radiation and that ATM promotes radiation induced apoptosis in post-mitotic, neural stem cell (NSC) (Gosink et al. 1999; Herzog et al. 1998), and in subventricular zone cells after low doses of radiation; NSC populations in ATM deficient embryos and adult mice exhibit radioresistance (Barazzuol et al. 2015; Gatz et al. 2011). All these studies may suggest that a potentially wide therapeutic window may exist between normal and brain tumour tissue. Furthermore, in assessing CP466722, Nadkarni et al. (2012), determined that glioblastoma cells sensitive to temozolomide could be further sensitised by combination with ATM inhibition as a route to achieving a greater impact on tumour growth inhibition through combination therapy.

AstraZeneca disclosed AZ32 at the 2016 AACR Annual Meeting (Durant et al. 2016), as a specific inhibitor of ATM possessing good blood-brain barrier (BBB) penetration in mouse. Based on these data, AstraZeneca continues to invest in developing a BBB-penetrating ATM inhibitor for clinical use in combination with radiotherapy for the treatment of primary malignancies of the brain and CNS as well as brain metastases. To this end, further optimisation of a molecule active in mice has resulted in the discovery of AZD1390, a potent and selective ATM inhibitor which is anticipated to efficiently cross the BBB in man. AZD1390 affords excellent efficacy in preclinical orthotopic brain tumour models and represents an exciting addition to the candidate drug portfolio for ATM inhibition. The structure of AZD1390 has yet to be disclosed but as clinical development continues then more information on this agent is expected to be released.

8.7   Concluding Remarks

Early molecules that enabled exploration of the in vivo activity of ATM inhibitors and the potential for chemo- and radio-sensitisation of tumour cells, were flawed and failed with poor selectivity. The improvement in selectivity and design of ATM specific inhibitors such as KU-55933, substantially improved the understanding of the in vitro properties, phenotypes and complex biology of ATM inhibition but were compromised by poor potency, selectivity or pharmacokinetic properties that restricted their utility as in vivo probes. However, in the past decade, a number of substantial improvements have been made and the availability of molecules, including AZ31 and Compound 14, have enabled both selective inhibition of ATM and exploration of the in vivo consequence of ATM inhibition, enhancement of tumour killing from combination therapies and a lack of obvious toxicity to normal tissues. In the context of combination with chemotherapy, it is perhaps the transient nature of ATM inhibition that provides a therapeutic window between the killing of tumour cells and normal cell toxicity – intermittent scheduling of chemotherapy or olaparib with AZD0156 were shown to be tolerated and efficacious in vivo suggesting scheduling may also result in clinically tolerated combinations. Together with the inherent sensitivity of genetically unstable tumours, that may lack e.g. p53 could further separate tumour sensitivity as it would not be constrained by the checkpoints and DNA damage responses afforded to normal tissue. In the case of combinations with irradiation, the exposure of normal tissue to ionising radiation in the presence of ATM inhibitors may be more toxic than radiation alone (Kahn et al. 2017; Vendetti et al. 2017), but targeted delivery of therapy may avoid such collateral toxicity (Kahn et al. 2017). In addition, studies in ATM knock-out mice have shown normal brain tissue to be relatively radio-resistant, in fact, potentially protected from the effects of radiation compared with wild type mice, suggesting a wide therapeutic window may exist particularly in brain.

Further improvements to increase pharmacokinetic half-life and thereby reduce clinical dose has resulted in the discovery of AZD0156, an extremely potent and selective ATM inhibitor with good physicochemical properties and preclinical pharmacokinetics. AZD0156 has allowed more detailed in vivo target validation and has now entered clinical trials. The initial stages of the clinical evaluation of AZD0156 will be to establish a tolerated dose as a single agent and in combination with olaparib and with cytotoxic chemotherapies, in a typical Phase I patient population of patients with advanced disease in a range of tumour indications. Secondary endpoints will determine if biomarker changes and enhancement of therapeutic effect of PARP inhibition or combination therapies can be detected in circulating tumours cells or circulating tumour DNA. One of the key challenges facing the successful clinical development of ATM inhibitors will be to understand how best to combine with the variety of DSB inducing agents, and which patients will respond best to such combinations. The earlier molecules and the data generated with these can help guide such combinations, but as the use of AZD0156 further develops our understanding of the biology and potential of ATM inhibition, additional opportunities for rational combinations or even for monotherapy treatment may well emerge (Morgado-Palacin et al. 2016).

The potential for ATM inhibition to combine with radiotherapy is also an area of active research and the importance of the blood-brain barrier in the potential to treat patients with brain tumours (such as GBM), will need to be established to ensure that clinical agents with suitable profiles can be developed. The biology of ATM is known to include its activation by ROS and the emergence of high quality ATM inhibitors will allow more detailed investigations into additional therapeutic areas, potentially beyond cancer. Early work with KU-55933 gave evidence to a role in the inhibition of HIV infection (Lau et al. 2005), the virus requires host cell mechanisms to integrate into the genome and prevention of homologous recombination by inhibition of ATM prevents viral propagation. More recently, it has been shown that ATM inhibition may have therapeutic potential in Huntingdon's disease due to alleviation of persistent and elevated activation of ATM by the mutant Huntingtin protein (Lu et al. 2014). Both approaches are still anchored in the role of ATM in homologous recombination repair but show scope well beyond the role of the target in cancer biology. The ultimate scope of therapeutic ATM inhibition awaits further experimentation, enabled by the chemistry described here.

References

Aguilar-Quesada R, Muñoz-Gámez JA, Martín-Oliva D, Peralta A, Valenzuela MT, Matínez-Romero R, Quiles-Pérez R, Menissier-de Murcia J, de Murcia G, Ruiz de Almodóvar M, Oliver FJ (2007) Interaction between ATM and PARP-1 in response to DNA damage and sensitization of ATM deficient cells through PARP inhibition. BMC Mol Biol 8:29–37

Ajaz M, Jefferies S, Brazil L, Watts C, Chalmers A (2014) Current and investigational drug strategies for glioblastoma. Clin Oncol 26:419–430

Andrs M, Korabecny J, Jun D, Hodny Z, Bartek J, Kuca K (2015) Phosphatidylinositol 3-kinase (PI3K) and phosphatidylinositol 3-kinase-related kinase (PIKK) inhibitors: importance of the morpholine ring. J Med Chem 58:41–71

Bakkenist CJ, Kastan MB (2003) DNA damage activates ATM through intermolecular autophosphorylation and dimer dissociation. Nature 421:499–506

Banin S, Moyal I, Shieh SY, Taya Y, Anderson CW, Chessa L, Smorodinsky NI, Prives C, Reiss Y, Shiloh Y, Ziv Y (1998) Enhanced phosporylation of p53 by ATM in response to DNA damage. Science 281:1674–1677

Barazzuol L, Rickett N, Ju L, Jeggo PA (2015) Low levels of endogenous or X-ray-induced DNA double-strand breaks activate apoptosis in adult neural stem cells. Cell Sci 128:3597–3606

Batey MA, Zhao Y, Kyle S, Richardson C, Slade A, Martin NMB, Lau A, Newell DR, Curtin NJ (2013) Preclinical evaluation of a novel ATM inhibitor, KU59403, in vitro and in vivo in p53 functional and dysfunctional models of human cancer. Mol Cancer Ther 12:959–967

Beamish H, Lavin MF (1994) Radiosensitivity in ataxia-telangiectasia: anomalies in radiation-induced cell cycle delay. Int J Radiat Biol 65:175–184

Bennetzen MV, Larsen DH, Bunkenborg J, Bartek J, Lukas J, Anderson JS (2010) Site-specific phosphorylationdynamics of the nuclear proteome during the DNA damage response. Mol Cell Proteomics 9:1314–1323

Biddlestone-Thorpe L, Sajjad M, Rosenberg E, Beckta JM, Valerie NCK, Tokarz M, Adams BR, Wagner AF, Khalil A, Gilfor D, Golding SE, Deb S, Temesi DG, Lau A, O'Connor MJ, Choe KS, Parada LF, Lim SK, Mukhopadhyay ND, Valerie K (2013) ATM kinase inhibition preferentially sensitizes p53-mutant glioma to ionizing radiation. Clin Cancer Res 19:3189–3200

Blasina A, Price BD, Turenne GA, McGowan CH (1999) Caffeine inhibits the checkpoint kinase ATM. Curr Biol 9:1135–1138

Bracey TS, Williams AC, Paraskeva C (1997) Inhibition of radiation-induced G2 delay potentiates cell death by apoptosis and/or the induction of giant cells in colorectal tumor cells with disrupted p53 function. Clin Cancer Res 3:1371–1381

Bryant HE, Schultz N, Thomas HD, Parker KM, Flower D, Lopez E, Kyle S, Meuth M, Curtin NJ, Helleday T (2005) Specific killing of BRCA2-deficient tumours with inhibitors of poly(ADP-ribose) polymerase. Nature 434:913–917

Choi S, Gamper AM, White JS, Bakkenist CJ (2010) Inhibition of ATM kinase activity does not phenocopy ATM protein disruption: implications for the clinical utility of ATM kinase inhibitors. Cell Cycle 9:4052–4057

Choi S, Toledo LI, Fernandez-Capetillo O, Bakkenist CJ (2011) CGK733 does not inhibit ATM or ATR kinase activity in H460 human lung cancer cells. DNA Repair 10:1000–1001

Daniel JA, Pellegrini M, Lee B-S, Guo Z, Filsuf D, Belkina NV, You Z, Paull TT, Sleckman BP, Feigenbaum L, Nussenzweig A (2012) Loss of ATM kinase activity leads to embryonic lethality in mice. J Cell Biol 198:295–304

Degorce SL, Barlaam B, Cadogan E, Dishington A, Ducray R, Glossop SC, Hassall LA, Lach F, Lau A, McGuire TM, Nowak T, Ouvry G, Pike KG, Thomason AG (2016) Discovery of novel 3-quinline carboxamides as potent, selective and orally bioavailable inhibitors of ataxia telangiectasia mutated (ATM) kinase. J Med Chem 59:6281–6292

Delgado-López PD, Corrales-García EM (2016) Survival in glioblastoma: a review on the impact of treatment modalities. Clin Transl Oncol 18:1062–1071

Ding X, Rose JP, Van Gelder J (2012) Developability assessment of clinical drug products with maximum absorbable doses. Int J Pharm 427:260–269

Durant ST, Karlin J, Pike K, Colclough N, Mukhopadhyay N, Ahmad SF, Bekta JM, Tokarz M, Bardelle C, Hughes G, Patel B, Thomason A, Cadogan E, Barrett I, Lau A, Pass M, Valerie K (2016) Blood-brain barrier penetrating ATM inhibitor (AZ32) radiosensitises intracranial gliomas in mice. Cancer Res 76(suppl):3041

Farmer H, McCabe N, Lord CJ, Tutt ANJ, Johnson DA, Richardson TB, Santarosa M, Dillon KJ, Hickson I, Knights C, Martin NMB, Jackson SP, Smith GCM, Ashworth A (2005) Targeting the DNA repair defect in BRCA mutant cells as a therapeutic strategy. Nature 434:917–921

Fedier A, Schlamminger M, Schwarz VA, Haller U, Howell SB, Fink D (2003) Loss of atm sensitises p53-deficient cells to topoisomerase poisons and antimetabolites. Ann Oncol 14:938–945

Foray N, Priestley A, Alsbeih G, Badie C, Capulas EP, Arlett CF, Malaise EP (1997) Hypersensitivity of ataxia telangiectasia fibroblasts to ionizing radiation is associated with a repair deficiency of DNA double-strand breaks. Int J Radiat Biol 72:271–283

Fruman DA, Meyers RE, Cantley LC (1998) Phosphoinositide kinases. Annu Rev Biochem 67:481–507

Furet P, Caravatti G, Guagnano V, Lang M, Meyer T, Schoepfer J (2008) Entry into a new class of protein kinase inhibitors by pseudo ring design. Bioorg Med Chem Lett 18:897–900

Gatz SA, Ju L, Gruber R, Hoffmann E, Carr AM, Wang ZQ, Liu C, Jeggo PA (2011) Requirement for DNA ligase IV during embryonic neuronal development. J Neurosci 31:10088–10100

Golding SE, Rosenberg E, Valerie N, Hussaini I, Frigerio M, Cockcroft XF, Chong WY, Hummersone M, Rigoreau L, Menear KA, O'Connor MJ, Povirk LF, van Meter T, Valerie K (2009) Improved ATM kinase inhibitor KU-60019 radiosensitizes glioma cells, compromises insulin, AKT and ERK prosurvival signaling, and inhibits migration and invasion. Mol Cancer Ther 8:2894–2902

Golding SE, Rosenberg E, Adams BR, Wignarajah S, Beckta JM, O'Connor MJ, Valerie K (2012) Dynamic inhibition of ATM kinase provides a strategy for glioblastoma multiforme radiosensitization and growth control. Cell Cycle 11:1167–1173

Gosink EC, Chong MJ, McKinnon PJ (1999) Ataxia telangiectasia mutated deficiency affects astrocyte growth but not radiosensitivity. Cancer Res 59:5294–5298

Guo K, Shelat A, Guy RK, Kastan MB (2014) Development of a cell-based, high-throughput screening assay for ATM kinase inhibitors. J Biomol Screen 19:538–546

Herzog KH, Chong MJ, Kapsetaki M, Morgan JI, McKinnon PJ (1998) Requirement for Atm in ionizing radiation-induced cell death in the developing central nervous system. Science 280:1089–1091

Hickson I, Zhao Y, Richardson CJ, Green SJ, Martin NMB, Orr AI, Reaper PM, Jackson SP, Curtin NJ, Smith GC (2004) Identification and characterization of a novel and specific inhibitor of the ataxia-telangiectasia mutated kinase ATM. Cancer Res 64:9152–9159

Hilgers AR, Smith DP, Biermacher JJ, Day JS, Jensen JL, Sims SM, Adams WJ, Friis JM, Palandra J, Hosley JD, Shobe EM, Burton PS (2003) Predicting oral absorption of drugs: a case study with a novel class of antimicrobial agents. Pharm Res 20:1149–1155

Hollick JJ, Rigoreau LJM, Cano-Soumillac C, Cockcroft X, Curtin NJ, Frigerio M, Golding BT, Guiard S, Hardcastle IR, Hickson I, Hummersone MG, Menear KA, Martin NMB, Matthews I, Newell DR, Ord R, Richardson CJ, GCM S, Griffin RJ (2007) Pyranone, thiopyranone, and pyridone inhibitors of phosphatidylinositol 3-kinase related kinases. Structure-activity relationships for DNA-dependent protein kinase inhibition, and identification of the first potent and selective inhibitor of the ataxia telangiectasia mutated kinase. J Med Chem 50:1958–1972

Houldsworth J, Lavin M (1980) Effect of ionizing radiation on DNA synthesis in ataxia teleangiectasia cells. Nucleic Acids Res 8:3709–3720

Izzard RA, Jackson SP, Smith GCM (1999) Competitive and non-competitive inhibition of the DNA dependent protein kinase. Cancer Res 59:2581–2586

Johnson KC, Swindell AC (1996) Guidance in the setting of drug particle size specification to minimize variability in absorption. Pharm Res 3:1795–1798

Kaelin WGJ (2005) The concept of synthetic lethality in the context of anticancer therapy. Nat Rev Cancer 5:689–698

Kahn J, Allen J, Karlin JD, Ahmad S, Sule A, Tokarz M, Henderson A, Mukhopadhyay ND, Pike K, Colclough N, Pass M, Durant S, Valerie K (2017) Next-generation ATM kinase inhibitors under development radiosensitize glioblastoma with conformal radiation in a mouse orthotopic model. Int J Rad Oncol 99:E600–E601

Karve S, Werner ME, Sukumar R, Cummings ND, Copp JA, Wang EC, Li C, Sethi M, Chen RC, Pacold ME, Wang AZ (2012) Revival of the abandoned therapeutic wortmannin by nanoparticle drug delivery. Proc Natl Acad Sci U S A 109:8230–8235

Kastan MB, Zhan Q, El-Deiry WS, Carrier F, Jacks T, Walsh WV, Plunkett BS, Vogelstein B, Fornace AJJ (1992) A mammalian cell cycle checkpoint pathway utilizing p53 and GADD45 is defective in ataxia-telangiectasia. Cell 71:587–597

Kim SY, Rhee JG, Song X, Prochownik EV, Spitz DR, Lee YJ (2012) Breast cancer stem cell-like cells are more sensitive to ionizing radiation than non-stem cells: role of ATM. PLoS One 7:e50423

Knight ZA, Shokat KM (2005) Features of selective kinase inhibitors. Chem Biol 12:621–637

Knight ZA, Chiang GG, Alaimo PJ, Kenski DM, Ho CB, Coan K, Abraham RT, Shokat KM (2004) Isoform-specific phosphoinositide 3-kinase inhibitors from an arylmorpholine scaffold. Bioorg Med Chem 12:4749–4759

Knight ZA, Gonzalez B, Feldman ME, Zunder ER, Goldenberg DD, Williams O, Loewith R, Stokoe D, Balla A, Toth B, Balla T, Weiss WA, Williams RL, Shokat KM (2006) A pharmacological map of the PI3-K family defines a role for p110alpha in insulin signaling. Cell 125:733–747

Köcher S, Rieckmann T, Rohaly G, Mansour WY, Dikomey E, Dornreiter I, Dahm-Daphi J (2012) Radiation-induced double-strand breaks require ATM but not Artemis for homologous recombination during S-phase. Nucleic Acids Res 40:8336–8347

Köcher S, Spies-Naumann A, Kriegs M, Dahm-Daphi J, Dornreiter I (2013) ATM is required for the repair of Topotecan-induced replication-associated double-strand breaks. Radiother Oncol 108:409–414

Konstantinidou G, Bey EA, Rabellino A, Schuster K, Maira MS, Gazdar AF, Amici A, Boothman DA, Scaglioni PP (2009) Dual phosphoinositide 3-kinase/mammalian target of rapamycin blockade is an effective radiosensitizing strategy for the treatment of non-small cell lung cancer harboring K-RAS mutations. Cancer Res 69:7644–7652

Kubota E, Williamson CT, Ye R, Elegbede A, Peterson L, Lees-Miller SP, Bebb DG (2014) Low ATM protein expression and depletion of p53 correlates with olaparib sensitivity in gastric cancer cell lines. Cell Cycle 13:2129–2137

Kühne M, Riballo E, Rief N, Ku M, Rothkamm K, Jeggo PA, Löbrich M (2004) A double-strand break repair defect in ATM-deficient cells contributes to radiosensitivity. Cancer Res 64:500–508

Lau A, Swinbank KM, Ahmed PS, Taylor DL, Jackson SP, Smith GC, O'Connor MJ (2005) Suppression of HIV-1 infection by a small molecule inhibitor of the ATM kinase. Nat Cell Biol 7:493–500

Lavin MF (2008) Ataxia-telangiectasia: from a rare disorder to a paradigm for cell signalling and cancer. Nat Rev Mol Cell Biol 9:759–769

Lavin MF, Shiloh Y (1997) The genetic defect in ataxia-telangiectasia. Annu Rev Immunol 15:177–202

Lee J-H, Paull TT (2005) ATM Activation by DNA Double-Strand Breaks Through the Mre11-Rad50-Nbs1 Complex. Science 308:551–554

Lin X, DeAngelis LM (2015) Treatment of brain metastases. J Clin Oncol 33:3475–3484

Lu XH, Mattis VB, Wang N, Al-Ramahi I, van den Berg N, Fratantoni SA, Waldvogel H, Greiner E, Osmand A, Elzein K, Xiao J, Dijkstra S, de Pril R, Vinters HV, Faull R, Signer E, Kwak S, Marugan JJ, Botas J, Fischer DF, Svendsen CN, Munoz-Sanjuan I, Yang XW (2014) Targeting ATM ameliorates mutant Huntingtin toxicity in cell and animal models of Huntington's disease. Sci Transl Med 6:268ra178

Maira S-M, Stauffer F, Brueggen J, Furet P, Schnell C, Fritsch C, Brachmann S, Chène P, De Pover A, Schoemaker K, Fabbro D, Gabriel D, Simonen M, Murphy L, Finan P, Sellers W, García-Echeverría C (2008) Identification and characterization of NVP-BEZ235, a new orally available dual phosphatidylinositol 3-kinase/mammalian target of rapamycin inhibitor with potent in vivo antitumor activity. Mol Cancer Ther 7:1851–1863

Marine JC, Lozano G (2010) Mdm2-mediated ubiquitylation: p53 and beyond. Cell Death Differ 17:93–102

Matsuoka S, Huang M, Elledge SJ (1998) Linkage of ATM to cell cycle regulation by the Chk2 protein kinase. Science 282:1893–1897

Morgado-Palacin I, Day A, Murga M, Lafarga V, Anton ME, Tubbs A, Chen HT, Ergan A, Anderson R, Bhandoola A, Pike KG, Barlaam B, Cadogan E, Wang X, Pierce AJ, Hubbard C, Armstrong SA, Nussenzweig A, Fernandez-Capetillo O (2016) Targeting the kinase activities of ATR and ATM exhibits antitumoral activity in mouse models of MLL-rearranged AML. Sci Signal 9:ra91

Murai J, Huang SY, Das BB, Renaud A, Zhang Y, Doroshow JH, Ji J, Takeda S, Pommier Y (2012) Trapping of PARP1 and PARP2 by clinical PARP inhibitors. Cancer Res 72:5588–5599

Nadkarni A, Shrivastav M, Mladek AC, Schwingler PM, Grogan PT, Chen J, Sarkaria JN (2012) ATM inhibitor KU-55933 increases the TMZ responsiveness of only inherently TMZ sensitive GBM cells. J Neuro-Oncol 110:349–357

Page KM (2016) Validation of early human dose prediction: a key metric for compound progression in drug discovery. Mol Pharm 13:609–620

Painter RB, Young BR (1980) Radiosensitivity in ataxia-telangiectasia: a new explanation. Proc Natl Acad Sci U S A 77:7315–7317

Pike K, Barlaam B, Cadogan E, Campbell A, Colclough N, Davies N, de Almeida C, Degorce S, Didelot M, Dishington A, Ducray R, Durant S, Hassall L, Holmes J, Hughes G, MacFaul P, Mulholland K, McGuire T, Ouvry G, Pass M, RobB G, Stratton N, Wang Z, Wilson J, Zhai B, Zhao K (2018) The Identification of Potent, Selective and Orally Available Inhibitors of Ataxia Telangiectasia Mutated (ATM) Kinase: The Discovery of AZD0156 (8-{6-[3-(dimethylamino)propoxy]pyridin-3-yl}-3-methyl-1-(tetrahydro-2H-pyran-4-yl)-1,3-dihydro-2H-imidazo[4,5-c]quinolin-2-one). J Med Chem, submitted

Powell SN, DeFrank JS, Connell P, Eogan M, Preffer F, Dombkowski D, Tang W, Friend S (1995) Differential sensitivity of p53(−) and p53(+) cells to caffeine-induced radiosensitization and override of G2 delay. Cancer Res 55:1643–1648

Powis G, Bonjouklian R, Berggren MM, Gallegos A, Abraham R, Ashendel C, Zalkow L, Matter WF, Dodge J, Grindey G, Vlahos CJ (1994) Wortmannin, a potent and selective inhibitor of phosphatidylinositol-3-kinase. Cancer Res 54:2419–2423

Price BD, Youmell MB (1996) The phosphatidylinositol 3-kinase inhibitor wortmannin sensitizes murine fibroblasts and human tumor cells to radiation and blocks induction of p53 following DNA damage. Cancer Res 56:246–250

Rainey MD, Charlton ME, Stanton RV, Kastan MB (2008) Transient inhibition of ATM kinase is sufficient to enhance cellular sensitivity to ionizing radiation. Cancer Res 68:7466–7474

Reaper PM, Griffiths MR, Long JM, Charrier J-D, Maccormick S, Charlton PA, Golec JMC, Pollard JR (2011) Selective killing of ATM- or p53-deficient cancer cells through inhibition of ATR. Nat Chem Biol 7:428–430

Redfern WS, Carlsson L, Davis AS, Lynch WG, MacKenzie I, Palethorpe S, Siegl PKS, Strang I, Sullivan AT, Wallis R, Camm AJ, Hammond TG (2003) Relationships between preclinical cardiac electrophysiology, clinical QT interval prolongation and torsade de pointes for a broad range of drugs: evidence for a provisional safety margin in drug development. Cardiovasc Res 58:32–45

Rotman G, Shiloh Y (1998) ATM: from gene to function. Hum Mol Genet 7:1555–1563

Roy K, Wang L, Makrigiorgos GM, Price BD (2006) Methylation of the ATM promoter in glioma cells alters ionizing radiation sensitivity. Biochem Biophys Res Commun 344:821–826

Sarkaria JN, Eshleman JS (2001) ATM as a target for novel radiosensitizers. Semin Radiat Oncol 11:316–327

Sarkaria JN, Tibbetts RS, Busby EC, Kennedy AP, Hill DE, Abraham RT (1998) Inhibition of phosphoinositide 3-kinase related kinases by the radiosensitizing agent wortmannin. Cancer Res 58:4375–4382

Sarkaria JN, Busby EC, Tibbetts RS, Roos P, Taya Y, Karnitz LM, Abraham RT (1999) Inhibition of ATM and ATR kinase activities by the radiosensitizing agent, caffeine. Cancer Res 59:4375–4382

Shiloh Y (2003) ATM and related protein kinases: safeguarding genome integrity. Nat Rev Cancer 3:155–168

Smith DA, Beaumont K, Maurer TS, Di L (2015) Volume of distribution in drug design. J Med Chem 58:5691–5698

Sullivan KD, Gallant-Behm CL, Henry RE, Fraikin JL, Espinosa JM (2012) The p53 circuit board. Biochim Biophys Acta 1825:229–244

Sultana R, McNeill DR, Abbotts R, Mohammed MZ, Zdzienicka MZ, Qutob H, Seedhouse C, Laughton CA, Fischer PM, Patel PM, Wilson DM, Madhusudan S (2012) Synthetic lethal targeting of DNA double-strand break repair deficient cells by human apurinic/apyrimidinic endonuclease inhibitors. Int J Cancer 131:2433–2444

Sultana R, Abdel-Fatah T, Abbotts R, Hawkes C, Albarakati N, Seedhouse C, Ball G, Chan S, E a R, Ellis IO, Madhusudan S (2013) Targeting XRCC1 deficiency in breast cancer for personalized therapy. Cancer Res 73:1621–1634

Taylor AMR, Harnden DG, Arlett CF, Harcourt SA, Lehmann AR, Stevens S, Bridges BA (1975) Ataxia teleangiectasia: a human mutation with abnormal radiation sensitivity. Nature 258:427–429

Teng P, Bateman NW, Darcy KM, Hamilton CA, Larry G, Bakkenist CJ, Conrads TP (2015) Pharmacologic inhibition of ATR and ATM offers clinically important distinctions to enhancing platinumor radiation response in ovarian, endometrial, and cervical cancer cells. Gynecol Oncol 136:554–561

Toledo LI, Murga M, Zur R, Soria R, Rodriguez A, Martinez S, Oyarzabal J, Pastor J, Bischoff JR, Fernandez-Capetillo O (2011) A cell-based screen identifies ATR inhibitors with synthetic lethal properties for cancer-associated mutations. Nat Struct Mol Biol 18(6):721–727

Ui M, Okada T, Hazeki K, Hazeki O (1995) Wortmannin as a unique probe for an intracellular signalling protein, phosphoinositide 3-kinase. Trends Biochem Sci 20:303–307

Vendetti FP, Leibowitz BJ, Barnes J, Schamus S, Kiesel BF, Abberbock S, Conrads T, Clump DA, Cadogan E, O'Connor MJ, Yu J, Beumer JH, Bakkenist CJ (2017) Pharmacologic ATM but not ATR kinase inhibition abrogates p21-dependent G1 arrest and promotes gastrointestinal syndrome after total body irradiation. Sci Rep 7:41892

Vlahos CJ, Matter WF, Hui KY, Brown RF (1994) A specific inhibitor of phosphatidylinositol 3-kinase, 2-(4-morpholinyl)-8-phenyl-4H-1-benzopyran-4-one. J Biol Chem 269:5241–5248

Walker EH, Pacold ME, Perisic O, Stephens L, Hawkins PT, Wymann MP, Williams RL (2000) Structural determinants of phosphoinositide3-kinase inhibition by wortmannin, LY294002, quercetin, myricetin, and staurosporine. Mol Cell 6:909–919

Waring MJ, Johnstone C, McKerrecher D, Pike KG, Robb G (2011) Matrix-based multiparameter optimisation of glucokinase activators: the discovery of AZD1092. Med Chem Commun 2:775–779

Weber AM, Ryan AJ (2015) ATM and ATR as therapeutic targets in cancer. Pharmacol Ther 149:124–138

Weston VJ, Oldreive CE, Skowronska A, Oscier DG, Pratt G, Dyer MJS, Smith G, Powell JE, Rudzki Z, Kearns P, Moss PAH, Taylor AMR, Stankovic T (2010) The PARP inhibitor olaparib induces significant killing of ATM-deficient lymphoid tumor cells in vitro and in vivo. Blood 116:4578–4587

White JS, Choi S, Bakkenist CJ (2010) Transient ATM kinase inhibition disrupts DNA damage-induced sister chromatid exchange. Sci Signal 3:ra44

Won J, Kim M, Kim N, Ahn JH, Lee WG, Kim SS, Chang KY, Yi YW, Kim TK (2006) Small molecule-based reversible reprogramming of cellular lifespan. Nat Chem Biol 2:369–374

Won J, Kim M, Kim N, Ahn JH, Lee WG, Kim SS, Chang KY, Yi YW, Kim TK (2008) Retraction: small molecule–based reversible reprogramming of cellular lifespan. Nat Chem Biol 4:431. retracted 17 June 2008

Yamamoto K, Wang Y, Jiang W, Liu X, Dubois RL, Lin C-S, Ludwig T, Bakkenist CJ, Zha S (2012) Kinase-dead ATM protein causes genomic instability and early embryonic lethality in mice. J Cell Biol 198:305–313

Yang H, Rudge DG, Koos JD, Vaidialingham B, Yang HJ, Pavletich NP (2013) mTOR kinase structure, mechanism and regulation. Nature 497:217–223

Yao S-L, Akhtar AJ, McKenna KA, Bedi GC, David S, Mack M, Rajani R, Collector MI, Jones RJ, Sharkis SJ, Fuchs EJ, Bedi A (1996) Selective radiosensitization of p53-deficient cells by caffeine-mediated activation of p34 cdc2 kinase. Nat Med 2:1140–1143

Chapter 9
Targeting CHK1 for Cancer Therapy: Rationale, Progress and Prospects

David A. Gillespie

Abstract During the past 20 years or so the serine-threonine protein kinase CHK1 has emerged as a key regulator of genome stability in vertebrate cells. When cells sustain acute DNA damage, or when DNA replication is impeded, CHK1 is activated to mitigate against the lethal consequences of cell division with damaged or incompletely replicated genomes. To achieve this CHK1 acts to delay cell cycle progression, stimulate DNA repair, and to promote the accurate completion of genome duplication. Collectively, these checkpoint responses are crucial for cell survival under conditions of genotoxic stress, and numerous pre-clinical studies have shown that inhibition of CHK1 can enhance tumour cell killing by radiation and genotoxic chemotherapeutic agents with diverse mechanisms of action. As a result, a number of small-molecule CHK1 inhibitor drugs have been developed, some of which have reached clinical trials in combination with existing chemo-therapies. CHK1 inhibitors have also been shown to synergise with non-genotoxic inhibitors targeting other checkpoint regulators, such as Wee1 kinase, whilst other evidence suggests that certain tumour cell types may be inherently sensitive to CHK1 inhibition alone, perhaps reflecting underlying defects in DNA repair or replication processes. Despite these promising advances, rational strategies for the targeted deployment of CHK1 inhibitor drugs remain at a relatively early stage of development, whilst the important issues of therapeutic index and normal tissue toxicity remain to be fully explored.

Keywords Cancer therapy · CHK1 · DNA damage · Checkpoint · DNA repair · Mitosis · Chemotherapy · Cell cycle · Protein kinase · Inhibitor drug

D. A. Gillespie (✉)
Institute of Biomedical Technologies, Canary Islands Centre for Biomedical Research, Faculty of Medicine, University of La Laguna, Tenerife, Spain
e-mail: dgillesp@ull.es

© Springer International Publishing AG, part of Springer Nature 2018   209
J. Pollard, N. Curtin (eds.), *Targeting the DNA Damage Response for Anti-Cancer Therapy*, Cancer Drug Discovery and Development, https://doi.org/10.1007/978-3-319-75836-7_9

9.1   Introduction

Checkpoint kinase 1 (CHK1), a serine/threonine protein kinase, was originally discovered as a "Checkpoint Rad" gene in fission yeast whose genetic inactivation conferred sensitivity to DNA damage induced by ultraviolet light or ionising radiation (Walworth and Bernards 1996). The subsequent realisation that CHK1, as well as many other key biochemical components of what has subsequently come to be referred to as the "DNA Damage Response" (DDR) signal transduction pathway (Harper and Elledge 2007), was highly conserved in humans raised the obvious question of whether inhibition of CHK1 would render tumour cells similarly sensitive to genotoxic damage. If so, then clearly CHK1 inhibitor drugs might provide a means of enhancing the potency of conventional genotoxic therapies, a concept that had previously motivated the initial development of Poly(ADP)ribose polymerase (PARP) inhibitors (Curtin 2005).

Numerous basic and pre-clinical studies using diverse technical approaches have subsequently confirmed that CHK1 inhibition can indeed enhance tumour cell killing by radiation and diverse genotoxic chemotherapies (McNeely et al. 2014). In addition, evidence suggests that some tumour cells may overexpress and potentially rely on CHK1 for successful proliferation to a greater extent than normal cells, even in the absence of exogenous genotoxic stress, while this dependence may be even more pronounced in a subset of tumours with inherent genome stability defects (Al-Ahmadie et al. 2014). Thus, a substantial body of evidence argues that in principle CHK1 is indeed a rational drug target for anticancer therapy. As a result, a number of CHK1 inhibitor drugs have been developed or are currently under development (McNeely et al. 2014; O'Connor 2015).

At present however, we still lack clear, rational insights as to which specific genotoxic therapies will synergise optimally with CHK1 inhibitors, or in which specific tumour types or individual patients they should be deployed, either in combination or as single agents (Garrett and Collins 2011). To answer these questions, we need to understand the molecular consequences of CHK1 inhibition and how these interact with specific kinds of DNA damage lesions, or tumour genotypes, in order to elicit selective tumour cell death. This review therefore begins with a very brief overview of our current understanding of CHK1 activation and functions in cells exposed to genotoxic stress before turning more specifically to the consequences of CHK1 inhibition and potential mechanisms of tumour cell killing in various biological contexts. Readers who may wish to learn more about the functions and regulation of CHK1 in detail are referred to recent reviews on this specific topic (Smits and Gillespie 2015; Goto et al. 2015).

9.2   CHK1 Activation and Checkpoint Functions;
A Thumbnail Sketch

Radiation and genotoxic chemotherapies can both damage DNA and inhibit DNA replication, sometimes concurrently, and each of these pathological conditions elicits activation of CHK1 via a relatively well-defined molecular mechanism

(Smits and Gillespie 2015). Key in both cases is the initial formation of single-stranded DNA (ssDNA) that rapidly becomes coated with the ssDNA binding protein RPA (Fig. 9.1). When DNA synthesis is inhibited ssDNA is created directly when the replicative helicase becomes "uncoupled" from, or runs ahead of, the inhibited DNA polymerase (Zeman and Cimprich 2014). This leads to unwinding of the undamaged double-stranded template to form tracts of ssDNA that then associate with RPA (Fig. 9.1). Small amounts of ssDNA are normally associated with active replication forks, particularly the lagging strand, however DNA synthesis inhibition amplifies this enormously (Zeman and Cimprich 2014). DNA polymerase inhibitors, such as hydroxyurea or aphidicolin, are therefore potent activators of CHK1.

The situation with DNA damage is somewhat more complicated owing to the plethora of possible DNA damage lesions and the distinct DNA repair mechanisms that effect their repair (Hoeijmakers 2009). It is generally accepted however that

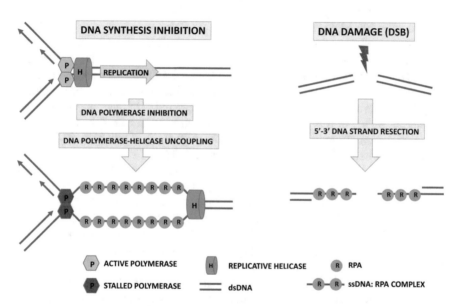

Fig. 9.1 Formation of ssDNA: RPA complexes in response to DNA synthesis inhibition and DNA damage. Active DNA polymerases (P) at replication forks are preceded by a replicative helicase complex (H) which unwinds the double-stranded DNA template to allow synthesis on the leading and lagging strands. During unperturbed replication the DNA polymerase and helicase move in concert, minimising exposure of ssDNA at active replication forks. When DNA polymerase catalytic activity is inhibited, for example through nucleotide precursor depletion or direct inhibition, helicase activity outstrips polymerisation leading to template unwinding and exposure of extensive tracts of ssDNA that rapidly associate with RPA. DNA double-strand breaks by contrast are subject to 5′ to 3′ nucleolytic strand resection to leave overhanging 3′ tails of ssDNA that again associate with RPA. In addition to serving as a platform for checkpoint activation these structures serve to initiate DNA repair by homologous recombination. Strand resection is a highly cell cycle-dependent process that occurs only in S and G2 phase when sister chromatids are available for homology-directed repair

DNA double strand breaks (DSBs) are amongst the most toxic lesions created either directly or indirectly by radiation and genotoxic chemotherapies. DSBs are subject to nucleolytic resection in a 5′ to 3′ direction to create overhanging 3′ ssDNA tails which associate with RPA and serve both to activate checkpoint signalling and to initiate DNA repair by homologous recombination [Fig. 9.1: (Symington and Gautier 2011)]. Resection is a highly regulated process that is largely confined to the S and G2 phases of the cell cycle when sister chromatids are available to template recombinational repair (Symington and Gautier 2011).

Variable amounts of ssDNA can also be generated through the action of other repair mechanisms such as, for example, nucleotide excision repair and some forms of base excision repair. In general, it is considered that the intensity of CHK1 activation is proportional to amount of ssDNA generated (MacDougall et al. 2007).

Regardless of how it is formed, ssDNA: RPA within the context of chromatin then acts as a platform to nucleate the formation of a large complex of proteins, including ATR, ATRIP, Claspin, Rad9, Rad1, and Hus1, within which CHK1 becomes activated (Fig. 9.2; Smits and Gillespie 2015).

The assembly of this complex is a highly regulated process involving multiple protein-protein interactions, many of which are dependent on specific phosphorylation events (Smits and Gillespie 2015). Notable amongst these are the recruitment of TopBP1 by phosphorylated Rad9 and of CHK1 by the adaptor protein Claspin following phosphorylation within several "CHK1-activation" (CKA) motifs (Fig. 9.2, Smits and Gillespie 2015). A detailed description of these interactions lies outside the scope of this review, however ultimately CHK1 itself is activated via phosphorylation of multiple serine- glutamine (SQ) residues within the C-terminal regulatory domain (Fig. 9.2; Smits and Gillespie 2015).

Phosphorylation of these sites is catalysed by the upstream kinase ATR (Smits and Gillespie 2015), and modification of one SQ residue in particular, serine 345 (S345), is crucial as phosphorylation of this single site is essential for CHK1 function (Walker et al. 2009). Phosphorylation of S345 also correlates well with the extent and duration of checkpoint activation and has thus served as the most widely used surrogate marker for CHK1 activity measured using phospho-specific antibodies (Smits and Gillespie 2015; Walker et al. 2009).

Phosphorylation of CHK1 S345 also promotes release of CHK1 from the chromatin- associated activation complex and creates a binding site for 14-3-3 proteins (Fig. 9.2; Smits et al. 2006). Evidence suggests that 14-3-3 protein binding is required for activation and may also play a role in retaining CHK1 within the nucleus and facilitating interactions with certain substrates (Smits and Gillespie 2015). Once released from chromatin, activated CHK1 disperses through the nucleoplasm to trigger multiple, distinct, DNA damage and replication checkpoint responses by phosphorylating a variety of substrates (Smits and Gillespie 2015). Although this general scheme is well-accepted, some uncertainties remain over the relative importance of increased CHK1 catalytic activity versus alterations in subcellular localisation for triggering checkpoint activation (Smits and Gillespie 2015).

As depicted in Fig. 9.3, DNA damage triggers cell cycle arrest in the G1 and G2 phases of the cell cycle (the G1 and G2 checkpoints) in genetically normal cells,

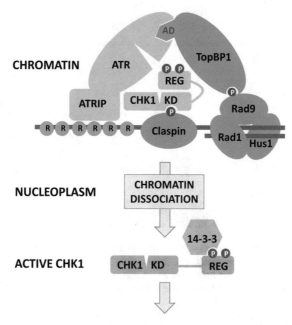

DNA DAMAGE AND REPLICATION CHECKPOINTS

Fig. 9.2 ssDNA: RPA serves as a platform for CHK1 activation by ATR. CHK1 activation occurs within a large multi-protein signalling complex that assembles at sites of ssDNA: RPA formation within the context of chromatin. Some of the components of this complex, such as the adaptor protein Claspin, may also be normal constituents of active replication complexes, whereas others, such as the Rad9:Rad1:Hus1 (9:1:1) complex and TopBP1, are loaded onto DNA specifically in response to genotoxic stress. ATR kinase is recruited via its targeting subunit, ATRIP, which interacts directly with ssDNA:RPA, whilst TopBP1 is recruited through a phosphorylation-dependent interaction with the Rad9 component of the 9:1:1 complex. TopBP1 stimulates the catalytic activity of ATR via a direct interaction with its "ATR activation domain" (AD). This in turn leads to ATR-dependent phosphorylation of Claspin within two short repeated "CHK1 activation" (CKA) peptide motifs. CHK1 can then bind to CKA-phosphorylated Claspin, thereby enabling ATR to efficiently phosphorylate CHK1 at multiple serine-glutamine (SQ) residues within the C-terminal regulatory domain, notably serine 317 and 345 (S317/S345). Phosphorylation of S345 promotes dissociation from the chromatin-bound activation complex, enabling CHK1 to disperse throughout the nucleoplasm, and also creates a binding site for 14-3-3 proteins

together with a rapid but transient decrease in the rate of DNA synthesis in replicating cells (the intra-S checkpoint). These responses have three biological objectives: by blocking entry to S phase the G1 checkpoint effectively prevents the replication of damaged genomes, while by slowing DNA synthesis the intra-S phase checkpoint facilitates the repair and accurate replication of damaged genomes in cells that have already committed to S phase when the damage is incurred. Finally, the G2 checkpoint prevents cells with damaged chromosomes from initiating mitosis, providing time for repair and preventing immediate mitotic catastrophe or permanent loss of genetic material (Fig. 9.3, Smits and Gillespie 2015).

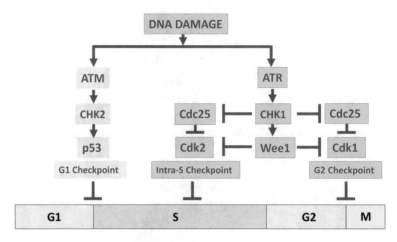

Fig. 9.3 DNA damage checkpoint responses. DNA damage evokes cell cycle arrests in G1 (the G1 checkpoint) and G2 (the G2 checkpoint) phases that prevent the replication and division of damaged genomes respectively. In addition the rate at which damaged DNA is replicated in S phase cells is slowed (intra-S checkpoint). CHK1 is a key effector in all of these responses with the exception of the G1 checkpoint, which is imposed through ATM-CHK2-mediated activation of the p53 tumor suppressor protein and its downstream target the cyclin-dependent kinase inhibitor, p21^{CIP1}. The ultimate target of the G2 checkpoint is Cdk1, whose rapid activation through removal of inhibitory tyrosine 15 (Y15) phosphorylation normally initiates the onset of mitosis. CHK1 phosphorylates and inhibits the Cdc25 family phosphatases that remove Cdk1 Y15 phosphorylation and phosphorylates and stimulates the catalytic activity of Wee1, a Cdk1 Y15 kinase. The net result is to maintain Cdk1 in its inactive, Y15-phosphorylated state whilst damage persists and CHK1 is active

G2 arrest is mechanistically the best understood of the DNA damage checkpoints (Fig. 9.4; Smits and Gillespie 2015). Under normal circumstances mitosis is initiated when Cdk1 is activated via rapid removal of inhibitory tyrosine 15 (Y15) phosphorylation, a reaction catalysed by Cdc25 family phosphatases (Cdc25A, B, C; Lindqvist et al. 2009). However, when activated in response to DNA damage, CHK1 phosphorylates and inhibits Cdc25 family phosphatases via multiple mechanisms including degradation and sequestration through association with 14-3-3 proteins (Fig. 9.4; Mailand et al. 2000; Chen et al. 2003; Peng et al. 1997). CHK1 also phosphorylates and stimulates the catalytic activity of Wee1, a dual specificity kinase that contributes to Cdk1 Y15 phosphorylation (Lee et al. 2001). The combined effect of these actions is to ensure that whilst damage persists and CHK1 is active, Cdk1 Y15 phosphorylation is maintained at high levels and entry to mitosis is effectively blocked (Fig. 9.4; Smits and Gillespie 2015). In addition to precluding mitotic entry with damage, CHK1-mediated arrest in G2 is considered to facilitate repair. In part this is simply a consequence of cell cycle arrest, since the error-free mechanism of homologous recombination repair (HRR) is highly active in G2 phase (Symington and Gautier 2011). CHK1 however is also thought to promote HRR directly, by phosphorylating and promoting recruitment of the Rad51 recombinase and its loading factor Brca2, which are required for HRR, to ssDNA at sites of damage (Sorensen et al. 2005).

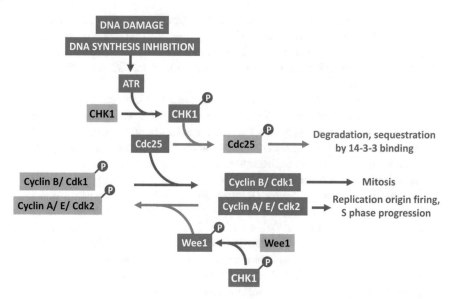

Fig. 9.4 Mechanism of regulation of Cdc25 and Cdk family proteins by CHK1. In response to DNA damage or DNA synthesis inhibition CHK1 is activated through phosphorylation by ATR (activated components are depicted in red, inactive in grey). CHK1 phosphorylates Cdc25 family proteins leading to their inhibition via degradation and sequestration by 14-3-3 proteins. CHK1 also phosphorylates and stimulates the activity of Wee1, a tyrosine kinase that catalyses inhibitory Y15 phosphorylation of Cdk1 and Cdk2. The net effect of Cdc25 inhibition and Wee1 activation is to prevent activation of Cdk1 and reduce the basal activity of Cdk2 by maintaining, or increasing, the levels of inhibitory Y15 phosphorylation, thus blocking entry to mitosis and suppressing replication origin firing

Finally, CHK1 also controls the intra-S checkpoint which acts to slow the replication of damaged templates (Fig. 9.3; Sorensen et al. 2003). This is achieved, at least in part, through inhibition of Cdk2, which is required for DNA replication origin firing. Cdk2 is also subject to inhibitory tyrosine Y15 phosphorylation catalysed by Wee1 (Fig. 9.4), and, although this modification is regulated very differently to Cdk1, inhibition of Cdc25 phosphatase activity by CHK1 leads to suppression of basal Cdk2 catalytic activity and thus a decrease in DNA synthesis rate, most likely as a result of late replication origin suppression (Sorensen et al. 2003).

Genetically normal cells can also arrest in G1 phase in response to DNA damage (Fig. 9.3). G1 arrest prevents cells from replicating damaged DNA templates and, in some cases at least, is irreversible, a phenotype also referred to as replicative senescence (von Zglinicki et al. 2005). CHK1 is not thought to be involved in triggering DNA damage-induced G1 arrest (Smits and Gillespie 2015), which instead is imposed via the Ataxia Telangiectasia Mutated (ATM)—Checkpoint kinase 2 (CHK2) pathway activating the p53 tumour suppressor protein to induce expression of its downstream effector the p21 Cyclin-dependent kinase Inhibitor Protein 1 (p21 CIP1; Fig. 9.3). It is important to note however that the G1 checkpoint is absent or compromised in many, although not all, tumour cells owing to functional inactivation of components within the ATM/CHK2/p53 pathway (most frequently p53 itself; Muller and Vousden 2013). G1 checkpoint deficiency seems to alter the overall cellular response to DNA damage, and under some circumstances may increase dependence on the CHK1-mediated damage checkpoints acting in S and G2 phase for adequate repair and cell survival.

Cells experiencing replication stress, which can result from nucleotide depletion through the action of antimetabolite drugs, or direct DNA polymerase inhibition in the case of chain terminating agents, face a different set of problems (Fig. 9.5). When DNA synthesis is slowed but not completely blocked it is vital that the onset of mitosis is delayed until genome replication is complete, since any attempt to divide a partially duplicated genome would obviously be disastrous. CHK1 is the key effector of the mitotic delay triggered by DNA synthesis inhibition, a response generally referred to as the S-M checkpoint to distinguish it from the G2 arrest induced by DNA damage (Zachos et al. 2005). As with G2 arrest, the S-M checkpoint depends at least in part on blocking activation of Cdk1 via inhibition of Cdc25 family phosphatases, although other mechanisms may also contribute (Smits and Gillespie 2015).

When DNA synthesis inhibition is sufficiently severe to prevent replication fork progression completely the paused forks are said to be "stalled" and require a CHK1-dependent process of stabilization to prevent irreversible functional inactivation or

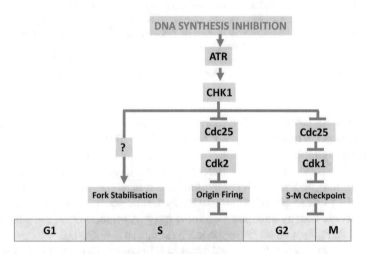

Fig. 9.5 DNA replication checkpoint responses. When DNA replication is impeded responses are triggered that maintain the viability of stalled replication forks (fork stabilisation), prevent the formation of new forks (suppression of origin firing), and block entry to mitosis until genome duplication is complete (the S-M checkpoint). Cdk2 activity is required for replication origin firing and, as with Cdk1, Cdk2 is subject to inhibitory Y15 phosphorylation. When DNA synthesis is inhibited activated CHK1 phosphorylates and inhibits the activity of cdc25 phosphatases leading to a decrease in basal Cdk2 activity and suppression of replication origin firing. CHK1-mediated phosphorylation of an additional effector protein, Treslin, likely also contributes to inhibition of replication origin firing. As with DNA damage, activation of Cdk1 is blocked through inhibition of Cdc25 phosphatases, although other mechanisms may also contribute. The mechanisms of replication fork stabilisation are currently less well understood

"collapse" (Fig. 9.5; Paulsen and Cimprich 2007). Replication fork collapse is associated with the formation of DNA damage lesions at the sites of fork demise that are marked by accumulation of γ-H2AX (Paulsen and Cimprich 2007). Exactly how CHK1 prevents or slows this process of replication fork collapse during acute DNA synthesis inhibition remains relatively unclear, however collapse is associated with accumulation and cleavage of naked ssDNA structures through the action of nucleases such as Mus81/Mre11 (Forment et al. 2011; Thompson et al. 2012) to form DSBs and possibly also with changes in the composition of fork-associated replisome components. Exhaustion of the pool of RPA available for association with ssDNA may also render stalled forks particularly vulnerable to nucleolytic attack (Toledo et al. 2013). Ultimately, collapsed forks are frequently thought to form "single-ended" DSBs that can only be repaired through recombination (Allen et al. 2011).

Finally, when DNA synthesis is severely inhibited cells attempt to prevent the problem of stalled replication forks escalating by blocking the firing of further licensed replication origins (Fig. 9.5). As with the intra-S DNA damage checkpoint CHK1 achieves this partly by suppressing Cdk2 activity through CdcC25 inhibition and increased Y15 phosphorylation, but also by inhibiting the origin firing activity of a protein called Treslin (Smits and Gillespie 2015). Collectively, via this combination of mitotic delay, fork stabilization, and origin suppression, the replication checkpoints "freeze" cells in S phase so that genome duplication can ultimately be achieved in an orderly fashion if and when DNA synthesis can resume (Smits and Gillespie 2015).

These canonical DNA damage and replication checkpoint responses represent the best characterised functions of CHK1, and as discussed in more detail below, failure of one or more of these responses is likely to contribute to the toxicity of CHK1 inhibition in many biological situations. Nevertheless, it is important to bear in mind that CHK1 also participates in a number of other, less well-characterised aspects of cell cycle progression and cell division such as spindle checkpoint proficiency, cytokinesis, and gene regulation, and it is possible that suppression of these functions could also lead to, or enhance, cell death under specific conditions (Smits and Gillespie 2015).

9.3 CHK1 as a Therapeutic Target: Theoretical Considerations

To be a valid therapeutic target for cancer therapy candidates clearly need to meet certain general criteria. Amongst these might be; (1) is the target present and active in tumour cells? (2) is the target amenable to pharmacological inhibition? (3) can target inhibition lead to tumour cell death by a specific mechanism? (4) is target inhibition more toxic to tumour cells than cells in normal tissues; i.e. is there a therapeutic index?

Published expression surveys indicate that CHK1 is generally, and possibly invariably, expressed in human tumours and tumour cell lines (Bartek and Lukas

2003). In addition, reports of tumour- specific mutations affecting CHK1 are exceedingly rare and remain of unknown functional significance (Bertoni et al. 1999). It therefore appears that a certain level of functional CHK1 expression is generally either required for or beneficial for tumour cell proliferation and/ or survival (Bartek and Lukas 2003). This conclusion is further borne out by experimental studies in conditional CHK1 knockout (KO) mice which show that complete loss of CHK1 is incompatible with tumour formation in both the skin and intestine (Tho et al. 2012; Greenow et al. 2014). In addition, a limited number of attempts to delete CHK1 in human cancer cell lines have been uniformly unsuccessful, again suggesting that CHK1 is required for survival (Wilsker et al. 2008). Based on these observations, and the fact that CHK1 is essential for mouse embryogenesis (Liu et al. 2000), it is often stated emphatically that CHK1 is indispensable for metazoan cell survival. Whilst this may be true in human and mouse cells, and even here there may be room for some residual doubt, CHK1 was successfully deleted by gene targeting in avian DT40 B-lymphoma cells (Zachos et al. 2003). The CHK1 KO lymphoma cells grow less vigorously than their wild-type parents (Zachos et al. 2003), indicating a significant loss of fitness even in the absence of exogenous genotoxic stress, yet this example proves that CHK1 is not always indispensable in tumour cells in metazoans. Unfortunately, the genetic factors that presumably allow DT40 cells to tolerate loss of CHK1 have not yet been defined (Zachos et al. 2003).

How frequently CHK1 is overexpressed in tumour cells compared to normal cells is less clear. The gene encoding CHK1 is under transcriptional control by the Retinoblastoma protein (Rb)-E2F transcription repressor system (Carrassa et al. 2003), which coordinates the cell cycle- dependent expression of many genes required for DNA replication and cell division. In genetically normal cells Rb-E2F regulation restricts CHK1 expression to the proliferative phase and expression is extinguished upon cell cycle exit to quiescence (Kaneko et al. 1999). This predicts that CHK1 is likely not expressed in the quiescent, terminally-differentiated functional cells that make up a large proportion of many normal tissues in vivo, although this topic has not received much direct study. Deregulation of Rb-E2F control may also explain reports of CHK1 overexpression in tumour cell lines (Verlinden et al. 2007), since this pathway is frequently compromised by oncogenic mutations in cancer leading to upregulation or constitutive expression of Rb-E2F target genes. Interestingly, a number of recent studies have demonstrated a correlation between the level of both total or activated (S345-phosphoryated) CHK1 protein expression in tumour samples with clinical outcomes in breast cancer, with higher expression associated with more rapid recurrence and poorer overall survival (Al-Kaabi et al. 2015; Alsubhi et al. 2016).

Assessing CHK1 function in vivo is more complicated, however where examined inhibition of CHK1 in diverse tumour cell lines using siRNA depletion or small molecule inhibitors generally results in checkpoint defects that are broadly consistent with failure or override of the DNA damage response and replication functions that have been defined in model systems (Smith et al. 2010). Perhaps surprisingly, given its central importance in genome stability, CHK1 has no closely-related kinase relatives that can compensate for loss of function, as evidenced by the complete lack of residual checkpoint proficiency in CHK1 KO DT40 cells (Zachos et al. 2003). Some limited functional overlap or redundancy in checkpoint regulation with other DDR components, such as CHK2 and p53, or other signalling pathways, such as p38 MAPK, has been reported in certain cell types, however in most tumour cell lines CHK1 seems to be the dominant regulator of the DNA damage and replication checkpoints (with the exception of p53-mediated G1 arrest; Smith et al. 2010). In marked contrast to p53, there is little or no evidence that CHK1 actively promotes cell death by apoptosis or any other mechanism in response to genotoxic stress, in fact the converse has been reported (Meuth 2010).

Where tested experimentally, all CHK1 functions in the DNA damage and replication checkpoints have been shown to depend on kinase catalytic activity, although such tests have necessarily been confined to tractable experimental systems (Walker et al. 2009). Protein kinases are in general of course readily "druggable" with the caveat that many inhibitors compete with ATP for binding to the kinase catalytic site. This can limit specificity, as exemplified by UCN-01, the first CHK1 inhibitor identified, which is also active against many other protein kinases (Akinaga et al. 1993). However, as discussed below, several effective and more selective CHK1 inhibitors have subsequently been isolated and characterised. In addition to targeted drug-development efforts based on empirical knowledge, CHK1 has also been identified in several unbiased high-throughput "kinome" screens as a target whose inhibition enhances cell killing by specific chemotherapeutics or under conditions of replication stress (Azorsa et al. 2009; Arora et al. 2010).

The consequences of loss or inhibition of CHK1 function in various contexts have been studied using siRNA-mediated depletion, small molecule inhibitors, and gene deletion to temporarily or permanently ablate CHK1 function. In general, the assumption guiding these studies has been that checkpoint responses are protective; in other words that checkpoint abrogation as a result of CHK1 inhibition should escalate the level of spontaneous or exogenously induced DNA damage, promote the formation of more lethal secondary lesions, or trigger some new mechanism of cell death that would otherwise not occur. Such studies have been performed using tumour cell lines in culture or as xenografts, but also to a lesser extent using mouse models and primary human patient material, and now constitute a large and rapidly growing body of literature. The discussion that follows will therefore seek to summarise the consequences of CHK1 inhibition using selected examples in three main areas; synergy with radiation and conventional chemotherapy agents, synergy with other molecularly targeted agents, and finally inherent toxicity of CHK1 inhibition as monotherapy.

9.4 Potentiation of Radiation and Conventional Chemotherapy Agents by CHK1 Inhibition

The principle of chemo-sensitisation as a result of checkpoint override was first demonstrated using caffeine in combination with nitrogen mustard in baby hamster kidney cells almost 40 years ago (Lau and Pardee 1982). Although the molecular mechanism was not understood at the time, it is probable that the effect of caffeine in these experiments was to block activation of CHK1, and thus G2 arrest, by inhibiting the upstream kinase ATR. The result was that damaged cells were impelled to enter mitosis from G2 with lethal levels of chromosome damage (Lau and Pardee 1982). Unfortunately, the therapeutic potential of this novel concept could not be pursued as caffeine was too toxic for in vivo studies.

Nonetheless, some decades after the advent of detailed knowledge of CHK1 and cell cycle checkpoint mechanisms at the molecular level, the consequences of checkpoint suppression have been revisited in great detail. Enhanced tumour cell killing as a result of CHK1 inhibition using small molecule inhibitors or siRNA-mediated depletion has been reported for a wide range of genotoxic agents, including radiation, alkylating agents, topoisomerase poisons, and anti-metabolites. In addition, radio- or chemo-sensitisation has been observed in cell lines derived from a wide range of cancer types, including breast, colon, head and neck squamous carcinoma (HNSCC), leukaemia, lung, melanoma, neuroblastoma, ovarian, pancreatic, prostate, and others. It seems therefore that, in principle at least, adjuvant CHK1 inhibition could represent a generic approach to improving existing conventional genotoxic cancer therapies.

A significant number of small molecule CHK1 inhibitors with different chemical characteristics have been described, including the previously mentioned UCN-01 (Graves et al. 2000), but also Go6976 (Kohn et al. 2003), ICP-1 (Eastman et al. 2002), debromohymendialisine (Curman et al. 2001), isogranulatimide (Jiang et al. 2004), CEP-3891 (Syljuasen et al. 2004), CHIR-124 (Tse et al. 2007), XL844 (Matthews et al. 2007), SAR-020106 (Walton et al. 2010), CCT244747 (Walton et al. 2012), AZD7762 (Zabludoff et al. 2008), MK-8776 (Guzi et al. 2011) (formerly SCH900776), LY2603618 (Weiss et al. 2013), LY2606368 (King et al. 2015), PF-00477736 (Blasina et al. 2008), GNE-900 (Blackwood et al. 2013), and AR458323 (Davies et al. 2011a). Some of these compounds, such as UCN-01 and Go6976, were originally isolated as inhibitors of protein kinase C (PKC; Akinaga et al. 1993) and are known to inhibit numerous other protein kinases, whilst for many others information on specificity is highly limited. Of the CHK1 inhibitors that are considered to be selective, the most extensively studied are AZD7762, MK-8776, LY2603618, and PF-00477736.

Although its lack of specificity potentially complicates interpretation of toxicity studies, UCN-01 is worth briefly reviewing since it is an effective CHK1 inhibitor and has been very widely used, particularly in early pre-clinical studies. Once it was established that CHK1 was indeed a target of UCN-01 (Graves et al. 2000), potentiation of radiation (Yu et al. 2002a), topisomerase poisons (Tse and Schwartz 2004), anti-metabolites (Shao et al. 2004), and alkylating agents (Hirose et al. 2001; Perez et al. 2006) was quickly demonstrated.

Interactions between UCN-01 and a number of non-genotoxic molecularly targeted agents were also documented, most notably the Raf/MEK/ERK, Akt, and JNK pathways (Yu et al. 2002b; Jia et al. 2003; Dai et al. 2005; Hahn et al. 2005). It is likely that CHK1 was the biologically significant target of UCN-01 in these studies, although in most cases some contribution from "off-target" effects could not be ruled out.

AZD7762 is an ATP-competitive dual CHK1/CHK2 inhibitor that was initially shown to enhance the potency of gemcitabine and topoisomerase poisons in vitro and using xenogaft models (Zabludoff et al. 2008). AZD7762 also enhanced cell killing by fractionated radiotherapy in clonogenic and xenograft assays, whilst little effect was observed in normal fibroblasts (Mitchell et al. 2010). In pancreatic cancer cell lines or patient-derived xenografts AZD7762 was shown to potentiate a combination of radiation and gemcitabine, an effect that was linked to inhibition of HRR as well as G2 checkpoint override (Morgan et al. 2010). Synergy with radiation or genotoxic chemotherapies using AZD7762 has also been observed in cell lines or patient material derived from neuroblastoma, leukaemia, HNSCC, and lung, breast, and ovarian cancer (Xu et al. 2011; Yang et al. 2011; Bartucci et al. 2012; Vance et al. 2011; Didier et al. 2012; Itamochi et al. 2014). Where tested, the potentiating effects of AZD7762 were observed to be greater in cells with loss of p53 function and thus a defect in G1 checkpoint proficiency (Xu et al. 2011; Vance et al. 2011). Although not tested in many cases, most of the available evidence suggests that the biologically significant target of AZD7762 that underlies synergistic cell killing is CHK1 rather than CHK2. Although it was initially thought that the functions of CHK1 and CHK2 were overlapping, it is now accepted that CHK1 plays a dominant role in the pro-survival DNA damage and replication checkpoints (Smith et al. 2010). The precise functions of CHK2 have been less well defined, however it has been implicated in p53 activation and apoptosis regulation under conditions of genotoxic stress (Smith et al. 2010). Whether there would be any consistent therapeutic advantage in inhibiting CHK1 and CHK2 simultaneously to enhance genotoxic stress-induced cell death therefore remains unclear.

MK-8776 was isolated using a high-content, cell-based screen that assayed for formation of γ-H2AX foci, a surrogate marker of DSBs (Guzi et al. 2011). This screen was used in combination with medicinal chemistry to modify existing kinase inhibitor compounds in order to maximise selectivity and potency against CHK1. MK-8776 was initially shown to phenocopy the effects of CHK1 inhibition by siRNA depletion and to synergise with hydroxyurea and the anti-metabolites gemcitabine and pemetrexed both in vitro and in xenograft assays (Guzi et al. 2011). MK-8776 also significantly enhanced the toxicity of cytarabine but had little effect in combination with cisplatin, 5-fluorouracil, or 6-thioguanine (Montano et al. 2012). In combination with the topoisomerase I inhibitor, SN38, MK-8776 accelerated the rate but not the overall incidence of cell death, and was observed to be significantly toxic as a single agent to a subset of cell lines (Guzi et al. 2011; Montano et al. 2012). In human acute myeloid leukaemia (AML) cell lines in vitro and patient samples ex vivo MK-8776 enhanced the cytotoxicity of cytarabine but had negligible effect on the sensitivity of normal myeloid progenitors (Schenk et al. 2012). MK-8776 was also found to enhance the toxicity of a gemcitabine-radiation combination in HRR-proficient pancreatic cancer cell lines but had little effect in HRR-deficient lines (Engelke et al. 2013).

LY2603618 is a potent and selective CHK1 inhibitor that was shown to phenocopy the effects of CHK1 inhibition by siRNA depletion and to enhance the toxicity of doxorubicin and gemcitabine in colon and pancreatic cell lines and xenografts, with greater effects observed in p53-deficient cell lines than wild-type (King et al. 2014). LY2603618 was also shown to be significantly toxic as a single agent in lung cancer cell lines, inducing DNA damage, cell cycle arrest, and increased levels of autophagy (Wang et al. 2014). Interaction between LY2603618 and gemcitabine was also studied in xenografts formed from human colon, lung, and pancreatic cell lines, where significantly greater tumour growth inhibition was obtained when gemcitabine was combined with LY2603618 over gemcitabine alone (Barnard et al. 2016). Interestingly, a significantly more potent growth inhibitory effect was obtained when LY2603618 was administered 24 h after gemcitabine, indicating that drug scheduling can significantly modify the toxic consequences of checkpoint suppression (Barnard et al. 2016).

PF-00477736 is a potent, selective inhibitor of CHK1 (Blasina et al. 2008) that was initially reported to synergise with docetaxel, which induces DNA damage and CHK1 activation at high doses, to suppress the growth of xenografts formed using human COLO205 colon cancer cells (Zhang et al. 2009).

Growth inhibition resulted from a combination of increased apoptosis and antiproliferative effects. Synergism between PF-00477736 and topotecan was subsequently observed in a panel of ovarian cancer cell lines (Kim et al. 2015). PF-00477736 also exhibited significant toxicity as a single agent in mouse lymphoma cells derived from a model where tumourigenesis is driven by overexpression of the c-Myc oncogene (Eµ-Myc) and p53 status can be controlled genetically (Ferrao et al. 2012). Treatment with PF-00477736 resulted in spontaneous DNA damage in Eµ-Myc lymphoma cells in vitro, leading ultimately to cell death by caspase-dependent apoptosis (Ferrao et al. 2012). Perhaps surprisingly, p53 wild-type Eµ-Myc lymphoma cells were more sensitive to PF00477736 than p53-null, in contrast to what has been observed in a variety of human cancer cell lines (Ferrao et al. 2012). Single agent toxicity with PF-00477736 has also been observed in triple-negative breast cancer and ovarian cancer cell lines (Bryant et al. 2014a), acute lymphoblastic leukaemia (ALL) (Derenzini et al. 2015; Iacobucci et al. 2015) and leukaemia cell lines (Bryant et al. 2014b), in each case associated with accumulation of spontaneous DNA damage and apoptosis. Finally, PF00477736 synergised with gemcitabine to kill human non-small cell lung cancer cells (NSCLC) cultured as spheroids in order to enrich for cancer stem cell-like cells (CSCs) (Fang et al. 2013).

As must be apparent from this brief overview, the preclinical characterisation of the four most selective and best-characterised CHK1 inhibitors has utilised many different cancer cell types in combination with many different genotoxic agents, dose and scheduling regimens. Despite this effort, clearly innumerable possible combinations still remain unexplored. Is it possible therefore to discern general principles of synergy and mechanisms of cell killing to guide future development of rational therapeutic strategies based on CHK1 inhibition?

Clearly this is a complex issue and there will likely be substantial mechanistic variations according to the exact biological context. Many different downstream markers have been studied in connection with CHK1 inhibition, either to obtain biochemical evidence of drug efficacy or insights into specific mechanisms of cell killing. In the former category stabilisation of Cdc25A, together with the resulting decrease in Y15 phosphorylation and increase in activity of Cdk1 and Cdk2, has been fairly widely documented together with increased phosphorylation of CHK1 at S345 or serine 296 [S296, a site of auto-phosphorylation (Rawlinson and Massey 2014)].

In the latter, formation of γ-H2AX foci as a surrogate marker for replication fork collapse or DSB formation (Rawlinson and Massey 2014) and measurements of apoptosis and premature entry to mitosis predominate. The picture remains incomplete; nevertheless, by interpreting the findings of these disparate preclinical studies in the light of knowledge of checkpoint mechanisms it is possible to propose that CHK1 inhibition can enhance exogenous or elicit de novo toxicity through at least four mechanisms; (1) by escalating exogenously-induced DNA damage, (2) by eliciting spontaneous DNA damage, (3) by inhibiting DNA repair, and (4) by promoting the division of lethally damaged or un-replicated genomes that are incapable of sustaining subsequent cell survival (Fig. 9.6).

For example, in cells exposed to topoisomerase poisons, suppression of the intra-S checkpoint escalates the formation of DSBs during S phase by releasing the brakes on DNA replication, whilst simultaneous override of the G2 checkpoint permits cells bearing damage to enter a lethal mitosis (Fig. 9.6). In cells treated with anti-metabolites, CHK1 inhibition causes stalled replication forks to collapse to generate DSBs during S phase, whilst uncontrolled origin firing amplifies this damage by increasing the number of replication forks that ultimately undergo collapse (Fig. 9.6). Replication fork collapse and deregulated origin firing is also likely a significant source of spontaneous DNA damage in cells ablated for CHK1 function alone. With concurrent S-M checkpoint suppression, cells bearing DNA damage arising from fork collapse ultimately enter mitosis with both damaged and partially-replicated genomes (Fig. 9.6). In the case of radiation, G2 checkpoint suppression primarily results in division with lethal levels of DNA damage. In each of these scenarios diminished proficiency for HRR due either to direct inhibition of CHK1 suppressing Rad51 recruitment or as a consequence of checkpoint override is likely to further enhance the accumulation of damage lesions. How cells that divide with damaged or un-replicated DNA ultimately die is not entirely clear, in some cases they may progress to apoptosis, but senescence, necrosis, or a combination of all three may also contribute.

9.5   Interactions with Other Molecularly Targeted Agents

Synergy with conventional genotoxic cancer therapies has been the principal focus of efforts to target CHK1 for cancer therapy, however interactions with several other categories of molecularly targeted agents have also been documented. Wee1 is a Cdk1 Y15 kinase that is the target of an experimental anti-cancer drug, MK-1775. As with CHK1, inhibition of Wee1 with MK-1775 can potentiate cell killing by radiation and genotoxic chemotherapies, often showing greater potency in cells with defects in p53 function (Hirai et al. 2009, 2010; Sarcar et al. 2011; Bridges et al.

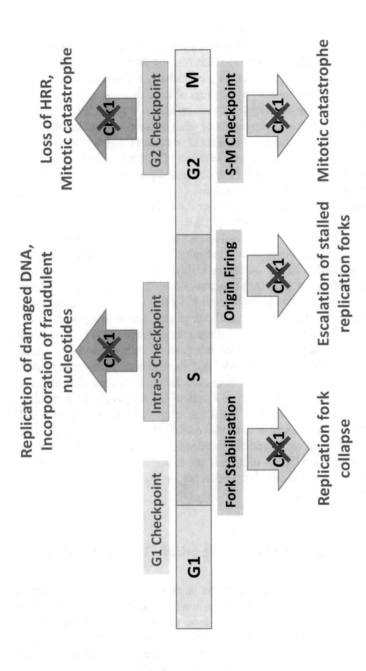

Fig. 9.6 Consequences of checkpoint suppression as a result of CHK1 inhibition. Cells exposed to DNA damaging agents or DNA synthesis inhibitors trigger different combinations of checkpoint responses that are controlled by CHK1 as depicted in Figs. 9.3 and 9.5. Checkpoint suppression as a result of CHK1 inhibition can enhance cell killing by multiple mechanisms according to cell cycle position and the nature of the genotoxic insult. Please refer to the text for additional information and explanation

2011). Interestingly however, simultaneous inhibition of CHK1 and Wee1 alone in the absence of any exogenous genotoxic stress can also be extremely toxic to cancer cells.

siRNA-mediated depletion of Wee1 was initially found to enhance the toxicity of two small molecule inhibitors of CHK1, AR458323 and PF-00477736, an effect that could be reproduced using multiple cancer cell lines and xenografts when the CHK1 inhibitors were combined with the Wee1 inhibitor MK-1775 (Davies et al. 2011a). Conversely, siRNA-mediated depletion of CHK1 was shown to enhance the toxicity of MK-1775 in acute myeloid leukaemia (AML) cell lines in vitro (Chaudhuri et al. 2014). This effect too could be reproduced by combining the CHK1 and Wee1 inhibitors, MK-8776 and MK-1775, in both AML cell lines and AML tumour cells derived from primary patient material (Chaudhuri et al. 2014). Interestingly, normal myeloid progenitors were less susceptible to combined Wee1/CHK1 inhibition, suggesting a degree of tumour specificity (Chaudhuri et al. 2014). Subsequently, combined inhibition of Wee1 and CHK1 has been shown to be synergistically toxic in neuroblastoma cell lines and xenografts (Russell et al. 2013), mantle cell lymphoma (Chila et al. 2015), nasopharyngeal carcinoma cell lines (Mak et al. 2015), and malignant melanoma cell lines and xenografts (Magnussen et al. 2015).

Cell death as a result of combined Wee1/CHK1 inhibition has been variously associated with increased levels of apoptosis, premature mitotic entry, mitotic catastrophe, spontaneous DNA damage, and inhibition of DNA synthesis (Chaudhuri et al. 2014; Russell et al. 2013; Chila et al. 2015; Mak et al. 2015; Magnussen et al. 2015). The proximal cause(s) of these effects is not completely understood, however deregulation of Cdk activity is likely to play an important role. Decreased inhibitory Y15 phosphorylation and increased Cdk1 and Cdk2 activity has been documented following combined inhibition of Wee1 and CHK1, and in some cases concurrent inhibition of Cdk activity by siRNA depletion or using pan-specific inhibitors such as roscovitine has been shown to diminish toxicity (Chaudhuri et al. 2014; Qi et al. 2014).

Premature activation of Cdk1 may plausibly explain mitotic abnormalities induced by combined Wee1/CHK1 inhibition, whilst increased Cdk2 activity could amplify DNA damage resulting from the replication fork collapse that occurs in CHK1 inhibited cells by promoting excessive origin firing and possibly activating nucleases such as Mre11 (Thompson et al. 2012). Deregulated origin firing combined with replication fork collapse and ssDNA cleavage may also explain a strong synergistic toxicity that has been documented when cells are treated with a combination of CHK1 and ATR inhibitors (Sanjiv et al. 2016).

Catalytic inhibitors of PARP1, such as olaparib (AZD2281), exhibit selective toxicity for cells deficient in HRR (Farmer et al. 2005). PARP1 is required for base excision repair and PARP1 inhibitors are thought to kill HRR-deficient cells through a "synthetic lethal" mechanism whereby simultaneous loss or inhibition of two major DNA repair mechanisms leads to spontaneous DNA damage and ultimately cell death (Lord et al. 2015). Evidence suggests that inhibition of CHK1 adversely affects HRR proficiency (Sorensen et al. 2005), and several studies have reported synergistic cell killing as a result of combined CHK1 and PARP1 inhibition both in the presence and absence of exogenous DNA damage. In pancreatic cancer cell lines combined inhibition of CHK1 and PARP1 resulted in radio-sensitisation that was associated with escalation of DNA damage due to a decrease in HRR proficiency (Vance et al. 2011). Sensitisation was greater in p53 mutant than p53 wild-type cell lines and was not observed in normal intestinal epithelial cells (Vance et al. 2011). Synergistic cell killing has also been documented in mammary carcinoma cells exposed to combinations of multiple PARP1 and CHK1 inhibitors, an effect that was associated with increased DNA damage (Tang et al. 2012). It is plausible that diminished HRR as a result of CHK1 inhibition sensitises cancer cells to PARP1 inhibitors, however whether this is the only mechanism involved remains unknown.

Several studies have shown that CHK1 inhibition sensitises cells to spindle poisons.

This was first shown using siRNA-mediated depletion of CHK1 in combination with docetaxel, an effect that was ascribed mechanistically to more rapid entry to mitosis after CHK1 downregulation leading to mitotic catastrophe and apoptosis (Zhang et al. 2009). Although these findings were quite unexpected at the time, it was later shown that CHK1 is required for optimal spindle checkpoint proficiency through modulation of Aurora B kinase (Zachos et al. 2007). Subsequent to this, PF-00477736 was independently shown to potentiate tumour cell killing by docetaxel in cells in culture and xenografts (Ren et al. 2005; Xiao et al. 2005; Carrassa et al. 2009). Spindle poisons do not activate CHK1 as judged by conventional criteria such as S345 phosphorylation (Zachos et al. 2007), although evidence suggests that CHK1 is active at some basal level during unperturbed mitosis and cytokinesis and affects multiple aspects of these processes (Smits and Gillespie 2015). Despite this, the exact mechanistic basis of sensitisation to spindle poisons upon CHK1 inhibition remains unclear.

Drug-induced depletion of CHK1 protein expression levels provides another means of compromising CHK1 function. CHK1 is known to be a client of HSP90 and several studies have demonstrated that HSP90 inhibitors, such as 17-N-Allylamino-17-demethoxygeldanamycin (17AAG; also known as geldanamycin), lead to decreased expression levels as a result of enhanced degradation. This effect was first demonstrated in the context of replication stress, where 17AAG-induced CHK1 depletion led to increased Cdc25A levels and potentiated cell death in response to gemcitabine treatment in diverse tumour cell lines (Arlander et al. 2003). Subsequently, 17AAG was shown to deplete CHK1 leading to checkpoint override and enhanced cell killing in acute myeloid leukaemia cells exposed to cytarabine (Mesa et al. 2005), and in FLT3(+) leukaemia cells treated with etoposide (Yao et al. 2007). Interestingly, Wee1 is also an HSP90 client (Aligue et al. 1994) and co-depletion of both CHK1 and Wee1 was shown to potentiate cell killing by irinotecan in colon cancer cells, an effect that showed selectivity for cells lacking p53 function (Tse et al. 2009).

CHK1 inhibitors (UCN-01, AZD7762, and CHIR-124) were found to synergise with HDAC inhibitors (vorinostat, romidempsin, entinostat) to induce cell killing in the absence of exogenous genotoxic stress that was associated with increased levels of DNA damage and chromosomal and mitotic abnormalities (Lee et al. 2011).

The HDAC inhibitor panobinostat was shown to markedly enhance the cytotoxicity of cytarabine and daunorubicin in acute myeloid leukaemia cells (Xie et al. 2013), an effect that was attributed to downregulation of CHK1 (but also BRCA1 and Rad51) expression at the level of gene transcription through attenuation of E2F transcriptional activity. CHK1 inhibition has also been shown to synergise with Src and MEK1/2 inhibitors to induce spontaneous cell killing and radio-sensitisation in mammary carcinoma cells and transformed murine fibroblasts (Mitchell et al. 2011). Interestingly, quiescent multiple myeloma cells were very sensitive to simultaneous inhibition of CHK1 and MEK1/2 using a combination of AZD7762 and selumetinib (AZD6244). Cell death was associated with increased DNA damage, as judged by γ-H2AX staining, and upregulation of the pro-apoptotic Bcl2-family protein, Bim (Pei et al. 2011). Combined inhibition of CHK1 and PDK1 has also been shown to enhance the toxicity of temozolomide in glioblastoma stem cell lines in culture and xenograft assays (Signore et al. 2014), whilst a combination of CHK1 inhibitor PF-004777 and gemcitabine was extremely effective in eliminating pancreatic xenografts in combination with radiolabelled anti-EGFR antibodies (Al-Ejeh et al. 2014). Finally, oncolytic adenoviruses encoding CHK1 siRNA have been shown to be markedly more potent in killing tumour cells in xenograft assays in combination with cisplatin than the corresponding parent vectors (Gao et al. 2006).

9.6 CHK1 Inhibition as Monotherapy

Although genetic deletion of CHK1 is generally incompatible with cell survival, indicative of a long-term requirement for function, short-term inhibition of CHK1 using either siRNA depletion or small molecule inhibitors has generally been found to be much less toxic. As a result it was not generally anticipated that CHK1 inhibitors could be deployed as a monotherapy. As already mentioned, during the past few years a number of studies have noted that CHK1 inhibition alone can result in significant anti-cancer activity in certain tumour cell lines (King et al. 2015; Bryant et al. 2014a, b; Iacobucci et al. 2015; Davies et al. 2011b; Sakurikar et al. 2016; Walton et al. 2016; Murga et al. 2011), spurring interest in identifying the factors that determine such single agent sensitivity.

One important candidate mechanism is DNA replication stress (Brooks et al. 2013). It is thought that many cancers suffer from high levels of replication stress that arise from the activation of growth-promoting oncogenes such as c-Myc (Hills and Diffley 2014). The exact molecular cause of oncogene-induced replication stress remain poorly defined, however it appears that nucleotide precursor depletion, either as a result of decreased ribonucleotide reductase activity and/or deregulated replication origin firing, is an important component (Hills and Diffley 2014).

Precursor depletion results in replication fork slowing or stalling and leads to activation of ATR-CHK1. Under these conditions CHK1 (and ATR) inhibition can result in replication fork collapse, accumulation of DNA damage, and premature entry to mitosis (Brooks et al. 2013). An attractive feature of this scenario is that the vulnerability to CHK1 inhibition created by replication stress is in principle tightly linked to the oncogenic driver mutations that are responsible for the abnormal proliferation of the tumour cells. Although this paradigm has been clearly demonstrated in experimental model systems (Puigvert et al. 2016), it remains uncertain how widespread the occurrence of analogous replication stress is in human tumours in vivo.

Other factors may also create sensitivity to CHK1 monotherapy. A recent systematic survey of a large number of tumour cell lines showed that a majority (85%) were able to grow normally for up to a week in the continued presence of the CHK1 inhibitor MK-8776, despite clear evidence that CHK1 function was effectively compromised throughout that time (Sakurikar et al. 2016). In marked contrast, the remaining 15% of cell lines were extremely sensitive to MK-8776, showing a combination of severe growth inhibition and increased cell death. Subsequent investigations established that sensitivity to MK-8776 correlated with high levels of spontaneous DSBs, whose formation depended in turn on increased activity of cyclin A/Cdk2, probably acting to stimulate Mre11 nuclease activity (Sakurikar et al. 2016). Activation of Cdk2 was traced to accumulation of Cdc25A under conditions of CHK1 inhibition, which occurred in sensitive but not in resistant lines (Sakurikar et al. 2016). Interestingly, MK-8776-resistant cells were sensitive to inhibition of Wee1, which resulted in de-phosphorylation and activation of Cdk2 even when Cdc25A expression did not increase. It appears therefore that in a subset of tumour cell lines CHK1 plays a crucial role in restraining dangerous over-activation of Cdk2 during unperturbed growth by limiting the levels of Cdc25A expression and activity (Sakurikar et al. 2016).

Again, although clearly established using tumour cell lines in vitro, whether this principle can be extended to human tumours in vivo remains uncertain at this point.

9.7   Clinical Trials

Drug development candidates typically suffer from a high rate of attrition during the transition from pre-clinical "proof-of-principle" evaluation to demonstration of safety and ultimately therapeutic benefit in patients owing either to unacceptable toxicity profiles and/or lack of efficacy. Multiple early stage trials of CHK1 inhibitors have been reported or are currently in progress, primarily in combination with genotoxic chemotherapies but also as a mono-therapy. Some positive results have been reported, however problems with toxicity have also featured prominently and development of several candidate CHK1 inhibitor drugs has been discontinued either at the pre-clinical or early clinical stage.

Initial Phase I Clinical trials with UCN-01 focused on combination with cisplatin and topotecan in advanced solid tumours in relatively small numbers of patients (Perez et al. 2006; Lara Jr. et al. 2005; Hotte et al. 2006; Sampath et al. 2006). Significant dose-limiting toxicities were observed in each of these studies, although these were in some cases mitigated by adjusting the dose of UCN-01 administered. Analysis of specific markers of CHK1 inhibition was either lacking or minimal in these initial studies and, although tolerable combination regimens were identified, little or no clear evidence for beneficial therapeutic responses was obtained (Perez et al. 2006; Lara Jr. et al. 2005; Hotte et al. 2006; Sampath et al. 2006). Subsequently a Phase II study of UCN-01 in combination with irinotecan in triple-negative breast cancer (TNBC) was reported (Ma et al. 2013). Interesting features of this trial include assessment of the p53 mutation status of individual tumours and in vivo analysis of specific markers of CHK1 inhibition and DNA damage. Combined treatment with UCN-01 and irinotecan conferred measureable clinical benefit on a minority of patients (12%), with no evidence that there was a better response to UCN-01 in patients bearing tumours with mutant p53 (Ma et al. 2013). Evidence for increased DNA damage and inhibition of CHK1 as a result of UCN-01 exposure was obtained from biomarker analysis, however this was seen only in a subset of tumours (Ma et al. 2013). Although UCN-01 is an effective CHK1 inhibitor it also targets many other important protein kinases. It is therefore unclear whether either the toxicities or limited therapeutic benefits observed in these trials were really due to inhibition of CHK1 or some other kinase target. In addition, UCN-01 exhibits adverse pharmacodynamics characteristics in humans (Fuse et al. 2005). As a result, UCN-01 is not currently undergoing further development as a CHK1 inhibitor drug.

Significantly more encouraging results have been obtained with more selective second generation CHK1 inhibitors. In a Phase I trial of MK-8776 in combination with cytosine arabinoside in relapsed and refractory acute leukaemia complete remission was observed in 33% of patients, most of whom were in the group that received the highest dose of MK-8776, with minimal adverse side-effects (Karp et al. 2012). The activity of MK-8776 has also been examined in diverse advanced, pre-treated solid tumours both as a mono-therapy and in combination with gemcitabine (Daud et al. 2015). MK-8776 was well-tolerated as a mono-therapy although more toxicity was observed with gemcitabine, with 50% of patients overall exhibiting evidence of clinical benefit as evidenced by partial responses or stable disease (Daud et al. 2015).

The selective CHK1 inhibitor AZD7762 has also been evaluated alone and in combination with gemcitabine in advanced solid tumours (Seto et al. 2013; Sausville et al. 2014). Modest responses characterised by partial responses or stable disease were observed specifically in lung cancer patients, however AZD7762 treatment also resulted in unpredictable cardiotoxicity problems which have led to discontinuation of its clinical development (Seto et al. 2013; Sausville et al. 2014).

LY2603618 is a selective CHK1 inhibitor that has been evaluated in combination with pemetrexed and cisplatin in patients with advanced cancer (Calvo et al. 2014). This regimen demonstrated an acceptable safety profile and 10 out of 14 patients exhibited some evidence of clinical benefit as evidenced by partial responses or stable disease (Calvo et al. 2014). A subsequent Phase I study of LY2603618 in combination with gemcitabine in a group of 50 patients with diverse solid tumours noted a partial response in one of three NSCLC whilst 22 patients achieved stable disease (Calvo et al. 2016). In a Phase I study of Japanese patients with solid tumors partial responses to a combination of gemcitabine and LY2603618 were observed in

24% of cases and in each case these were associated with decreases in circulating tumour DNA (Doi et al. 2015). In comparison, a Phase II study of LY2603618 in combination with pemetrexed in advanced or metastatic NSCLC led to partial response in 9% of patients with stable disease in 36%, however the combination was not judged to be superior to pemetrexed alone based on comparison with historical data (Scagliotti et al. 2016). Interestingly, in this study p53 mutation status was evaluated by both immunocytochemistry and exome sequencing, however it was not found to correlate with response (Scagliotti et al. 2016). Neither was clear clinical benefit observed in a Phase II study of LY2603618 in combination with gemcitabine in pancreatic cancer (Laquente et al. 2017). Finally, a very recent Phase II study of LY2603618 in combination with pemetrexed and cisplatin in NSCLC detected a clear increase in progression-free survival but concluded that a marked increase in the incidence of adverse thromboembolic events precluded further development of this combination (Wehler et al. 2017).

In addition to these published studies, a number of clinical trials involving CHK1 inhibitor drugs are currently active or recruiting patients (O'Connor 2015). These include several involving the selective dual CHK1/CHK2 inhibitor, LY2606368; Phase I trials as mono-therapy in advanced squamous (ClinicalTrials.gov; NCT01115790) and solid (NCT02514603) tumours, and a Phase II trial as mono-therapy in BRCA1/BRCA2-mutant breast and ovarian cancer, TNBC, and advanced serous ovarian cancer (NCT022203513). A Phase II trial of MK-8876 in combination with cytosine arabinoside in AML is also currently active (NCT01870596), although further development of this compound may be discontinued for business reasons (Sakurikar and Eastman 2015). Finally, a new CHK1 inhibitor, GDC-0575, whose specificity has not yet been reported, has been trialled in combination with gemcitabine in solid tumours (Infante et al. 2017), and is currently under investigation as a mono therapy in leukaemias (NCT01564251). The outcome of these latter studies is awaited with interest.

9.8 Issues and Future Prospects

Despite considerable progress since it was first postulated that CHK1 might represent a rational anti-cancer drug target a number of fundamental issues still remain poorly explored. Firstly, does a therapeutic index exist for CHK1 inhibitor drugs in combination with genotoxic therapies; that is, are tumour cells more readily killed than normal? Anecdotal findings from a small number of pre-clinical studies using matched transformed and non-transformed cells suggest that this could be true, at least in some cases. However, even if this is the case, we still have little concrete insight into the basis of this distinction.

Because CHK1 expression is thought to be restricted to proliferating cells inhibitors seem unlikely to impact terminally-differentiated cells and tissues. The side-effects of conventional genotoxic therapies however are most acute in dose-limiting proliferative tissues such as bone marrow and digestive tract. An important question therefore is—do tumour-specific alterations create an exploitable distinction between tumour cells and normal proliferating cells in terms of CHK1 inhibition in these tissues? Deficiency for p53 has been widely postulated to confer vulnerability to CHK1 inhibition by increasing dependence on the S and G2 checkpoints after damage. Because p53 function is lost or impaired in more than 50% of human cancers, this could potentially create a generic therapeutic index for CHK1 inhibition. As already discussed, many pre-clinical studies have indeed observed greater toxicity as a result of CHK1 inhibition in p53-deficient backgrounds, however others have not for reasons that remain unclear (Yu et al. 2002a; Tse and Schwartz 2004; Hirose et al. 2001). Admittedly, p53 function is notoriously complex and pleiotropic, controlling both cell cycle arrest and apoptosis in response to DNA damage, and it may be that the functional interactions between p53 and CHK1 that influence cell survival are cell type-dependent. Further study into this issue and other possible determinants of sensitivity to combination therapy are warranted.

Secondly, why is CHK1 inhibition inherently toxic to some cancer cells in the absence of exogenous damage? It seems clear now that this is the case, at least in cells in culture (Sakurikar et al. 2016), however again the reasons remain incompletely understood. Replication stress in cancer cells is one potential cause of increased dependence on CHK1 function, however the exact cause and prevalence of this phenomenon outside of experimental model systems remains unclear (Puigvert et al. 2016). Tumour cell-specific variations in the relative importance of CHK1 in restraining over-activation of Cdk2 via regulation of Cdc25A represent another potential mechanism (Sakurikar et al. 2016), however again we lack a full molecular explanation for this phenomenon. The issue of therapeutic index in the context of mono-therapy also needs to be assessed.

It will be important to understand the molecular basis for variations in tumour cell sensitivity to CHK1 inhibitors, either in combination or mono-therapy contexts, since this could lead to the identification of biomarkers that would allow patient stratification and targeting in clinical trials. It is interesting that the initial development of PARP1 inhibitors was guided by the combination therapy paradigm, yet their greatest potency has been achieved as a mono-therapy in tumours which are specifically deficient for HRR. It seems possible that the development of CHK1 inhibitor drugs could follow an analogous path.

Finally, a word of caution; studies in genetically modified mice have shown that tissue-specific homozygous deletion of CHK1 in the skin and intestine blocked the formation of tumours in these tissues. Both of these studies however also found that deletion of one allele of CHK1 accelerated tumour progression (Tho et al. 2012; Greenow et al. 2014), presumably because CHK1 haplo-insufficiency promotes genetic instability and thus more rapid accumulation of oncogenic mutations. It is generally believed that tissues in adult humans contain many "initiated" cells that bear oncogenic mutations but do not progress owing to the action of multiple tumour-suppressor mechanisms (Martincorena et al. 2015). It will be important therefore to rule out the possibility that CHK1 inhibitor drugs might promote the outgrowth of such initiated cells to form therapy-related cancers by promoting genetic instability, an issue that so far has received little attention.

Acknowledgements D.A.G. acknowledges the IMBRAIN Project (FP7-REGPOT-2012-CT2012-31637-IMBRAIN: EU FP7 and Gobierno de Canarias) and World Wide Cancer Research Project Grant 12-0149 for financial support.

Conflict of Interest There are no conflicts of interest.

References

Akinaga S, Nomura K, Gomi K, Okabe M (1993) Enhancement of antitumor activity of mitomycin C in vitro and in vivo by UCN-01, a selective inhibitor of protein kinase C. Cancer Chemother Pharmacol 32:183–189

Al-Ahmadie H, Iyer G, Hohl M, Asthana S, Inagaki A, Schultz N, Hanrahan AJ, Scott SN, Brannon AR, McDermott GC, Pirun M, Ostrovnaya I, Kim P, Socci ND, Viale A, Schwartz GK, Reuter V, Bochner BH, Rosenberg JE, Bajorin DF, Berger MF, Petrini JH, Solit DB, Taylor BS (2014) Synthetic lethality in ATM-deficient RAD50-mutant tumors underlies outlier response to cancer therapy. Cancer Discov 4:1014–1021

Al-Ejeh F, Pajic M, Shi W, Kalimutho M, Miranda M, Nagrial AM, Chou A, Biankin AV, Grimmond SM, Brown MP, Khanna KK, Australian Pancreatic Cancer Genome Initiative (2014) Gemcitabine and CHK1 inhibition potentiate EGFR-directed radioimmunotherapy against pancreatic ductal adenocarcinoma. Clin Cancer Res 20:3187–3197

Aligue R, Akhavan-Niak H, Russell P (1994) A role for Hsp90 in cell cycle control: Wee1 tyrosine kinase activity requires interaction with Hsp90. EMBO J 13:6099–6106

Al-Kaabi MM, Alshareeda AT, Jerjees DA, Muftah AA, Green AR, Alsubhi NH, Nolan CC, Chan S, Cornford E, Madhusudan S, Ellis IO, Rakha EA (2015) Checkpoint kinase1 (CHK1) is an important biomarker in breast cancer having a role in chemotherapy response. Br J Cancer 112:901–911

Allen C, Ashley AK, Hromas R, Nickoloff JA (2011) More forks on the road to replication stress recovery. J Mol Cell Biol 3:4–12

Alsubhi N, Middleton F, Abdel-Fatah TM, Stephens P, Doherty R, Arora A, Moseley PM, Chan SY, Aleskandarany MA, Green AR, Rakha EA, Ellis IO, Martin SG, Curtin NJ, Madhusudan S (2016) Chk1 phosphorylated at serine(345) is a predictor of early local recurrence and radioresistance in breast cancer. Mol Oncol 10:213–223

Arlander SJ, Eapen AK, Vroman BT, McDonald RJ, Toft DO, Karnitz LM (2003) Hsp90 inhibition depletes Chk1 and sensitizes tumor cells to replication stress. J Biol Chem 278:52572–52577

Arora S, Bisanz KM, Peralta LA, Basu GD, Choudhary A, Tibes R, Azorsa DO (2010) RNAi screening of the kinome identifies modulators of cisplatin response in ovarian cancer cells. Gynecol Oncol 118:220–227

Azorsa DO, Gonzales IM, Basu GD, Choudhary A, Arora S, Bisanz KM, Kiefer JA, Henderson MC, Trent JM, Von Hoff DD, Mousses S (2009) Synthetic lethal RNAi screening identifies sensitizing targets for gemcitabine therapy in pancreatic cancer. J Transl Med 7:43

Barnard D, Diaz HB, Burke T, Donoho G, Beckmann R, Jones B, Barda D, King C, Marshall M (2016) LY2603618, a selective CHK1 inhibitor, enhances the anti-tumor effect of gemcitabine in xenograft tumor models. Invest New Drugs 34:49–60

Bartek J, Lukas J (2003) Chk1 and Chk2 kinases in checkpoint control and cancer. Cancer Cell 3:421–429

Bartucci M, Svensson S, Romania P, Dattilo R, Patrizii M, Signore M, Navarra S, Lotti F, Biffoni M, Pilozzi E, Duranti E, Martinelli S, Rinaldo C, Zeuner A, Maugeri-Sacca M, Eramo A, De Maria R (2012) Therapeutic targeting of Chk1 in NSCLC stem cells during chemotherapy. Cell Death Differ 19:768–778

Bertoni F, Codegoni AM, Furlan D, Tibiletti MG, Capella C, Broggini M (1999) CHK1 frameshift mutations in genetically unstable colorectal and endometrial cancers. Genes Chromosomes Cancer 26:176–180

Blackwood E, Epler J, Yen I, Flagella M, O'Brien T, Evangelista M, Schmidt S, Xiao Y, Choi J, Kowanetz K, Ramiscal J, Wong K, Jakubiak D, Yee S, Cain G, Gazzard L, Williams K, Halladay J, Jackson PK, Malek S (2013) Combination drug scheduling defines a "window of opportunity" for chemopotentiation of gemcitabine by an orally bioavailable, selective ChK1 inhibitor, GNE-900. Mol Cancer Ther 12:1968–1980

Blasina A, Hallin J, Chen E, Arango ME, Kraynov E, Register J, Grant S, Ninkovic S, Chen P, Nichols T, O'Connor P, Anderes K (2008) Breaching the DNA damage checkpoint via PF-00477736, a novel small-molecule inhibitor of checkpoint kinase 1. Mol Cancer Ther 7:2394–2404

Bridges KA, Hirai H, Buser CA, Brooks C, Liu H, Buchholz TA, Molkentine JM, Mason KA, Meyn RE (2011) MK-1775, a novel Wee1 kinase inhibitor, radiosensitizes p53-defective human tumor cells. Clin Cancer Res 17:5638–5648

Brooks K, Oakes V, Edwards B, Ranall M, Leo P, Pavey S, Pinder A, Beamish H, Mukhopadhyay P, Lambie D, Gabrielli B (2013) A potent Chk1 inhibitor is selectively cytotoxic in melanomas with high levels of replicative stress. Oncogene 32:788–796

Bryant C, Rawlinson R, Massey AJ (2014a) Chk1 inhibition as a novel therapeutic strategy for treating triple-negative breast and ovarian cancers. BMC Cancer 14:570

Bryant C, Scriven K, Massey AJ (2014b) Inhibition of the checkpoint kinase Chk1 induces DNA damage and cell death in human leukemia and lymphoma cells. Mol Cancer 13:147

Calvo E, Chen VJ, Marshall M, Ohnmacht U, Hynes SM, Kumm E, Diaz HB, Barnard D, Merzoug FF, Huber L, Kays L, Iversen P, Calles A, Voss B, Lin AB, Dickgreber N, Wehler T, Sebastian M (2014) Preclinical analyses and phase I evaluation of LY2603618 administered in combination with pemetrexed and cisplatin in patients with advanced cancer. Invest New Drugs 32:955–968

Calvo E, Braiteh F, Von Hoff D, McWilliams R, Becerra C, Galsky MD, Jameson G, Lin J, McKane S, Wickremsinhe ER, Hynes SM, Bence Lin A, Hurt K, Richards D (2016) Phase I study of CHK1 inhibitor LY2603618 in combination with gemcitabine in patients with solid tumors. Oncology 91:251–260

Carrassa L, Broggini M, Vikhanskaya F, Damia G (2003) Characterization of the 5' flanking region of the human Chk1 gene: identification of E2F1 functional sites. Cell Cycle 2:604–609

Carrassa L, Sanchez Y, Erba E, Damia G (2009) U2OS cells lacking Chk1 undergo aberrant mitosis and fail to activate the spindle checkpoint. J Cell Mol Med 13:1565–1576

Chaudhuri L, Vincelette ND, Koh BD, Naylor RM, Flatten KS, Peterson KL, McNally A, Gojo I, Karp JE, Mesa RA, Sproat LO, Bogenberger JM, Kaufmann SH, Tibes R (2014) CHK1 and WEE1 inhibition combine synergistically to enhance therapeutic efficacy in acute myeloid leukemia ex vivo. Haematologica 99:688–696

Chen MS, Ryan CE, Piwnica-Worms H (2003) Chk1 kinase negatively regulates mitotic function of Cdc25A phosphatase through 14-3-3 binding. Mol Cell Biol 23:7488–7497

Chila R, Basana A, Lupi M, Guffanti F, Gaudio E, Rinaldi A, Cascione L, Restelli V, Tarantelli C, Bertoni F, Damia G, Carrassa L (2015) Combined inhibition of Chk1 and Wee1 as a new therapeutic strategy for mantle cell lymphoma. Oncotarget 6:3394–3408

Curman D, Cinel B, Williams DE, Rundle N, Block WD, Goodarzi AA, Hutchins JR, Clarke PR, Zhou BB, Lees-Miller SP, Andersen RJ, Roberge M (2001) Inhibition of the G2 DNA damage checkpoint and of protein kinases Chk1 and Chk2 by the marine sponge alkaloid debromohymenialdisine. J Biol Chem 276:17914–17919

Curtin NJ (2005) PARP inhibitors for cancer therapy. Expert Rev Mol Med 7:1–20

Dai Y, Rahmani M, Pei XY, Khanna P, Han SI, Mitchell C, Dent P, Grant S (2005) Farnesyltransferase inhibitors interact synergistically with the Chk1 inhibitor UCN-01 to induce apoptosis in human leukemia cells through interruption of both Akt and MEK/ERK pathways and activation of SEK1/JNK. Blood 105:1706–1716

Daud AI, Ashworth MT, Strosberg J, Goldman JW, Mendelson D, Springett G, Venook AP, Loechner S, Rosen LS, Shanahan F, Parry D, Shumway S, Grabowsky JA, Freshwater T, Sorge C, Kang SP, Isaacs R, Munster PN (2015) Phase I dose-escalation trial of checkpoint kinase 1 inhibitor MK-8776 as monotherapy and in combination with gemcitabine in patients with advanced solid tumors. J Clin Oncol Off J Am Soc Clin Oncol 33:1060–1066

Davies KD, Cable PL, Garrus JE, Sullivan FX, von Carlowitz I, Huerou YL, Wallace E, Woessner RD, Gross S (2011a) Chk1 inhibition and Wee1 inhibition combine synergistically to impede cellular proliferation. Cancer Biol Ther 12:788–796

Davies KD, Humphries MJ, Sullivan FX, von Carlowitz I, Le Huerou Y, Mohr PJ, Wang B, Blake JF, Lyon MA, Gunawardana I, Chicarelli M, Wallace E, Gross S (2011b) Single-agent inhibition of Chk1 is antiproliferative in human cancer cell lines in vitro and inhibits tumor xenograft growth in vivo. Oncol Res 19:349–363

Derenzini E, Agostinelli C, Imbrogno E, Iacobucci I, Casadei B, Brighenti E, Righi S, Fuligni F, Ghelli Luserna Di Rora A, Ferrari A, Martinelli G, Pileri S, Zinzani PL (2015) Constitutive activation of the DNA damage response pathway as a novel therapeutic target in diffuse large B-cell lymphoma. Oncotarget 6:6553–6569

Didier C, Demur C, Grimal F, Jullien D, Manenti S, Ducommun B (2012) Evaluation of checkpoint kinase targeting therapy in acute myeloid leukemia with complex karyotype. Cancer Biol Ther 13:307–313

Doi T, Yoshino T, Shitara K, Matsubara N, Fuse N, Naito Y, Uenaka K, Nakamura T, Hynes SM, Lin AB (2015) Phase I study of LY2603618, a CHK1 inhibitor, in combination with gemcitabine in Japanese patients with solid tumors. Anticancer Drugs 26:1043–1053

Eastman A, Kohn EA, Brown MK, Rathman J, Livingstone M, Blank DH, Gribble GW (2002) A novel indolocarbazole, ICP-1, abrogates DNA damage-induced cell cycle arrest and enhances cytotoxicity: similarities and differences to the cell cycle checkpoint abrogator UCN-01. Mol Cancer Ther 1:1067–1078

Engelke CG, Parsels LA, Qian Y, Zhang Q, Karnak D, Robertson JR, Tanska DM, Wei D, Davis MA, Parsels JD, Zhao L, Greenson JK, Lawrence TS, Maybaum J, Morgan MA (2013) Sensitization of pancreatic cancer to chemoradiation by the Chk1 inhibitor MK8776. Clin Cancer Res 19:4412–4421

Fang DD, Cao J, Jani JP, Tsaparikos K, Blasina A, Kornmann J, Lira ME, Wang J, Jirout Z, Bingham J, Zhu Z, Gu Y, Los G, Hostomsky Z, Vanarsdale T (2013) Combined gemcitabine and CHK1 inhibitor treatment induces apoptosis resistance in cancer stem cell-like cells enriched with tumor spheroids from a non-small cell lung cancer cell line. Front Med 7:462–476

Farmer H, McCabe N, Lord CJ, Tutt AN, Johnson DA, Richardson TB, Santarosa M, Dillon KJ, Hickson I, Knights C, Martin NM, Jackson SP, Smith GC, Ashworth A (2005) Targeting the DNA repair defect in BRCA mutant cells as a therapeutic strategy. Nature 434:917–921

Ferrao PT, Bukczynska EP, Johnstone RW, McArthur GA (2012) Efficacy of CHK inhibitors as single agents in MYC-driven lymphoma cells. Oncogene 31:1661–1672

Forment JV, Blasius M, Guerini I, Jackson SP (2011) Structure-specific DNA endonuclease Mus81/Eme1 generates DNA damage caused by Chk1 inactivation. PLoS One 6:e23517

Fuse E, Kuwabara T, Sparreboom A, Sausville EA, Figg WD (2005) Review of UCN-01 development: a lesson in the importance of clinical pharmacology. J Clin Pharmacol 45:394–403

Gao Q, Zhou J, Huang X, Chen G, Ye F, Lu Y, Li K, Zhuang L, Huang M, Xu G, Wang S, Ma D (2006) Selective targeting of checkpoint kinase 1 in tumor cells with a novel potent oncolytic adenovirus. Mol Ther 13:928–937

Garrett MD, Collins I (2011) Anticancer therapy with checkpoint inhibitors: what, where and when? Trends Pharmacol Sci 32:308–316

Goto H, Kasahara K, Inagaki M (2015) Novel insights into Chk1 regulation by phosphorylation. Cell Struct Funct 40:43–50

Graves PR, Yu L, Schwarz JK, Gales J, Sausville EA, O'Connor PM, Piwnica-Worms H (2000) The Chk1 protein kinase and the Cdc25C regulatory pathways are targets of the anticancer agent UCN-01. J Biol Chem 275:5600–5605

Greenow KR, Clarke AR, Williams GT, Jones R (2014) Wnt-driven intestinal tumourigenesis is suppressed by Chk1 deficiency but enhanced by conditional haploinsufficiency. Oncogene 33:4089–4096

Guzi TJ, Paruch K, Dwyer MP, Labroli M, Shanahan F, Davis N, Taricani L, Wiswell D, Seghezzi W, Penaflor E, Bhagwat B, Wang W, Gu D, Hsieh Y, Lee S, Liu M, Parry D (2011) Targeting the replication checkpoint using SCH 900776, a potent and functionally selective CHK1 inhibitor identified via high content screening. Mol Cancer Ther 10:591–602

Hahn M, Li W, Yu C, Rahmani M, Dent P, Grant S (2005) Rapamycin and UCN-01 synergistically induce apoptosis in human leukemia cells through a process that is regulated by the Raf-1/MEK/ERK, Akt, and JNK signal transduction pathways. Mol Cancer Ther 4:457–470

Harper JW, Elledge SJ (2007) The DNA damage response: ten years after. Mol Cell 28:739–745

Hills SA, Diffley JF (2014) DNA replication and oncogene-induced replicative stress. Curr Biol 24:R435–R444

Hirai H, Iwasawa Y, Okada M, Arai T, Nishibata T, Kobayashi M, Kimura T, Kaneko N, Ohtani J, Yamanaka K, Itadani H, Takahashi-Suzuki I, Fukasawa K, Oki H, Nambu T, Jiang J, Sakai T, Arakawa H, Sakamoto T, Sagara T, Yoshizumi T, Mizuarai S, Kotani H (2009) Small-molecule inhibition of Wee1 kinase by MK-1775 selectively sensitizes p53-deficient tumor cells to DNA-damaging agents. Mol Cancer Ther 8:2992–3000

Hirai H, Arai T, Okada M, Nishibata T, Kobayashi M, Sakai N, Imagaki K, Ohtani J, Sakai T, Yoshizumi T, Mizuarai S, Iwasawa Y, Kotani H (2010) MK-1775, a small molecule Wee1 inhibitor, enhances anti-tumor efficacy of various DNA-damaging agents, including 5-fluorouracil. Cancer Biol Ther 9:514–522

Hirose Y, Berger MS, Pieper RO (2001) Abrogation of the Chk1-mediated G(2) checkpoint pathway potentiates temozolomide-induced toxicity in a p53-independent manner in human glioblastoma cells. Cancer Res 61:5843–5849

Hoeijmakers JH (2009) DNA damage, aging, and cancer. N Engl J Med 361:1475–1485

Hotte SJ, Oza A, Winquist EW, Moore M, Chen EX, Brown S, Pond GR, Dancey JE, Hirte HW (2006) Phase I trial of UCN-01 in combination with topotecan in patients with advanced solid cancers: a Princess Margaret Hospital Phase II Consortium study. Ann Oncol 17:334–340

Iacobucci I, Di Rora AG, Falzacappa MV, Agostinelli C, Derenzini E, Ferrari A, Papayannidis C, Lonetti A, Righi S, Imbrogno E, Pomella S, Venturi C, Guadagnuolo V, Cattina F, Ottaviani E, Abbenante MC, Vitale A, Elia L, Russo D, Zinzani PL, Pileri S, Pelicci PG, Martinelli G (2015) In vitro and in vivo single-agent efficacy of checkpoint kinase inhibition in acute lymphoblastic leukemia. J Hematol Oncol 8:125

Infante JR, Hollebecque A, Postel-Vinay S, Bauer TM, Blackwood EM, Evangelista M, Mahrus S, Peale FV, Lu X, Sahasranaman S, Zhu R, Chen Y, Ding X, Murray ER, Schutzman JL, Lauchle JO, Soria JC, LoRusso PM (2017) Phase I study of GDC-0425, a checkpoint kinase 1 inhibitor, in combination with gemcitabine in patients with refractory solid tumors. Clin Cancer Res 23:2423–2432

Itamochi H, Nishimura M, Oumi N, Kato M, Oishi T, Shimada M, Sato S, Naniwa J, Sato S, Kudoh A, Kigawa J, Harada T (2014) Checkpoint kinase inhibitor AZD7762 overcomes cisplatin resistance in clear cell carcinoma of the ovary. Int J Gynecol Cancer 24:61–69

Jia W, Yu C, Rahmani M, Krystal G, Sausville EA, Dent P, Grant S (2003) Synergistic antileukemic interactions between 17-AAG and UCN-01 involve interruption of RAF/MEK- and AKT-related pathways. Blood 102:1824–1832

Jiang X, Zhao B, Britton R, Lim LY, Leong D, Sanghera JS, Zhou BB, Piers E, Andersen RJ, Roberge M (2004) Inhibition of Chk1 by the G2 DNA damage checkpoint inhibitor isogranulatimide. Mol Cancer Ther 3:1221–1227

Kaneko YS, Watanabe N, Morisaki H, Akita H, Fujimoto A, Tominaga K, Terasawa M, Tachibana A, Ikeda K, Nakanishi M (1999) Cell-cycle-dependent and ATM-independent expression of human Chk1 kinase. Oncogene 18:3673–3681

Karp JE, Thomas BM, Greer JM, Sorge C, Gore SD, Pratz KW, Smith BD, Flatten KS, Peterson K, Schneider P, Mackey K, Freshwater T, Levis MJ, McDevitt MA, Carraway HE, Gladstone DE, Showel MM, Loechner S, Parry DA, Horowitz JA, Isaacs R, Kaufmann SH (2012) Phase I and pharmacologic trial of cytosine arabinoside with the selective checkpoint 1 inhibitor Sch 900776 in refractory acute leukemias. Clin Cancer Res 18:6723–6731

Kim MK, James J, Annunziata CM (2015) Topotecan synergizes with CHEK1 (CHK1) inhibitor to induce apoptosis in ovarian cancer cells. BMC Cancer 15:196

King C, Diaz H, Barnard D, Barda D, Clawson D, Blosser W, Cox K, Guo S, Marshall M (2014) Characterization and preclinical development of LY2603618: a selective and potent Chk1 inhibitor. Invest New Drugs 32:213–226

King C, Diaz HB, McNeely S, Barnard D, Dempsey J, Blosser W, Beckmann R, Barda D, Marshall MS (2015) LY2606368 causes replication catastrophe and antitumor effects through CHK1-dependent mechanisms. Mol Cancer Ther 14:2004–2013

Kohn EA, Yoo CJ, Eastman A (2003) The protein kinase C inhibitor Go6976 is a potent inhibitor of DNA damage-induced S and G2 cell cycle checkpoints. Cancer Res 63:31–35

Laquente B, Lopez-Martin J, Richards D, Illerhaus G, Chang DZ, Kim G, Stella P, Richel D, Szcylik C, Cascinu S, Frassineti GL, Ciuleanu T, Hurt K, Hynes S, Lin J, Lin AB, Von Hoff D, Calvo E (2017) A phase II study to evaluate LY2603618 in combination with gemcitabine in pancreatic cancer patients. BMC Cancer 17:137

Lara PN Jr, Mack PC, Synold T, Frankel P, Longmate J, Gumerlock PH, Doroshow JH, Gandara DR (2005) The cyclin-dependent kinase inhibitor UCN-01 plus cisplatin in advanced solid tumors: a California cancer consortium phase I pharmacokinetic and molecular correlative trial. Clin Cancer Res 11:4444–4450

Lau CC, Pardee AB (1982) Mechanism by which caffeine potentiates lethality of nitrogen mustard. Proc Natl Acad Sci U S A 79:2942–2946

Lee J, Kumagai A, Dunphy WG (2001) Positive regulation of Wee1 by Chk1 and 14-3-3 proteins. Mol Biol Cell 12:551–563

Lee JH, Choy ML, Ngo L, Venta-Perez G, Marks PA (2011) Role of checkpoint kinase 1 (Chk1) in the mechanisms of resistance to histone deacetylase inhibitors. Proc Natl Acad Sci U S A 108:19629–19634

Lindqvist A, Rodriguez-Bravo V, Medema RH (2009) The decision to enter mitosis: feedback and redundancy in the mitotic entry network. J Cell Biol 185:193–202

Liu Q, Guntuku S, Cui XS, Matsuoka S, Cortez D, Tamai K, Luo G, Carattini-Rivera S, DeMayo F, Bradley A, Donehower LA, Elledge SJ (2000) Chk1 is an essential kinase that is regulated by Atr and required for the G(2)/M DNA damage checkpoint. Genes Dev 14:1448–1459

Lord CJ, Tutt AN, Ashworth A (2015) Synthetic lethality and cancer therapy: lessons learned from the development of PARP inhibitors. Annu Rev Med 66:455–470

Ma CX, Ellis MJ, Petroni GR, Guo Z, Cai SR, Ryan CE, Craig Lockhart A, Naughton MJ, Pluard TJ, Brenin CM, Picus J, Creekmore AN, Mwandoro T, Yarde ER, Reed J, Ebbert M, Bernard PS, Watson M, Doyle LA, Dancey J, Piwnica-Worms H, Fracasso PM (2013) A phase II study of UCN-01 in combination with irinotecan in patients with metastatic triple negative breast cancer. Breast Cancer Res Treat 137:483–492

MacDougall CA, Byun TS, Van C, Yee MC, Cimprich KA (2007) The structural determinants of checkpoint activation. Genes Dev 21:898–903

Magnussen GI, Emilsen E, Giller Fleten K, Engesaeter B, Nahse-Kumpf V, Fjaer R, Slipicevic A, Florenes VA (2015) Combined inhibition of the cell cycle related proteins Wee1 and Chk1/2 induces synergistic anti-cancer effect in melanoma. BMC Cancer 15:462

Mailand N, Falck J, Lukas C, Syljuasen RG, Welcker M, Bartek J, Lukas J (2000) Rapid destruction of human Cdc25A in response to DNA damage. Science 288:1425–1429

Mak JP, Man WY, Chow JP, Ma HT, Poon RY (2015) Pharmacological inactivation of CHK1 and WEE1 induces mitotic catastrophe in nasopharyngeal carcinoma cells. Oncotarget 6:21074–21084

Martincorena I, Roshan A, Gerstung M, Ellis P, Van Loo P, McLaren S, Wedge DC, Fullam A, Alexandrov LB, Tubio JM, Stebbings L, Menzies A, Widaa S, Stratton MR, Jones PH, Campbell PJ (2015) Tumor evolution. High burden and pervasive positive selection of somatic mutations in normal human skin. Science 348:880–886

Matthews DJ, Yakes FM, Chen J, Tadano M, Bornheim L, Clary DO, Tai A, Wagner JM, Miller N, Kim YD, Robertson S, Murray L, Karnitz LM (2007) Pharmacological abrogation of S-phase checkpoint enhances the anti-tumor activity of gemcitabine in vivo. Cell Cycle 6:104–110

McNeely S, Beckmann R, Bence Lin AK (2014) CHEK again: revisiting the development of CHK1 inhibitors for cancer therapy. Pharmacol Ther 142:1–10

Mesa RA, Loegering D, Powell HL, Flatten K, Arlander SJ, Dai NT, Heldebrant MP, Vroman BT, Smith BD, Karp JE, Eyck CJ, Erlichman C, Kaufmann SH, Karnitz LM (2005) Heat shock protein 90 inhibition sensitizes acute myelogenous leukemia cells to cytarabine. Blood 106:318–327

Meuth M (2010) Chk1 suppressed cell death. Cell Div 5:21

Mitchell JB, Choudhuri R, Fabre K, Sowers AL, Citrin D, Zabludoff SD, Cook JA (2010) In vitro and in vivo radiation sensitization of human tumor cells by a novel checkpoint kinase inhibitor, AZD7762. Clin Cancer Res 16:2076–2084

Mitchell C, Hamed HA, Cruickshanks N, Tang Y, Bareford MD, Hubbard N, Tye G, Yacoub A, Dai Y, Grant S, Dent P (2011) Simultaneous exposure of transformed cells to SRC family inhibitors and CHK1 inhibitors causes cell death. Cancer Biol Ther 12:215–228

Montano R, Chung I, Garner KM, Parry D, Eastman A (2012) Preclinical development of the novel Chk1 inhibitor SCH900776 in combination with DNA-damaging agents and antimetabolites. Mol Cancer Ther 11:427–438

Morgan MA, Parsels LA, Zhao L, Parsels JD, Davis MA, Hassan MC, Arumugarajah S, Hylander-Gans L, Morosini D, Simeone DM, Canman CE, Normolle DP, Zabludoff SD, Maybaum J, Lawrence TS (2010) Mechanism of radiosensitization by the Chk1/2 inhibitor AZD7762 involves abrogation of the G2 checkpoint and inhibition of homologous recombinational DNA repair. Cancer Res 70:4972–4981

Muller PA, Vousden KH (2013) p53 mutations in cancer. Nat Cell Biol 15:2–8

Murga M, Campaner S, Lopez-Contreras AJ, Toledo LI, Soria R, Montana MF, D'Artista L, Schleker T, Guerra C, Garcia E, Barbacid M, Hidalgo M, Amati B, Fernandez-Capetillo O (2011) Exploiting oncogene-induced replicative stress for the selective killing of Myc-driven tumors. Nat Struct Mol Biol 18:1331–1335

O'Connor MJ (2015) Targeting the DNA damage response in cancer. Mol Cell 60:547–560

Paulsen RD, Cimprich KA (2007) The ATR pathway: fine-tuning the fork. DNA Repair 6:953–966

Pei XY, Dai Y, Youssefian LE, Chen S, Bodie WW, Takabatake Y, Felthousen J, Almenara JA, Kramer LB, Dent P, Grant S (2011) Cytokinetically quiescent (G0/G1) human multiple myeloma cells are susceptible to simultaneous inhibition of Chk1 and MEK1/2. Blood 118:5189–5200

Peng CY, Graves PR, Thoma RS, Wu Z, Shaw AS, Piwnica-Worms H (1997) Mitotic and G2 checkpoint control: regulation of 14-3-3 protein binding by phosphorylation of Cdc25C on serine-216. Science 277:1501–1505

Perez RP, Lewis LD, Beelen AP, Olszanski AJ, Johnston N, Rhodes CH, Beaulieu B, Ernstoff MS, Eastman A (2006) Modulation of cell cycle progression in human tumors: a pharmacokinetic and tumor molecular pharmacodynamic study of cisplatin plus the Chk1 inhibitor UCN-01 (NSC 638850). Clin Cancer Res 12:7079–7085

Puigvert JC, Sanjiv K, Helleday T (2016) Targeting DNA repair, DNA metabolism and replication stress as anti-cancer strategies. FEBS J 283:232–245

Qi W, Xie C, Li C, Caldwell JT, Edwards H, Taub JW, Wang Y, Lin H, Ge Y (2014) CHK1 plays a critical role in the anti-leukemic activity of the wee1 inhibitor MK-1775 in acute myeloid leukemia cells. J Hematol Oncol 7:53

Rawlinson R, Massey AJ (2014) gammaH2AX and Chk1 phosphorylation as predictive pharmacodynamic biomarkers of Chk1 inhibitor-chemotherapy combination treatments. BMC cancer 14:483

Ren Q, Liu R, Dicker A, Wang Y (2005) CHK1 affects cell sensitivity to microtubule-targeted drugs. J Cell Physiol 203:273–276

Russell MR, Levin K, Rader J, Belcastro L, Li Y, Martinez D, Pawel B, Shumway SD, Maris JM, Cole KA (2013) Combination therapy targeting the Chk1 and Wee1 kinases shows therapeutic efficacy in neuroblastoma. Cancer Res 73:776–784

Sakurikar N, Eastman A (2015) Will targeting Chk1 have a role in the future of cancer therapy? J Clin Oncol Off J Am Soc Clin Oncol 33:1075–1077

Sakurikar N, Thompson R, Montano R, Eastman A (2016) A subset of cancer cell lines is acutely sensitive to the Chk1 inhibitor MK-8776 as monotherapy due to CDK2 activation in S phase. Oncotarget 7:1380–1394

Sampath D, Cortes J, Estrov Z, Du M, Shi Z, Andreeff M, Gandhi V, Plunkett W (2006) Pharmacodynamics of cytarabine alone and in combination with 7-hydroxystaurosporine (UCN-01) in AML blasts in vitro and during a clinical trial. Blood 107:2517–2524

Sanjiv K, Hagenkort A, Calderon-Montano JM, Koolmeister T, Reaper PM, Mortusewicz O, Jacques SA, Kuiper RV, Schultz N, Scobie M, Charlton PA, Pollard JR, Berglund UW, Altun M, Helleday T (2016) Cancer-specific synthetic lethality between ATR and CHK1 kinase activities. Cell Rep 14:298–309

Sarcar B, Kahali S, Prabhu AH, Shumway SD, Xu Y, Demuth T, Chinnaiyan P (2011) Targeting radiation-induced G(2) checkpoint activation with the Wee-1 inhibitor MK-1775 in glioblastoma cell lines. Mol Cancer Ther 10:2405–2414

Sausville E, Lorusso P, Carducci M, Carter J, Quinn MF, Malburg L, Azad N, Cosgrove D, Knight R, Barker P, Zabludoff S, Agbo F, Oakes P, Senderowicz A (2014) Phase I dose-escalation study of AZD7762, a checkpoint kinase inhibitor, in combination with gemcitabine in US patients with advanced solid tumors. Cancer Chemother Pharmacol 73:539–549

Scagliotti G, Kang JH, Smith D, Rosenberg R, Park K, Kim SW, Su WC, Boyd TE, Richards DA, Novello S, Hynes SM, Myrand SP, Lin J, Smyth EN, Wijayawardana S, Lin AB, Pinder-Schenck M (2016) Phase II evaluation of LY2603618, a first-generation CHK1 inhibitor, in combination with pemetrexed in patients with advanced or metastatic non-small cell lung cancer. Invest New Drugs 34:625–635

Schenk EL, Koh BD, Flatten KS, Peterson KL, Parry D, Hess AD, Smith BD, Karp JE, Karnitz LM, Kaufmann SH (2012) Effects of selective checkpoint kinase 1 inhibition on cytarabine cytotoxicity in acute myelogenous leukemia cells in vitro. Clin Cancer Res 18:5364–5373

Seto T, Esaki T, Hirai F, Arita S, Nosaki K, Makiyama A, Kometani T, Fujimoto C, Hamatake M, Takeoka H, Agbo F, Shi X (2013) Phase I, dose-escalation study of AZD7762 alone and in combination with gemcitabine in Japanese patients with advanced solid tumours. Cancer Chemother Pharmacol 72:619–627

Shao RG, Cao CX, Pommier Y (2004) Abrogation of Chk1-mediated S/G2 checkpoint by UCN-01 enhances ara-C-induced cytotoxicity in human colon cancer cells. Acta Pharmacol Sin 25:756–762

Signore M, Pelacchi F, di Martino S, Runci D, Biffoni M, Giannetti S, Morgante L, De Majo M, Petricoin EF, Stancato L, Larocca LM, De Maria R, Pallini R, Ricci-Vitiani L (2014) Combined PDK1 and CHK1 inhibition is required to kill glioblastoma stem-like cells in vitro and in vivo. Cell Death Dis 5:e1223

Smith J, Tho LM, Xu N, Gillespie DA (2010) The ATM-Chk2 and ATR-Chk1 pathways in DNA damage signaling and cancer. Adv Cancer Res 108:73–112

Smits VA, Gillespie DA (2015) DNA damage control: regulation and functions of checkpoint kinase 1. FEBS J 282:3681–3692

Smits VA, Reaper PM, Jackson SP (2006) Rapid PIKK-dependent release of Chk1 from chromatin promotes the DNA-damage checkpoint response. Curr Biol 16:150–159

Sorensen CS, Syljuasen RG, Falck J, Schroeder T, Ronnstrand L, Khanna KK, Zhou BB, Bartek J, Lukas J (2003) Chk1 regulates the S phase checkpoint by coupling the physiological turnover and ionizing radiation-induced accelerated proteolysis of Cdc25A. Cancer Cell 3:247–258

Sorensen CS, Hansen LT, Dziegielewski J, Syljuasen RG, Lundin C, Bartek J, Helleday T (2005) The cell-cycle checkpoint kinase Chk1 is required for mammalian homologous recombination repair. Nat Cell Biol 7:195–201

Syljuasen RG, Sorensen CS, Nylandsted J, Lukas C, Lukas J, Bartek J (2004) Inhibition of Chk1 by CEP-3891 accelerates mitotic nuclear fragmentation in response to ionizing radiation. Cancer Res 64:9035–9040

Symington LS, Gautier J (2011) Double-strand break end resection and repair pathway choice. Annu Rev Genet 45:247–271

Tang Y, Hamed HA, Poklepovic A, Dai Y, Grant S, Dent P (2012) Poly(ADP-ribose) polymerase 1 modulates the lethality of CHK1 inhibitors in mammary tumors. Mol Pharmacol 82:322–332

Tho LM, Libertini S, Rampling R, Sansom O, Gillespie DA (2012) Chk1 is essential for chemical carcinogen-induced mouse skin tumorigenesis. Oncogene 31:1366–1375

Thompson R, Montano R, Eastman A (2012) The Mre11 nuclease is critical for the sensitivity of cells to Chk1 inhibition. PLoS One 7:e44021

Toledo LI, Altmeyer M, Rask MB, Lukas C, Larsen DH, Povlsen LK, Bekker-Jensen S, Mailand N, Bartek J, Lukas J (2013) ATR prohibits replication catastrophe by preventing global exhaustion of RPA. Cell 155:1088–1103

Tse AN, Schwartz GK (2004) Potentiation of cytotoxicity of topoisomerase I poison by concurrent and sequential treatment with the checkpoint inhibitor UCN-01 involves disparate mechanisms resulting in either p53-independent clonogenic suppression or p53-dependent mitotic catastrophe. Cancer Res 64:6635–6644

Tse AN, Rendahl KG, Sheikh T, Cheema H, Aardalen K, Embry M, Ma S, Moler EJ, Ni ZJ, Lopes de Menezes DE, Hibner B, Gesner TG, Schwartz GK (2007) CHIR-124, a novel potent inhibitor of Chk1, potentiates the cytotoxicity of topoisomerase I poisons in vitro and in vivo. Clin Cancer Res 13:591–602

Tse AN, Sheikh TN, Alan H, Chou TC, Schwartz GK (2009) 90-kDa heat shock protein inhibition abrogates the topoisomerase I poison-induced G2/M checkpoint in p53-null tumor cells by depleting Chk1 and Wee1. Mol Pharmacol 75:124–133

Vance S, Liu E, Zhao L, Parsels JD, Parsels LA, Brown JL, Maybaum J, Lawrence TS, Morgan MA (2011) Selective radiosensitization of p53 mutant pancreatic cancer cells by combined inhibition of Chk1 and PARP1. Cell Cycle 10:4321–4329

Verlinden L, Vanden Bempt I, Eelen G, Drijkoningen M, Verlinden I, Marchal K, De Wolf-Peeters C, Christiaens MR, Michiels L, Bouillon R, Verstuyf A (2007) The E2F-regulated gene Chk1 is highly expressed in triple-negative estrogen receptor/progesterone receptor/HER-2 breast carcinomas. Cancer Res 67:6574–6581

Walker M, Black EJ, Oehler V, Gillespie DA, Scott MT (2009) Chk1 C-terminal regulatory phosphorylation mediates checkpoint activation by de-repression of Chk1 catalytic activity. Oncogene 28:2314–2323

Walton MI, Eve PD, Hayes A, Valenti M, De Haven Brandon A, Box G, Boxall KJ, Aherne GW, Eccles SA, Raynaud FI, Williams DH, Reader JC, Collins I, Garrett MD (2010) The preclinical pharmacology and therapeutic activity of the novel CHK1 inhibitor SAR-020106. Mol Cancer Ther 9:89–100

Walton MI, Eve PD, Hayes A, Valenti MR, De Haven Brandon AK, Box G, Hallsworth A, Smith EL, Boxall KJ, Lainchbury M, Matthews TP, Jamin Y, Robinson SP, Aherne GW, Reader JC, Chesler L, Raynaud FI, Eccles SA, Collins I, Garrett MD (2012) CCT244747 is a novel potent and selective CHK1 inhibitor with oral efficacy alone and in combination with genotoxic anticancer drugs. Clin Cancer Res 18:5650–5661

Walton MI, Eve PD, Hayes A, Henley AT, Valenti MR, De Haven Brandon AK, Box G, Boxall KJ, Tall M, Swales K, Matthews TP, McHardy T, Lainchbury M, Osborne J, Hunter JE, Perkins ND, Aherne GW, Reader JC, Raynaud FI, Eccles SA, Collins I, Garrett MD (2016) The clinical development candidate CCT245737 is an orally active CHK1 inhibitor with preclinical activity in RAS mutant NSCLC and Emicro-MYC driven B-cell lymphoma. Oncotarget 7:2329–2342

Walworth NC, Bernards R (1996) rad-dependent response of the ChK1-encoded protein kinase at the DNA damage checkpoint. Science 271:353–356

Wang FZ, Fei HR, Cui YJ, Sun YK, Li ZM, Wang XY, Yang XY, Zhang JG, Sun BL (2014) The checkpoint 1 kinase inhibitor LY2603618 induces cell cycle arrest, DNA damage response and autophagy in cancer cells. Apoptosis 19:1389–1398

Wehler T, Thomas M, Schumann C, Bosch-Barrera J, Vinolas Segarra N, Dickgreber NJ, Dalhoff K, Sebastian M, Corral Jaime J, Alonso M, Hynes SM, Lin J, Hurt K, Bence Lin A, Calvo E, Paz-Ares L (2017) A randomized, phase 2 evaluation of the CHK1 inhibitor, LY2603618, administered in combination with pemetrexed and cisplatin in patients with advanced nonsquamous non-small cell lung cancer. Lung Cancer 108:212–216

Weiss GJ, Donehower RC, Iyengar T, Ramanathan RK, Lewandowski K, Westin E, Hurt K, Hynes SM, Anthony SP, McKane S (2013) Phase I dose-escalation study to examine the safety and tolerability of LY2603618, a checkpoint 1 kinase inhibitor, administered 1 day after pemetrexed 500 mg/m(2) every 21 days in patients with cancer. Invest New Drugs 31:136–144

Wilsker D, Petermann E, Helleday T, Bunz F (2008) Essential function of Chk1 can be uncoupled from DNA damage checkpoint and replication control. Proc Natl Acad Sci U S A 105:20752–20757

Xiao Z, Xue J, Semizarov D, Sowin TJ, Rosenberg SH, Zhang H (2005) Novel indication for cancer therapy: Chk1 inhibition sensitizes tumor cells to antimitotics. Int J Cancer 115:528–538

Xie C, Drenberg C, Edwards H, Caldwell JT, Chen W, Inaba H, Xu X, Buck SA, Taub JW, Baker SD, Ge Y (2013) Panobinostat enhances cytarabine and daunorubicin sensitivities in AML cells through suppressing the expression of BRCA1, CHK1, and Rad51. PLoS One 8:e79106

Xu H, Cheung IY, Wei XX, Tran H, Gao X, Cheung NK (2011) Checkpoint kinase inhibitor synergizes with DNA-damaging agents in G1 checkpoint-defective neuroblastoma. Int J Cancer 129:1953–1962

Yang H, Yoon SJ, Jin J, Choi SH, Seol HJ, Lee JI, Nam DH, Yoo HY (2011) Inhibition of checkpoint kinase 1 sensitizes lung cancer brain metastases to radiotherapy. Biochem Biophys Res Commun 406:53–58

Yao Q, Weigel B, Kersey J (2007) Synergism between etoposide and 17-AAG in leukemia cells: critical roles for Hsp90, FLT3, topoisomerase II, Chk1, and Rad51. Clin Cancer Res 13:1591–1600

Yu Q, La Rose J, Zhang H, Takemura H, Kohn KW, Pommier Y (2002a) UCN-01 inhibits p53 up-regulation and abrogates gamma-radiation-induced G(2)-M checkpoint independently of p53 by targeting both of the checkpoint kinases, Chk2 and Chk1. Cancer Res 62:5743–5748

Yu C, Dai Y, Dent P, Grant S (2002b) Coadministration of UCN-01 with MEK1/2 inhibitors potently induces apoptosis in BCR/ABL+ leukemia cells sensitive and resistant to ST1571. Cancer Biol Ther 1:674–682

Zabludoff SD, Deng C, Grondine MR, Sheehy AM, Ashwell S, Caleb BL, Green S, Haye HR, Horn CL, Janetka JW, Liu D, Mouchet E, Ready S, Rosenthal JL, Queva C, Schwartz GK, Taylor KJ, Tse AN, Walker GE, White AM (2008) AZD7762, a novel checkpoint kinase inhibitor, drives checkpoint abrogation and potentiates DNA-targeted therapies. Mol Cancer Ther 7:2955–2966

Zachos G, Rainey MD, Gillespie DA (2003) Chk1-deficient tumour cells are viable but exhibit multiple checkpoint and survival defects. EMBO J 22:713–723

Zachos G, Rainey MD, Gillespie DA (2005) Chk1-dependent S-M checkpoint delay in vertebrate cells is linked to maintenance of viable replication structures. Mol Cell Biol 25:563–574

Zachos G, Black EJ, Walker M, Scott MT, Vagnarelli P, Earnshaw WC, Gillespie DA (2007) Chk1 is required for spindle checkpoint function. Dev Cell 12:247–260

Zeman MK, Cimprich KA (2014) Causes and consequences of replication stress. Nat Cell Biol 16:2–9

von Zglinicki T, Saretzki G, Ladhoff J, d'Adda di Fagagna F, Jackson SP (2005) Human cell senescence as a DNA damage response. Mech Ageing Dev 126:111–117

Zhang C, Yan Z, Painter CL, Zhang Q, Chen E, Arango ME, Kuszpit K, Zasadny K, Hallin M, Hallin J, Wong A, Buckman D, Sun G, Qiu M, Anderes K, Christensen JG (2009) PF-00477736 mediates checkpoint kinase 1 signaling pathway and potentiates docetaxel-induced efficacy in xenografts. Clin Cancer Res 15:4630–4640

Chapter 10
Preclinical Profiles and Contexts for CHK1 and CHK2 Inhibitors

Ian Collins and Michelle D. Garrett

Abstract CHK1 and CHK2 are two structurally distinct serine/threonine kinases that are key components of the DNA damage response (DRR). The DDR allows cancer cells to react to DNA damage caused by exogenous agents such as genotoxic chemotherapy and endogenous insults exemplified by oncogene-driven replication stress. The importance of CHK1 and CHK2 in the DDR provided the initial therapeutic rationale for pharmacological blockade of these two kinases: to enhance the effectiveness of cancer therapies that induce DNA damage. In this chapter we will review CHK1 and CHK2 tool compounds and clinical candidates and explain how they have been used preclinically to define therapeutic contexts and to drive identification of candidate biomarkers for patient stratification in the clinic.

Keywords CHK1 · CHK2 · Checkpoint · Kinase · DNA damage · Replication stress · Preclinical · Biomarkers

10.1 Introduction

The checkpoint kinases CHK1 and CHK2 are components of the DNA damage response (DDR) pathway, a complex intracellular signalling network that executes and coordinates the cellular activities required to detect and repair damaged DNA (Dai and Grant 2010; Antoni et al. 2007). CHK1 and CHK2, although similarly named, are structurally distinct kinases with different but overlapping roles in the DDR (Fig. 10.1) (Garrett and Collins 2011). The result of checkpoint kinase activity

I. Collins
Cancer Research UK Cancer Therapeutics Unit at The Institute of Cancer Research, London, UK
e-mail: ian.collins@icr.ac.uk

M. D. Garrett (✉)
School of Biosciences, University of Kent, Kent, UK
e-mail: m.d.garrett@kent.ac.uk

© Springer International Publishing AG, part of Springer Nature 2018   241
J. Pollard, N. Curtin (eds.), *Targeting the DNA Damage Response for Anti-Cancer Therapy*, Cancer Drug Discovery and Development, https://doi.org/10.1007/978-3-319-75836-7_10

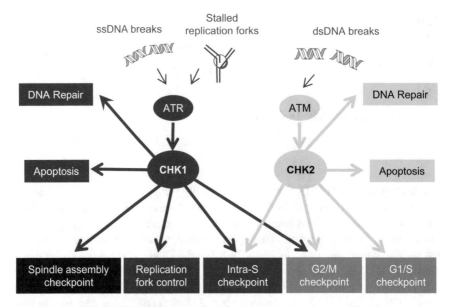

Fig. 10.1 The roles of CHK1 and CHK2 in the DNA damage response. Adapted from (Garrett and Collins 2011)

is to halt cell growth and division at several possible checkpoints in the cell cycle and to initiate different DNA repair processes depending on the nature of the damage e.g., single *versus* double strand breaks. The cell cycle checkpoints allow time for repair of the damaged DNA and re-entry into the cell cycle, or will induce cell death if DNA repair cannot be achieved (Stracker et al. 2009). CHK1 and CHK2 therefore have important roles in normal and transformed cell growth and division, in particular in responding to DNA damage arising during DNA replication (Lecona and Fernández-Capetillon 2014).

The DDR is also critical to the cell's response to exogenous DNA-damaging agents, including ionising radiation and the many cancer chemotherapies that cause DNA strand breaks or cross links. Thus the checkpoint kinases are part of an intrinsic resistance mechanism to DNA-damaging cancer treatments (Zhang and Hunter 2014). Inhibition of checkpoint kinases presents two broad opportunities for therapeutic intervention: first, to enhance the effectiveness of classical cancer therapies that damage DNA, and second, to impair the survival of cancer cells with intrinsically high levels of DNA damage that rely on the DDR for survival (Garrett and Collins 2011). While checkpoint kinase signalling and DNA damage repair are also features of normal cells, cancer cells often have defects in one or more components of the multiple cell cycle checkpoints or DNA repair mechanisms, thus making them dependent on the remaining functional arms of the DDR and providing a window for selective effects on cancer cells (Ma et al. 2011).

In the past decade there has been significant progress in the discovery and development of selective inhibitors of CHK1 and/or CHK2 (Janetka et al. 2007;

Garrett and Collins 2011; Chen et al. 2012; Maugeri-Sacca et al. 2013). Multiple compounds have entered clinical trials, although no agent has yet reached regulatory approval. In tandem with the success in preclinical drug discovery, there has been an ongoing reassessment of the appropriate clinical contexts for CHK1 and CHK2 inhibition. This has been supported by the availability of more structurally diverse and refined, selective inhibitors of the enzymes for use as pharmacological tools (Matthews et al. 2013). As more selective inhibitors have become available, the distinctions between the roles of CHK1 and CHK2 in the DDR and cell cycle checkpoint control have become clearer. A large body of evidence exists to confirm the long-standing proposed combinations of CHK1 inhibitors with DNA-damaging chemotherapies or ionising radiation, as discussed in this chapter. This remains the most clearly developed preclinical context for CHK1 inhibition, while the relevance of CHK2 in this setting is much less supported.

At the same time as pharmacological studies have accumulated, RNA interference techniques have continued to provide critical insight into the roles that CHK1 and CHK2 inhibition may play in cancer therapy. The combination of siRNA screens with selective CHK1 or CHK2 inhibitors has proved especially powerful in identifying potential new combinations with molecularly targeted agents and in defining tumor genetic backgrounds that offer the possibility of efficacious synthetic lethal interactions with checkpoint kinase inhibitors. Most notable has been the strengthening understanding of the potential for single agent activity of CHK1 inhibitors in specific tumor types (McNeely et al. 2014), and the emergence of a synthetic lethal context for CHK2 inhibition in combination with inhibition of PARP-dependent DNA repair (Anderson et al. 2011; Höglund et al. 2011a).

Alongside the increased pharmacological understanding of checkpoint kinase inhibition there have been advances in the knowledge and measurement of biomarkers in the DNA damage response pathways. Assays to confirm target engagement and modulation of the DDR by CHK1 and CHK2 inhibitors have been critical in interpreting preclinical and clinical studies. The quantification of the DDR status in tumors and the corresponding sensitivity to CHK1 and/or CHK2 inhibition is also essential in building strategies to select which patients may benefit from checkpoint inhibitor therapy. In this chapter, we review recent pharmacological data from cellular and in vivo preclinical models using CHK1 and CHK2 preclinical chemical tools and clinical candidates, and how that informs current expectations of the most promising clinical contexts for checkpoint kinase inhibition.

10.2 Small-Molecule Inhibitors of Checkpoint Kinases

While the first inhibitors of CHK1 and CHK2 have been known for over 15 years, the pace of discovery of new molecules has been especially fast in the past 5 years. Multiple checkpoint kinase inhibitors have progressed to early clinical studies, and many more small molecule inhibitors of the enzymes are available as preclinical tools. A selection of these inhibitors is shown in Table 10.1, focused on compounds

Table 10.1 Structures and biochemical activities of selected checkpoint kinase inhibitors[a]

Compound	Structure	Inhibitory activity	Ref.	In vivo dosing route[b]
CHK1/CHK2				
AZD7762		CHK1 K_i = 5 nM CHK2 IC$_{50}$ < 10 nM 38 kinases <10-fold selective	Zabludoff et al. 2008; Oza et al. 2012	IV
LY2606368 (prexasertib)		CHK1 K_i = 0.9 nM CHK2 IC$_{50}$ = 8 nM CDK1 IC$_{50}$ > 10,000 nM CDK2 IC$_{50}$ > 10,000 nM RSK1 IC$_{50}$ = 9 nM	King et al. 2015	IV/IP[c]
V158411		CHK1 IC$_{50}$ = 4.4 nM CHK2 IC$_{50}$ = 4.5 nM CDK1 IC$_{50}$ > 50,000 nM	Massey et al. 2015	IV
CHK1				
PF00477736		CHK1 K_i = 0.5 nM CHK2 K_i = 47 nM	Blasina et al. 2008	IV/IP[c]
CHIR124		CHK1 IC$_{50}$ = 0.3 nM CHK2 IC$_{50}$ = 697 nM	Tse et al. 2007	PO[d]
MK8776 (SCH900776)[e]		CHK1 IC$_{50}$ = 3 nM CHK2 IC$_{50}$ = 1500 nM CDK2 IC$_{50}$ = 160 nM	Guzi et al. 2011	IV/IP[c]
LY2603618		CHK1 IC$_{50}$ = 7 nM CHK2 IC$_{50}$ = 12,000 nM CDK1 IC$_{50}$ > 20,000 nM CDK2 IC$_{50}$ > 20,000 nM	King et al. 2014	IV/PO[f]
SAR020106		CHK1 IC$_{50}$ = 13 nM CHK2 IC$_{50}$ > 10,000 nM CDK1 IC$_{50}$ > 1000 nM	Walton et al. 2010; Reader et al. 2011	IP
CCT244747		CHK1 IC$_{50}$ = 8 nM CHK2 IC$_{50}$ > 10,000 nM CDK1 IC$_{50}$ > 10,000 nM	Walton et al. 2012; Lainchbury et al. 2012	PO
CCT245737 (SRA737)[g]		CHK1 IC$_{50}$ = 1.3 nM CHK2 IC$_{50}$ = 2440 nM CDK1 IC$_{50}$ = 9030 nM CDK2 IC$_{50}$ = 3850 nM	Walton et al. 2016	PO

(continued)

Table 10.1   (continued)

Compound	Structure	Inhibitory activity	Ref.	In vivo dosing route[b]
GNE783		CHK1 IC_{50} = 1 nM CHK2 IC_{50} = 444 nM CDK1 IC_{50} = 528 nM CDK2 IC_{50} = 456 nM AuroraB IC_{50} = 840 nM	Xiao et al. 2013	–
GNE900		CHK1 IC_{50} = 1.1 nM CHK2 IC_{50} = 1500 nM CDK1 IC_{50} = 706 nM CDK2 IC_{50} = 366 nM	Blackwood et al. 2013; Gazzard et al. 2015	PO
S1181		CHK1 IC_{50} = 2.5 nM CHK2 IC_{50} > 1000 nM CDK1 IC_{50} > 1000 nM CDK2 IC_{50} > 1000 nM	Koh et al. 2015	–
CHK2				
CHK2 inhibitor II (C3742)		CHK1 IC_{50} > 10,000 nM CHK2 K_i = 37 nM	Arienti et al. 2005	–
VRX0466617		CHK1 IC_{50} = 10,000 nM CHK2 K_i = 11 nM	Carlessi et al. 2007	–
PV10109		CHK1 IC_{50} = 15,730 nM CHK2 IC_{50} = 3 nM	Jobson et al. 2009	–
CCT241533		CHK1 IC_{50} = 190 nM CHK2 IC_{50} = 3 nM	Caldwell et al. 2011	–

[a]Adapted and extended from (Garrett and Collins 2011); [b] Intravenous (IV), intraperitoneal (IP) or oral (PO) administration in vivo, where reported; [c] Clinical formulation IV, preclinical IP dosing reported; [d] Preclinical PO dosing reported at high frequency (4× daily); [e] SCH900776 renamed MK8776 subsequent to change of ownership; [f] Clinical formulation IV, preclinical PO dosing reported; [g] CCT245737 renamed SRA737 subsequent to licensing

with fully disclosed structures and for which extensive preclinical data have been published. Where known, the routes of administration of the compounds for pre-clinical in vivo experiments and clinical studies have been included. It is notable that several of the dual CHK1/2 or CHK1-selective inhibitors are suitable for in vivo administration by systemic, intraperitoneal or oral dosing (Table 10.1), but in contrast there are no current CHK2-selective inhibitors similarly well-characterised for in vivo studies.

The discovery of this array of checkpoint kinase inhibitors has been underpinned by extensive structural biology studies on both CHK1 and CHK2 (Matthews et al. 2013).

For both enzymes, high selectivity has been achieved in several examples by exploiting unusual bound water molecules. In the case of CHK1 a network of tightly bound water molecules in a pocket adjacent to the ATP-binding site differentiates CHK1 from CHK2 and other kinases and is known to be targeted by several inhibitor chemical scaffolds. For CHK2, the highest selectivity over CHK1 has resulted from scaffolds that make use of, or replace, a water molecule bound to the hinge-region of the kinase ATP-binding site.

These considerations notwithstanding, a broad spectrum of selectivities for CHK1 and CHK2 inhibition are exhibited by the molecules commonly used to probe cellular and in vivo biology. Many studies continue to use earlier discovered inhibitors based on the indole-maleimide natural product staurosporine, such as UCN01 (Busby et al. 2000; Yu et al. 2002) or SB218078 (Jackson et al. 2000), where the risk of significant off-target kinase inhibition is high. This can confound interpretation of the cellular biology, since the effects on the cell cycle checkpoints of CHK1 and CHK2 inhibition can be masked by inhibition of other kinases involved in cell cycle progression, for example the cyclin dependent kinases. Subsequent inhibitors have been reported with improved selectivity for CHK1 and/ or CHK2 over other kinases which arguably offer better defined and more reliable reagents for probing checkpoint kinase biology (Workman and Collins 2010). The subsequent sections of this chapter will focus on results obtained using the compounds shown in Table 10.1. For many of the compounds, kinome profiles have been published that allow an estimation of the likelihood of off-target kinase inhibition leading to cellular or in vivo effects at a given concentration (e.g. see references cited in Table 10.1 for details of the inhibition of between 100 and 400 kinases for the majority of compounds described).

As more evidence of the difference between the biological functions of CHK1 and CHK2 has become available it has become more important to differentiate between them in preclinical studies (Pommier et al. 2005; Xiao et al. 2006; Antoni et al. 2007; Guzi et al. 2011). In this regard, the clinical candidates and tool compounds fall mainly into two classes: dual CHK1/CHK2 inhibitors such as AZD7762, LY2606368 and V158411, and those with biochemical specificity for one of the checkpoint kinases. In interpreting the preclinical activity of the compounds, it is important to note that some of the most potent CHK1 inhibitors with >tenfold selectivity over CHK2 still have significant affinity (10–100 nM) for the less potently inhibited enzyme, and may therefore inhibit CHK2 at compound concentrations used in cellular assays or achieved in vivo. The clinical candidate LY2606368 is unusual among the more recent checkpoint kinase inhibitors in that it showed potent inhibition of proliferation across a wide range of cancer cell lines, as well as single agent efficacy in vivo in tumor xenografts (King et al. 2015) (see Sect. 3.2).

The differences in the potency and selectivity profiles of the available agents, and their application in different cellular contexts, can lead to fragmentary and often contradictory biological findings. The use of multiple inhibitors from different chemical classes in pharmacological studies can address the issue of off-target inhibition (Workman and Collins 2010), and the observation of consistent behaviours with different compounds across several experimental contexts gives confidence in the generality of the phenomena. In the following section, we particularly highlight where multiple studies using different pharmacological probes in different cellular or tumor models have converged on similar findings of relevance to the translation of checkpoint kinase inhibitors to the clinic.

10.3 Preclinical Contexts for Checkpoint Kinase Inhibitors

The most established preclinical contexts for checkpoint kinase inhibitors are combinations with DNA-damaging chemotherapies and ionising radiation, and this has informed many of the early clinical trials (Bucher and Britten 2008; Chen et al. 2012). CHK1-dependent contexts are best evidenced in most cases, with CHK2 inhibition so far offering different and far fewer opportunities for anti-tumor activity (Fig. 10.2). Increasingly, attention has turned to combinations of checkpoint kinase inhibitors

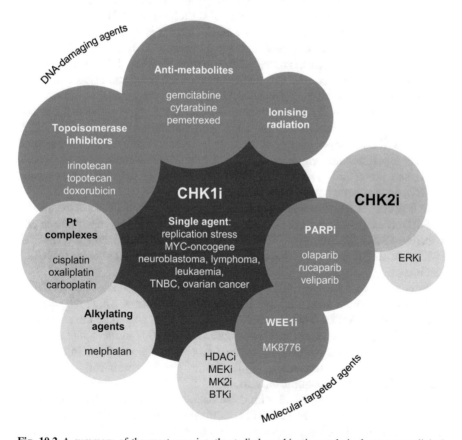

Fig. 10.2 A summary of the most prominently studied combination and single agent preclinical contexts for CHK1 and CHK2 inhibition. Drugs, clinical candidates and chemical probes most commonly used in preclinical studies in combination with checkpoint kinase inhibitors are indicated

with other molecular targeted agents, especially those involved in the same or complementary DDR pathways as CHK1 and CHK2. Single agent activity of CHK1 inhibitors is a topic of considerable current interest, with much data emerging to show that a variety of tumors may be dependent on the CHK1-mediated DDR for survival and thus susceptible to CHK1 inhibitor monotherapy (McNeely et al. 2014).

10.3.1 Combination Contexts for Checkpoint Kinase Inhibition

10.3.1.1 Combinations with Antimetabolites

Combinations of CHK1 inhibition with antimetabolites such as gemcitabine, cytarabine, pemetrexed and cladribine have consistently emerged as the most synergistic pairings for checkpoint kinase inhibition with DNA-damaging chemotherapy. A kinase siRNA synthetic lethal screen with gemcitabine in pancreatic cancer cells identified silencing of CHK1, but not CHK2, as giving the most sensitization to inhibition of cell growth (Azorsa et al. 2009). The selective CHK1 inhibitor GNE783 was used to screen a library of 51 DNA-damaging drugs, spanning alkylating agents, anthracyclines, antimetabolites, DNA cross-linkers, topoisomerase inhibitors, and antimitotic agents, for synergistic effects on HT29 colon cancer cell viability (Xiao et al. 2013). The antimetabolites showed the highest synergy, particularly gemcitabine and cladribine, and a repeat of the screen using AZD7762 generated a very similar pattern. Similarly, MK8776 more strongly potentiated the efficacy of nucleoside DNA antimetabolites and antifolates compared to either topoisomerase inhibitors or melphalan in U2OS sarcoma cells (Guzi et al. 2011) and preferentially sensitized MDA-MB-231 triple negative breast cancer (TNBC) cells to gemcitabine and cytarabine, but not SN38 or 5-fluorouracil (5-Fu) (Montano et al. 2012). Stronger potentiation of gemcitabine or 5-fluoro-deoxyuridine (5-FdU) efficacy than for other DNA-damaging agents was also seen with the highly selective CHK1 inhibitors CCT244747 (Walton et al. 2012) and CCT245737 (Walton et al. 2016) in colon, pancreatic and non-small cell lung cancer (NSCLC) cell lines.

In contrast to selective CHK1 and CHK1/2 dual inhibitors, selective CHK2 inhibitors have often shown no synergy with antimetabolites. Thus, the selective CHK2 inhibitors VRX0466617 and CCT241533 did not potentiate the efficacy of gemcitabine in several cancer cell lines (Carlessi et al. 2007; Anderson et al. 2011) and the selective CHK2 inhibitor II gave no chemosensitization to 5-FU in colorectal cancer cells expressing truncations of the adenomatous polyposis coli (APC) gene, while CHK1 inhibitors significantly increased 5-FU-induced apoptosis (Martino-Echarri et al. 2014). Consistent with these data, studies using CHK1 and CHK2 single and dual siRNA in the context of hydroxyurea-induced DNA damage found that while CHK1 siRNA significantly increased DNA damage, CHK2 siRNA alone gave no increase and the combination of CHK1 and CHK2 siRNAs was less effective than CHK1 siRNA alone (Guzi et al. 2011).

Gemcitabine has been the most intensively studied anti-metabolite in combination with checkpoint kinase inhibitors, with in vitro and in vivo potentiation of gemcitabine efficacy shown by both CHK1 selective and dual CHK1/CHK2 inhibitors, including PF-00477736 (Blasina et al. 2008), AZD7762 (Zabludoff et al. 2008), SAR020106 (Walton et al. 2010), CCT244747 (Walton et al. 2012), CCT245737 (Walton et al. 2016), GNE900 (Blackwood et al. 2013) and MK8776 (Guzi et al. 2011; Montano et al. 2013). Gemcitabine is used clinically in regimens to treat pancreatic and lung cancers, and most reported in vivo preclinical experiments have involved pancreatic cancer, NSCLC and colon cancer tumor xenografts. Chemo-potentiation of gemcitabine has also been reported in TNBC and ovarian cancer cell lines for VER158411, AZD7762 and PF00477736 (Bryant et al. 2014a) and in TNBC cells and tumor xenografts for AZD7762 (Bennett et al. 2012), while MK8776 also sensitized ovarian cancer xenografts to gemcitabine (Guzi et al. 2011).

As expected from the proposed mechanism of action, requiring external DNA damage before abrogation of the CHK1-mediated cell cycle checkpoint will affect cell survival, the CHK1 inhibitors generally showed minimal single agent cytotoxicity or tumor growth inhibition in these models. The nucleoside analogue is incorporated into replicating DNA to give single-strand breaks and also depletes the nucleotide intermediate pool through inhibition of ribonucleotide reductase, leading to a CHK1-dependent S-phase arrest. A common molecular signature for pharmacological CHK1 inhibition in the combinations has been observed consisting of concentration-dependent inhibition of gemcitabine-induced CHK1 pSer296 autophosphorylation, inhibition of depletion of CDC25A, a decrease in pTyr15 CDK1, and increases in γH2AX signals and PARP cleavage.

While various dosing schedules have been used for the combination of CHK1 inhibitors and gemcitabine in preclinical models, the schedule dependence has been investigated in detail in several studies. In vivo studies with gemcitabine and GNE900 in HT29 colon cancer xenografts showed that chemo-potentiation was most effective with a 16–36 h delay between the administration of gemcitabine and the start of CHK1 inhibitor therapy (Blackwood et al. 2013). The refined schedule also improved the efficacy in chemo-resistant xenografts. In HT29 cells the CHK1-dependent checkpoints were found to lie downstream of gemcitabine triphosphate incorporation into DNA following gemcitabine treatment, implicating the timing of release from gemcitabine-mediated replication arrest as a critical determinant of an effective dosing schedule. In HT29 cell culture studies with gemcitabine and CCT244747 the greatest potentiation of chemotherapeutic efficacy was associated with delayed administration of CCT244747 until 24 h after gemcitabine with subsequent maintenance of CHK1 inhibition for 24–48 h required to achieve full chemo-potentiation (Walton et al. 2012). Both CCT244747 and CCT245737 gave in vivo efficacy in xenograft tumors on this schedule (Walton et al. 2012, 2016).

Cellular studies with MK8776 and gemcitabine, using bolus administration of the compounds to better mimic the clinical pharmacokinetic profiles of the IV agents, found that gemcitabine rapidly induced cell cycle arrest, but the stalled replication forks were not dependent on CHK1 activity for stability until 18 h after the genotoxic was given (Montano et al. 2013). At this point, treatment with

MK8776 invoked replication fork collapse and cell death. The delayed in vitro schedule translated to in vivo activity in two pancreatic cancer xenografts, with MK8776 given 18 h after gemcitabine causing significantly delayed tumor growth compared to either drug alone, or when both drugs were administered with only a 30 min interval between them. The enhanced activity with the delayed schedule may reflect an increased number of cells arrested in S-phase before the checkpoint abrogation is effected or a need for the arrested cells to have adequate time to initiate CHK1-dependent DNA repair.

While there is an apparent consensus from several studies on the benefit of a sequential, delayed dosing schedule for gemcitabine and potentially other antimetabolites acting in S-phase, the underlying mechanisms may be complex. Studies with AZD7762 indicated that chemo-sensitisation to gemcitabine involved both deregulation of DNA replication origin firing and replication fork stabilisation in S-phase as well as checkpoint abrogation (McNeely et al. 2010). Using different ratios of gemcitabine and the selective CHK1 inhibitor S1181 in pancreatic cancer cells, a range of mechanistic effects were observed dependent on the concentrations of the two drugs (Koh et al. 2015). This study suggested that CHK1 inhibition synergized with lower concentrations of gemcitabine not predominantly through abrogation of a frank S- or G2/M-phase cell cycle arrest but by disrupting DNA replication leading to cumulative genotoxicity occurring at later points in the cell cycle. At high concentrations of gemcitabine the observed synergy was ascribed to checkpoint activation leading to a cell cycle synchronisation that accelerated the onset of cytotoxicity when the CHK1 inhibitor was added to override the checkpoint. The authors proposed that metronomic administration of low doses of gemcitabine in combination with a CHK1 inhibitor might take advantage of this mechanism.

As well as the mechanistic aspects underlying efficacy, the scheduling of antimetabolites and CHK1 inhibitors has implications for their tolerability in patients. While the typical, dose-limiting myelosuppressive effects of antimetabolites occur sometime after dosing, the delayed, sequential administration of CHK1 inhibitors with the genotoxic drugs in the first few days of treatment presents an opportunity to mitigate other acute toxicities of the drug combinations. Moreover, the apparent benefit in cellular and in vivo models of maintaining inhibitor concentrations so as to achieve continuous and sustained CHK1 inhibition to elicit maximal chemo-potentiation of antimetabolites emphasizes the importance of tailoring the schedules to the pharmacokinetic and pharmacodynamic profiles of the clinical candidates. While the first generation of CHK1 and CHK1/2 inhibitors were intravenously administered, several oral compounds are now available (Table 10.1) and may be advantageous for prolonged administration over several days. It is also important to note that the optimum schedule for combinations with other classes of genotoxic drugs may be significantly different (Massey et al. 2015).

Issues of tolerability may be important considerations for combinations involving checkpoint kinase inhibitors and more than one other agent. Successful preclinical efficacy for triple chemotherapy combinations has been reported for the selective oral CHK1 inhibitor CCT245737 with gemcitabine and cisplatin in RAS mutant NSCLC xenografts (Walton et al. 2016), while the intravenous clinical candidate

LY2603618 sensitized NSCLC cell lines and xenografts to the antifolate pemetrexed, and was subsequently taken into a Phase I clinical trial in a triple combination with pemetrexed and cisplatin (Calvo et al. 2014). Triple combinations of checkpoint kinase inhibitors with gemcitabine and radiotherapy modalities have been extensively explored. Thus, in MiaPaCa-2 pancreatic cancer cells and xenografts, and also two patient-derived pancreatic cancer xenografts, a triple combination of AZD7762, gemcitabine and ionising radiation was more effective for tumor growth delay than any of the corresponding doublet regimens (Morgan et al. 2010). The triple combination of MK8776, gemcitabine and radiotherapy in pancreatic cancer cells showed that homologous recombination repair (HRR)-proficient cells were sensitized by the CHK1 inhibitor (Engelke et al. 2013). Encouragingly, in an HRR-proficient xenograft of MiaPaCa-2 pancreatic cancer cells, efficacy was observed from the combination with no observable toxicity to the small intestine, which is typically the dose-limiting organ for chemo-radiation in pancreatic cancer. PF00477736 potentiated the effects of gemcitabine and radioimmunotherapy using a radiolabelled anti-EGFR antibody (anti-EGFR-177Lu) in pancreatic cancer cell lines and in vivo, including in patient-derived pancreatic tumor xenografts, with complete responses obtained to the triple therapy (Al-Ejeh et al. 2014). It was also found that there was a loss of tumorigenicity when cells from the treated tumors were used to establish new tumors in vivo and a concomitant reduction of tumor-initiating stem-like cells in the treated tumors.

This last effect of gemcitabine and CHK1 inhibitors on stem-like cancer cells has been demonstrated in other contexts. AZD7762 was found to sensitize two patient-derived pancreatic cancer xenografts to gemcitabine with a reduction in the number of pancreatic cancer stem cell marker positive cells, and a delay in secondary tumor initiation compared to control or gemcitabine-treated tumors (Venkatesha et al. 2012). Stem cells from NSCLC patient tumors were found to undergo CHK1-mediated cell cycle arrest following DNA-damaging chemotherapy, whereas differentiated NSCLC cells did not, and a combination of AZD7762 and gem-citabine was effective against NSCLC stem cells in vitro and reduced the proportion of NSCLC stem cells in treated xenografts (Bartucci et al. 2012).

Apart from gemcitabine and pemetrexed in solid tumors, the next most explored combinations of CHK1 inhibition with antimetabolite chemotherapy have been for cytarabine in the context of acute myeloid leukaemia (AML). AZD7762 chemo-sensitized isolated primary AML samples from patients to cytarabine, and in particular was found to target the primitive leukemic progenitor cells which are responsible for the majority of AML patient relapses (Didier et al. 2012). In another study, paired bone marrow aspirates sampled from AML patients before and 48 h after treatment with cytarabine showed an increase in CHK1 activation in 5/9 of the samples with detectable CHK1 expression, as measured by immunoblotting for pSer317 CHK1 (Schenk et al. 2012). MK8776 sensitized 10/14 AML patient samples to cytarabine while no effect was seen on normal myeloid precursors isolated from healthy volunteers. The CHK1 inhibitor also abrogated cytarabine-induced cell cycle arrest and enhanced apoptosis and anti-proliferative effects in clonogenic assays in human AML cell lines.

10.3.1.2   Combinations with Topoisomerase Inhibitors

The combination of checkpoint kinase inhibitors with topoisomerase I and II inhibitors has been well studied. While topoisomerase I inhibition by such drugs as camptothecin, irinotecan and topotecan causes single-strand breaks in DNA and intra-S-phase arrest, topisomerase II inhibitors e.g. etoposide and doxorubicin, lead to cell cycle arrest in late S and G2/M phases. Irinotecan is often part of combination chemotherapies for colon cancer, while topotecan is used to treat ovarian and lung cancers, and doxorubicin is widely applied to treat solid tumors and haematological malignancies. There is plentiful evidence that both dual CHK1/2 and CHK1-selective inhibitors abrogate the cell cycle arrests caused by topoisomerase inhibitors in vitro and potentiate their DNA-damaging effects (Tse et al. 2007; Zabludoff et al. 2008; Blasina et al. 2008; Walton et al. 2010; Aris and Pommier 2012; Walton et al. 2012; Xiao et al. 2013; Walton et al. 2016; Kim et al. 2015; Massey et al. 2015). It should be noted that SN38, the active metabolite of irinotecan, is used in place of the drug in cellular studies.

In general, a lower potentiating effect has been observed in vitro for topoisomerase inhibitors and CHK1 inhibitors than for combinations with gemcitabine and related antimetabolites (Guzi et al. 2011; Xiao et al. 2013; Montano et al. 2012; Walton et al. 2012; Walton et al. 2016). Interestingly, an exception was noted for the CHK1/2 dual inhibitor V158411 which showed a generally stronger in vitro potentiation of topoisomerase I inhibitors than antimetabolites in colon cancer cell lines (Massey et al. 2015). Although chemo-sensitization in tumor xenograft models has been demonstrated for multiple checkpoint kinase inhibitors in combination with topoisomerase I or II inhibitors (Tse et al. 2007; Walton et al. 2010; Ma et al. 2012; Walton et al. 2012; Walton et al. 2016; Massey et al. 2015), including regressions for AZD7762 in combination with irinotecan (Zabludoff et al. 2008), there have also been instances where the translation to in vivo efficacy has been disappointing. While not exhibiting as effective synergy as seen with antimetabolites, the CHK1-selective inhibitor GNE783 nevertheless potentiated the activity of topoisomerase I inhibitors in HT29 colon cancer cells, but no robust potentiation of the effect of CPT-11 was observed in vivo in HT29 colon cancer xenografts with the oral analogue GNE900, despite this compound showing synergy in vivo with gemcitabine (Xiao et al. 2013).

The status of the *TP53* tumor suppressor pathway and its relation to synergy between checkpoint kinase inhibitors and topoisomerase inhibitors has been probed in several studies. In TNBC patient-derived xenograft tumors, AZD7762 strongly potentiated irinotecan-induced checkpoint abrogation, apoptosis and tumor growth delay in *TP53* deficient but not in *TP53* wild type cells, and RNAi knockdown of *TP53* in a wild type xenograft rendered it more sensitive to the combination (Ma et al. 2012). AZD7762 was also found to synergize with SN38, topotecan and etoposide in G1-checkpoint deficient neuroblastoma cell lines, but not in checkpoint proficient cells (Xu et al. 2011). This contrasted with the combination of gemcitabine and AZD7762 which synergized across all the cell lines tested. Likewise V158411 preferentially synergized with SN38 and camptothecin in five *TP53*-deficient but not three *TP53*-proficient cell lines (Massey et al. 2015).

The optimum schedule for combinations of topoisomerase inhibitors and CHK1 inhibitors may be strikingly different from that for combinations with gemcitabine. Thus, while delayed dosing of VER158411 gave greater in vitro synergy with gemcitabine, a minimal dependence on scheduling was seen with topoisomerase I inhibitors, and simultaneous dosing in vivo enhanced tumor growth delay of Colo205 and SW620 colon cancer xenografts (Massey et al. 2015). Similarly, simultaneous treatment of high-grade serous ovarian cancer cells with PF00477736 and topotecan was the same or more effective than sequential exposure, regardless of the order of dosing or time of exposure, in contrast to results with gemcitabine (Kim et al. 2015).

In contrast to CHK1 inhibition, there is less evidence that selective pharmacological inhibition of CHK2 in combination with topoisomerase inhibitors offers an anti-tumor benefit. While the CHK2-selective inhibitor PV1019 synergised with topotecan and camptothecin in OVCAR-4 ovarian cancer cells (Jobson et al. 2009), the CHK2 inhibitor CCT241533 showed no potentiation of SN38, etoposide or doxorubicin cytotoxicity in HeLa or HT29 cells (Anderson et al. 2011) and VRX0466617 did not potentiate the cytotoxicity of doxorubicin in BJ-hTERT cells (Carlessi et al. 2007). In a panel of colon cancer cell lines with genetic alterations in CHK2, the potentiation of topoisomerase inhibition by the dual CHK1/2 inhibitor AZD7762 was found to be independent of the CHK2 status and not related to the potential for CHK2 inhibition (Aris and Pommier 2012).

An important reverse-translational finding was made concerning checkpoint kinase and topoisomerase inhibitor combinations following the observation of a singular curative response in the clinical trial of AZD7762 and irinotecan in a patient with invasive small-cell cancer of the ureter (Al-Ahmadie et al. 2014). Whole genome sequencing of the tumor and matched normal tissue identified a mis-sense mutation in the DNA repair protein RAD50. Subsequent cell line studies using RAD50 mutations showed that RAD50 L1237F-mutant cells were highly dependent on the remaining CHK1-dependent checkpoint for survival of topoisomerase inhibitor-induced DNA damage. It was notable that in this case 95% of all the somatic mutations identified were present in the dominant tumor clone, giving a clonal architecture dominated by one well-defined genotype and providing an ideal context for an effective synthetic lethal interaction.

10.3.1.3 Combinations with Platinum Complexes

Cisplatin, carboplatin and oxaliplatin are widely used anticancer drugs that cross-link DNA, and are in part cytotoxic through resulting inhibition of DNA replication and transcription. The drugs are especially important in ovarian, testicular, colon, lung and breast cancer treatments. Unlike combinations with antimetabolites and topoisomerase inhibitors, the evidence for productive chemo-sensitization of platinum complexes by checkpoint kinase inhibitors is equivocal. Most comparative studies have shown that where in vitro potentiation of platinum complex efficacy by CHK1 inhibitors is observed in cancer cell lines, the effect is significantly less strong than that seen for antimetabolites (Xu et al. 2011; Walton et al. 2012; Xiao et al. 2013; Massey et al. 2015; Bryant et al. 2014a). In some cases, no in vitro synergy has been seen, as for AZD7762 with cisplatin in HeLa cervical cancer cells (Wagner and Karnitz 2009) and MK8776 with cisplatin in TNBC cells (Montano et al. 2012). On the other hand, CHK1 was identified as one of the top hits in an siRNA screen for sensitizers of cisplatin in SKOV4 ovarian cancer cells (Arora et al. 2010) and synergistic effects leading to apoptotic cell death were observed in four human ovarian clear cell (OCC) cancer cell lines and an OCC tumor xenograft with the combination of AZD7762 and cisplatin (Itamochi et al. 2014). AZD7762 also potentiated the efficacy of cisplatin against patient-derived NSCLC stem-like cells in viability and colony forming assays, and in vivo in a patient-derived xenograft of NSCLC stem-like cells (Bartucci et al. 2012). In this context, it is informative to note that the CHK1-selective inhibitor CCT245737 potentiated the efficacy of a gemcitabine and cisplatin combination in a NSCLC xenograft (Walton et al. 2016). Thus while combinations of platinum complexes alone with CHK1 inhibitors may not always give clear chemo-sensitization, this should not impede the addition of CHK1 inhibitors to chemotherapy regimens where the platinum agent is given with an antimetabolite or topoisomerase inhibitor.

As with the topoisomerase inhibitors, it has been suggested that the combination of CHK1 inhibition and platinum complexes will be most effective in *TP53*-deficient cell lines (Xu et al. 2011; Massey et al. 2015). In head and neck squamous cell cancer (HNSCC) cell lines, wild type *TP53* was found to be associated with sensitivity to cisplatin treatment, whereas mutation or loss of *TP53* was associated with cisplatin resistance (Gadhikar et al. 2013). Treatment of *TP53*-deficient HNSCC cells with AZD7762 re-sensitized them to cisplatin cytotoxicity.

The therapeutic benefit of specific CHK2 inhibition in combination with platinum complexes is unclear. RNAi studies showed that depletion of CHK1, but not CHK2, enhanced the cytotoxicity of cisplatin in *TP53*-deficient compared to wild-type tumor cells (Carrassa et al. 2004). Selective inhibition of CHK2 by VRX0466617 or CCT241533 failed to potentiate cisplatin cytotoxicity in cancer cells (Carlessi et al. 2007; Anderson et al. 2011), and in HCT116 colon cancer cells, CHK2 Inhibitor II antagonized oxaliplatin-induced apoptosis (Pires et al. 2010). However, it has also been reported that wild-type *TP53* plays a role in the regulation of CHK2 activation in response to cisplatin in ovarian cancer cell lines, and in this context the combination with CHK2 Inhibitor II increased cisplatin cytotoxicity in both *TP53*-wild type and deficient ovarian cancer cells (Liang et al. 2011).

10.3.1.4   Combinations with Alkylating Agents

As with platinum complexes, comparisons of the chemo-potentiation achieved with different DNA-damaging agents have generally ranked combinations of checkpoint kinase inhibitors with DNA alkylating agents below those with antimetabolites or topoisomerase inhibitors. Thus, low or no synergy was seen between the CHK1-selective inhibitor GNE783 and alkylating agents in HT29 colon cancer cells (Xiao et al. 2013). Across a panel of 24 cancer cell lines, combining GNE783 with temozolomide showed some chemo-potentiation in *TP53*-deficient cell lines.

Weak potentiation of melphalan cytotoxicity by AZD7762 was seen in G1 checkpoint-deficient, but not proficient, neuroblastoma cell lines (Xu et al. 2011), and AZD7762 also potentiated the anti-proliferative effects of melphalan and bendamustine in *TP53*-deficient multiple myeloma cell lines (Landau et al. 2012). AZD7762, PF00477736 and LY2603618 all potentiated the cytotoxicity of the hypoxia-activated mustard pro-drug TH-302 in HT29 colon cancer cells, and comparisons using isogenic pairs of *TP53* +/+ and *TP53* −/− cell lines showed the magnitude of the potentiation to be highest in the *TP53*-deficient background (Meng et al. 2015). The schedule dependence of the combination was investigated for AZD7762, but no difference in the potentiation of cytotoxicity was seen for simultaneous or sequential dosing. In vivo, AZD7762 moderately potentiated the tumor growth delay due to TH-302 treatment in HT29 colon cancer xenografts.

10.3.1.5 Combinations with Ionising Radiation

There is substantial evidence of a beneficial interaction between CHK1 inhibitors and ionising radiation (IR). Thus, CHIR124 moderately sensitized HCT116 colon cancer cells to IR (Tao et al. 2009) and AZD7762 has been reported to sensitize many cell lines to IR (Mitchell et al. 2010a; Morgan et al. 2010; Yang et al. 2011; Hasvold et al. 2013; Kleiman et al. 2013; Williams et al. 2013; Grabauskiene et al. 2014; Patel et al. 2017). In many, but not all, of these studies preferential sensitization of *TP53*-deficient over *TP53*-proficient cells was noted. For example, AZD7762 sensitized *TP53* mutant, but not *TP53* wild type, glioblastoma cell lines to radiation (Williams et al. 2013). In vivo in a PDGF-driven genetically modified mouse model of glioblastoma, the combination of AZD7762 and IR gave greater tumor growth delay than either agent alone. The selective CHK1 inhibitor SAR020106 potentiated fractionated IR and reduced clonogenic survival in *TP53*-deficient head and neck cancer cell lines and in a HNCC xenograft tumor (Borst et al. 2013). Whereas SAR020106 promoted mitotic entry for both radiation-arrested *TP53* wild type and deficient cells, only *TP53* deficient cells underwent apoptosis or became aneuploid, while *TP53* wild type cells arrested in G1 post-mitosis and then re-entered a normal cell cycle. In vivo radio-sensitization has also been demonstrated with triple combinations of gemcitabine and IR (or radio-immunotherapy) with AZD7762 (Morgan et al. 2010), MK8776 (Engelke et al. 2013) and PF00477736 (Al-Ejeh et al. 2014). The potential for combination of CHK1 inhibition with external beam radiotherapy and virus-guided radiovirotherapy has also been explored (Touchefeu et al. 2013).

The role of CHK2 in combination with ionising radiation is generally opposite to that of CHK1. Thus, CHK2-selective inhibitors are consistently found to protect normal human and mouse T cells from IR-mediated toxicity (Arienti et al. 2005; Carlessi et al. 2007; Jobson et al. 2009; Caldwell et al. 2010). CHK2 shRNA radioprotected MYC-driven mouse lymphoma cells (Höglund et al. 2011b) and CHK2 knock-out mice are radio-resistant (Takai et al. 2002). The CHK2 selective inhibitor PV1019 sensitized human gliomblastoma cancer cells to IR (Jobson et al. 2009), but RNAi studies have generally found that CHK2 depletion in cancer cell lines is not radio-sensitizing (Morgan et al. 2010; Yang et al. 2011; Wu et al. 2012) and the selective CHK2 inhibitor CT241533 did not potentiate the toxicity of bleomycin, which creates double-strand breaks in DNA similar to IR (Anderson et al. 2011).

10.3.1.6 Combinations with Molecular-Targeted Agents

Combinations with WEE1 Inhibitors

Considerable preclinical data has emerged in the past 5 years to support the combination of CHK1 inhibition and inhibitors of the DDR tyrosine kinase WEE1, with multiple siRNA screens identifying synthetic lethality between the two targets (Aarts et al. 2015; Carrassa et al. 2012; Chaudhuri et al. 2014; Davies et al. 2011). The selective WEE1 inhibitor MK1775 has been used ubiquitously as a pharmacological tool in these studies (Hirai et al. 2009).

An siRNA screen of 195 cell cycle or DNA damage repair related genes for synthetic lethality with the CHK1 inhibitor AR458323 in three cancer cell lines identified WEE1 siRNA as one of the most consistent hits (Davies et al. 2011). The inhibitors MK1775 and AR458323 were shown to have a synergistic effect on cell viability and induction of apoptosis in multiple cell lines. A screen using siRNA to 719 human kinase genes in combination with CHK1 siRNA in an ovarian cancer cell line resistant to CHK1 inhibitors also found WEE1 gave the most significant synthetic lethality (Carrassa et al. 2012). Studies using non-toxic concentrations of PF00477736 and MK1775 confirmed the synergistic effects of dual inhibition in breast, ovarian, colon and prostate cancer cell lines, independent of their *TP53* status, and showed the cells to undergo premature entry into mitosis before the completion of DNA replication. The combination gave increased tumor growth delay over either single agent in an OVCAR5 ovarian tumor xenograft. CHK1 was also identified from a screen of 1206 siRNAs to sensitize WiDr cells to WEE1 inhibition by MK1775 (Aarts et al. 2015) and the effects on cell viability of the combination were confirmed in a panel of breast and colon cancer cell lines. Synthetic lethality between CHK1 siRNA and MK1775 was seen in four myeloid leukemia cell lines (Chaudhuri et al. 2014). The selective CHK1 inhibitor MK8776 sensitized AML cell lines and patient leukemia cells ex vivo to MK1775, with evidence of increased apoptosis, whereas smaller effects of the combination were observed in normal myeloid progenitor cells.

In vitro and in vivo activity of combined CHK1 and WEE1 inhibition has been demonstrated in several other studies. PF00477736 and MK1775 together gave partial regression of JeKo-1 mantle cell lymphoma xenografts (Chila et al. 2015), while a combination of LY2603618 and MK1775 synergised in AML cell lines and patient tumor cells assayed ex vivo (Qi et al. 2014). The cytotoxicity of MK1775 was potentiated between two and tenfold by the selective CHK1 inhibitor MK8776 in eight cancer cell lines from various tissues, with accumulation of DNA damage observed, and this combination decreased the growth of a LoVo colorectal cancer xenograft (Guertin et al. 2012). Combinatorial inhibition with MK8776 and MK1775 was also effective in neuroblastoma tumor xenografts (Russell et al. 2013), while the CHK1/2 inhibitor AZD7762 gave synergy in combination with MK1775 in nasopharyngeal carcinoma cells (Mak et al. 2015). The combination of AZD7762 and MK1775 was effective in vitro in melanoma cell lines, with decreased viability and increased DNA damage, but no significant benefit was seen for the combination over AZD7762 as a single agent in vivo in a patient-derived melanoma xenograft (Magnussen et al. 2015). The combination of CHK1 inhibitors MK8776 or LY2603618 with MK1775 sensitized HPV-positive head and neck squamous cell cancer cell lines to ionising radiation (Busch et al. 2017).

The combination of CHK1 and WEE1 inhibition is potentially attractive as it elicits the lethal effects of DNA double strand breaks in the cancer cells induced by the combined targeting of the two components of the DDR. Mechanistic studies using MK1775 and various CHK1 inhibitors have suggested that the two drug targets interact synergistically through their regulation of CDK1 activity, causing increased S-phase DNA damage (Guertin et al. 2012; Hauge et al. 2017). A therapeutic index over non-tumor cells has been shown (Guertin et al. 2012; Chaudhuri et al. 2014) but the general extent of the cancer cell selectivity of this combination remains to be fully determined.

Combinations with PARP Inhibitors

Continuing the theme of combining checkpoint kinase inhibition with modulation of other components of the DDR, the connection between CHK1, CHK2 and inhibitors of the DNA repair enzyme poly (ADP-ribose) polymerase (PARP) is becoming increasingly studied. CHK1 inhibition prevents phosphorylation of the DNA binding protein RAD51 and impairs its recruitment to single strand DNA, an early step in the HRR pathway (Bahassi et al. 2008; Thompson and Eastman 2013). Separately, inhibition of PARP prevents single strand break repair through the base-excision repair (BER) pathway, and is synthetically lethal with existing cancer defects in HRR, notably mutations in the BRCA proteins (Curtin 2014). Dual inhibition of CHK1 and PARP is an attractive strategy as the CHK1 inhibitor component induces the HRR deficiency required for synthetic lethality of the PARP inhibitor. Inhibition of multiple DNA repair pathways has the potential to overcome intrinsic redundancy and resistance. However, it appears that both CHK1 and CHK2 have potential interactions with PARP function, thus this is an area where a lack of specificity in the checkpoint kinase inhibitor used may complicate interpretation of preclinical data.

Several PARP1 inhibitors were reported to synergise with the CHK1/2 inhibitor AZD7762 for cytotoxicity toward a panel of breast and pancreatic cancer cell lines (Mitchell et al. 2010b), and AZD7762 and the PARP1 inhibitor olaparib (AZD2281) gave greater than additive cell kill in estrogen-dependent and triple-negative breast cancer cell lines (Tang et al. 2012). This latter in vitro activity was duplicated with dominant negative CHK1 expression combined with the PARP inhibitor, and would therefore seem to be CHK1-driven. In vivo, BT549 and BT474 breast cancer xeno-grafts treated with the AZD7762 and olaparib combination showed significant tumor growth delays and survival advantages over either agent used alone. Four PARP1 inhibitors were found to potentiate the cytotoxicity of AZD7762 or the CHK1-selective inhibitor LY2603618 and to increase activity in the intrinsic apoptosis pathway in mammary carcinoma cells (Booth et al. 2013). The combination of AZD7762 and olaparib sensitized pancreatic cancer cells to ionising radiation, with no effect seen on normal intestinal epithelial cells (Vance et al. 2011). LY2606368 potentiated the efficacy of the PARP inhibitor BMN63 in gastric cancer cell lines and in a patient-derived gastric cancer xenograft model (Yin et al. 2017).

The therapeutic potential of dual CHK2 and PARP inhibition was first shown using siRNA for CHK2 (McCabe et al. 2006). Consistent with this, the selective CHK2 inhibitor CCT241533 potentiated the efficacy of the PARP inhibitors AG14447 and olaparib in HeLa cervical cancer and HT29 colon cancer cells (Anderson et al. 2011). The PARP inhibitors activated signalling through CHK2, presumably as a result of increased double strand breaks occurring upon inhibition of PARP-dependent base excision repair. A comparison of the combinations of either a CHK1/2 or a CHK1-selective inhibitor with the PARP1 inhibitor velapirib (ABT888) in MYC-driven mouse lymphoma cells found robust synergistic increases in apoptotic cell number occurred only with the dual CHK1/2 inhibitor, suggesting that CHK2 inhibition was the dominant effect for synergy in this model (Höglund et al. 2011b).

Combinations with Microtubule-Targeting Agents

CHK1 plays a role in the mitotic checkpoint (Tang et al. 2006) and an interaction with microtubule-targeting agents, e.g., paclitaxel and docetaxel, might be anticipated but results from pharmacological and genetic studies are so far equivocal. CHK1 siRNA sensitized HeLa cells to paclitaxel (Xiao et al. 2005) but CHK1-deficient DT40 avian lymphoma cells were less sensitive to paclitaxel treatment than the wild-type cells (Zachos et al. 2007). A wide cellular screen of the chemo-potentiating activity of MK8776 and AZD7762 found negligible potentiation of anti-mitotic agents (Xiao et al. 2013). However, PF00477736 was found to enhance the efficacy of docetaxel in Colo205 colon cancer cells in vitro and in vivo in two xenograft tumors (Zhang et al. 2009). The combination of AZD7762 and paclitaxel was effective against NSCLC stem-like cells in vitro in colony forming assays where each single agent had minimal effect (Bartucci et al. 2012). There appears to be no role for selective CHK2 inhibition in combination with tubulin-targeting agents (Carlessi et al. 2007).

Combinations with Other Molecular Targeted Agents

So far, there are only a limited number of publications of preclinical combinations of checkpoint kinase inhibitors with molecular targeted agents other than those discussed above. Recent reports may, however, indicate new potential avenues for study, particularly as checkpoint kinase inhibitors advance through clinical development.

DNA repair pathways may be a mechanism of resistance to DNA damage caused by histone deacetylase (HDAC) inhibition, and AZD7762 and CHIR124 increased the sensitivity of both normal human foreskin fibroblasts and tumor cells to the HDAC inhibitors vorinostat, romedepsin and entinostat with evidence of extensive mitotic disruption (Lee et al. 2011). While this study might suggest a poor therapeutic window for the combination, it has also been reported that the CHK1-selective inhibitor MK8776 synergised with vorinostat to kill FLT3-ITD-driven AML cell lines and patient primary AML blasts, without toxicity to normal cord-blood cells (Dai et al. 2013). Certain class I HDAC inhibitors inhibit HRR and non-homologous end joining (NHEJ) DNA repair pathways, although these effects vary with the inhibitor studied (Fukuda et al. 2015), potentially complicating interpretation of the pharmacology of CHK1 and HDAC inhibitor combinations.

In vivo combinatorial activity has been reported for CHK1 and MK2 inhibition in KRAS mutant cancer cell lines and multiple human tumor xenografts, as well as in a genetically modified mouse model of KRAS-driven NSCLC (Dietlein et al. 2015). CHK1 inhibition was effective in combination with MEK1/2 inhibition in proteasome inhibitor-resistant multiple myeloma cells expressing high levels of the anti-apoptotic protein MCL-1 (Pei et al. 2014) and with BTK inhibition in tyrosine kinase-resistant, BCR/ABL-positive leukaemia cells (Nguyen et al. 2015). The CHK1 inhibitor LY2603618 overcame MCL-1 dependent intrinsic resistance to the BCL-2 inhibitor ABT-199 in AML cell lines and primary patient samples (Zhao et al. 2016). The potential for combined CHK2 and ERK1/2 inhibition in diffuse large B-cell lymphoma (DLBCL) has been described (Dai et al. 2011). Inhibition of mTOR has also recently been shown to have synergistic cytotoxicity with the CHK1 inhibitor V158411 in p53 mutant colon cancer cell lines (Massey et al. 2016). Recent findings showed additive or synergistic effects of AZD7762 and the androgen receptor (AR) signalling inhibitor enzalutamide in AR-positive prostate cancer xenograft tumors (Karanika et al. 2017). The combination of AZD7762 and an ATR inhibitor gave a synergistic anti-tumour effect in a lung cancer xenograft model (Sanjiv et al. 2016).

10.3.2   Single Agent Contexts for Checkpoint Kinase Inhibition

Selective inhibitors of the checkpoint kinases have generally not shown potent anti-proliferative activity as single agents against wide panels of cancer cell lines from tumors of different origins. As previously noted (Sect. 2), an exception is LY2606368 (prexasertib) which has broad anti-proliferative activity (King et al. 2015; Lowery et al. 2017). The compound was shown to induce DNA damage and replication catastrophe in the absence of exogenous genotoxic agents.

There is mounting data that selective inhibition of CHK1 has the potential to be an effective monotherapy in cancer cells with high replication stress. In this scenario, oncogene-induced genomic instability and/or associated hyper-replicative states are proposed to render the cancer cells reliant on a constitutive DDR to cope with the replication stress, and in particular with DNA damage arising in S-phase that is repaired dependent on CHK1 activation. The single agent sensitivity can therefore be considered as a form of synthetic lethality with the replication stressed phenotype, leading to replication catastrophe through exhaustion of rate-limiting regulators of replication (Toledo et al. 2017). There is consistent evidence that MYC-driven cancers are sensitive to CHK1 inhibitors (Murga et al. 2011; Höglund et al. 2011a; Ferrao et al. 2012; Walton et al. 2012, 2016; Sen et al. 2017). In particular, this has been demonstrated in vitro and in vivo in preclinical models of MYC-driven lymphoma and neuroblastoma. The link between the DDR and c-MYC has also been explored in nasopharyngeal carcinoma cell lines, which were found to be radio-resistant due to MYC transcription factor-controlled over-expression of CHK1 and CHK2 (Wang et al. 2013). More recently, LY2606368 was shown to have single agent efficacy in xenograft models of cMYC-overexpressing small-cell lung cancer (Sen et al. 2017) and colorectal cancer stem cells with markers of ongoing replication stress had increased sensitivity to LY2606368 (Manic et al. 2017).

A number of studies have focussed on the effects of checkpoint kinase inhibitors on human lymphoma cell lines or genetically modified mouse models of lymphoma. B-cell lymphoma cell lines with endogenous activation of the DDR, and also a genetically modified mouse model of MYC-driven lymphoma, were sensitive to the selective CHK1 inhibitor "Checkin" (Höglund et al. 2011a). Degradation of CHK1 was seen in response to the inhibitor. Mouse Eµ-myc lymphoma cells treated with PF04777376 and AZD7762 showed increased DNA damage and activation of DDR signalling, followed by caspase-dependent apoptosis and cell death (Ferrao et al. 2012). No effect of the agents on normal B cells was detected. The selective oral CHK1 inhibitor CCT245737 was efficacious in vivo as a single agent in the Eµ-myc lymphoma transgenic mouse transplant model of B-cell lymphoma. Significant reduction in the tumor infiltration of the lymph nodes was observed after nine days of inhibitor treatment, with minimal effects on normal tissues such as lung, bone marrow and kidney (Walton et al. 2016). Activity has also been reported for other, earlier checkpoint kinase inhibitors in this model (Murga et al. 2011). An immuno-histochemical analysis of 99 DLBCL patient samples found that all expressed CHK1, CHK2 and the DDR phosphatase CDC25, with 38% expressing activated phospho-CHK1, compared to only 5% expressing phospho-CHK2 (Derenzini et al. 2015). The checkpoint inhibitors PF04777376 and AZD7762 had sub-micromolar activity against these cell lines in viability assays, whereas a Hodgins lymphoma cell line (KMH2) with no elevated DDR was insensitive to either agent, and normal bone marrow cells were also unaffected. A panel of leukaemia and lymphoma cell lines showed equivalent patterns of sub-micromolar sensitivity to the checkpoint inhibitors VER158411 and PF04777376, which were 10 to 100-fold less potent for cytotoxicity against solid tumor cell lines (Bryant et al. 2014b). CHK1 inhibition by VER158411 induced CHK1 degradation, DNA fragmentation and increased γH2Ax phosphorylation, with cell death occurring through caspase dependent and independent mechanisms. However, the sensitive leukaemia and lymphoma cell lines in this study did not have consistently elevated levels of phospho-CHK1.

CHK1 was identified from a siRNA screen as a target protein whose depletion was cytotoxic to paediatric neuroblastoma cell lines (Cole et al. 2011). The neuroblastoma cell lines were sensitive to inhibition of CHK1 by SB128078, and PF00477736 inhibited the growth of subcutaneous NB1643 and NB1691 neuroblastoma xenografts. The selective oral CHK1 inhibitor CCT244747 showed single agent efficacy in a genetically modified mouse model of MYCN-driven neuroblastoma, with a reduction in tumor size demonstrated by magnetic resonance imaging before and after treatment (Walton et al. 2012), and similar oral efficacy was seen with the clinical candidate CCT245737 (SRA737) (Osborne et al. 2016). The in vivo efficacy studies in lymphoma and neuroblastoma models draw attention to the more continuous dosing schedules anticipated for single agent CHK1 inhibition compared to the combinations with genotoxic chemotherapies, although in vivo efficacy in neuroblastoma xenograft models has been shown for the intravenous inhibitor LY2606368 on an intermittent schedule (Lowery et al. 2017).

Beyond MYC-driven tumors, other oncogenic drivers of genomic instability and replication stress have been identified as potential contexts for single agent CHK1 inhibition. Sensitivity to CHK1 siRNA and checkpoint kinase inhibition was identified in complex karyotype AML cells with elevated levels of DNA damage and DDR activation (Cavelier et al. 2009). The checkpoint inhibitors AZD7762, CHIR124 and SCH900776 inhibited the growth of FLT3-ITD positive MV411 AML cells, but not the FLT3-ITD negative K562 leukaemia cell line (Yuan et al. 2014). AZD7762 and CHIR124 were found to inhibit FLT3 directly while SCH900776 was selective for CHK1 over this kinase. Importantly, SCH900776 decreased the clonogenic growth of leukemic progenitor cells isolated from primary patient samples. CHK1 was found to be overexpressed and constitutively activated in a majority of T-cell acute lymphoblastic leukemia (T-ALL) cell lines and primary patient samples, associated with an intrinsically high level of replication stress (Sarmento et al. 2015). PF00477736 potently inhibited the viability of the T-ALL cell lines, enhanced apoptosis in ex vivo primary T-ALL patient cells, and gave a tumor growth delay in a T-ALL subcutaneous xenograft.

A screen of the sensitivity of breast cancer cell lines to PF00477736 found that TNBC cells, but not luminal or HER2-positive breast cancer cells, were sensitive to the inhibitor in viability and clonogenic assays (Shibata et al. 2011). The sensitivity was correlated with high expression of activated phospho-CHK1. The potential for checkpoint kinase inhibition in TNBC cells was also demonstrated in vitro using V158411, PF00477736 and AZD7762, which inhibited cell proliferation (Bryant et al. 2014a). TNBC cells were found to be more sensitive than estrogen receptor positive breast cancer or other solid tumor cell lines. The same authors also showed single agent sensitivity of some ovarian cancer cell lines to V158411, PF00477736 and AZD7762. CHK1 inhibition by two compounds (structures not disclosed) was reported to be effective against melanoma cell lines (Brooks et al. 2013). Thus while the range and impact of single agent CHK1 inhibition is still being defined, it is clear that the use of the inhibitors is likely to extend beyond combination therapies and present potential opportunities for single agent clinical investigation.

10.4 Preclinical Biomarkers for Checkpoint Kinase Inhibitors

Biomarkers have been an important component of both the discovery and development of checkpoint kinase inhibitors (Garrett and Collins 2011). They can be divided into two major types; those that detect target engagement (proof-of-mechanism biomarkers) and those that will predict response to target engagement (predictive biomarkers). Biomarkers to detect on-target activity of an inhibitor can be correlated with pharmacokinetic and tumour efficacy data (preclinical or clinical) to provide the evidence that the inhibitor is responsible for antitumour efficacy through target engagement, a concept originally defined as the Pharmacological Audit Trail (Workman 2003). This concept has been further developed to take account of other factors including predictive biomarkers (Tan et al. 2009; Yap and Workman 2012). The ability to identify those patients who will respond to a drug, can provide the most effective and rapid clinical development route to registration and so predictive biomarkers are now also seen as a critical component of the pharmacological audit trail.

10.4.1 Biomarkers of Target Engagement

For any drug target, the availability of biomarkers that are either on or proximal to the target will provide the highest level of confidence that biomarker changes reflect a change in its activity and thereby demonstrate proof-of mechanism for the drug. In the case of kinases, the most proximal biomarker of target engagement is autophosphorylation by the target itself and this is indeed the case for both CHK1 and CHK2.

Site-specific autophosphorylation of human CHK1 was initially detected and confirmed at serine 296 on the protein (Clarke and Clarke 2005). The availability of phospho-specific antibodies that detect this signal has allowed its use as a biomarker of CHK1 activity by many researchers involved in the discovery and development of CHK1 inhibitors. In particular, induction of the pSer296 signal in response to DNA damage with classical chemotherapeutics and subsequent signal loss through CHK1 kinase inhibition has been extensively reported (Walton et al. 2010, 2012, 2016; Morgan et al. 2010; Wang et al. 2014; Ma et al. 2013). This biomarker has also been used to demonstrate high intrinsic CHK1 activity in cancer cells and subsequent signal loss on addition of a CHK1 inhibitor (Cole et al. 2011; Bryant et al. 2014a).

Two other keys sites of phosphorylation on CHK1 are Serine 317 (pSer317) and Serine 345 (pSer345) found in the C-terminal regulatory domain of CHK1. Both are phosphorylated by the upstream kinase ATR and required for full activation of CHK1, although serine 345 appears to be the more critical residue (Walker et al. 2009). Published data on the use of these two phospho-signals as biomarkers of target engagement is varied, in particular for the combination setting. Studies with the dual CHK1/2 inhibitor AZD7762 have reported upregulation of pSer345 in response to gemcitabine alone and in combination with ionising radiation, with further enhancement of this signal in the presence of AZD7762 (Morgan et al. 2010). The primary cause of pSer345 CHK1 induction was proposed to be enhanced DNA damage due to CHK1 inhibition causing a subsequent increase in ATR. It was also proposed that a secondary contributor to induction of pSer345 was inhibition of the CHK1 phosphatase PP2A (Morgan et al. 2010; Parsels et al. 2011). In contrast, Rawlinson and Massey reported down regulation of both pSer317 and pSer345 with all cytotoxics in combination with the CHK1 inhibitor V158411 (Rawlinson and Massey 2014). Studies with other structurally unrelated CHK1 inhibitors in combination with classical chemotherapeutic agents has shown no consistent enhancement of pSer317 or pSer345 when the CHK1 inhibitor is combined with a chemotherapeutic agent (Walton et al. 2012, 2016). The differences in these reports may be due to the fact that phosphorylation on Ser317 and Ser345 is a dynamic event, the use of different cell lines or possibly that the effects seen are inhibitor specific. A number of studies which include the use of a CHK1 inhibitor as a single agent have reported induction of pSer345 and/or pSer317 on CHK1, suggesting that in this context, up regulation of these signals may be a biomarker of response to target inhibition (Morgan et al. 2010; Parsels et al. 2011; Walton et al. 2012, 2016).

CHK1 substrate phosphorylation also provides the opportunity for additional biomarkers of target engagement. A number of human CHK1 substrates have been identified including the CDC25 family of phosphatases and the DNA repair protein Rad51 (Sanchez et al. 1997; Peng et al. 1997; Sørensen et al. 2005). Screening activities have identified additional substrates of CHK1 including the transcriptional co-repressor, KAP1 phosphatase and the tumour suppressor and DNA repair protein BRCA1 (O'Neill et al. 2002; Clarke and Clarke 2005; Kim et al. 2007; Blasius et al. 2011). The CDC25 family of phosphatases are the most comprehensively studied and extensively used CHK1 substrate biomarkers of CHK1 activity. CDC25A is phosphorylated by CHK1 on multiple sites, which target it for ubiquitin-mediated proteolysis (Sørensen et al. 2003). Therefore inhibition of CHK1 alone is predicted to lead to CDC25A accumulation and when combined with genotoxic chemotherapy to block DNA damage induced turnover of CDC25A. Indeed a number CHK1 inhibitors have been shown to induce or stabilise CDC25A expression alone or in combination with DNA damaging agents respectively (Morgan et al. 2010; King et al. 2015; Sakurikar et al. 2016). Phosphorylation of CDC25C at serine 216 has also been used as a biomarker of CHK1 activity although not as extensively as CDC25A stabilisation (Graves et al. 2000; Zhang et al. 2009).

Detection of CHK2 activity and its inhibition has mainly focussed on autophosphorylation at serine 516. Phospho-specific antibodies that detect the pS516 signal are available commercially and have been used by a number of researchers to monitor the activity of CHK2 inhibitors in cells (Jobson et al. 2009; Anderson et al. 2011; Nguyen et al. 2012; Duong et al. 2013). A number of substrates have also been identified for CHK2, therefore offering the potential for additional biomarkers of CHK2 activity. However there is significant overlap with CHK1 substrates including KAP1, BRCA1, p53 and the CDC25 family of phosphatases,

(O'Neill et al. 2002; Pommier et al. 2006; Kim et al. 2007; Blasius et al. 2011; Seo et al. 2003). Their use, therefore, as biomarkers of either CHK1 or CHK2 activity must be carefully considered. Other substrates which appear to be specific for CHK2 are E2F1, HDMX, and PML (Yang et al. 2002; Stevens et al. 2003; Buscemi et al. 2006; Pommier et al. 2006). Active CHK2 phosphorylates HDMX at serine 367, which leads to ubiquitin mediated proteolysis of this protein. A number of selective CHK2 inhibitors have been shown to block DNA damage induced turnover of HDMX, which could therefore be considered a biomarker of CHK2 activity (Carlessi et al. 2007; Jobson et al. 2009; Anderson et al. 2011).

10.4.2   Predictors of Sensitivity

In the preclinical setting, the ability to predict which cell lines or in vivo tumour models will respond to inhibitors of a particular drug target can be of great value. This is especially true during lead optimisation when multiple compounds are being evaluated. The greatest value however, is in the clinical setting where being able to identify those patients who will respond to a new agent, can greatly speed up clinical development and time to registration. A case in point is imatinib mesylate, which was granted accelerated approval by the FDA in 2001, based on the results of three single-arm Phase II studies conducted in CML patients identified as being Philadelphia chromosome–positive, a predictive biomarker of response for the drug (Cohen et al. 2002). In this context, a predictive biomarker can therefore save time, money and most importantly, patient lives. Studies in the preclinical setting to identify predictive biomarkers for a particular drug target are therefore an important component of drug discovery and development.

There has been extensive research on predictive biomarkers of cellular sensitivity to CHK1 inhibition, both alone and in combination with genotoxic cancer agents. The combination setting was the first therapeutic strategy proposed for CHK1 and the tumour suppressor *TP53* has been the focus of much of the research in this area. *TP53* has an essential role in the G1 DNA damage induced cell cycle checkpoint where it upregulates expression of the CDK inhibitor p21CIP1/WAF1 to block CDK activity leading to G1 arrest (Lane 1992; Bartek and Lukas 2001). The *TP53* gene is often found mutated in cancer, leading to a defective DNA damage induced G1 checkpoint and a reliance by cancer cells on S and G2 checkpoints, where CHK1 is required. This led to the hypothesis that inhibition of CHK1 in combination with a genotoxic chemotherapeutic would be more effective in cells where *TP53* is defective (Dixon and Norbury 2002). Thus mutation of the *TP53* gene would potentially predict sensitivity to CHK1 inhibition in this combination setting. This hypothesis was supported in studies using the dual CHK1/2 inhibitor UCN-01 where it was found that the combination of UCN-01 with chemotherapeutic agents showed greater efficacy in *TP53* deficient versus wild-type cancer cells (Wang et al. 1996; Shao et al. 1997; Sugiyama et al. 2000). There is also evidence that in certain disease types, for example head and neck cancer and triple negative breast cancer, that this hypothesis holds true (Borst et al. 2013; Ma et al. 2012). Other studies however, have shown that both wild-type and *TP53* deficient cancers cells can be similarly sensitive to the combination of CHK1 inhibitor with genotoxic anti-cancer agent (Barnard et al. 2016; Xiao et al. 2013). It is possible that these wild-type *TP53* cancer cells have other defects in the *TP53* signalling pathway. For example, amplification of MDM2, an E3 ligase and negative regulator of *TP53*, or mutation of p14ARF, a negative regulator of MDM, causing the G1 DNA damaged induced checkpoint to be functionally defective (Gallagher et al. 2006). Alternatively, they may harbour mutations in other DNA damage response or DNA repair pathways that are essential, when a cell is subjected to DNA damage, and CHK1 is inhibited. An example of this is the curative response of a patient with metastatic small cell cancer to the CHK1/2 inhibitor AZD7762 in combination with weekly irinotecan (Al-Ahmadie et al. 2014). The patient was subsequently shown to have a hemizygous mutation in the Mre11 complex gene *RAD50* that caused reduced ATM signalling. Loss of ATM signalling in the presence of CHK1 inhibition was a synthetic lethal event leading to extreme tumour versus normal cell sensitivity to irinotecan.

An additional factor to be considered when predicting sensitivity to CHK1 inhibition in combination with chemotherapy or IR is the type of genotoxic agent used. For example, it has been reported by several groups that the greatest synergy seen with CHK1 inhibitors is in combination with antimetabolites, and in particular with gemcitabine (See Sect. 3.1: Combinations with anti-metabolites). In this context, synergy has been reported to be associated with high levels of replication stress and DNA damage leading to accumulation of tumour cells in S phase, and replication catastrophe rather than G2 checkpoint abrogation. It may be that that the level of intrinsic replication stress in a tumour cell, can predict sensitivity to combined CHK1/gemcitabine treatment. One study has also reported that elevated levels of the ribonuclease reductase M1 protein (RRM1), the regulatory sub-unit of ribonucleotide reductase (RNR), predicts sensitivity to combined treatment with gemcitabine and a CHK1 inhibitor (Zhou et al. 2013). RNR catalyzes the reduction of ribonucleotides to generate deoxyribonucleotides (dNTPs), which are required for DNA replication and DNA repair processes and it is also a target of gemcitabine, which covalently binds to and inhibits the RRM1 sub-unit. The proposed rationale for sensitivity to combined CHK1/gemcitabine treatment is that CHK1 inhibition leads to a decrease in expression of RRM1, a target of gemcitabine, thus allowing greater efficacy of the drug. However the authors also report that their previous work (Gautam and Bepler 2006), identified a delayed G2 progression when RRM1 is overexpressed and therefore CHK1 inhibition may overcome this. A more recent study (Taricani et al. 2014) has shown a direct association between CHK1 and RNR sub-units in cells, which may represent a close relationship between the DNA replication machinery (RNR) and effectors of the replication checkpoint (CHK1). In summary, sensitivity to CHK1 inhibition in combination with chemotherapy or IR may be dependent on a number factors including, the presence of a specific biomarker, the specific disease type and also on the type of genotoxic treatment given. The potential that one biomarker will therefore predict sensitivity to CHK1 inhibition in all disease types with all drug combinations is unrealistic.

As discussed earlier there are now multiple studies that report single agent efficacy in the preclinical setting with potent and selective CHK1 inhibitors. The leading hypothesis for sensitivity to CHK1 inhibition is that instead of extrinsic DNA damage being provided by chemotherapy or ionising radiation, the DNA damage is intrinsic to the tumour with two key sources being oncogenes and defects in DNA damage and repair genes that can both induce genomic instability and/or replication stress (Toledo et al. 2011). In many cases this will lead to reliance on CHK1 activity, in particular with DNA damage arising in S-phase (due to replication stress) that is repaired dependent on CHK1 activation. The reliance of these cellular DNA damage phenotypes on CHK1 could therefore be considered a form of synthetic lethality. Thus potential biomarkers of CHK1 inhibitor sensitivity may include gene changes that induce genome instability and replication stress and known biomarkers of these cell phenotypes, examples of which are given below.

One gene family, which when overexpressed in cancer cells causes replication stress and induces sensitivity to CHK1 inhibition, is MYC. In particular, preclinical models of MYC-driven lymphoma and neuroblastoma have shown sensitivity to CHK1 inhibitors both in vitro and in vivo (Murga et al. 2011; Höglund et al. 2011a; Ferrao et al. 2012; Walton et al. 2016). However, whilst MYC gene amplification may drive CHK1 inhibitor sensitivity (through higher levels of replication stress), it is already clear that testing for *MYC* gene amplification alone may not be sufficient to identify all patient tumours in a particular disease population that may be sensitive to CHK1 inhibition. For example, Cole et al. reported that CHK1 inhibitor sensitivity in neuroblastoma correlated with total MYC (MYCN and c-MYC) protein expression and not just *MYCN* gene amplification alone (Cole et al. 2011). Further evidence of this is a recent study in small-cell lung cancer where it was found that high cMYC protein expression was the top biomarker of sensitivity to two CHK1 inhibitors. High cMYC protein expression was observed in both *cMYC*-amplified and non-amplified cell lines (Sen et al. 2017), leading to the proposal that the optimal biomarker would be detection of cMYC protein expression and not gene amplification.

There are now multiple reports of defects in DNA damage and repair genes that are synthetically lethal with CHK1 inhibition and therefore may also be biomarkers of sensitivity to CHK1 inhibitors. One key example is the study by Chen et al., which showed that Fanconi Anemia (FA) deficient cell lines were hypersensitive to CHK1 loss using both independent siRNAs and CHK1 pharmacologic inhibition with Gö6976 and UCN-01 (Chen et al. 2009). More recently the loss of the DNA polymerase POLD1 demonstrated synthetic lethality with pharmacological inhibition of both ATR and CHK1 (Hocke et al. 2016). Thus POLD1 deficiency, which is seen in some cancers, may represent a predictive biomarker for treatment response with either ATR or CHK1 inhibitors. Another example of synthetic lethality with CHK1 inhibition is loss of the trimethyl mark found on lysine 36 of histone H3 (H3K36me3). In a recent study it was shown that cancers which exhibit loss of the H3K36me3 signal are sensitive to both WEE1 and CHK1 inhibition (Pfister et al. 2015). This appears to be due to loss of expression of the ribonuclease reductase subunit 2 (RRM2), which is positively regulated by H3K36me3 facilitated transcription initiation factor recruitment and WEE1/CHK1 signalling. Therefore potential biomarkers of CHK1 inhibitor sensitivity in tumours are low H3K36me3 signal, mutation/loss of the H3K36 methyl transferase SETD2 or overexpression of the H3K36 demethylase, KDM4A. Recently, expression of functional DNA-PKcs has been found to correlate with sensitivity to the CHK1 inhibitor V158411 (Massey et al. 2016). In this study mTOR inhibition caused down regulation of proteins involved in HRR and interstrand crosslink repair and increased sensitivity to CHK1 inhibition. Unexpectedly, it was also reported that cells with defective DNA-PKcs were, paradoxically, resistant to CHK1 inhibition whilst cells with functional DNA-PKcs were more sensitive. There was also a positive correlation between CHK1 and DNA-PKcs expression in several tumour types including lung and hepatocellular carcinoma. Thus high DNA-PKcs expression (which correlates with high CHK1 expression) may be a predictor of sensitivity to CHK1 inhibition in specific tumour types.

Moving on to biomarkers of DNA damage and replication stress, both γH2AX (pSer139H2AX) and replication protein A (RPA) have been proposed as potential biomarkers of sensitivity to CHK1 inhibition. There are now reports that elevated γH2AX correlates with sensitivity to CHK1 inhibition in a number of tumour types including luminal breast cancer, melanoma and T-cell acute lymphoblastic leukemia (T-ALL) (Bryant et al. 2014a; Brooks et al. 2013; Sarmento et al. 2015). A further study in a panel of lung, leukemia and lymphoma cell lines also reported a weak correlation between the level of γH2AX in these cell lines and sensitivity to the CHK1 inhibitor V158411, but this relationship was lost if the leukemia and lymphoma cell lines were removed (Bryant et al. 2014b). A recent report also suggests that elevated phosphorylation of histone H3.3 at serine 31 may predict sensitivity to CHK1 inhibition of human Alternative Lengthening of Telomeres (ALT) cancers, through CHK1 acting as a H3.3 kinase at this site (Chang et al. 2015). For RPA, direct evidence for correlation of CHK1 inhibitor sensitivity with elevated total or phosphorylated RPA protein is limited. Sarmento and colleagues reported that T-ALL cells exhibit high levels of replication stress including elevated phospho-RPA32 and are sensitive to the CHK1 inhibitor PF-004777736 (Sarmento et al. 2015). There has also been a report that cancer cells with activated replication stress are dependent on ATR and CHK1 to prevent exhaustion of nuclear RPA and therefore sensitive to CHK1 inhibition by UCN-01 (Toledo et al. 2013). However, this study did not provide evidence of correlation between phosphorylation status of RPA and sensitivity to CHK1 inhibition. However, interest in RPA as a potential biomarker of CHK1 inhibitor sensitivity will most surely be re-ignited with the recent review by Toledo and colleagues, which brings together the concepts of replication stress, RPA exhaustion and replication catastrophe and proposes how inhibitors of ATR/CHK1/WEE1 may trigger replication catastrophe (Toledo et al. 2017).

Finally, the status of CHK1 itself may be a biomarker of sensitivity to inhibition of this protein as a drug target. This can currently be defined by the level of total CHK1 expression, autophosphorylation at pSer296 or the phosphorylation status of the ATR target sites Ser317 and Ser345. In the in T-ALL study that reported high levels of H2AX and phospho-RPA32 and sensitivity to the CHK1 inhibitor PF00477736, CHK1 itself was found to be overexpressed and exhibited high levels of phosphorylation on both Ser296 and Ser317 in the majority of the T-ALL cell lines and primary patient samples (Sarmento et al. 2015). High CHK1 expression has also been highlighted as an adverse prognostic marker, and potential predictive biomarker of CHK1 inhibitor sensitivity in MYC-driven medulloblastoma (Prince et al. 2016). An in vitro study in multiple cancer types using V158411, PF00477736 and AZD7762 demonstrated potent inhibition of cell proliferation in TNBC and ovarian cancer cell lines, which correlated with high levels of pSer296 CHK1 (Bryant et al. 2014a). A correlation between high pSer317CHK1 levels in TNBC and sensitivity to CHK1 inhibition (PF00477736) has also been reported (Shibata et al. 2011). Unfortunately the pSer296CHK1 signal was not investigated in this study. In contrast, the study in lung cancer, leukemia and lymphoma cell lines with V158411 found no correlation between the levels of pSer345CHK1 and sensitivity to this inhibitor (Bryant et al. 2014b). In conclusion, data on the phosphorylation status of CHK1 and correlation with CHK1 inhibitor sensitivity is limited. Further evaluation of these candidate biomarkers should help define their potential use for patient stratification before CHK1 inhibitor treatment in the clinic.

10.5   Conclusion

Over the past two decades, research on CHK1 and CHK2 has been interwoven with the discovery and development of ATP competitive inhibitors of these two kinases. Studies using both gene knockdown technologies and pharmacological intervention have consistently shown that loss of CHK1 function sensitises cancer cells to a variety of chemotherapeutic agents and CHK1 inhibitors are currently undergoing clinical evaluation in this setting. There is also strong preclinical evidence for the use of CHK1 inhibitors as radiosensitisers, but this remains to be tested in the clinic. In contrast to CHK1, the majority of loss-of-CHK2 function studies demonstrate a lack of sensitisation to either chemotherapeutic agents (apart from PARP inhibitors) or ionising radiation. Indeed loss of CHK2 function appears to act as a radioprotector rather than a radiopotentiator. Thus, a number of CHK1 inhibitors have proceeded into the clinic, whilst to date, no selective CHK2 inhibitors have progressed to this stage. Single agent activity has also been demonstrated with multiple CHK1 inhibitors in a number of tumour types. However, unlike the synthetically lethal combination of PARP inhibition with deficiency in BRCA gene function, to date there is no one clear biomarker of sensitivity to single agent CHK1 inhibition. Indeed, it may be that different tumour types will each reveal distinct biomarkers of sensitivity to CHK1 inhibition that may each depend on a specific gene change in that disease context. A key question for the next decade therefore is can we identify the best way to use CHK1 and CHK2 inhibitors, be it as single agents, chemo/radio-sensitisors or even as radioprotectors?

References

Aarts M, Bajrami I, Herrera-Abreu MT et al (2015) Functional genetic screen identifies increased sensitivity to WEE1 inhibition in cells with defects in Fanconi Anemia and HR pathways. Mol Cancer Ther 14:865–876

Al-Ahmadie H, Iyer G, Hohl M et al (2014) Synthetic lethality in ATM-deficient RAD50-mutant tumors underlies outlier response to cancer therapy. Cancer Discov 4:1014–1021

Al-Ejeh F, Pajic M, Shi W et al (2014) Gemcitabine and CHK1 inhibition potentiate EGFR-directed radioimmunotherapy against pancreatic ductal adenocarcinoma. Clin Cancer Res 20:3187–3197

Anderson VE, Walton MI, Eve PD et al (2011) CCT241533 is a potent and selective inhibitor of CHK2 that potentiates the cytotoxicity of PARP inhibitors. Cancer Res 71:463–472

Antoni L, Sodha N, Collins I et al (2007) CHK2 kinase: cancer susceptibility and cancer therapy – two sides of the same coin? Nat Rev Cancer 7:925–936

Arienti KL, Brunmark A, Axe FU et al (2005) Checkpoint kinase inhibitors: SAR and radioprotective properties of a series of 2-arylbenzimidazoles. J Med Chem 48:1873–1885

Aris SM, Pommier Y (2012) Potentiation of the novel topoisomerase I inhibitor indenoisoquinoline LMP-400 by the cell checkpoint and Chk1-Chk2 inhibitor AZD7762. Cancer Res 72:979–989

Arora S, Bisanz KM, Peralta LA et al (2010) RNAi screening of the kinome identifies modulators of cisplatin response in ovarian cancer cells. Gynecol Oncol 118:220–227

Azorsa DO, Gonzales IM, Basu GD et al (2009) Synthetic lethal RNAi screening identifies sensitizing targets for gemcitabine therapy in pancreatic cancer. J Transl Med 7:43

Bahassi EM, Ovesson JL, Riesenberg AL et al (2008) The checkpoint kinases Chk1 and Chk2 regulate the functional associations between hBRCA2 and Rad51 in response to DNA damage. Oncogene 27:3977–3985

Barnard D, Diaz HB, al BT (2016) LY2603618, a selective CHK1 inhibitor, enhances the antitumor effect of gemcitabine in xenograft tumor models. Investig New Drugs 34(1):49–60

Bartek J, Lukas J (2001) Pathways governing G1/S transition and their response to DNA damage. FEBS Lett 490:117–122

Bartucci M, Svensson S, Romania P et al (2012) Therapeutic targeting of Chk1 in NSCLC stem cells during chemotherapy. Cell Death Differ 19:768–788

Bennett CN, Tomlinson CC, Michalowski AM et al (2012) Cross-species genomic and functional analyses identify a combination therapy using a CHK1 inhibitor and a ribonucleotide reductase inhibitor to treat triple-negative breast cancer. Breast Cancer Res 14:R109

Blackwood E, Epler J, Yen I, Flagella M et al (2013) Combination drug scheduling defines a "window of opportunity" for chemopotentiation of gemcitabine by an orally bioavailable, selective ChK1 inhibitor, GNE-900. Mol Cancer Ther 12:1968–1980

Blasina A, Hallin J, Chen E et al (2008) Breaching the DNA damage checkpoint via PF-00477736, a novel small-molecule inhibitor of checkpoint kinase 1. Mol Cancer Ther 7:2394–2404

Blasius M, Forment JV, Thakkar N et al (2011) A phospho-proteomic screen identifies substrates of the checkpoint kinase Chk1. Genome Biol 12:R78

Booth L, Cruickshanks N, Ridder T et al (2013) PARP and CHK inhibitors interact to cause DNA damage and cell death in mammary carcinoma cells. Cancer Biol Ther 14:458–465

Borst GR, McLaughlin M, Kyula JN et al (2013) Targeted radiosensitization by the Chk1 inhibitor SAR-020106. Int J Radiat Oncol Biol Phys 85:1110–1118

Brooks K, Oakes V, Edwards B et al (2013) A potent Chk1 inhibitor is selectively cytotoxic in melanomas with high levels of replicative stress. Oncogene 32:788–796

Bryant C, Rawlinson R, Massey AJ (2014a) Chk1 Inhibition as a novel therapeutic strategy for treating triple-negative breast and ovarian cancers. BMC Cancer 14:570

Bryant C, Scriven K, Massey AJ (2014b) Inhibition of the checkpoint kinase Chk1 induces DNA damage and cell death in human Leukemia and Lymphoma cells. Mol Cancer 13:147

Bucher N, Britten CD (2008) G2 checkpoint abrogation and checkpoint kinase-1 targeting in the treatment of cancer. Br J Cancer 98:523–528

Busby EC, Leistritz DF, Abraham RT et al (2000) The radiosensitizing agent 7-hydroxystaurospo-rine (UCN-01) inhibits the DNA damage checkpoint kinase hChk1. Cancer Res 60:2108–2112

Buscemi G, Carlessi L, Zannini L et al (2006) DNA damage-induced cell cycle regulation and function of novel Chk2 phosphoresidues. Mol Cell Biol 26:7832–7845

Busch CJ, Kröger MS, Jensen J et al (2017) G2-checkpoint targeting and radiosensitization of HPV/p16-positiveHNSCC cells through the inhibition of Chk1 and Wee1. Radiother Oncol 122:260–266

Caldwell JJ, Welsh EJ, Matijssen C et al (2010) Structure-based design of potent and selective 2-(quinazolin-2-yl)phenol inhibitors of checkpoint kinase 2. J Med Chem 54:580–590

Calvo E, Chen VJ, Marshall M et al (2014) Preclinical analyses and phase I evaluation of LY2603618 administered in combination with Pemetrexed and cisplatin in patients with advanced cancer. Investig New Drugs 32:955–968

Carlessi L, Buscemi G, Larson G et al (2007) Biochemical and cellular characterization of VRX0466617, a novel and selective inhibitor for the checkpoint kinase Chk2. Mol Cancer Ther 6:935–944

Carrassa L, Broggini M, Erba E et al (2004) Chk1, but not Chk2, is involved in the cellular response to DNA damaging agents: differential activity in cells expressing or not p53. Cell Cycle 3:1177–1181

Carrassa L, Chilà R, Lupi M et al (2012) Combined inhibition of Chk1 and Wee1: in vitro syner-gistic effect translates to tumor growth inhibition in vivo. Cell Cycle 11:2507–2517

Cavelier C, Didier C, Prade N et al (2009) Constitutive activation of the DNA damage signalling pathway in acute myeloid leukaemia with complex karyotype: potential importance in check-point targeting therapy. Cancer Res 69:8652–8661

Chang FT, Chan FL, R McGhie JD et al (2015) CHK1-driven histone H3.3 serine 31 phosphory-lation is important for chromatin maintenance and cell survival in human ALT cancer cells. Nucleic Acids Res 43:2603–2614

Chaudhuri L, Vincelette ND, Koh BD et al (2014) CHK1 and WEE1 inhibition combine synergistically to enhance therapeutic efficacy in acute myeloid leukemia ex vivo. Haematologica 99:688–696

Chen CC, Kennedy RD, Sidi S et al (2009) CHK1 inhibition as a strategy for targeting Fanconi Anemia (FA) DNA repair pathway deficient tumors. Mol Cancer 8:24

Chen T, Stephens PA, Middleton FK et al (2012) Targeting the S and G2 checkpoint to treat cancer. Drug Discov Today 17:194–202

Chila R, Basana A, Lupi M et al (2015) Combined inhibition of Chk1 and Wee1 as a new therapeu-tic strategy for mantle cell lymphoma. Oncotarget 6:3394–3408

Clarke CA, Clarke PR (2005) DNA-dependent phosphorylation of Chk1 and Claspin in a human cell-free system. Biochem J 388:705–712

Cohen MH, Williams G, Johnson JR et al (2002) Approval summary for imatinib mesylate cap-sules in the treatment of chronic myelogenous leukemia. Clin Cancer Res 8:935–942

Cole KA, Huggins J, Laquaglia M et al (2011) RNAi screen of the protein kinome identifies checkpoint kinase 1 (CHK1) as a therapeutic target in neuroblastoma. Proc Natl Acad Sci U S A 108:3336–3341

Curtin N (2014) PARP inhibitors for anticancer therapy. Biochem Soc Trans 42:82–88

Dai B, Zhao XF, Mazan-Mamczarz K et al (2011) Functional and molecular interactions between ERK and CHK2 in diffuse large B-cell lymphoma. Nat Commun 2:402

Dai Y, Chen S, Kmieciak M et al (2013) The novel Chk1 inhibitor MK-8776 sensitizes human leukemia cells to HDAC inhibitors by targeting the intra-S checkpoint and DNA replication and repair. Mol Cancer Ther 12:878–889

Dai Y, Grant S (2010) New insights into checkpoint kinase 1 in the DNA damaging response signalling network. Clin Cancer Res 16:376–383

Davies KD, Cable PL, Garrus JE et al (2011) Chk1 inhibition and Wee1 inhibition combine synergistically to impede cellular proliferation. Cancer Biol Ther 12:788–796

Derenzini E, Agostinelli C, Imbrogno E et al (2015) Constitutive activation of the DNA damage response pathway as a novel therapeutic target in diffuse large B-cell lymphoma. Oncotarget 6:6553–6569

Didier C, Demur C, Grimal F et al (2012) Evaluation of checkpoint kinase targeting therapy in acute myeloid leukemia with complex karyotype. Cancer Biol Ther 13:307–313

Dietlein F, Kalb B, Jokic M et al (2015) A synergistic interaction between Chk1- and MK2 inhibitors in KRAS-mutant cancer. Cell 162:146–159

Dixon H, Norbury CJ (2002) Therapeutic exploitation of checkpoint defects in cancer cells lacking p53 function. Cell Cycle 1:362–368

Duong HQ, Hong YB, Kim JS, Lee HS, Yi YW, Kim YJ, Wang A, Zhao W, Cho CH, Seong YS, Bae I (2013) Inhibition of checkpoint kinase 2 (CHK2) enhances sensitivity of pancreatic adenocarcinoma cells to gemcitabine. J Cell Mol Med 17:1261–1270

Engelke CG, Parsels LA, Qian Y et al (2013) Sensitization of pancreatic cancer to chemoradiation by the chk1 inhibitor MK8776. Clin Cancer Res 19:4412–4421

Ferrao PT, Bukczynska EP, Johnstone RW et al (2012) Efficacy of CHK inhibitors as single agents in MYC-driven lymphoma cells. Oncogene 31:1661–1672

Fukuda T, Wu W, Okada M et al (2015) Class I histone deacetylase inhibitors inhibit the retention of BRCA1 and 53BP1 at the site of DNA damage. Cancer Sci 106:1050–1056

Gadhikar MA, Sciuto MR, Alves MV et al (2013) Chk1/2 inhibition overcomes the cisplatin resistance of head and neck cancer cells secondary to the loss of functional p53. Mol Cancer Ther 12:1860–1873

Gallagher SJ, Kefford RF, Rizos H (2006) The ARF tumour suppressor. Int J Biochem Cell Biol 38:1637–1641

Garrett MD, Collins I (2011) Anticancer therapy with checkpoint inhibitors: what, where and when? Trends Pharmacol Sci 32:308–316

Gautam A, Bepler G (2006) Suppression of lung tumor formation by the regulatory subunit of ribonucleotide reductase. Cancer Res 66:6497–6502

Gazzard L, Williams K, Chen H et al (2015) Mitigation of acetylcholine esterase activity in the 1,7-diazacarbazole series of inhibitors of checkpoint kinase 1. J Med Chem 58:5053–5074

Grabauskiene S, Bergeron EJ, Chen G et al (2014) Checkpoint kinase 1 protein expression indicates sensitization to therapy by checkpoint kinase 1 inhibition in non-small cell lung cancer. J Surg Res 187:6–13

Graves PR, Yu L, Schwarz JK, Gales J et al (2000) The Chk1 protein kinase and the Cdc25C regulatory pathways are targets of the anticancer agent UCN-01. J Biol Chem 275:5600–5605

Guertin AD, Martin MM, Roberts B et al (2012) Unique functions of CHK1 and WEE1 underlie synergistic anti-tumor activity upon pharmacologic inhibition. Cancer Cell Int 12:45

Guzi TJ, Paruch K, Dwyer MP et al (2011) Targeting the replication checkpoint using SCH 900776, a potent and functionally selective CHK1 inhibitor identified via high content screening. Mol Cancer Ther 10:591–602

Hasvold G, Nähse-Kumpf V, Tkacz-Stachowska K et al (2013) The efficacy of CHK1 inhibitors is not altered by hypoxia, but is enhanced after reoxygenation. Mol Cancer Ther 12:705–716

Hauge S, Naucke C, Hasvold G et al (2017) Combined inhibition of Wee1 and Chk1 gives synergistic DNA damage in S-phase due to distinct regulation of CDK activity and CDC45 loading. Oncotarget 8:10966–10979

Hirai H, Iwasawa Y, Okada M et al (2009) Small-molecule inhibition of Wee1 kinase by MK-1775 selectively sensitizes p53-deficient tumor cells to DNA-damaging agents. Mol Cancer Ther 8:2992–3000

Höglund A, Nilsson LM, Muralidharan SV et al (2011a) Therapeutic implications for the induced levels of Chk1 in Myc-expressing cancer cells. Clin Cancer Res 17:7067–7079

Höglund A, Strömvall K, Li Y et al (2011b) Chk2 deficiency in Myc overexpressing lymphoma cells elicits a synergistic lethal response in combination with PARP inhibition. Cell Cycle 10:3598–3607

Hocke S, Guo Y, Job A et al (2016) A synthetic lethal screen identifies ATR-inhibition as a novel therapeutic approach for POLD1-deficient cancers. Oncotarget 7(6):7080–7095. https://doi.org/10.18632/oncotarget.6857. [Epub ahead of print]

Itamochi H, Nishimura M, Oumi N et al (2014) Checkpoint kinase inhibitor AZD7762 overcomes cisplatin resistance in clear cell carcinoma of the ovary. Int J Gynecol Cancer 24:61–69

Jackson JR, Gilmartin A, Imburgia C et al (2000) An indolocarbazole inhibitor of human check-point kinase (Chk1) abrogates cell cycle arrest caused by DNA damage. Cancer Res 60:566–572

Janetka JW, Ashwell S, Zabludoff S et al (2007) Inhibitors of checkpoint kinases: from discovery to the clinic. Curr Opin Drug Discov Devel 10:473–486

Jobson AG, Lountos GT, Lorenzi PL et al (2009) Cellular inhibition of checkpoint kinase 2 (Chk2) and potentiation of camptothecins and radiation by the novel Chk2 inhibitor PV1019 [7-nitro-1H-indole-2-carboxylic acid {4-[1-(guanidinohydrazone)-ethyl]-phenyl}-amide]. J Pharmacol Exp Ther 331:816–826

Karanika S, Karantanos T, Li L et al (2017) Targeting DNA damage response in prostate cancer by inhibiting androgen receptor-CDC6-ATR-Chk1 signaling. Cell Rep 18:1970–1981

Kim MA, Kim HJ, Brown AL et al (2007) Identification of novel substrates for human checkpoint kinase Chk1 and Chk2 through genome-wide screening using a consensus Chk phosphorylation motif. Exp Mol Med 39:205–212

Kim MK, James J, Annunziata CM (2015) Topotecan synergizes with CHEK1 (CHK1) inhibitor to induce apoptosis in ovarian cancer cells. BMC Cancer 28:15

King C, Diaz H, Barnard D et al (2014) Characterization and preclinical development of LY2603618: a selective and potent Chk1 inhibitor. Investig New Drugs 32:213–226

King C, Diaz HB, McNeely S et al (2015) LY2606368 causes replication catastrophe and anti-tumor effects through CHK1-dependent mechanisms. Mol Cancer Ther 14:2004–2013

Kleiman LB, Krebs AM, Kim SY et al (2013) Comparative analysis of radiosensitizers for K-RAS mutant rectal cancers. PLoS One 8:e82982

Koh SB, Courtin A, Boyce RJ et al (2015) CHK1 inhibition synergizes with gemcitabine initially by destabilizing the DNA replication apparatus. Cancer Res 75:3583–3593

Lane DP (1992) Cancer. p53, guardian of the genome. Nature 358:15–16

Lainchbury M, Matthews TP, McHardy T et al (2012) Discovery of 3-alkoxyamino-5-(pyridin-2-ylamino)pyrazine-2-carbonitriles as selective, orally bioavailable CHK1 inhibitors. J Med Chem 55:10229–10240

Landau HJ, McNeely SC, Nair JS et al (2012) The checkpoint kinase inhibitor AZD7762 potentiates chemotherapy-induced apoptosis of p53-mutated multiple myeloma cells. Mol Cancer Ther 11:1781–1788

Lecona E, Fernández-Capetillon O (2014) Replication stress and cancer: it takes two to tango. Exp Cell Res 329:26–34

Lee JH, Choy ML, Ngo L et al (2011) Role of checkpoint kinase 1 (Chk1) in the mechanisms of resistance to histone deacetylase inhibitors. Proc Natl Acad Sci U S A 108:19629–19634

Liang X, Guo Y, Figg WD et al (2011) The role of wild-type p53 in cisplatin-induced Chk2 phosphorylation and the inhibition of platinum resistance with a Chk2 inhibitor. Chemother Res Pract 2011:715469

Lowery CD, VanWye AB, Dowless M et al (2017) The checkpoint kinase 1 inhibitor prexasertib induces regression of preclinical models of human neuroblastoma. Clin Cancer Res 23(15):4354–4363. https://doi.org/10.1158/1078-0432.CCR-16-2876

Ma CX, Janetka JW, Piwnica-Worms H (2011) Death by releasing the breaks: Chk1 inhibitors as cancer therapeutics. Trends Mol Med 17:88–96

Ma CX, Cai S, Li S et al (2012) Targeting Chk1 in p53-deficient triple-negative breast cancer is therapeutically beneficial in human-in-mouse tumor models. J Clin Invest 122:1541–1552

Ma CX, Ellis MJ, Petroni GR et al (2013) A phase II study of UCN-01 in combination with irinotecan in patients with metastatic triple negative breast cancer. Breast Cancer Res Treat 137:483–492

Magnussen GI, Emilsen E, Giller Fleten K et al (2015) Combined inhibition of the cell cycle related proteins Wee1 and Chk1/2 induces synergistic anti-cancer effect in melanoma. BMC Cancer 15:462

Mak JP, Man WY, Chow JP et al (2015) Pharmacological inactivation of CHK1 and WEE1 induces mitotic catastrophe in nasopharyngeal carcinoma cells. Oncotarget 6:21074–21084

Manic G, Signore M, Sistigu A et al (2017) CHK1-targeted therapy to deplete DNA replication-stressed, p53-deficient, hyperdiploid colorectal cancer stem cells. Gut. https://doi.org/10.1136/gutjnl-2016-312623

Martino-Echarri E, Henderson BR, Brocardo MG (2014) Targeting the DNA replication checkpoint by pharmacologic inhibition of Chk1 kinase: a strategy to sensitize APC mutant colon cancer cells to 5-fluorouracil chemotherapy. Oncotarget 5:9889–9900

Massey AJ, Stokes S, Browne H et al (2015) Identification of novel, in vivo active Chk1 inhibitors utilizing structure guided drug design. Oncotarget 6:35797–35812

Massey AJ, Stephens P, Rawlinson R et al (2016) mTORC1 and DNA-PKcs as novel molecular determinants of sensitivity to Chk1 inhibition. Mol Oncol 10:101–121

Matthews TP, Jones AM, Collins I (2013) Structure-based design, discovery and development of checkpoint kinase inhibitors as potential anticancer therapies. Expert Opin Drug Discov 8:621–640

Maugeri-Sacca M, Bartucci M, De Maria R (2013) Checkpoint kinase 1 inhibitors for potentiating systemic anticancer therapy. Cancer Treat Rev 39:525–533

McCabe N, Turner NC, Lord CJ et al (2006) Deficiency in the repair of DNA damage by homologous recombination and sensitivity to poly(ADP-ribose) polymerase inhibition. Cancer Res 66:8109–8115

McNeely S, Conti C, Sheikh T, Patel H, Zabludoff S, Pommier Y, Schwartz G, Tse A (2010) Chk1 inhibition after replicative stress activates a double strand break response mediated by ATM and DNA-dependent protein kinase. Cell Cycle 9:995–1004

McNeely S, Beckmann R, Bence Lin AK (2014) CHEK again: revisiting the development of CHK1 inhibitors for cancer therapy. Pharmacol Ther 142:1–10

Meng F, Bhupathi D, Sun JD et al (2015) Enhancement of hypoxia-activated prodrug TH-302 anti-tumor activity by Chk1 inhibition. BMC Cancer 15:422

Mitchell JB, Choudhuri R, Fabre K et al (2010a) In vitro and in vivo radiation sensitization of human tumour cells by a novel checkpoint kinase inhibitor, AZD7762. Clin Cancer Res 16:2076–2084

Mitchell C, Park M, Eulitt P et al (2010b) Poly(ADP-ribose) polymerase 1 modulates the lethality of CHK1 inhibitors in carcinoma cells. Mol Pharmacol 78:909–917

Montano R, Chung I, Garner KM et al (2012) Preclinical development of the novel Chk1 inhibitor SCH900776 in combination with DNA-damaging agents and antimetabolites. Mol Cancer Ther 11:427–438

Montano R, Thompson R, Chung I et al (2013) Sensitization of human cancer cells to gemcitabine by the Chk1 inhibitor MK-8776: cell cycle perturbation and impact of administration schedule in vitro and in vivo. BMC Cancer 13:604

Morgan MA, Parsels LA, Zhao L et al (2010) Mechanism of radiosensitization by the Chk1/2 inhibitor AZD7762 involves abrogation of the G2 checkpoint and inhibition of homologous recombinational DNA repair. Cancer Res 70:4972–4981

Murga M, Campaner S, Lopez-Contreras AJ et al (2011) Exploiting oncogene-induced replicative stress for the selective killing of Myc-driven tumors. Nat Struct Mol Biol 18:1331–1335

Nguyen TN, Saleem RS, Luderer MJ et al (2012) Radioprotection by hymenialdisine-derived checkpoint kinase 2 inhibitors. ACS Chem Biol 7:172–184

Nguyen T, Hawkins E, Kolluri A et al (2015) Synergism between bosutinib (SKI-606) and the Chk1 inhibitor (PF-00477736) in highly imatinib-resistant BCR/ABL+ leukemia cells. Leuk Res 39:65–71

O'Neill T, Giarratani L, Chen P et al (2002) Determination of substrate motifs for human Chk1 and hCds1/Chk2 by the oriented peptide library approach. J Biol Chem 277:16102–16115

Osborne JD, Matthews TP, McHardy T et al (2016) Multiparameter lead optimization to give an oral checkpoint kinase 1 (CHK1) inhibitor clinical candidate: (R)-5-((4-((morpholin-2-ylmethyl)amino)-5-(trifluoromethyl)pyridin-2-yl)amino)pyrazine-2-carbonitrile (CCT245737). J Med Chem 59:5221–5237

Oza V, Ashwell S, Brassil P et al (2012) Discovery of checkpoint kinase inhibitor (S)-5-(3-fluorophenyl)-N-(piperidin-3-yl)-3-ureidothiophene-2-carboxamide (AZD7762) by structure based design and optimization of thiophene carboxamide ureas. J Med Chem 55:5130–5142

Parsels LA, Qian Y, Tanska DM et al (2011) Assessment of chk1 phosphorylation as a pharmacodynamic biomarker of chk1 inhibition. Clin Cancer Res 17:3706–3715

Patel R, Barker HE, Kyula J et al (2017) An orally bioavailable Chk1 inhibitor, CCT244747, sensitizes bladder and head and neck cancer cell lines to radiation. Radiother Oncol 122:470–475

Pei XY, Dai Y, Felthousen J et al (2014) Circumvention of Mcl-1-dependent drug resistance by simultaneous Chk1 and MEK1/2 inhibition in human multiple myeloma cells. PLoS One 9:e89064

Peng CY, Graves PR, Thoma RS et al (1997) Conservation of the Chk1 checkpoint pathway in mammals: linkage of DNA damage to Cdk regulation through Cdc25. Science 277:1501–1505

Pfister SX, Markkanen E, Jiang Y et al (2015) Inhibiting WEE1 selectively kills histon e H3K36me3-deficient cancers by dNTP starvation. Cancer Cell 28:557–568

Pires IM, Ward TH, Dive C et al (2010) Oxaliplatin responses in colorectal cells are modulated by CHK2 kinase inhibitors. Br J Pharmacol 159:1326–1338

Pommier Y, Sordet O, Rao VA et al (2005) Chk2 molecular interaction map and rationale for Chk2 inhibitors. Clin Cancer Res 12:2657–2661

Pommier Y, Weinstein JN, Aladjem MI et al (2006) Chk2 molecular interaction map and rationale for Chk2 inhibitors. Clin Cancer Res 12:265726–265761

Prince EW, Balakrishnan I, Shah M et al (2016) Checkpoint kinase 1 expression is an adverse prognostic marker and therapeutic target in MYC-driven medulloblastoma. Oncotarget 7:53881–53894

Qi W, Xie C, Li C et al (2014) CHK1 plays a critical role in the anti-leukemic activity of the wee1 inhibitor MK-1775 in acute myeloid leukemia cells. J Hematol Oncol 7:53

Rawlinson R, Massey AJ (2014) γH2AX and Chk1 phosphorylation as predictive pharmacodynamic biomarkers of Chk1 inhibitor-chemotherapy combination treatments. BMC Cancer 14:483

Reader JC, Matthews TP, Klair S et al (2011) Structure-guided evolution of potent and selective CHK1 inhibitors through scaffold morphing. J Med Chem 54:8328–8342

Russell MR, Levin K, Rader J et al (2013) Combination therapy targeting the Chk1 and Wee1 kinases shows therapeutic efficacy in neuroblastoma. Cancer Res 73:776–784

Sakurikar N, Thompson R, Montano R et al (2016) A subset of cancer cell lines is acutely sensitive to the Chk1 inhibitor MK-8776 as monotherapy due to CDK2 activation in S phase. Oncotarget 7:1380–1394

Sanchez Y, Wong C, Thoma RS et al (1997) Conservation of the Chk1 checkpoint pathway in mammals: linkage of DNA damage to Cdk regulation through Cdc25. Science 277:1497–1501

Sanjiv K, Hagenkort A, Calderon-Montano JM et al (2016) Cancer-specific synthetic lethality between ATR and CHK1 kinase activities. Cell Rep 14:298–309

Sarmento LM, Póvoa V, Nascimento R et al (2015) CHK1 overexpression in T-cell acute lymphoblastic leukemia is essential for proliferation and survival by preventing excessive replication stress. Oncogene 34:2978–2990

Schenk EL, Koh BD, Flatten KS et al (2012) Effects of selective checkpoint kinase 1 inhibition on cytarabine cytotoxicity in acute myelogenous leukemia cells in vitro. Clin Cancer Res 18:5364–5373

Sen T, Tong P, Stewart CA et al (2017) CHK1 inhibition in small-cell lung cancer produces single-agent activity in biomarker-defined disease subsets and combination activity with cisplatin or olaparib. Cancer Res 77(14):3870–3884. https://doi.org/10.1158/0008-5472.CAN-16-3409

Seo GJ, Kim SE, Lee YM et al (2003) Determination of substrate specificity and putative substrates of Chk2 kinase. Biochem Biophys Res Commun 304:339–343

Shibata H, Miuma S, Saldivar JC et al (2011) Response of subtype-specific human breast cancer-derived cells to poly(ADP-ribose) polymerase and checkpoint kinase 1 inhibition. Cancer Sci 102:1882–1888

Shao RG, Cao CX, Shimizu T et al (1997) Abrogation of an S-phase checkpoint and potentiation of camptothecin cytotoxicity by 7-hydroxystaurosporine (UCN-01) in human cancer cell lines, possibly influenced by p53 function. Cancer Res 57:4029–4035

Sørensen CS, Syljuåsen RG, Falck J et al (2003) Chk1 regulates the S phase checkpoint by coupling the physiological turnover and ionizing radiation-induced accelerated proteolysis of Cdc25A. Cancer Cell 3:247–258

Sørensen CS, Hansen LT, Dziegielewski J et al (2005) The cell-cycle checkpoint kinase Chk1 is required for mammalian homologous recombination repair. Nat Cell Biol 7:195–201

Stevens C, Smith L, La Thangue NB (2003) Chk2 activates E2F-1 in response to DNA damage. Nat Cell Biol 5:401–409

Stracker TH, Usui T, Petrini JH (2009) Taking the time to make important decisions: the checkpoint effector kinases Chk1 and Chk2 and the DNA damage response. DNA Repair 8:1047–1054

Sugiyama K, Shimizu M, Akiyama T et al (2000) UCN-01 selectively enhances mitomycin C cytotoxicity in p53 defective cells which is mediated through S and/or G(2) checkpoint abrogation. Int J Cancer 85:703–709

Takai H, Naka K, Okada Y et al (2002) Chk2-deficient mice exhibit radioresistance and defective p53-mediated transcription. EMBO J 21:5195–5205

Tan DS, Thomas GV, Garrett MD et al (2009) Biomarker-driven early clinical trials in oncology: a paradigm shift in drug development. Cancer J 15:406–420

Tang J, Erikson RL, Liu X et al (2006) Checkpoint kinase 1 (Chk1) is required for mitotic progression through negative regulation of polo-like kinase 1 (Plk1). Proc Natl Acad Sci U S A 103:11964–11969

Tang Y, Hamed HA, Poklepovic A et al (2012) Poly(ADP-ribose) polymerase 1 modulates the lethality of CHK1 inhibitors in mammary tumors. Mol Pharmacol 82:322–332

Tao Y, Leteur C, Yang C et al (2009) Radiosensitization by Chir-124, a selective CHK1 inhibitor. Effects of p53 and cell cycle checkpoints. Cell Cycle 8:1196–1205

Taricani L, Shanahan F, Malinao MC et al (2014) A functional approach reveals a genetic and physical interaction between ribonucleotide reductase and CHK1 in mammalian cells. PLoS One 9(11):e111714

Thompson R, Eastman A (2013) The cancer therapeutic potential of Chk1 inhibitors: how mechanistic studies impact on clinical trial design. Br J Pharmacol 76:358–369

Toledo LI, Murga M, Fernandez-Capetillo O (2011) Targeting ATR and Chk1 kinases for cancer treatment: a new model for new (and old) drugs. Mol Oncol 5:368–373

Toledo LI, Altmeyer M, Rask MB et al (2013) ATR prohibits replication catastrophe by preventing global exhaustion of RPA. Cell 155:1088–1103

Toledo L, Neelsen KJ, Lukas J (2017) Replication catastrophe: when a checkpoint fails because of exhaustion. Mol Cell 66:735–749

Touchefeu Y, Khan AA, Borst G et al (2013) Optimising measles virus-guided radiovirotherapy with external beam radiotherapy and specific checkpoint kinase 1 inhibition. Radiother Oncol 108:24–31

Tse AN, Rendahl KG, Sheikh T et al (2007) CHIR-124, a novel potent inhibitor of Chk1, potentiates the cytotoxicity of topoisomerase I poisons in vitro and in vivo. Clin Cancer Res 13:591–602

Vance S, Liu E, Zhao L et al (2011) Selective radiosensitization of p53 mutant pancreatic cancer cells by combined inhibition of Chk1 and PARP1. Cell Cycle 10:4321–4329

Venkatesha VA, Parsels LA, Parsels JD et al (2012) Sensitization of pancreatic cancer stem cells to gemcitabine by Chk1 inhibition. Neoplasia 14:519–525

Wagner JM, Karnitz LM (2009) Cisplatin-induced DNA damage activates replication checkpoint signalling components that differentially affect tumour cell survival. Mol Pharmacol 76:208–214

Walker M, Black EJ, Oehler V et al (2009) Chk1 C-terminal regulatory phosphorylation mediates checkpoint activation by de-repression of Chk1 catalytic activity. Oncogene 28:2314–2323

Walton MI, Eve PD, Hayes A et al (2010) The preclinical pharmacology and therapeutic activity of the novel CHK1 inhibitor SAR-020106. Mol Cancer Ther 9:89–100

Walton MI, Eve PD, Hayes A et al (2012) CCT244747 is a novel potent and selective CHK1 inhibitor with oral efficacy alone and in combination with genotoxic anticancer drugs. Clin Cancer Res 18:5650–5661

Walton MI, Eve PD, Hayes A et al (2016) The clinical development candidate CCT245737 is an orally active CHK1 inhibitor with preclinical activity in RAS mutant NSCLC and Eμ-MYC driven B-cell lymphoma. Oncotarget 7:2329–2342

Wang Q, Fan S, Eastman A et al (1996) UCN-01: a potent abrogator of G2 checkpoint function in cancer cells with disrupted p53. J Natl Cancer Inst 88:956–965

Wang WJ, Wu SP, Liu JB et al (2013) MYC regulation of CHK1 and CHK2 promotes radio-resistance in a stem cell-like population of nasopharyngeal carcinoma cells. Cancer Res 73:1219–1231

Wang FZ, Fei HR, Cui YJ et al (2014) The checkpoint 1 kinase inhibitor LY2603618 induces cell cycle arrest, DNA damage response and autophagy in cancer cells. Apoptosis 19:1389–1398

Williams TM, Galbán S, Li F et al (2013) DW-MRI as a predictive biomarker of radiosensitization of GBM through targeted inhibition of checkpoint kinases. Transl Oncol 6:133–142

Workman P (2003) How much gets there and what does it do?: The need for better pharmacokinetic and pharmacodynamic endpoints in contemporary drug discovery and development. Curr Pharm Des 9:891–902

Workman P, Collins I (2010) Probing the probes: fitness factors for small molecule tools. Chem Biol 17:561–577

Wu J, Lai G, Wan F et al (2012) Knockdown of checkpoint kinase 1 is associated with the increased radiosensitivity of glioblastoma stem-like cells. Tohoku J Exp Med 226:267–274

Xiao Y, Ramiscal J, Kowanetz K et al (2013) Identification of preferred chemotherapeutics for combining with a CHK1 inhibitor. Mol Cancer Ther 12:2285–2295

Xiao Z, Xue J, Semizarov D et al (2005) Novel indication for cancer therapy: Chk1 inhibition sensitizes tumor cells to antimitotics. Int J Cancer 115:528–538

Xiao Z, Xue J, Sowin TJ et al (2006) Differential roles of checkpoint kinase 1, checkpoint kinase 2, and mitogen-activated protein kinase-activated protein kinase 2 in mediating DNA damage-induced cell cycle arrest: implications for cancer therapy. Mol Cancer Ther 5:1935–1943

Xu H, Cheung IY, Wei XX et al (2011) Checkpoint kinase inhibitor synergizes with DNA-damaging agents in G1 checkpoint-defective neuroblastoma. Int J Cancer 129:1953–1962

Yin Y, Shen Q, Zhang P et al (2017) Chk1 inhibition potentiates the therapeutic efficacy of PARP inhibitor BMN673 in gastric cancer. Am J Cancer Res 7:473–483

Yang H, Yoon SJ, al JJ (2011) Inhibition of checkpoint kinase 1 sensitizes lung cancer brain metastases to radiotherapy. Biochem Biophys Res Commun 406:53–58

Yang S, Kuo C, Bisi JE et al (2002) PML-dependent apoptosis after DNA damage is regulated by the checkpoint kinase hCds1/Chk2. Nat Cell Biol 4:865–870

Yap TA, Workman P (2012) Exploiting the cancer genome: strategies for the discovery and clinical development of targeted molecular therapeutics. Annu Rev Pharmacol Toxicol 52:549–573

Yu Q, La Rose J, Zhang H et al (2002) UCN-01 inhibits p53 up-regulation and abrogates gamma-radiation-induced G2–M checkpoint independently of p53 by targeting both of the checkpoint kinases, Chk2 and Chk1. Cancer Res 62:5743–5748

Yuan LL, Green A, David L et al (2014) Targeting CHK1 inhibits cell proliferation in FLT3-ITD positive acute myeloid leukemia. Leuk Res 38:1342–1349

Zabludoff SD, Deng C, Grondine MR et al (2008) AZD7762, a novel checkpoint kinase inhibitor, drives checkpoint abrogation and potentiates DNA targeted therapies. Mol Cancer Ther 7:2955–2966

Zachos G, Black EJ, Walker M et al (2007) Chk1 is required for spindle checkpoint function. Dev Cell 12:247–260

Zhang C, Yan Z, Painter CL et al (2009) PF-00477736 mediates checkpoint kinase 1 signaling pathway and potentiates docetaxel-induced efficacy in xenografts. Clin Cancer Res 15:4630–4640

Zhang Y, Hunter T (2014) Roles of Chk1 in cell biology and cancer therapy. Int J Cancer 134:1013–1023

Zhao J, Niu X, Li X et al (2016) Inhibition of CHK1 enhances cell death induced by the Bcl-2-selective inhibitor ABT-199 in acute myeloid leukemia cells. Oncotarget 7:34785–34799

Zhou J, Chen Z, Malysa A et al (2013) A kinome screen identifies checkpoint kinase 1 (CHK1) as a sensitizer for RRM1-dependent gemcitabine efficacy. PLoS One 8(3):e58091

Chapter 11
Clinical Development of CHK1 Inhibitors

Alvaro Ingles Garces and Udai Banerji

Abstract Checkpoint kinase 1 (CHK1) is an intracellular multifunctional serine/threonine kinase and an important component in the regulation of the DNA damage response (DDR) (Dai and Grant 2010; Hong et al. 2016). Broadly, its function is to maintain the integrity of cellular DNA from intrinsic or genotoxic agent-induced DNA damage i.e. single- or double-strand breaks and stalled replication forks by interrupting progression of a cell through the cell cycle. The validation of CHK1 as a target in cancer therapeutics has been discussed in previous chapters.

Keywords Checkpoint · CHK1 inhibitors · CHK1 clinical trials · Biomarkers · AZD7762 · GDC-0425 · LY2606368 · MK-8776 · PF-736 · SRA737

11.1 Introduction

Checkpoint kinase 1 (CHK1) is an intracellular multifunctional serine/threonine kinase and an important component in the regulation of the DNA damage response (DDR) (Dai and Grant 2010; Hong et al. 2016). Broadly, its function is to maintain the integrity of cellular DNA from intrinsic or genotoxic agent-induced DNA damage i.e. single- or double-strand breaks and stalled replication forks by interrupting progression of a cell through the cell cycle. The validation of CHK1 as a target in cancer therapeutics has been discussed in previous chapters.

In this chapter, we will cover the clinical contexts of CHK1 inhibitors currently undergoing clinical evaluation. Broadly, CHK1 inhibitors can be used as single agents, in combination with other anticancer drugs, and in combination with radiotherapy. The most advanced evaluation of CHK1 inhibitors is as combination with chemotherapeutic agents targeting the S phase in the cell cycle. To some extent,

A. Ingles Garces · U. Banerji (✉)
Drug Development Unit, The Institute of Cancer Research and The Royal Marsden,
London, UK
e-mail: alvaro.inglesrusso@icr.ac.uk; udai.banerji@icr.ac.uk

© Springer International Publishing AG, part of Springer Nature 2018
J. Pollard, N. Curtin (eds.), *Targeting the DNA Damage Response
for Anti-Cancer Therapy*, Cancer Drug Discovery and Development,
https://doi.org/10.1007/978-3-319-75836-7_11

the eventual clinical use of these combinations is directed by the current use of the partner chemotherapeutic agent e.g. gemcitabine in pancreatic cancer and pemetrexed in lung cancer. Within these indications, later development will require stratification of patients into biomarker-defined subgroups such as *TP53* mutant and *TP53* wild type cohorts.

Over the last decade, there have been significant developments in the field of drugs targeting DDR. Many agents, such as PARP, ATR and Wee1 inhibitors, are either licensed or undergoing clinical evaluation: combination therapies of CHK1 inhibitors with such agents in biomarker-defined populations are potential areas for development. Radiotherapy (RT) has been a pillar of curative and palliative anticancer therapy and while there are challenges in evaluating investigational agents with radiotherapy, there remain opportunities for the use of CHK1 inhibitors in this setting (Janetka et al. 2007; Morgan et al. 2008; Seto et al. 2013). The role CHK1 plays in response to replication stress, coupled with the emerging understanding of how to quantify replicative stress may lead to opportunities for single agent use of CHK1 inhibitors in the treatment of cancer patients.

11.2   CHK1 Inhibition and Chemotherapy

CHK1 inhibitors are being developed primarily as chemo-potentiators, as a result of the important role in the DDR through regulation of the cell cycle (Hong et al. 2016) (Table 11.1). The development of rational combinations of agents targeting cell cycle checkpoints with chemotherapy is supported by extensive preclinical data (Daud et al. 2015; Montano et al. 2012), as reported in the previous chapter. Before discussing the clinical progress of combinations of chemotherapy and CHK1 inhibitors, it is important to describe briefly the partner chemotherapeutic agent in the combination. While a range of anticancer agents targeting S phase in the cell cycle have been tested in combination with CHK1 agents in the preclinical setting, gemcitabine has been reproducibly identified as the drug that is most effectively potentiated by CHK1 inhibitors (Daud et al. 2015; Karnitz et al. 2005; Venkatesha et al. 2012). However, the basis for this preferential potentiation is not well established. Clinical experience with the combination of various CHK1 inhibitors and gemcitabine has highlighted exacerbation of chemotherapy-induced myelotoxicity as a predominant hurdle. Optimizing the dosing schedules of CHK1 inhibitors led by pharmacokinetic (PK) and pharmacodynamic (PD) studies and the use of supportive measures such as granulocyte colony-stimulating factor (GCSF) will be crucial to help further evaluate these agents.

Table 11.1 CHK1 inhibitors currently in clinical development

Drug	Phase	Form of administration	No. patients/tumour type	Combination therapy	G3/G4 toxicity	Response
AZD7762 (Sausville et al. 2014) NCT00937664	I	IV	38 evaluable patients/solid tumours (Western population)	Gemcitabine	G3 chest pain G4 neutropaenia G3 troponin I increase G3 myocardial ischaemia G3 nausea/vomiting	PR: two patients SD: nine patients
AZD7762 (Seto et al. 2013) NCT00413686	I	IV	20/solid tumours (Japanese population)	Gemcitabine	G4 neutropaenia G3 increased troponin T G4 neutropaenia—five patients G4 hyponatraemia G4 thrombocytopaenia	No objective responses reported SD: five patients
AZD7762 (Ho et al. 2011) NCT00473616	I	IV	68/solid tumours	Irinotecan	Myocardial infarction with G4 ventricular G3/4 troponin increase G4 febrile neutropaenia G3 diarrhoea	CR: one patient PR: one patient
GDC-0425 (Infante et al. 2015) NCT01359696	I	PO	40/solid tumours	Gemcitabine	G3/4 thrombocytopaenia G3/4 neutropaenia	PR: two patients
GDC-0575 (ClinicalTrials.Gov 2018) NCT01564251	I	PO	Ongoing/solid tumours or lymphoma	Gemcitabine	Data not published	Data not published
LY2606368 (Hong et al. 2016) NCT02778126	I	IV	45/solid tumours	Single agent	G3/4 neutropaenia (88.9%), predominantly G4 (73.3%). G3/4 thrombocytopaenia (28.9%)	PR: 4.4% SD: 33.3%

(continued)

Table 11.1 (continued)

Drug	Phase	Form of administration	No. patients/ tumour type	Combination therapy	G3/G4 toxicity	Response
LY2606368 (Lee et al. 2016) NCT02203513	II	IV	22/HGSOC	Single agent	G3/4 neutropaenia: 91% G3/G4 thrombocytopaenia: 27% G3/G4 febrile neutropaenia: 9% G3/G4 diarrhea: 9%	PR: five patients
LY2606368 (Yang et al. 2016) NCT2555644	Ib	IV	Ongoing HNSCC	Cisplatin or cetuximab and RT	Data not published.	Data not available
LY2606368 (Karzai et al. 2016) NCT02203513	II	IV	9/TNBC	Single agent	G3/4 neutropaenia: 89% G3/4 anaemia: 33% G3/4 thrombocytopaenia: 22%	PR: 1 SD: 4
LY2603618 (Weiss et al. 2013) NCT00415636	I	IV	31/solid tumours	Pemetrexed	G3 anaemia G3 pneumonia G3 diarrhoea G3/4 myelotoxicity	PR: one patients SD: nine patients
LY2603618 (Calvo et al. 2014) NCT01139775	I	IV	14/solid tumours	Pemetrexed and cisplatin	Fatigue, nausea, pyrexia, neutropaenia and vomiting	PR: two patients SD: eight patients
LY2603618 (Wehler et al. 2017) NCT01139775	II	IV	62/non-squamous NSCLC	Pemetrexed and cisplatin	Thromboembolic events: 8 patients	OS: 12.9 (experimental arm) × 6.6 (control arm). P = 0.229
LY2603618 (Doi et al. 2015) NCT01341457	I	IV	50/solid tumours	Gemcitabine	Fatigue: 44% Thrombocytopaenia: 42% Neutropaenia: 32% Nausea: 26% Anaemia: 20%	PR: one patient SD: 22 patients

Drug (reference)	Phase	Route	N/tumour type	Combination	G3/4 toxicities	Efficacy
LY2603618 (Laquente et al. 2017) NCT00839332	II	IV	99/pancreatic cancer	Gemcitabine	G3 anaemia: 3.1% G3 neutropaenia: 7.7% G3 thrombocytopaenia: 10.8% G3/4 fatigue: 3% G3 hyponatraemia: 3.1%	PR: 21.5% (experimental arm) × 8.8 (control arm). SD: 33.8% (experimental arm) × 55.9% (control arm)
LY2603618 (Scagliotti et al. 2016) NCT00988858	II	IV	55/NSCLC	Pemetrexed	G3/4 neutropaenia: 21.8%	PR: 9.1% SD: 36.4%
MK-8776 (Daud et al. 2015) NCT00779584	I	IV	43/solid tumours	Gemcitabine	G3/4 neutropaenia (14%) G3/4 thrombocytopaenia (12%) G3/4 fatigue (10%) G3 QTc prolongation (5%)	PR 7% SD 43%
MK-8776 (Karp et al. 2012) NCT01870596	I	IV	24/acute leukaemia	Cytarabine	G3 QTcF prolongation G3 palmer-plantar dysaesthaesia G3 hyperbilirubinaemia G3/4 infectious complications	Complete tumour clearance: 50%
PF-00477736 (PF-736) (Brega et al. 2010) NCT00437203		IV	36/solid tumours	Gemcitabine	G3 neutropaenia: 42% DLT of thrombocytopaenia, sudden death, mucositis, and elevated lipase	PR: three patients
SRA737 (formerly CCT245737) (ClincalTrials.Gov 2016b) NCT02797977	I	PO	Ongoing/solid tumours	Gemcitabine ± cisplatin	Data not published	Data not published
SRA737 (formerly CCT245737) (ClincalTrials.Gov 2016a) NCT02797964	I	PO	Ongoing/solid tumours	Single agent	Data not published	Data not published

11.2.1 Gemcitabine

Gemcitabine, a nucleoside analogue antimetabolite, is currently in use for the treatment of pancreatic cancer, non-small cell lung cancer (NSCLC), breast cancer, ovarian cancer, bladder cancer, soft tissue sarcoma and lymphoma. The most common toxicities are myelosuppression (neutropaenia and thrombocytopaenia), mild-to-moderate nausea, vomiting, diarrhoea, mucositis, transient hepatic dysfunction and drug-induced pneumonitis. Gemcitabine is being assessed in Phase I studies in combination with various CHK1 inhibitors including AZD7762 (Seto et al. 2013; Sausville et al. 2014), GDC-0425 (Infante et al. 2015), MK-8776 (Daud et al. 2015), PF-00477736 (Brega et al. 2010) and SRA737 (ClincalTrials.Gov 2016a; ClincalTrials.Gov 2016b).

11.2.2 Pemetrexed

The antifolate pemetrexed is indicated for the treatment of NCSLC and mesothelioma. Examples of its toxicities are myelosuppression (neutropaenia and thrombocytopaenia most commonly observed); skin rash, mucositis, diarrhoea and fatigue are other common examples. Phase I and phase II studies in combination with pemetrexed have been carried out with LY2603618, for example (Scagliotti et al. 2016; Weiss et al. 2013).

11.2.3 Cytarabine

Cytarabine is another nucleoside analogue antimetabolite agent. It is commonly used in the treatment of leukaemia (acute myelogenous leukaemia, acute lymphocytic leukaemia, chronic myelogeneous leukaemia). Adverse effects (AEs) commonly associated with this drug are myelosuppression (leukopenia and thrombocytopaenia are common), mild-to-moderate nausea, vomiting, neurotoxicity, conjunctivitis and keratitis, erythema, acute pancreatitis and transient hepatic dysfunction. A phase I study of the CHK1 inhibitor, MK-8776, (Karp et al. 2012) has been carried out in combination with cytarabine.

11.2.4 Irinotecan

Preclinical data also support the combination of CHK1 inhibitors with topoisomerase I inhibitors (camptothecin, irinotecan and topotecan). Topoisomerase I inhibitors cause single-strand breaks in DNA and lead to S-phase arrest. The main side-effects of irinotecan are myelosuppression, diarrhoea, aesthenia, and transient elevation of serum transaminases, alkaline phosphatase and bilirubin. Irinotecan is currently used in the treatment of colorectal cancer and metastatic gastric cancer. A phase I study of the CHK1 inhibitor AZD7762, in combination with irinotecan has been carried out (Ho et al. 2011).

11.3   CHK1 Inhibitors and RT

Radiation therapy acts by causing extensive DNA damage including DNA double- and single-strand breaks, base modification and replication stress. The survival of the cancer cells depends on effective DDR mechanisms. There is abundant preclinical evidence for radiosensitisation with CHK1 inhibitors as has been discussed in previous chapters (Morgan et al. 2008; Barker et al. 2016; Borst et al. 2013; Bridges et al. 2016; Tao et al. 2009).

Curative radiotherapy is often given over a 6-week period as 30 fractions administered on each weekday and is used in two ways: combined with chemotherapy as the primary cancer treatment, such as cervical and head and neck cancers; or, as an adjuvant treatment with other curative treatments, such as surgery for breast and endometrial cancers. Clinical trials of combinations with CHK1 inhibitors in this setting are challenging, as the cure rates with radiation alone are high. Furthermore, any intervention (e.g. combination with a CHK1 inhibitor) that requires a reduction in the dose intensity of radiotherapy could compromise patient care. Accordingly, early phase clinical trials assessing the tolerability of combinations of radiation therapy and novel agents are often carried out in the setting of palliative radiotherapy over one week making the transition of novel agents such as CHK1 inhibitors into curative radiotherapy schedules complicated. Preclinical studies of CHK1 inhibitors have shown promise. As the DNA damage delivered with radiotherapy is local and not systemic, combination with CHK1 inhibitors often do not cause significant myelosuppression (Barker et al. 2016; Bridges et al. 2016; Tao et al. 2009; Benada and Macurek 2015). Future clinical trials of CHK1 inhibitors in combination with radiotherapy are awaited.

11.4   CHK1 Inhibitors and DDR Targeted Drugs

ATR and CHK1 kinases maintain cancer cell survival under replication stress. ATR phosphorylates CHK1 and inhibitors of both kinases are currently undergoing clinical trials (Sanjiv et al. 2016). Combinations of CHK inhibitors and drugs targeting the DDR have been explored in the preclinical setting. Wee1 kinase is an enzyme that is active during S and G2 phases of the cell cycle and is required for sustained ATR/CHK1 activity upon replication stress (Chaudhuri et al. 2014). There is increasing evidence that combined inhibition of Wee1 and CHK1 leads to synergistic cytotoxicity. Inhibition of both CHK1 and Wee1 has been shown to cause aberrant replication, an impaired G2/M checkpoint, premature entry to mitosis before completion of replication, abnormal mitosis and cell death. Combined inhibition of Wee1 and CHK1 efficiently inhibited tumour growth in various preclinical models, including acute myeloid leukaemia, ovarian cancer, neuroblastoma, mantle cell lymphoma, and melanoma (Guertin et al. 2012; Lu et al. 2006).

Combinations of CHK1 inhibitors and poly(ADP-ribose) polymerase (PARP) inhibitors have been explored and have been demonstrated to enhance the cytotoxicity of ionising radiation in clonogenic assays. Other studies have shown that CHK1 siRNA sensitised BRCA mutant cells to ionising radiation in mouse embryonic fibroblasts (MEF) models (Cole et al. 2011; Kulkarni et al. 2016). The common side-effects of DDR inhibitors such as Wee1 and PARP inhibitors when used in combination is myelotoxicity (Leijen et al. 2010; Oza et al. 2015). However, careful attention to PK-PD data and intermittent dosing schedules can help to circumvent some of these challenges.

11.5   CHK1 Inhibitors as a Single Agent

The inhibition of checkpoint kinases alone may exploit existing synthetic lethality with existing endogenous defects in tumour cells with specific genetic backgrounds. As single agents, CHK1 emerged as the most potent hit for which depletion was cytotoxic in pediatric neuroblastoma cell lines (Garrett and Collins 2011; Zabludoff et al. 2008). CHK1 mRNA expression was high in MYC-neuroblastoma-related (MYCN) amplified tumours and high-risk primary tumours, accompanied by constitutive activation of the ATR–CHK1 pathway, whereas non-neuroblastoma cell lines and low-risk primary tumour cells generally showed lower CHK1 expression and no pathway activation. Preliminary data from a different CHK1 inhibitor—PF-00477736—have shown that it inhibits the growth of subcutaneous neuroblastoma xenografts (Garrett and Collins 2011; Walton et al. 2012). Carefully designed, biomarker stratified clinical trials will be necessary in the development of CHK1 inhibitors in a single agent setting.

11.6   Clinical Trial Design of CHK1 Inhibitors

11.6.1   CHK1 Inhibitors in Combination with Chemotherapy

Early clinical trials need to incorporate an adaptable study design to allow multiple doses of chemotherapy so that dose escalation of the CHK1 inhibitor reaches a level that will inhibit CHK1. The development of biomarkers of CHK1 inhibition has been a challenge and has led to minimal pharmacodynamic data from the clinical trials. It is evident that myelotoxicity is limiting and early institution of growth factors such as GCSF should be administered. Responses will almost certainly be seen in phase I combination studies as the chemotherapy agents have activity on their own, thus making PK and PD end-points in phase I trials critical. Phase II studies of CHK1 chemotherapy combinations would benefit from being carried out in subpopulations that pre-clinical studies suggest may be most sensitive to the agents e.g. *TP53* mutant. This is an area that would benefit from substantial investment. As mentioned previously, because of the activity of the chemotherapy drugs alone, these studies need to be in a randomized setting.

11.6.2 CHK1 Studies in Combination with DDR Inhibitors

Because of the potential for myelotoxicity, trials should be designed with flexible dosing schedules that allow investigators to achieve a maximal therapeutic window and because of this potential for myelotoxicity, it is likely that continuous administration of both classes of agents may not be possible and early institution of growth factor support and intermittent dosing schedules may be necessary. If the partner DDR inhibitor is active in a certain biomarker-specified cohort e.g. PARP inhibitors are active in BRCA-mutated patients, then phase I expansions and phase II studies will have to be considered in a biomarker-stratified setting such as *BRCA1* mutations or other DDR defects such as *ATR/ATM* mutations. Randomized studies will be needed to evaluate the combinations.

11.6.3 CHK1 in Combination with Radiotherapy

Clinical trials of CHK1 inhibitors combined with RT should be guided by the tolerability, PK and PD data from single-agent studies and evaluated initially in a high-dose palliative and palliative setting before being trialed in a curative setting. As myelotoxicity has been well described in combinations with chemotherapy, attention to other normal tissue toxicity in the radiation field needs to be considered e.g. mucositis or diarrhoea. In addition to late side-effects, if the drugs are used in a curative setting, normal tissue toxicity such as fibrosis will need to be considered. Biomarker stratification such as *TP53* mutant tumours should be considered and because radiotherapy has activity on its own, phase II studies will need to be randomized.

11.6.4 CHK1 Inhibitors as Single Agents

Clinical trials of CHK1 inhibitors as single agents have tremendous potential. Although many are administered intravenously and dosing more than once a week is challenging, newer CHK1 inhibitors can be administered orally and make PK-PD-driven intermittent dosing possible. New strategies to evaluate tumour response to CHK1 inhibitors are necessary to be developed. The positron emission tomography (PET)-tracer, 18F-fluorine-L-thymidine (FLT), has been tested to monitor the effects of gemcitabine followed by PF477736 in nude mice harboring prostate cancer (PC-3) xenografts and this is promising to be used in the future to monitor response to target therapies, including CHK1 inhibitors (Ma et al. 2011).

Evaluation of efficacy in predictive biomarker-stratified cohorts can greatly accelerate the development of CHK1 inhibitors as single agents. Current candidate biomarkers could include oncogenes such as *MYC* or *KRAS* as surrogates for replicative stress or assays of replicative stress itself. Other candidate biomarkers include *BRCA*, *ATM* or *ATR* mutations, as some studies have shown that CHK1 inhibition synergizes with ATM loss in cells with Fanconi anaemia DNA repair defects and BRCA2-deficient cells—XRCC3 (X-ray repair cross complementing protein 3) are sensitized to the combination of gemcitabine and AZD7762 (Ma et al. 2011).

Several CHK1 inhibitors have been progressed to clinical studies. The majority of these are in combination with chemotherapy. However, the combination with DDR agents and single-agent studies are also being evaluated. The current CHK1 inhibitors assessed in clinical trials are discussed below.

11.7   AZD7762

AZD7762 (AstraZeneca) is an intravenous (IV) selective ATP-competitive CHK1/CHK2 kinase inhibitor that has shown, in *in vitro* and *in vivo* model systems, chemosensitizing activity with DNA-damaging agents, including gemcitabine and irinotecan (Sausville et al. 2014; ClinicalTrials.Gov 2018). This drug can enhance the response to DNA-damaging agents via different mechanisms of action, with gemcitabine arresting cells predominantly in the S phase and irinotecan in G2 (Seto et al. 2013; Zabludoff et al. 2008). Three phase I clinical trials evaluated this drug (Seto et al. 2013; Sausville et al. 2014; Ho et al. 2011):

11.7.1   Study 1

'Phase I dose-escalation study of AZD7762, a checkpoint kinase inhibitor, in combination with gemcitabine in US patients with advanced solid tumors' (Sausville et al. 2014)

This study was an open-label, multicenter dose-escalation phase I study using a standard 3 + 3 design. Patients received intravenous AZD7762 on day 1 and day 8 of a 14-day run-in cycle (cycle 0; AZD7762 monotherapy), followed by AZD7762 plus gemcitabine 750–1000 mg/m^2 on days 1 and 8, every 21 days, in ascending flat

AZD7762 doses (cycle 1; combination therapy). The AZD7762 dose cohorts were 6, 9, 14, 21, 32, 30, and 40 mg (Sausville et al. 2014).

Toxicity

Overall, the AEs most commonly observed were fatigue (41%), neutropaenia/leukopaenia (36%), anaemia (29%), and nausea, pyrexia, and ALT/AST increase (26% each). During cycle 0 (AZD7762 single agent), the most frequent AEs were fatigue (14%), vomiting (14%), and nausea (12%). One patient had grade 3 chest pain in the AZD7762 30 mg group and another patient developed grade 4 neutropaenia in the AZD7762 40 mg group (events in both patients were judged to be causally related to gemcitabine). The AZD7762 40 mg group had one patient with grade 3 myocardial ischaemia (Sausville et al. 2014).

The MTD of AZD7762 in combination with gemcitabine 1000 mg/m^2 was 30 mg (flat dose). In cycle 0, two patients had cardiac dose-limiting toxicities (DLTs): one at 32 mg of AZD7762 (asymptomatic grade 3 troponin I increase) and the other one at AZD7762 dose of 40 mg (grade 3 myocardial ischaemia associated with chest pain, ECG changes, decreased left ventricular ejection fraction, and increased troponin I). These events were reversible following permanent discontinuation of AZD7762 for both patients. In cycle 1, two additional patients reported non-cardiac DLTs: grade 3 nausea/vomiting at 32 mg of AZD7762 and grade 4 neutropaenia complicated by ≥ 38.5 °C fever at AZD7762 dose of 40 mg (Sausville et al. 2014).

Pharmacokinetics

AZD7762 exposure (C_{max}, C_{24h}, and AUC) increased in a dose-proportional manner over the dose range evaluated (from 6 to 40 mg). Following AZD7762 monotherapy, the mean half-life ranged from 8 to 15.5 h and mean clearance ranged from 35 to 73 l/h. During the first 48 h post-dosing, analysis of urine samples showed that across all dose levels, 11–20% of unchanged drug was excreted in the urine. Plasma concentrations of AZD7762 at doses >21 mg were compatible with those found to be biologically effective in preclinical studies (Sausville et al. 2014).

The peak plasma concentrations at the 30 mg dose was 291 ng/ml, consistent with those found to be biologically effective in preclinical studies. There was no evidence of pharmacological interaction of AZD7762 with the elimination of gemcitabine or vice versa (Sausville et al. 2014).

Biomarkers

The PD effect of AZD7762 as single agent and combined with gemcitabine was assessed in hair follicles from skin biopsies. There was a minimal degree of staining for both pChk1ser345 and pH2AX (<25%) and the range of H-scores for both biomarkers was from 0 to 3 out of 12. The non-significant pH2AX changes correlates with the lack of effectiveness of this drug (Sausville et al. 2014).

Efficacy

Thirty-eight patients were evaluable in this trial and two achieved a partial objective tumour response (AZD7762 6 mg + gemcitabine 750 mg/m² and AZD7762 9 mg cohort). Both patients had NSCLC and they had not received prior treatment with gemcitabine. A best response of stable disease (SD) for $\geq 6 \leq 12$ weeks was reported in five patients and four patients recorded stable disease for ≥ 12 weeks. Disease progression was reported as best response in 20 patients (Sausville et al. 2014).

In summary, the MTD of AZD7762 as a single agent was 30 mg, with reversible cardiac events. When combined with gemcitabine at doses >30 mg, nausea and neutropenic fever showed to be dose-limiting. The data suggest that a broad concentration-effect curve of a range of serious cardiovascular AEs would be associated with AZD7762 IV bolus administration in humans. This would make the use of AZD7762 IV bolus administration not feasible given the range of concomitant cardiovascular comorbidities presented by oncology population (Sausville et al. 2014).

AZD7762 study 2—'Phase I, dose-escalation study of AZD7762 alone and in combination with gemcitabine in Japanese patients with advanced solid tumours' (Seto et al. 2013).

This study in Japan evaluated Asian patients treated with AZD7762 at two doses one week apart as a run-in dose (cycle 0) and in combination with gemcitabine at 1000 mg/m² on day 1 and day 8 on a 21-day cycle (cycle 1). Twenty patients (14 male, 6 female) received at least one dose of AZD7762 (n = 3, 6 mg; n = 3, 9 mg; n = 6, 21 mg; n = 8, 30 mg) and were evaluable for safety and PK analysis (Seto et al. 2013).

This study was stopped prematurely due to the discontinuation of the AZD7762 clinical development program; however, the results were sufficiently mature to determine the MTD in Japanese patients with advanced solid tumours at 21 mg when used in combination with gemcitabine 1000 mg/m², based on the safety information from five evaluable patients at the time of study termination (Seto et al. 2013).

Toxicity

DLTs were observed in two patients in the 30 mg dose cohort, including one grade 3 increase in troponin T on day 1 of cycle 0 (AZD7762 single agent) (Seto et al. 2013).

The most common AEs reported during AZD7762 monotherapy were bradycardia (50%), hypertension (25%) and fatigue (15%). Overall (including the combination treatment), the most frequently reported AEs were bradycardia (55%), neutropaenia (45%), fatigue (30%), hypertension (30%) and rash (30%). The MTD of AZD7762 in combination with gemcitabine 1000 mg/m² was determined at 21 mg in Japanese patients (Seto et al. 2013).

Grade 3 AEs were reported in 11 patients and neutropaenia was the most common, occurring in 45% of patients (leukopenia in 25%). Only one grade 3 AE occurred during AZD7762 monotherapy (increased troponin T). Grade 4 AEs were neutropaenia (n = 1, 6 mg; n = 1, 21 mg; n = 3, 30 mg), leukopenia (n = 1 each, 6 mg and 30 mg), hyponatraemia (n = 1, 21 mg) and thrombocytopaenia (n = 1, 30 mg) (Seto et al. 2013).

Of the two DLTs in the 30 mg AZD7762 cohort, one was a cardiac DLT reported during AZD7762 monotherapy and the other was a liver function/haematological-related DLT during AZD7762 combination therapy. Both events resolved following discontinuation of treatment (Seto et al. 2013).

Other common AEs during monotherapy in this Japanese population were generally consistent with the previous studies in Western populations, predominantly fatigue and gastrointestinal effects (Seto et al. 2013).

Pharmacokinetics

Following a single-dose IV infusion, AZD7762 exposure increased in an approximately linear and dose-proportional way, achieving C_{max} approximately 1 h from the start of the infusion (Seto et al. 2013). At the end of the infusion, the disposition of AZD7762 may be described as multi-phasic with an initial rapid decline (distribution phase) followed by a slower elimination phase (Seto et al. 2013). AZD7762 was extensively distributed across all dose cohorts after single-dose administration (Seto et al. 2013).

The addition of gemcitabine does not seem to affect the PK of AZD7762. Between-subject variability was low to moderate with the coefficient of variation ranging from 10% to 45% (Seto et al. 2013). The PK profile reported in the Japanese population is generally consistent with the PK profile previously reported in Western patient populations (Seto et al. 2013).

Efficacy

No objective responses were reported during the Japanese study. A best response of SD was observed in five lung-cancer patients (n = 1, 9 mg; n = 2, 21 mg; n = 2, 30 mg) (Seto et al. 2013).

AZD7762 Study 3—'Phase I, open-label, dose-escalation study of AZD7762 in combination with irinotecan (irino) in patients (pts) with advanced solid tumors' (Ho et al. 2011).

A third study evaluating AZD7762 was performed. A 3 + 3 design trial evaluated the safety and PK of AZD7762 (6–144 mg IV) ± irinotecan (100 or 125 mg/m² IV) (NCT00473616). AZD7762 was given alone on day 1 and day 8 (cycle 0); after 7 days of observation, AZD7762 was given after irinotecan on days 1 and day 8 of 21-day cycles until disease progression/discontinuation for any reason. To further confirm safety, an expansion phase was conducted at the MTD (Ho et al. 2011).

Toxicity

During dose escalation, one patient had DLTs of myocardial infarction with G4 ventricular dysfunction during AZD7762 144 mg monotherapy (cycle 0). Three patients had non-cardiac DLTs during cycle 1: 6 mg (G3 diarrhoea/decreased appetite/dehydration); 14 mg (G3 increased ALT); 48 mg (G4 febrile neutropaenia). In the expansion phase (AZD7762 96 mg + irinotecan 100 mg/m^2), 3/11 evaluable patients had DLTs (G2 left ventricular systolic dysfunction/G4 troponin increase; G3 troponin increase; G3 cardiomyopathy)—all occurred during AZD7762 monotherapy. Overall, the most common AEs were diarrhoea, fatigue and nausea (Ho et al. 2011).

Pharmacokinetics

AZD7762 C_{max}, C24h, and AUC increased in a linear and dose-proportional manner. Irinotecan did not affect AZD7762 PK (Ho et al. 2011).

Results

Sixty-eight patients received AZD7762 (6 mg (n = 11); 9 mg (n = 3); 14 mg (n = 9); 21 mg (n = 4); 32 mg (n = 5); 48 mg (n = 7); 64 mg (n = 5); 96 mg (n = 19); 144 mg (n = 5)). Colorectal (n = 29) was the most common tumour site. Median exposure to AZD7762 was 43 days (range 1–520) (Ho et al. 2011).

One complete response (CR) was observed (48 mg; small cell carcinoma of the ureter; duration: 18 months) and one partial response (PR) (144 mg; colon with prior irinotecan treatment) (Ho et al. 2011).

Future Plans

Due to the incidence of cardiac toxicities reported in the overall phase I development programme, the balance between benefit and risk has been judged unfavorable and further clinical development of AZD7762 has been discontinued.

11.8   GDC-0425

GDC-0425 (Genentech) is an oral and selective CHK1 inhibitor. In tumour xenograft models, it has been shown to enhance gemcitabine efficacy and greater chemopotentiation was observed in cancer cell lines lacking p53 activity (Infante et al. 2015).

11.8.1 Phase 1

'Study of GDC-0425, a checkpoint kinase 1 inhibitor, in combination with gemcitabine in patients with refractory solid tumors' (Infante et al. 2015).

A phase I dose-escalation trial was performed including patients with refractory solid tumours. Patients received a single dose of GDC-0425 on day −7 for PK evaluation followed by 21-day cycles of gemcitabine on day 1 and day 8 and GDC-0425 on day 2 and day 9 at dose levels of 750 + 60, 1000 + 60, and 1000 + 80 of gemcitabine (mg/m^2) + GDC-0425 (mg) (Infante et al. 2015).

Forty patients were treated in this phase I trial. The most common tumour types were breast (n = 10), NSCLC (n = 5), and cancer of unknown primary (CUP; n = 4) (Infante et al. 2015).

Toxicity

Dose escalation was stopped at GDC-0425 80 mg with gemcitabine 1000 mg/m^2 as three of six patients experienced grade 4 thrombocytopaenia as a dose-limiting toxicity; one patient also had grade 3 neutropaenia that delayed cycle 2 (DLT). Blood counts recovered with treatment interruption. The MDT of GDC-0425 was 60 mg with gemcitabine 1000 mg/m^2. The most frequent AEs (all grades) related to GDC-0425 and/or gemcitabine were nausea (48%); anaemia, neutropaenia, vomiting (45% each); fatigue (43%); pyrexia (40%); and thrombocytopaenia (35%). Serious AEs related to GDC-0425 and/or gemcitabine occurred in eight patients: neutropaenia and thrombocytopaenia (=2 each); leukopaenia, ALT/AST/GGT increased, pyrexia, rash, dyspnoea, gastric ulcer, and gastroenteritis (n = 1 each). Median number of administered cycles was 3.5 (range 1–14) (Infante et al. 2015).

Pharmacokinetics

Maximum plasma concentrations of GDC-0425 were achieved within 4 h of dosing and its half-life was approximately 16 h. C_{max} following a 60 mg single dose of GDC-0425 was 100 ± 53.6 ng/mL and the mean C_{max} following 3 once-daily doses of 60 mg was approximately 1.6-fold higher than that. The single dose of 60 mg in humans exceeded the target exposures associated with checkpoint abrogation and anti-tumour activity in preclinical models. The exposure and half-life observed in humans were, respectively, six- and twofold higher than that predicted from nonclinical models. No PK interaction was observed with GDC-0425 and gemcitabine (Infante et al. 2015).

Response

There were three PRs: one patient with TNBC (*TP53* mutated), one melanoma, and one CUP, all of them at 60 mg of GDC-0425 (Infante et al. 2015).

Future Plans

The maximum tolerated dose of GDC-0425 was 60 mg, with gemcitabine 1000 mg/ m^2. At the doses assessed, bone marrow suppression was common but manageable and exposures exceeded those predicted by preclinical models to inhibit CHK1. Clinical activity was observed, including one patient with *TP53* mutated TNBC. In view of this, further clinical development is encouraged as it is important to evaluate tolerability and anti-tumour activity of GDC-0425 and gemcitabine in a less heavily treated population and to understand if tumours that lack functional p53 predict clinical benefit (Infante et al. 2015).

11.9   GDC-0575

A clinical trial (NCT01564251) of GDC-0575 (Genentech) as monotherapy and in combination with chemotherapy has been initiated but no results have been presented to date (ClinicalTrials.Gov 2018).

11.10   LY2606368 (Prexasertib)

LY2606368 monomesylate monohydrate (Eli Lilly) inhibits the enzymatic activity of CHK1, with a half-maximal inhibitory concentration (IC50) of 1 nM, and CHK2, with an IC50 of 8 nM, in cell-free assays (Hong et al. 2016). However, preclinical models have shown that the biologic effects of LY2606368 seem to be driven by CHK1. Several trials using this agent have been reported:

11.10.1   Study 1

LY2606368 Monotherapy - 'Phase I Study of LY2606368, a Checkpoint Kinase 1 Inhibitor, in Patients With Advanced Cancer' (Hong et al. 2016).

A phase I, non-randomized, multicenter, open-label clinical trial evaluating this molecule was performed and forty-five patients (schedule 1, n = 27; schedule 2, n = 18) were treated. LY2606368 was administered intravenously at 10–50 mg/m² on days 1–3 (schedule 1) or at 40–130 mg/m² on day 1 (schedule 2) every 14 days. Most patients had been treated with ≥3 systemic lines of therapy (69%), radiotherapy (56%), and/or surgery (82%). Colon/rectal (20%) and head and neck squamous cell carcinoma (HNSCC; 11%) were the two most common tumour types in this study (Hong et al. 2016).

Toxicity

The MTD in schedule 1 was 40 mg/m^2 and 105 mg/m^2 in schedule 2. Serious adverse events in schedule 1 were neutropaenia (n = 4), febrile neutropaenia (n = 2), leukopenia, anaemia, and lung infection (n = 1 each). In schedule 2, drug-related serious adverse events were neutropaenia, leukopenia, thrombocytopaenia, lung infection, and epistaxis, all occurring in a single patient. Only patients in schedule 1 had febrile neutropaenia (three patients in total).

The most common AEs related to study drug were neutropaenia (93.3%), leukopenia (82.2%), anaemia (68.9%), thrombocytopaenia (53.3%), and fatigue (31.1%). Grade 1 or 2 nausea (24.4%), oral mucositis (13.3%), and vomiting (11.1%) were also observed (Hong et al. 2016).

As reported above, neutropaenia was the most frequently observed toxicity and predominantly grade 4 (73.3%). Considering all grade 3/4 cases, 88.9% of patients developed this AE. The nadir occurred approximately 1 week after each dose and lasted for 5 days as a grade 4 event.

Cardiac events related to study treatment were not common, with only two events (grade 2 hypotension and grade 2 sinus tachycardia) (Hong et al. 2016).

Pharmacokinetics

LY2606368 exposure increased in a dose-dependent manner across the dose range of 10–130 mg/m^2 after a single dose (day 1) and multiple doses (day 3) in cycles 1 and 2 across both schedules (Hong et al. 2016). However, potential nonlinear PK behavior was observed after repeated administration on schedule 1 when decreases in clearance and volume of distribution at steady state were identified. This is probably related to an artifact of a shorter sampling duration on day 1 (only up to 24 h) compared with day 3 (up to 168 h). There was a moderate to large degree of inter-patient PK variability and the mean elimination half-life ($t_{1/2}$) varied across days and cycles of treatment. The mean LY2606368 $t_{1/2}$ range (11.4–27.1 h) across schedules, days, and cycles of treatment at the MTDs were similar and consistent with a $t_{1/2}$ suitable for achieving acceptable systemic exposure and minimizing intra- and inter-cycle accumulation of LY2606368 (Hong et al. 2016).

PK simulations also demonstrated that the LY2606368 systemic exposure correlating to CHK1 inhibition needed for maximal tumour response in preclinical xenograft models can be achieved and was similar for both the schedule 1 MTD and schedule 2 MTD (Hong et al. 2016).

Biomarkers

Changes in plasma concentrations of DNA and CK18 were not conclusive. Circulating tumour cells (CTCs) were detected in 29% of patients at low numbers and the observed change in CTCs positive for pH2A.X was not significant. The average post-dose and pre-dose pH2A.X levels measured in hair follicles were not statistically different. The absence of a direct PD biomarker to assess CHK1 modulation was a limitation of this study. In addition, changes in pH2A.X in hair may not be representative of modulation in the tumour (Hong et al. 2016).

CTC analysis was hindered by the limited numbers of cells obtained from this refractory population and the high proportion of patients with tumours not typically associated with releasing CTCs (Hong et al. 2016).

Efficacy

A total of 43 out of 45 patients were evaluable for efficacy in this trial. Two patients had PR (objective response rate, 4.4%) and SD was reported in 15 patients (33.3%). The clinical benefit rate was 33.3% in schedule 1 and 44.4% in schedule 2. Duration of clinical benefit for patients with PR or SD ranged from 1.2 to 7.2 months. Three patients (6.7%) had SD for at least 4 months (Hong et al. 2016).

The two PRs observed in this study are the first reports of single-agent activity for a CHK1/CHK2 inhibitor. Both patients with objective responses had SCC (one patient had SCC of the anus and the second one, SCCHN) (Hong et al. 2016).

11.10.2 Study 2

Monotherapy in triple negative breast cancer—'A phase II study of the cell cycle checkpoint kinases 1 and 2 (CHK1/2) inhibitor (LY2606368; prexasertib) in sporadic triple negative breast cancer (TNBC)' (Karzai et al. 2016).

LY2606368 is being evaluated in a group of patients diagnosed with TNBC without deleterious germline *BRCA* mutation or family history of hereditary breast and ovarian cancer syndrome. In this study, prexasertib is being administered at 105 mg/ m^2 IV once every 14 days on a 28-day cycle. Response is assessed every 2 cycles. An optimal two-stage design is being used; if ≥ 1 response is seen in the first nine patients, then accrual continues to 24 patients per cohort (Karzai et al. 2016).

Toxicity

Grade 3/4 AEs include neutropaenia (89%), anaemia (33%) and thrombocytopaenia (22%) (Karzai et al. 2016).

Efficacy

Nine patients with *BRCA* wild type TNBC patients were treated in the first stage. One PR was observed (overall response rate (ORR) = 11%). Four of nine evaluable patients attained SD >3 months (Karzai et al. 2016).

11.10.3 Study 3

LY2606368 monotherapy in patients with high grade serous ovarian cancer (HGSOC)—'A Phase II study of the cell cycle checkpoint kinases 1 and 2 inhibitor (LY2606368; Prexasertib monomesylate monohydrate) in sporadic high-grade serous ovarian cancer (HGSOC) and germline BRCA mutation-associated ovarian cancer (gBRCAm+ OvCa)' (Lee et al. 2016).

LY2606368 was evaluated in patients diagnosed with HGSOC. Subjects enrolled in this trial had recurrent HGSOC with negative *BRCA* testing or negative family history of hereditary breast and ovarian cancer syndrome (cohort 1) or a documented deleterious germline BRCA1/2 mutation (cohort 2). Patients received LY2606368 monotherapy at 105 mg/m^2 IV every 14 days per 28-day cycle (Lee et al. 2016).

Toxicity

Grade 3 or 4 treatment-emergent AEs include neutropaenia (91%), thrombocytopaenia (27%), febrile neutropaenia (9%) and diarrhoea (9%). Thirteen patients received growth factor support due to febrile neutropaenia or to avoid treatment delays (Lee et al. 2016).

Results

Twenty-two women (15 HGSOC/7 gBRCAmOvCa) have been treated. Five PRs have been seen in 13 evaluable cohort 1 patients (two with platinum-sensitive and three with platinum-resistant disease). Four of six evaluable cohort 2 patients presented SD ≥ 4 months, with 0/6 objective responses. Therefore, LY2606368 alone shows promising preliminary activity in BRCA wild type HGSOC patients (Lee et al. 2016). Further results of this trial are awaited.

11.10.4 Study 4

LY2606368 in head and neck cancers—'Phase Ib trial of LY2606368 in combination with chemoradiation in patients with locally advanced head and neck squamous cell cancer' (Yang et al. 2016).

LY2606368 is being assessed in a phase Ib, two-part multicenter, parallel, non-randomized, open-label trial with patients newly diagnosed with locally advanced untreated HNSCC. The primary objective is to determine the recommended phase II dose (RP2D) of LY2606368 in combination with either cisplatin and radiation therapy (RT) (Part A) or cetuximab and RT (Part B). All part A patients will receive

40 mg/m² cisplatin weekly for 7 weeks, while patients in Part B will receive cetuximab weekly at an initial dose of 400 mg/m² followed by 250 mg/m² for 7 weeks. All patients will receive 70 Gy of RT delivered as 5 fractions/week over 7 weeks and LY2606368 in 1-h infusions every 2 weeks. Dose escalation of LY2606368 will be performed using a modified time-to-event continual reassessment method. Following dose escalation and determination of the RP2D for each arm, dose expansion cohorts of approximately 15 patients will be enrolled to confirm the dose (Yang et al. 2016).

Toxicity and Efficacy

The safety and efficacy data from this trial have not been reported (Yang et al. 2016).

Future Development of LY2606368

There have been interesting responses observed in early clinical trials of LY2606368 as a single agent in biomarker-defined cohorts. In particular, 3/11 patients with HGSOC have had partial responses in a subset of patients with no *BRCA* mutations. Ovarian cancers are known to have multiple defects in DNA repair genes (Cancer Genome Atlas Research N 2011) and it is possible that further analysis of biomarkers will allow further enrichment of patient cohorts. Interestingly, one study found a response in patients with SCC; although the current biomarkers of sensitivity are not known, it is possible that further studies will help to elucidate biomarkers for the use of LY2606368 as monotherapy or in combination with chemotherapy or radiotherapy in this setting. Most preclinical studies have used gemcitabine as the chemotherapeutic partner and this has not been tested in combination with LY2606368.

11.11   LY2603618

LY2603618 (Eli Lilly) is an adenosine triphosphate-competitive inhibitor of CHK1, with more than 50-fold selectivity for CHK1 inhibition when evaluated in a 100-member protein-kinase panel (Weiss et al. 2013). This drug has shown to enhance the activity of cytotoxic chemotherapy agents, including gemcitabine, in *in vitro* and *in vivo* nonclinical efficacy studies (Laquente et al. 2017). Some phase I and phase II trials have been reported assessing this agent:

11.11.1   Study 1

'Phase I dose-escalation study to examine the safety and tolerability of LY2603618, a checkpoint 1 kinase inhibitor, administered 1 day after pemetrexed 500 mg/m² *every 21 days in patients with cancer'* (Infante et al. 2015).

This is an open-label, dose-escalation trial, which included patients with advanced solid tumours. Pemetrexed at the dose of 500 mg/m² was combined with increasing doses of LY2603618 (from 40 to 195 mg/m²). LY2603618 was administered on days 1 and 9 and pemetrexed on day 8 in a 28-day cycle during cycle 1. For the subsequent cycles, pemetrexed was administered on day 1 and LY2603618 on day 2 every 3 weeks. A total of six cohorts were enrolled. The MTD of LY2603618, when dosed in combination with pemetrexed 500 mg/m² on a 21-day schedule, was established at 150 mg/m² (Weiss et al. 2013).

Toxicity

A total of 31 patients were enrolled (3 at 40 mg/m² over 4.5-h infusion, 1-h infusion in subsequent cohorts: 3 each at 40, 70, and 195 mg/m²; 13 at 105 mg/m²; 6 at 150 mg/m²). Four patients experienced a DLT: diarrhoea (105 mg/m²); reversible infusion-related reaction (150 mg/m²); thrombocytopaenia (195 mg/m²); and fatigue (195 mg/m²) (Weiss et al. 2013).

The toxicity profile of LY2603618 in combination with pemetrexed is similar to pemetrexed as single-agent and is consistent with its non-clinical toxicology profile. Common adverse events were fatigue (61.3%), nausea (51.6%), vomiting (38.7%), diarrhoea (35.5%), dyspnoea (35.5%), and neutropaenia (32.3%). The majority of those events were mild or moderate and there was no correlation between the incidence of adverse events and the dose increase of LY2603618. SAEs related to both study drugs included Grade 3 anaemia, pneumonia, diarrhoea, blood/bone marrow events and Grade 2 fatigue and fever (Weiss et al. 2013).

Pharmacokinetics

LY2603618 showed dose-dependent increases in AUC and C_{max} after its administration on day 1 and day 9 of cycle 1 across the dose range from 40 to 195 mg/m². The PK data demonstrated that the exposure of LY2603618 was unaffected by the administration of pemetrexed. This study also showed that the majority of the calculated $t_{1/2}$ at doses >105 mg/m² (including the MTD of 150 mg/m²) are consistent with a $t_{1/2}$ (i.e., >10 and <24 h) suitable for achieving and maintaining acceptable human exposures while minimizing the intra-cycle accumulation of LY2603618 when given in combination with pemetrexed (Weiss et al. 2013).

Efficacy

Twenty-three patients were considered evaluable for best tumour response changes. One PR was observed in a patient with adenocarcinoma of the pancreas dosed on the 105 mg/m² cohort. Nine patients (39.1%) showed SD and 13 (56.5%) exhibited progressive disease (Weiss et al. 2013).

11.11.2   Study 2

'*Preclinical analyses and phase I evaluation of LY2603618 administered in combination with pemetrexed and cisplatin in patients with advanced cancer*' (Calvo et al. 2014).

Preclinical studies in NSCLC cell lines and *in vitro/in vivo* models treated with pemetrexed and LY2603618 provided the rationale for evaluating this combination in a clinical setting. These data informed the clinical assessment of LY2603618 in a phase I/II study, which administered pemetrexed at 500 mg/m² and cisplatin at 75 mg/m² and escalating doses of LY2603618, from 130 to 275 mg (Calvo et al. 2014).

Toxicity

In the phase I part, 14 patients were enrolled, and the most frequently AEs were: fatigue, nausea, pyrexia, neutropaenia and vomiting. No DLTs were observed at the tested doses. The combination of LY2603618, pemetrexed and cisplatin demonstrated acceptable safety profile (Calvo et al. 2014).

PK and Biomarkers

The systemic exposure of LY2603618 increased in a dose-dependent manner. PK parameters that correlate with the maximal pharmacodynamic effect in nonclinical xenograft models were achieved at doses ≥240 mg. No alteration was reported in the PKs of LY2603618, pemetrexed and cisplatin when used in combination (Calvo et al. 2014).

Efficacy

Two NSCLC patients achieved PR and eight patients had SD. The recommended phase II dose of LY2603618 was 275 mg (Calvo et al. 2014).

11.11.3 Study 3

'*Phase I study of LY2603618, a CHK1 inhibitor, in combination with gemcitabine in Japanese patients with solid tumors*' (Doi et al. 2015).

This phase I study evaluated patients with advanced solid tumours treated with LY2603618 at doses from 70 to 250 mg/m^2 or flat doses of 200 or 230 mg after administration of gemcitabine 1000 mg/m^2. Fifty patients were enrolled and the fixed LY2603618 dose of 230 mg combined with gemcitabine was selected as the recommended phase II dose (Doi et al. 2015).

Toxicity

Frequent adverse events possibly related to the study drug included fatigue (44%), thrombocytopaenia (42%), neutropaenia (32%), nausea (26%), and anaemia (20%) (Doi et al. 2015).

Pharmacokinetics and Biomarkers

Systemic exposure of LY2603618 increased dose dependently while clearance was relatively dose independent. The mean LY2603618 half-life varied; however, the durations were still suitable for maintaining exposures consistent with maximal pharmacodynamic effect in nonclinical models while minimizing accumulation. Of note, LY2603618 PK were not altered by gemcitabine administration (Doi et al. 2015).

Efficacy

One patient with NSCLC achieved a PR and other 22 patients had SD (Doi et al. 2015).

11.11.4 Study 4

'*A randomised, phase 2 evaluation of the CHK1 inhibitor, LY2603618, administered in combination with pemetrexed and cisplatin in patients with advanced nonsquamous non-small cell lung cancer*' (Wehler et al. 2017)

This is a phase II, multicenter, randomized, controlled, open-label study. Sixty-two patients were enrolled with histologically diagnosed stage IV, non-squamous NSCLC. They were randomized (2:1) to LY2603618 combined with pemetrexed and cisplatin (experimental arm) or pemetrexed and cisplatin. Patients received four 21-day cycles of induction therapy: day 1 (all patients), 500 mg/m^2 of pemetrexed IV and 75 mg/m^2 cisplatin IV (30 min after pemetrexed) and day 2 (experimental arm), 275 mg of LY2603618 IV. After induction, patients received maintenance therapy with pemetrexed on day 1 and in the experimental arm, on day 2, LY2603618 as per induction (Wehler et al. 2017).

Toxicity

In October 2012, a safety review of SAE data revealed an imbalanced rate of thromboembolic events in patients who received LY2603618 (rate = 23%, nine patients); therefore, enrollment was interrupted and permanently halted on 25 October 2012. Thereafter, patients in the experimental arm received only pemetrexed and cisplatin in the induction phase but they could continue with the LY2603618/pemetrexed in the maintenance phase (Wehler et al. 2017).

The thromboembolic events occurred within the first 3 months of treatment in eight patients. Seven patients experienced seven serious thromboembolic events: pulmonary embolism (n = 5, none related), ischemic stroke (n = 1, related) and cerebrovascular accident (n = 1, related). No thromboembolic events resulted in death or were reported after enrollment halting (Wehler et al. 2017).

The majority of patients had ≥1 treatment-related adverse event. The most common SAEs were thromboembolic events (experimental arm: 5/39 [12.8%]; pemetrexed + cisplatin: 0) and bone pain (experimental arm: 2/39 [5.1%]; pemetrexed + cisplatin: 1/22 [4.5%]). There were no marked differences/evidence of consistent changes in laboratory evaluations/vital signs (Wehler et al. 2017).

Pharmacokinetics and Biomarker

The LY2603618 exposure targets (AUC $\geq$ 21,000 ng·h/mL and $C_{max} \geq$ 2000 ng/mL), determined before clinical investigation and correlating with maximal pharmacodynaic effect in nonclinical HT-29 xenograft models, were achieved on a mean cohort basis after administration of LY2603618 at 275 mg. The PK results indicate that the recommended dose of 275 mg provides an elimination half-life suitable for achieving/maintaining optimal exposure while minimizing inter-cycle accumulation when combined with pemetrexed and cisplatin (Wehler et al. 2017).

Efficacy

This is the first phase II study to disclose the efficacy and safety of a CHK1 inhibitor combined with pemetrexed and cisplatin in patients with advanced non-squamous NSCLC. Bayesian analysis demonstrated that the probability of a PFS hazard ratio <1 for the experimental arm was 96% and frequentist analysis demonstrated that PFS was significantly longer for the experimental arm. Therefore, the primary endpoint of this study was met. In contrast with the primary efficacy outcome, there were no statistically significant differences between treatment arms among secondary efficacy outcomes (overall survival, duration of response, duration of disease control, clinical benefit rate, objective response rate, change in tumour size, and the proportion of patients who received maintenance therapy) (Wehler et al. 2017).

11.11.5   Study 5

'Phase II evaluation of LY2603618, a first-generation CHK1 inhibitor, in combination with pemetrexed in patients with advanced or metastatic non-small cell lung cancer' (Scagliotti et al. 2016)

This phase II trial assessed the ORR, safety and PK of the combination of LY2603618 and pemetrexed in patients with NSCLC. It was an open-label and single-arm trial with patients diagnosed with advanced or metastatic NSCLC progressing after prior first-line treatment regimen (not containing pemetrexed) and an Eastern Cooperative Oncology Group performance status ≤ 2. Patients received pemetrexed (500 mg/m^2, day 1) and LY2603618 (150 mg/m^2, day 2) every 21 days until disease progression (Scagliotti et al. 2016).

Toxicity

The most common study drug-related AEs were neutropaenia, nausea, anaemia, fatigue, and vomiting. The nature of these AEs was generally consistent with those reported for pemetrexed, suggesting that LY2603618 did not appreciably enhance toxicity when combined with pemetrexed. Grade 3/4 neutropaenia was reported in 29.1% of patients in this study. All study-drug-related serious AEs, except for one seizure event attributed to LY2603618 treatment, were consistent with the known toxicity profile of pemetrexed (Scagliotti et al. 2016).

Biomarkers

No evidence of an association between p53 status and ORR, PFS, or number of cycles administered was observed, regardless of the method used to determine p53 functionality. It is not known why LY2603618 did not result in improved outcomes in combination with pemetrexed. Since there was not a direct pharmacodynamic biomarker, it is possible that in humans LY2603618 does not have sufficient potency or duration of CHK1 inhibition for a significant therapeutic effect (Scagliotti et al. 2016).

Results

Of the 55 enrolled patients, 49 were evaluable for best overall response. All 55 patients were included in the overall analysis. No patients experienced a CR. PRs were observed in five patients (9.1%) and SD in 20 patients (36.4%). Twenty-four patients (43.6%) had progressive disease. The clinical benefit rate was 45.5%. The median progression-free survival (PFS) was 2.3 months (range as of data cut-off date, 0–27.1). Forty-six patients had PD or died. Therefore, in this study, the addition of LY2603618 to standard second-line therapy with pemetrexed did not improve outcomes relative to historical controls (Scagliotti et al. 2016).

11.11.6   Study 6

'*A phase II study to evaluate LY2603618 in combination with gemcitabine in pancreatic cancer patients*' (Laquente et al. 2017).

This phase II open-label, multicenter, randomized, 2-arm study evaluated patients with locally advanced or metastatic pancreatic cancer (stage II–IV). Ninety-nine patients (n = 65, LY2603618/gemcitabine; n = 34, gemcitabine alone) were enrolled (intent-to-treat population). Patients were randomized (2:1) to either LY2603618 at 230 mg and gemcitabine at 1000 mg/m^2 or gemcitabine as single agent at 1000 mg/m^2. Gemcitabine was administered on days 1, 8, and 15 of a 28-day cycle. LY2603618 (230 mg) was administered 24 h after administration of gemcitabine. OS, PFS, ORR, duration of response, PK and safety were evaluated in this study (Laquente et al. 2017).

Toxicity

The severity of AEs in the experimental arm was comparable to gemcitabine alone. The most frequently AEs in both arms were nausea, thrombocytopaenia, fatigue, and neutropaenia. Fewer patients experienced anaemia with LY2603618/gemcitabine (13.8%) than with gemcitabine (26.5%). On the other hand, a higher incidence of vomiting, loss of appetite and stomatitis was observed in the experimental arm. For each group, neutropaenia and thrombocytopaenia were the most common grade 3/4 AEs possibly related to treatment, in addition to anaemia, which was also common to gemcitabine. Fourteen patients (n = 8, LY2603618/gemcitabine; n = 6, gemcitabine) discontinued the study due to AEs. Of the 8 patients who discontinued in the LY2603618/gemcitabine arm, four events (grade 4 cerebrovascular accident, grade 1 left bundle branch block, grade 3 acute pulmonary oedema and grade 3 atrial fibrillation) were deemed possibly related to treatment. Of the six patients who discontinued in the gemcitabine arm, four possibly drug-related events occurred (grade 3 thrombotic microangiopathy, grade 4 acute renal failure, grade 2 thrombocytopaenia, and grade 3 hemolytic uraemic syndrome). The safety profiles were comparable between arms, indicating that the addition of LY2603618 did not significantly change the safety profile of gemcitabine (Laquente et al. 2017).

Pharmacokinetics

LY2603618 concentrations were quantified using a validated high-pressure liquid chromatography/mass spectrometry method. The LY2603618 exposure targets ($AUC_{0-\infty} \geq 21,000$ ng h/mL and $C_{max} \geq 2000$ ng/mL) predicted for maximum pharmacodynamic response were achieved after 230 mg of LY2603618 (Laquente et al. 2017).

The safety and PK profiles were comparable between treatment arms. More specifically, 87% and 73% of the individual PK profiles on days 2 and 16 of cycle 1 were above the targets for C_{max} and $AUC_{0-\infty,}$ respectively. Gemcitabine did not appear to affect the PK of LY2603618, as the PK parameters reported in this study were similar to the PK parameters calculated after LY2603618 monotherapy (Laquente et al. 2017).

Biomarkers

A nucleoside analog DNA incorporation assay method measured the amount of gemcitabine incorporated into genomic DNA. $2':2'$-difluorodeoxycytidine (dFdC) was incorporated into DNA following gemcitabine administration, with the levels declining to almost baseline by the end of each treatment cycle. The highest levels of dFdC incorporation were observed on days 8 and 15 across all doses. The increases in the amount of dFdC incorporation did not correspond to increasing doses of LY2603618 (Laquente et al. 2017).

Of the patients who had baseline CA19–9 levels > upper limit of normal, a similar percentage of patients (65.4% LY2603618/gemcitabine; 64% gemcitabine) experienced a >50% reduction from baseline in CA19–9 levels. Due to the lack of a clinically-validated pharmacodynamic marker to quantify direct CHK1 inhibition by LY2603618, the magnitude and duration of CHK1 target inhibition at 230 mg is neither known nor has it been correlated to clinical responses (Laquente et al. 2017).

Efficacy

OS was not improved with the addition of LY2603618/gemcitabine compared with gemcitabine alone: the median OS was 7.8 months (range: 0.3–18.9) with LY2603618/gemcitabine and 8.3 months (range: 0.8–19.1) with gemcitabine. Moreover, LY2603618/gemcitabine was not statistically superior to gemcitabine alone when PFS, duration of response, ORR and clinical benefit rate were assessed. No CR was observed with either treatment (Laquente et al. 2017).

Future Plans

LY2603618/gemcitabine will not be further developed for the treatment of patients with pancreatic cancer in the light of the results presented (Laquente et al. 2017). The combination of LY2606368 with pemetrexed in a phase II study has been disappointing. Regarding the combination of this CHK1 inhibitor with pemetrexed and cisplatin, although the primary endpoint of the phase II study was met, no further development will be done for treatment of advanced non-squamous NSCLC due to the potential increased risk of thromboembolic events (Wehler et al. 2017). This should not, however, be interpreted as a lack of efficacy of LY2606368 with S phase targeting agents.

11.12   MK-8776

Initially known as SCH900776, MK-8776 (Merck) is a pyrazolo [1,5-a]pyrimidine derivative with a potent and selective ATP-competitive CHK1 inhibition, low protein binding and adequate aqueous solubility (Daud et al. 2015; Guzi et al. 2011).

MK-8776 inhibits CHK1 without substantial effect on the potentially antagonistic checkpoint regulators CHK2 or CDK1. In preclinical models, this CHK1 inhibitor synergized with antimetabolites, including the nucleoside analogs cytarabine and gemcitabine, to induce apoptosis and long-lasting tumour regressions in ovarian and pancreatic tumour models, without apparent exacerbation of toxicity in normal tissues (Daud et al. 2015). Experiments in the A2780 human ovarian carcinoma xenograft model confirmed marked induction of γ-H2AX with the combination of MK-8776 and gemcitabine and a similar effect was shown in the MIAPaCa-2 xenograft with slow-growing gemcitabine-refractory pancreatic carcinoma cells (Daud et al. 2015).

11.12.1   Study 1

'Phase I Dose-Escalation Trial of Checkpoint Kinase 1 Inhibitor MK-8776 As Monotherapy and in Combination with Gemcitabine in Patients with Advanced Solid Tumors' (Daud et al. 2015).

This study evaluated MK-8776 as monotherapy and combined with gemcitabine. It was a phase I, open-label, dose-escalation clinical trial (Merck; protocol No. P05248). It was conducted in two parts: the first one, part A, gemcitabine 800 mg/m^2 was combined with MK-8776 at 10, 20, 40, 80, or 112 mg/m^2. In part B, gemcitabine 1000 mg/m^2 was combined with MK-8776 at 80, 112, or 150 mg/m^2 or a flat dose of 200 mg. Cycle 0 consisted of one dose of monotherapy with MK-8776 at the assigned dose level. The combination of gemcitabine and MK-8776 was administered on days

1 and 8 of a classic 21-day cycle. Cycles continued until progression of disease or treatment discontinuation for other reasons (Daud et al. 2015).

Dose escalation occurred for each treatment cohort based on demonstration of pharmacologically active exposures (PK/PD correlation) at the highest gemcitabine dose safely achievable in combination with MK-8776. The maximal administered dose of MK-8776 was 150 mg/m^2 and the RP2D was gemcitabine 1000 mg/m^2 plus MK-8776 200 mg as a flat dose (i.e., 112 mg/m^2 at a BSA of 1.8 m^2) on day 1 and day 8 of a 21-day cycle (Daud et al. 2015).

In this trial, a total of 43 patients (26 in part A and 17 in part B) were enrolled. Forty-one patients discontinued MK-8776 treatment as a result of disease progression (54%), AEs (17%), withdrawal of consent (15%), symptomatic deterioration (12%), or loss of follow-up (1, 2%) (Daud et al. 2015).

Toxicity

The most common MK-8776 monotherapy-related (cycle 0) AEs were QTc prolongation (19%), nausea (16%), constipation (14%), and fatigue (14%). The most common combination-therapy-related AEs were fatigue (63%), nausea (44%), decreased appetite (37%), thrombocytopaenia (32%), infections (29%), pyrexia (29%), abdominal pain (24%), and neutropaenia (24%). The most common (10% of patients) grade 3 or 4 AEs reported were neutropaenia (14%), thrombocytopaenia (12%), and fatigue (10%). Two patients (5%) experienced grade 3 QTc prolongation in the combination therapy (one patient during cycle 1 and the other one on day 344) (Daud et al. 2015).

Pharmacokinetics

There was a linear PK profile, with limited intra-patient variability. Age, sex, height, weight, body surface area (BSA), and creatinine clearance did not affect the PK parameters of MK-8776. BSA-based dosing was not associated with a significant reduction in inter-patient variability of drug clearance or volume of distribution (Daud et al. 2015).

MK-8776 is not highly protein bound (49% in human plasma) and exhibits a rapid distribution phase when administered as a 15–30 min IV infusion (plasma concentration declined in a multiphasic manner) (Daud et al. 2015).

MK-8776 cleared from plasma with mean terminal-phase half-life values ranging from 5.56 to 9.78 h in a dose-independent fashion. Individual dose-normalized MK-8776 plasma exposures were generally comparable when MK-8776 was given as monotherapy or in combination with gemcitabine. The infusion duration of MK-8776 was evaluated as 15 and 30 min. When increased from 15 to 30 min, mean C_{max} of MK-8776 decreased by 20% in both monotherapy and in combination with gemcitabine. Nevertheless, mean plasma exposure of MK-8776 was comparable between the 15- and 30-min infusions. Because of the small sample size, a correlation between C_{max} and absolute QTc could not be concluded (Daud et al. 2015).

Biomarkers

A direct correlation between administered dose of MK-8776 and penetrance of the γ-H2AX (number of γ-H2AX positive cells, expressed as percentage of total cell culture population) was reported. As observed in pharmacodynamic studies, serum levels of MK-8776 were sufficient to produce effective synergy with gemcitabine (Daud et al. 2015).

Efficacy

Of 43 patients treated, 30 were evaluable for response. Two (7%) showed PR (melanoma, n = 1; cholangiocarcinoma, n = 1) and 13 patients (43%) had SD, six of them for 4 months. One patient with previously gemcitabine-refractory cholangio-carcinoma had a sustained PR over 19 months. Clinical efficacy was observed even in patients previously refractory to gemcitabine, as expected from preclinical studies (Daud et al. 2015).

11.12.2   Study 2

MK-8776 in hematological malignancies—'Phase I and Pharmacologic Trial of Cytosine Arabinoside with the Selective Checkpoint 1 Inhibitor Sch 900776 in Refractory Acute Leukemias' (Karp et al. 2012).

In preclinical models, MK-8776 synergized with antimetabolites, including the nucleoside analogs cytarabine, inducing apoptosis and sustained tumour regressions in ovarian and pancreatic tumour models (Karp et al. 2012). It was shown that MK-8776 diminished cytarabine-induced S-phase arrest and enhanced cytarabine cytotoxicity in AML lines and AML clinical specimens ex vivo (Karp et al. 2012). Based on those preclinical findings, the present study evaluated MK-8776 in combination with cytarabine (Karp et al. 2012). A total of 24 adults with relapsed (37%) or refractory (63%) acute leukaemias were enrolled on study between September 2009 and January 2011. The majority had acute myeloid leukaemia (AML) that had not responded to the most recent therapy (refractory, 13/24, 54%), previous exposure to moderately high doses of cytarabine (15/24, 63%). In addition, 7 of 21 (33%) patients with AML had received prior allogeneic stem cell transplantation (SCT). Median time from SCT to relapse was 7 months (range, 3–16) (Karp et al. 2012).

In this trial, all patients received continuous infusion cytarabine 2 g/m² over 72 h (667 mg/m²/24 h) on days 1 and 10. MK-8776 was administered on days 2, 3, 11, and 12 at starting dose of 10 mg/m^2/dose. This dose was doubled on levels 2 and 3 (20 and 40 mg/m^2/dose, respectively) and increased by 40% thereafter (level 4, 56 mg/m^2/dose; level 5, 80 mg/m^2). At level 5, dosing calculations were changed to flat dosing—140 mg (Karp et al. 2012).

Toxicities

DLT occurred at a dose level of MK-8776 140 mg flat dosing (equivalent to 80 mg/ m^2), manifested by asymptomatic but extended (45 min) grade 3 QTcF prolongation in one patient and transient (<15 min) grade 3 QTcF prolongation in another patient. This effect on cardiac conduction was likely to be related directly to MK-8776, with no contribution from cytarabine. Prolonged (>7 days) grade 3 palmar-plantar erythodysesthesia observed in one patient represented an exacerbation of a known cytarabine toxicity. Another two patients had grade 2 (483–485 ms) QTcF prolongation at the end of the MK-8776 infusion and for 15 min thereafter with subsequent spontaneous resolution. All episodes of QTcF prolongation occurred in the setting of electrolyte optimization and avoidance of agents that could cause or exacerbate QTcF (Karp et al. 2012).

Grade 1–2 gastrointestinal symptoms were experienced by all patients during the trial but symptoms were transient with appropriate supportive care. Four patients had grade 3 hyperbilirubinaemia but it was short-lived and resolved completely within 48 h. The incidence of grade 3/4 infectious complications was consistent with cytarabine treatment across all dose levels (25%). Considering all those findings, the RP2D for MK-8776 was 100 mg/dose (equivalent to 56 mg/m^2/dose) on days 2, 3 11, and 12 in combination with cytarabine 2 g/m^2/72 h on days 1–3 and 10–12 (Karp et al. 2012).

Pharmacokinetics

Dose-related increases in MK-8776 plasma concentrations were reported in mean C_{max} and exposure values ($AUC_{0-8.25 h}$ for 15-min infusion or $AUC_{0-8.5h}$ for 30-min infusion) over the dose range evaluated. As dose increased in a ratio of 1:2:4:6 following 15-min infusions, mean C_{max} (day 2) increased in the ratio of 1:3:6:9 and exposure (day 2) increased in a ratio of 1:3:5:6. At each dose level, plasma C_{max} and exposure values were comparable for study days 2 and 3 (Karp et al. 2012).

Biomarkers

To evaluate the impact of MK-8776 given during the continuous cytarabine infusion on leukemic blast cell DNA damage, H2Ax phosphorylation was examined in bone marrow aspirates harvested sequentially before (day 0) and 24 h after the beginning of the cytarabine infusion but before the first MK-8776 dose (day 2) and 2 h after the end of the second MK-8776 infusion (day 3). An increase in H2Ax phosphorylation was observed after 24 h of continuous cytarabine infusion in 2 of 10 samples and a further robust increase in H2Ax phosphorylation in three of seven specimens 26 h later following the second MK-8776 dose. This marker of enhanced DNA damage was observed in three of five sets of samples from patients treated with 40 mg/m^2 MK-8776 or higher, showing that the action of MK-8776 detected in preclinical studies can also be identified in the clinical setting (Karp et al. 2012).

Efficacy

There is preliminary evidence of clinical activity in this small group of patients with relapsed and/or refractory acute leukaemias, including those who have had previous exposure to moderate-high-dose cytarabine. The achievement of complete tumour clearance by day 14 of therapy occurred across all dose levels in 50% of the patients, including two of six (17%) at MK-8776 doses of 20 mg/m^2 and at least three of six (50%) beginning at dose level 3 (40 mg/m^2). Similarly, the overall response rate (CR plus CRi) was 8 of 24 (33%), with 1 CRi (17%) of six patients treated with MK-8776 doses of ≤20 mg/m^2 and 7 (39%; 5 CR, 2 CRi) of 18 patients treated at dose level 3 (40 mg/m^2) or higher, with at least two of six (33%) in each of dose levels 3 through 5. All eight CR/CRi occurred in the 21 (38%) patients with AML. All CR/CRi were associated with cytogenetic clearance. CR/CRi occurred in 6 of 14 (43%) patients who had received prior high doses of cytarabine. Four (50%), including two who received additional post-CR cycles, were able to proceed to allo-SCT or donor lymphocyte infusion following achievement of CR/CRi. Median duration of response for all patients with CR/CRi was 10 months (Karp et al. 2012).

The notion that part of the responses might be related to the association of MK-8776 to the timed sequential cytarabine infusions is supported by the presence of a dose-response curve, with clinical responses to MK-8776 beginning at 40 mg/m^2, in conjunction with C$_{max}$ exceeding 1000 ng/mL (Karp et al. 2012). For patients who received <40 mg/m^2 MK-8776, the CR/CRi rate was one of six (17%) versus 7 of 18 (39%) for those receiving ≥40 mg/m^2 (P = 0.0005, Fisher exact test). Of the eight who responded, six had previously received moderate to high-dose cytarabine, two had undergone prior allo-SCT and two had primary refractory AML following moderate- to high-dose cytarabine (Karp et al. 2012).

Future Plans

MK-8776 as combination therapy with gemcitabine is well tolerated and shows a reproducibly effective degree of CHK1 inhibition. Marrow blasts obtained pretreatment and during therapy showed increased phosphorylation of H2Ax after MK-8776 beginning at 40 mg/m^2, consistent with unrepaired DNA damage, providing evidence that the action of MK-8776 observed in preclinical studies can also be detected in the clinical setting. However, given the small sample size of these dose-finding trials, further studies are necessary. Moreover, a larger cohort of relapsed and refractory patients with AML would be important to determine whether there is any relationship between prior cytarabine treatment, the presence of a complex karyotype or any other pretreatment parameter and response to this therapy (Karp et al. 2012).

11.13   PF-00477736 (PF-736)

PF-736 (Pfizer) is a selective inhibitor of CHK1, displaying >10-fold selectivity over CHK2. Preclinical studies have shown that PF-736 can enhance the response to gemcitabine. This is associated with abrogation of the S/G2 checkpoint with cells entering mitosis prematurely (Brega et al. 2010).

11.13.1   Phase 1

Clinical trial of gemcitabine (GEM) in combination with PF-00477736 (PF-736), a selective inhibitor of CHK1 kinase' (Brega et al. 2010).

A phase I trial was conducted to evaluate the combination of PF-736 with gemcitabine in sequential cohorts of 3–6 gemcitabine-naïve patients with advanced solid tumours. Patients received IV PF-736 alone on days 1 and 8 in cycle 0 (C0) and then started the combination of gemcitabine and PF-736 in C1, days 1 and 8 and 2 and 9 respectively, with PF-736 starting 20–24 h after completion of gemcitabine, in 21-day cycles. C0 and C1 were considered for DLT (Brega et al. 2010).

Toxicity

DLT of thrombocytopaenia, sudden death, mucositis, and elevated lipase were seen in C1. The MTD was 270 mg of PF-736 with gemcitabine 750 mg/m^2. One patient treated at PF-736 80 mg had abnormal elevated liver function tests on C10 and died from hepatic veno-occlusive disease 3 weeks later. Common drug-related AEs occurring in >30% patients were pyrexia, fatigue, neutropaenia, nausea, vomiting, and diarrhoea. Forty-two per cent of patients had dose delays due to G3 neutropaenia making days 1 and 8 of the schedule difficult to maintain (Brega et al. 2010).

Pharmacokinetics

The exposure of PF-736 increased proportionally with increased dose from 50 mg to 270 mg. Mean $T_{1/2}$ ranged from 8 to 20 h (Brega et al. 2010).

Response

Three PRs were observed in patients with SCC of the skin, NSCLC, and mesothelioma (Brega et al. 2010).

Future Plans

At the MTD of 270 mg of PF-736 in combination with gemcitabine 750 mg/m², clinical activity was demonstrated. However, hepatic veno-occlusive disease was seen for the first time (Brega et al. 2010). The trial was terminated prematurely due to a commercial decision (Brega et al. 2010).

11.14 SRA737

SRA737 (Sierra Oncology) is a potent, highly selective, orally bioavailable small molecule inhibitor of CHK1. This agent is being investigated in two parallel clinical contexts: as a single agent and in combination with standard-of-care chemotherapy in solid tumours (ClincalTrials.Gov 2016a, b).

In the combination scheme, SRA737 is being investigated in a dose escalation design in association with gemcitabine plus cisplatin and also with gemcitabine alone (NCT02797977) (ClincalTrials.Gov 2016b). A monotherapy study is also currently ongoing (NCT02797964) (ClincalTrials.Gov 2016a). Once PK-PD-driven doses and schedules have been defined, dose expansion into biomarker-enriched cohorts is planned.

11.15 Conclusions and Future Perspectives

Evaluation of CHK1 inhibitors is at an exciting stage in their clinical development. Early doubts about the 'on target' cardiac effects of CHK1 inhibitors, initially seen with AZD7762, have not been realized, with multiple new CHK1 inhibitors reaching pharmacologically active doses without being limited by cardiotoxicity. We have also learned that combinations of CHK1 inhibitors with chemotherapy are myelotoxic and early institution of intermittent schedules enabled by orally administered inhibitors and growth factor support can circumvent some of these toxicities. Exciting responses in cancers with possible DDR defects, such as ovarian cancer, have been seen (Lee et al. 2016; Kim et al. 2015; Kobayashi et al. 2015; Walton et al. 2016). In addition, responses in squamous cell cancers treated with a CHK1 inhibitor as monotherapy have been reported (Hong et al. 2016). Research focusing on finding biomarkers of replicative stress and DDR can capitalize on the knowledge that these early responses have brought to further enrich clinical trials. Importantly, preclinical studies have shown activity of CHK1 inhibitors as monotherapy in lymphoma (Garrett and Collins 2011; Walton et al. 2016; Bryant et al. 2014) and neuroblastoma (Cole et al. 2011; Garrett and Collins 2011): areas of high unmet need. In addition to monotherapy and combinations with chemotherapy/radiotherapy, a range of DDR inhibitors such as PARP, Wee and ATR inhibitors are now either licensed or undergoing clinical evaluation and CHK1 inhibitors may combine beneficially with these agents. Finally, there have been significant advances in immune oncology. The effects of CHK1-mediated cell death, either as a monotherapy or in combination with chemotherapy or radiotherapy on neo-antigen presentation, is not fully understood and further research into this area could leverage further activity from this class of agents.

References

Barker HE, Patel R, McLaughlin M, Schick U, Zaidi S, Nutting CM, Newbold KL, Bhide S, Harrington KJ (2016) CHK1 inhibition radiosensitizes head and neck cancers to paclitaxel-based chemoradiotherapy. Mol Cancer Ther 15:2042–2054

Benada J, Macurek L (2015) Targeting the checkpoint to kill cancer cells. Biomol Ther 5:1912–1937

Borst GR, McLaughlin M, Kyula JN, Neijenhuis S, Khan A, Good J, Zaidi S, Powell NG, Meier P, Collins I et al (2013) Targeted radiosensitization by the Chk1 inhibitor SAR-020106. Int J Radiat Oncol Biol Phys 85:1110–1118

Brega N, McArthur GA, Britten C, Wong SG, Wang E, Wilner KD, Blasina A, Schwartz GK, Gallo J, Tse AN (2010) Phase I clinical trial of gemcitabine (GEM) in combination with PF-00477736 (PF-736), a selective inhibitor of CHK1 kinase. In: ASCO annual meeting. Chicago, USA. J Clin Oncol 28:15s

Bridges KA, Chen X, Liu H, Rock C, Buchholz TA, Shumway SD, Skinner HD, Meyn RE (2016) MK-8776, a novel chk1 kinase inhibitor, radiosensitizes p53-defective human tumor cells. Oncotarget 7(44):71660–71672

Bryant C, Scriven K, Massey AJ (2014) Inhibition of the checkpoint kinase Chk1 induces DNA damage and cell death in human leukemia and lymphoma cells. Mol Cancer 13:147

Calvo E, Chen VJ, Marshall M, Ohnmacht U, Hynes SM, Kumm E, Diaz HB, Barnard D, Merzoug FF, Huber L et al (2014) Preclinical analyses and phase I evaluation of LY2603618 administered in combination with pemetrexed and cisplatin in patients with advanced cancer. Investig New Drugs 32:955–968

Cancer Genome Atlas Research N (2011) Integrated genomic analyses of ovarian carcinoma. Nature 474:609–615

Chaudhuri L, Vincelette ND, Koh BD, Naylor RM, Flatten KS, Peterson KL, McNally A, Gojo I, Karp JE, Mesa RA et al (2014) CHK1 and WEE1 inhibition combine synergistically to enhance therapeutic efficacy in acute myeloid leukemia ex vivo. Haematologica 99:688–696

ClincalTrials.Gov (2016a) ClincalTrials.Gov: a CRUK phase I trial of CCT245737 in patients with advanced cancer. https://clinicaltrials.gov/ct2/results?term=NCT02797964&Search=Search

ClincalTrials.Gov (2016b) ClincalTrials.Gov: a CRUK phase I trial of CCT245737 in combination with gemcitabine plus cisplatin or gemcitabine alone in patients with advanced cancer. https://clinicaltrials.gov/ct2/results?term=NCT02797977&Search=Search

ClinicalTrials.Gov (2018) A study of GDC-0575 alone and in combination with gemcitabine in patients with refractory solid tumors or lymphoma. https://clinicaltrials.gov/ct2/show/NCT01564251?term=GDC-0575&rank=1:

Cole KA, Huggins J, Laquaglia M, Hulderman CE, Russell MR, Bosse K, Diskin SJ, Attiyeh EF, Sennett R, Norris G et al (2011) RNAi screen of the protein kinome identifies checkpoint kinase 1 (CHK1) as a therapeutic target in neuroblastoma. Proc Natl Acad Sci U S A 108:3336–3341

Dai Y, Grant S (2010) New insights into checkpoint kinase 1 in the DNA damage response signaling network. Clin Cancer Res 16:376–383

Daud AI, Ashworth MT, Strosberg J, Goldman JW, Mendelson D, Springett G, Venook AP, Loechner S, Rosen LS, Shanahan F et al (2015) Phase I dose-escalation trial of checkpoint kinase 1 inhibitor MK-8776 as monotherapy and in combination with gemcitabine in patients with advanced solid tumors. J Clin Oncol 33:1060–1066

Doi T, Yoshino T, Shitara K, Matsubara N, Fuse N, Naito Y, Uenaka K, Nakamura T, Hynes SM, Lin AB (2015) Phase I study of LY2603618, a CHK1 inhibitor, in combination with gemcitabine in Japanese patients with solid tumors. Anti-Cancer Drugs 26:1043–1053

Garrett MD, Collins I (2011) Anticancer therapy with checkpoint inhibitors: what, where and when? Trends Pharmacol Sci 32:308–316

Guertin AD, Martin MM, Roberts B, Hurd M, Qu X, Miselis NR, Liu Y, Li J, Feldman I, Benita Y et al (2012) Unique functions of CHK1 and WEE1 underlie synergistic anti-tumor activity upon pharmacologic inhibition. Cancer Cell Int 12:45

Guzi TJ, Paruch K, Dwyer MP, Labroli M, Shanahan F, Davis N, Taricani L, Wiswell D, Seghezzi W, Penaflor E et al (2011) Targeting the replication checkpoint using SCH 900776, a potent and functionally selective CHK1 inhibitor identified via high content screening. Mol Cancer Ther 10:591–602

Ho AL, Bendell JC, Cleary JM, Schwartz GK, Burris HA, Oakes P, Agbo F, Barker PN, Senderowicz AM, Shapiro G (2011) Phase I, open-label, dose-escalation study of AZD7762 in combination with irinotecan (irino) in patients (pts) with advanced solid tumors. In: ASCO annual meeting, Chicago. J Clin Oncol 29(Suppl):3033–3033

Hong D, Infante J, Janku F, Jones S, Nguyen LM, Burris H, Naing A, Bauer TM, Piha-Paul S, Johnson FM et al (2016) Phase I study of LY2606368, a checkpoint kinase 1 inhibitor, in patients with advanced cancer. J Clin Oncol 34:1764–1771

Infante JR, Hollebecque A, Postel-Vinay S, Bauer T, Blackwood B, Evangelista M, Mahrus S, Peale F, Lu X, Sahasranaman S et al (2015) Phase I study of GDC-0425, a checkpoint kinase 1 inhibitor, in combination with gemcitabine in patients with refractory solid tumors. In: Proceedings of the 106th annual AACR meeting,18–22 Apr 2015, Philadelphia, PA, USA. Cancer Res 75(15 Suppl):abstract nr CT139

Janetka JW, Ashwell S, Zabludoff S, Lyne P (2007) Inhibitors of checkpoint kinases: from discovery to the clinic. Curr Opin Drug Discov Devel 10:473–486

Karnitz LM, Flatten KS, Wagner JM, Loegering D, Hackbarth JS, Arlander SJ, Vroman BT, Thomas MB, Baek YU, Hopkins KM et al (2005) Gemcitabine-induced activation of checkpoint signaling pathways that affect tumor cell survival. Mol Pharmacol 68:1636–1644

Karp JE, Thomas BM, Greer JM, Sorge C, Gore SD, Pratz KW, Smith BD, Flatten KS, Peterson K, Schneider P et al (2012) Phase I and pharmacologic trial of cytosine arabinoside with the selective checkpoint 1 inhibitor Sch 900776 in refractory acute leukemias. Clin Cancer Res 18:6723–6731

Karzai F, Zimmer A, Lipkowitz S, Annunziata CM, Parker B, Houston N, Ekwede I, Kohn EC, Lee J-M (2016) A phase II study of the cell cycle checkpoint kinases 1 and 2 (CHK1/2) inhibitor (LY2606368); prexasertib in sporadic triple negative breast cancer (TNBC). In: ESMO congress, Copenhagen, Denmark. Ann Oncol 27(Suppl 6):296–312

Kim MK, James J, Annunziata CM (2015) Topotecan synergizes with CHEK1 (CHK1) inhibitor to induce apoptosis in ovarian cancer cells. BMC Cancer 15:196

Kobayashi H, Shigetomi H, Yoshimoto C (2015) Checkpoint kinase 1 inhibitors as targeted molecular agents for clear cell carcinoma of the ovary. Oncol Lett 10:571–576

Kulkarni A, Natarajan SK, Chandrasekar V, Pandey PR, Sengupta S (2016) Combining immune checkpoint inhibitors and kinase-inhibiting supramolecular therapeutics for enhanced anticancer efficacy. ACS Nano 10(10): 9227–9242

Laquente B, Lopez-Martin J, Richards D, Illerhaus G, Chang DZ, Kim G, Stella P, Richel D, Szcylik C, Cascinu S et al (2017) A phase II study to evaluate LY2603618 in combination with gemcitabine in pancreatic cancer patients. BMC Cancer 17:137

Lee J-M, Karzai FH, Zimmer A, Annunziata CM, Lipkowitz S, Parker B, Houston N, Ekwede I, Kohn EC (2016) A phase II study of the cell cycle checkpoint kinases 1 and 2 inhibitor (LY2606368; Prexasertib monomestylate monohydrate) in sporadic high-grade serous ovarian cancer (gBRCAm+ OvCa). In: ESMO congress 2016. Copenhagen, Denmark. Ann Oncol 27(Suppl 6):296–312

Leijen S, Schellens JH, Shapiro G, Pavlick AC, Tibes R, Demuth T, Viscusi J, Cheng JD, Xu Y, Oza AM (2010) A phase I pharmacological and pharmacodynamic study of MK-1775, a Weel tyrosine kinase inhibitor, in monotherapy and combination with gemcitabine, cisplatin, or carboplatin in patients with advanced solid tumors. J Clin Oncol 28:3067–3067

Lu HR, Wang X, Wang Y (2006) A stronger DNA damage-induced G2 checkpoint due to over-activated CHK1 in the absence of PARP-1. Cell Cycle 5:2364–2370

Ma CX, Janetka JW, Piwnica-Worms H (2011) Death by releasing the breaks: CHK1 inhibitors as cancer therapeutics. Trends Mol Med 17:88–96

Montano R, Chung I, Garner KM, Parry D, Eastman A (2012) Preclinical development of the novel Chk1 inhibitor SCH900776 in combination with DNA-damaging agents and antimetabolites. Mol Cancer Ther 11:427–438

Morgan MA, Parsels LA, Maybaum J, Lawrence TS (2008) Improving gemcitabine-mediated radiosensitization using molecularly targeted therapy: a review. Clin Cancer Res 14:6744–6750

Oza AM, Cibula D, Benzaquen AO, Poole C, Mathijssen RH, Sonke GS, Colombo N, Spacek J, Vuylsteke P, Hirte H et al (2015) Olaparib combined with chemotherapy for recurrent platinum-sensitive ovarian cancer: a randomised phase 2 trial. Lancet Oncol 16:87–97

Sanjiv K, Hagenkort A, Calderon-Montano JM, Koolmeister T, Reaper PM, Mortusewicz O, Jacques SA, Kuiper RV, Schultz N, Scobie M et al (2016) Cancer-specific synthetic lethality between ATR and CHK1 kinase activities. Cell Rep 14:298–309

Sausville E, Lorusso P, Carducci M, Carter J, Quinn MF, Malburg L, Azad N, Cosgrove D, Knight R, Barker P et al (2014) Phase I dose-escalation study of AZD7762, a checkpoint kinase inhibitor, in combination with gemcitabine in US patients with advanced solid tumors. Cancer Chemother Pharmacol 73:539–549

Scagliotti G, Kang JH, Smith D, Rosenberg R, Park K, Kim SW, Su WC, Boyd TE, Richards DA, Novello S et al (2016) Phase II evaluation of LY2603618, a first-generation CHK1 inhibitor, in combination with pemetrexed in patients with advanced or metastatic non-small cell lung cancer. Investig New Drugs 34:625–635

Seto T, Esaki T, Hirai F, Arita S, Nosaki K, Makiyama A, Kometani T, Fujimoto C, Hamatake M, Takeoka H et al (2013) Phase I, dose-escalation study of AZD7762 alone and in combination with gemcitabine in Japanese patients with advanced solid tumours. Cancer Chemother Pharmacol 72:619–627

Tao Y, Leteur C, Yang C, Zhang P, Castedo M, Pierre A, Golsteyn RM, Bourhis J, Kroemer G, Deutsch E (2009) Radiosensitization by Chir-124, a selective CHK1 inhibitor: effects of p53 and cell cycle checkpoints. Cell Cycle 8:1196–1205

Venkatesha VA, Parsels LA, Parsels JD, Zhao L, Zabludoff SD, Simeone DM, Maybaum J, Lawrence TS, Morgan MA (2012) Sensitization of pancreatic cancer stem cells to gemcitabine by Chk1 inhibition. Neoplasia 14:519–525

Walton MI, Eve PD, Hayes A, Valenti MR, De Haven Brandon AK, Box G, Hallsworth A, Smith EL, Boxall KJ, Lainchbury M et al (2012) CCT244747 is a novel potent and selective CHK1 inhibitor with oral efficacy alone and in combination with genotoxic anticancer drugs. Clin Cancer Res 18:5650–5661

Walton MI, Eve PD, Hayes A, Henley AT, Valenti MR, De Haven Brandon AK, Box G, Boxall KJ, Tall M, Swales K et al (2016) The clinical development candidate CCT245737 is an orally active CHK1 inhibitor with preclinical activity in RAS mutant NSCLC and Emicro-MYC driven B-cell lymphoma. Oncotarget 7:2329–2342

Wehler T, Thomas M, Schumann C, Bosch-Barrera J, Vinolas Segarra N, Dickgreber NJ, Dalhoff K, Sebastian M, Corral Jaime J, Alonso M et al (2017) A randomized, phase 2 evaluation of the

CHK1 inhibitor, LY2603618, administered in combination with pemetrexed and cisplatin in patients with advanced nonsquamous non-small cell lung cancer. Lung Cancer 108:212–216

Weiss GJ, Donehower RC, Iyengar T, Ramanathan RK, Lewandowski K, Westin E, Hurt K, Hynes SM, Anthony SP, McKane S (2013) Phase I dose-escalation study to examine the safety and tolerability of LY2603618, a checkpoint 1 kinase inhibitor, administered 1 day after pemetrexed 500 mg/m(2) every 21 days in patients with cancer. Investig New Drugs 31:136–144

Yang E, William W, Fayette J, Zhang W, Fink A, Lin AB, Deutsch E (2016) Phase Ib trial of LY2606368 in combination with chemoradiation in patients with locally advanced head and neck squamous cell cancer. In: ESMO congress 2016. Ann Oncol 27(Suppl 6):1019TiP

Zabludoff SD, Deng C, Grondine MR, Sheehy AM, Ashwell S, Caleb BL, Green S, Haye HR, Horn CL, Janetka JW et al (2008) AZD7762, a novel checkpoint kinase inhibitor, drives checkpoint abrogation and potentiates DNA-targeted therapies. Mol Cancer Ther 7:2955–2966

Chapter 12
Established and Emerging Roles of the DNA-Dependent Protein Kinase Catalytic Subunit (DNA-PKcs)

Edward J. Bartlett and Susan P. Lees-Miller

Abstract The DNA-dependent protein kinase catalytic subunit (DNA-PKcs) is a large polypeptide of over 4000 amino acids with serine/threonine protein kinase activity that is enhanced in the presence of double stranded DNA and the Ku70/80 heterodimer. The discovery of this DNA activated protein kinase activity led to investigation of its role in DNA double-strand break repair and DNA-PKcs was shown to play important roles in repair of ionizing radiation-induced DNA double strand breaks and V(D)J recombination through the non-homologous end joining (NHEJ) pathway. However, recently, additional roles for DNA-PKcs in mitosis, transcription and cell migration have been suggested. Here, we review the structure, established and emerging roles of DNA-PKcs and its potential as a target for cancer therapy.

Keywords DNA-PKcs · Non-homologous end joining · DNA damage repair · Double strand break · V(D)J recombination

12.1 Introduction

DNA-dependent protein kinase catalytic subunit (DNA-PKcs) is the largest member of the phosphatidyl inositol-3 kinase-like (PIKK) family of serine/threonine protein kinases. Originally discovered as a protein kinase that phosphorylates its substrates

E. J. Bartlett
Department of Biochemistry and Molecular Biology and Robson DNA Science Centre, Arnie Charbonneau Cancer Institute, University of Calgary, Calgary, AB, Canada

Sir William Dunn School of Pathology, University of Oxford, Oxford, England, UK

S. P. Lees-Miller (✉)
Department of Biochemistry and Molecular Biology and Robson DNA Science Centre, Arnie Charbonneau Cancer Institute, University of Calgary, Calgary, AB, Canada
e-mail: leesmill@ucalgary.ca

© Springer International Publishing AG, part of Springer Nature 2018
J. Pollard, N. Curtin (eds.), *Targeting the DNA Damage Response for Anti-Cancer Therapy*, Cancer Drug Discovery and Development, https://doi.org/10.1007/978-3-319-75836-7_12

in the presence of double-stranded (ds) DNA, DNA-PKcs was subsequently shown to play important roles in DNA double strand break (DSB) repair via the process of non-homologous end joining (NHEJ) and, in the immune system, V(D)J recombination. More recently, roles for DNA-PKcs in transcription, mitosis and metastasis have also been indicated. Here we review the current state of understanding on DNA-PKcs, its roles in human disease and describe the potential for targeting DNA-PKcs for therapeutic advantage.

12.2   The PIKK Family

The human genome encodes over 500 putative protein kinases, the majority of which form the canonical AGC protein kinase family that includes protein kinase A, protein kinase B and protein kinase C, and are termed the eukaryotic protein kinases (ePKs) (Manning et al. 2002). In addition, there are about 40 human genes that bear resemblance to the ePK family but lack certain defining residues in the catalytic site. One of these "atypical protein kinase" families is that of the phosphatidyl-inositol-3 kinase-like (PIKK) serine/threonine protein kinases that includes DNA-PKcs (Hartley et al. 1995), ataxia telangiectasia mutated (ATM) (Savitsky et al. 1995; Lavin et al. 1995), ATM and Rad3-related (ATR), Suppressor with Morphological effect on Genitalia (SMG1), mammalian target of rapamycin (mTOR) and the

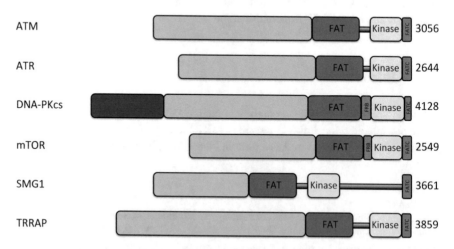

Fig. 12.1 Domain architecture of the PIKK family. The phosphatidyinositol 3-kinase (PI3K) like domain, which includes the active site for each member of the PIKK family, except TRRAP, which has a pseudo-kinase domain, is shown in yellow. The FAT and FATC domains are depicted in purple, whilst the N-terminal α-helical repeats are shown in green (DNA-PKcs has an additional N-terminal HEAT repeat region shown in blue). The FRB domains of DNA-PKcs and mTOR are indicated in orange. The amino acid length of each protein is noted at the C-terminal end of the domain representation. Adapted from (Shiloh 2003)

kinase inactive Transformation/transcription domain-associated protein (TRRAP) (Lavin et al. 1995; Hunter 1995; Shiloh 2003) (Fig. 12.1). As inferred from their name, the catalytic site of the PIKK proteins shares similarity to the lipid kinase, PI3K (Hartley et al. 1995; Hunter 1995), but to date no lipid kinase activity has been detected and the PIKKs appear to act instead as serine/threonine protein kinases. The PIKKs share the conserved catalytic aspartic acid in the sequence DXXXXN and the magnesium binding DXG motifs found in the canonical ePK protein kinase family, but lack the GXGXXG ATP binding motif (Fig. 12.2). However, the catalytic mechanism between the PIKKs and the ePKs is likely conserved as demonstrated by the similarity of the mTOR catalytic domain to that of canonical protein kinases (Yang et al. 2013). Like PI3K, the catalytic activity of the PIKKs is inhibited by wortmannin (Hartley et al. 1995; Hunter 1995; Canman et al. 1998; Banin et al. 1998), and recently, highly selective inhibitors have been generated that have enhanced our understanding of the roles of this important protein kinase family in the cell and

```
                                DXXXXN               DFG                 *
P78527|PRKDC   FASSHALICISHWILGIGDRHLNNFMVAMETGGVIGIDFGHAFGS---------ATQ-FLPVPELMPFR 3962
P42345|MTOR    YTRSLAVMSMVGYILGLGDRHPSNLMLDRLSGKILHIDFGDCFEV---------AMT-REKFPEKIPFR 2378
P42336|PK3CA   FTRSCAGYCVATFILGIGDRHNSNIMVK-DDGQLFHIDFGHFLDH---------KKKKFGYKRERVPFV 955
Q13315|ATM     YTRSVATSSIVGYILGLGDRHVQNILINEQSAELVHIDLGVAFEQ---------GKI--LPTPETVPFR 2909
Q13535|ATR     YCRSTAVMSMVGYILGLGDRHGENILFDSLTGECVHVDFNCLFNK---------GET--FEVPEIVPFR 2514
Q96Q15|SMG1    YARSTAVMSMVGYIIGLGDRHLDNVLIDMTTGEVVHIDYNVCFEK---------GKS--LRVPEKVPFR 2374
P17612|KAPCA   -----------------DLKPENLLIDQQGYIQV-TDFG--FAKRV---KGRTWTLCG-----------201
```

Fig. 12.2 Amino acid sequence alignment of the putative active site region of the kinase active PIKK family members. The putative catalytic site region of the PIKKs (human) compared to the amino acid sequences of PI3K (*PK3CA*) and PKA (*KAPCA*) are indicated. Conserved residues in this region of other PIKKs compared to DNA-PKcs/*PRKDC*, are shown in bold. Retrieval of sequences of PIKKs was carried out by Uniprot (uniprot.org) using Clustal Omega for sequence alignment. The amino acid residue numbers are indicated on the right and the Uniprot identifiers on the left. The amino acid sequence of PKA/*KAPCA* was manually inserted. The position of the active site DXXXXN and DFG residues is shown in blue in the sequence of PKA/*KAPCA* and above the PIKK sequences for comparison. Also shown is autophosphorylation site T3950 in DNA-PKcs (indicated by the asterisks. See (Block and Lees-Miller 2005) for details)

Table 12.1 Selective inhibitors of the PIKK family

PIKK	Inhibitor	IC50	Reference
DNA-PKcs	NU-7441	14 nM	(Leahy et al. 2004)
ATM	KU-55933	12.9 nM	(Hickson et al. 2004)
	KU-60019	6.3 nM	(Golding et al. 2009)
ATR	VE-821	13 nM	(Reaper et al. 2011)
	AZD6738	1 nM	(Checkley et al. 2015)
mTOR	Rapamycin	0.1 nM	(Edwards and Wandless 2007)
DNA-PKcs and mTOR	CC-115	DNA-PKcs 21 nM mTOR 13 nM	(Mortensen et al. 2015)

IC_{50}s were determined experimentally as follows; NU-7441, KU-55933, KU-60019 and VE-821 in cell-free assays, AZD-6738 in Kras mutant cell lines H23, H460, A549, and H358, Rapamycin in HEK293 cells, CC-115 in PC-3 cancer cells. This list is not exhaustive. In particular, additional inhibitors of mTOR and PI3K are in widespread use and, in some cases in clinic trials. Other DNA-PKcs inhibitors such as VX-984 (Boucher et al. 2016) and M3814 are referred to in the text opened the window for therapeutic opportunities (Zhao et al. 2006; Tavecchio et al. 2012; Davidson et al. 2013; Munck et al. 2012; Hickson et al. 2004) (Table 12.1).

12.3 PRKDC

The *PRKDC* gene (XRCC7) that encodes DNA-PKcs is located on chromosome 8 (8q11) (Sipley et al. 1995) (http://www.ncbi.nlm.nih.gov/gene/5591). DNA-PKcs is conserved in humans, *Mus musculus, Gallus gallus, Canis familiaris, Equus caballus, Xenopus laevis* and *Anopheles gambiae* (i.e., mouse, chicken, dog, horse, toad and mosquito) however, no putative homologues have been detected in *Caenorhabditis elegans, Arabidopsis thaliana, Drosophila melanogaster, Schizosaccharomyces pombe* or *Saccharomyces. cerevisiae* (Hudson et al. 2005). Curiously, however, a putative *PRKDC* gene has been detected in the slime mold, *Dictyostelium discoideum* (Block and Lees-Miller 2005; Hsu et al. 2006).

12.4 DNA-PKcs Protein

DNA-PKcs was first detected as a serine/threonine protein kinase activity in human cell extracts that was enhanced by the presence of double stranded (ds) DNA (Walker et al. 1985). The putative catalytic polypeptide ran at over 300 kDa on SDS PAGE gels, hence its early name of p350 (Carter et al. 1990; Lees-Miller et al. 1990). Highly purified extracts that contained DNA-PKcs/p350 as well as the Ku70/80 heterodimer were shown to phosphorylate the 90 kDa heat shock protein, hsp90 (Walker et al. 1985; Lees-Miller et al. 1990; Lees-Miller and Anderson 1989a), beta-casein (Carter et al. 1990), transcription factor Sp1 (Jackson et al. 1990), and the C-terminal domain of RNA polymerase II (Dvir et al. 1992, 1993). Subsequently, Ku was shown to stimulate the catalytic activity of DNA-PKcs in the presence of dsDNA ends, and the term DNA-PK (DNA-dependent protein kinase) was used to describe the catalytically active complex of DNA-PKcs and Ku in the presence of dsDNA (Dvir et al. 1993; Gottlieb and Jackson 1993).

A critical clue to the function of DNA-PK was the observation that catalytic activity required ends of dsDNA (Gottlieb and Jackson 1993). For example, circular dsDNA plasmid did not activate purified DNA-PK *in vitro*, but the same DNA after digestion by restriction enzyme did (Chan et al. 1996). It is now well established that while DNA-PKcs can interact weakly with dsDNA ends, it is recruited to DSBs through its interaction with the Ku70/80 heterodimer (discussed in more detail below). Interestingly, dsDNA with single stranded nucleotide extensions was shown to activate DNA-PKcs better than blunt ended dsDNA, leading to the suggestion that DNA-PKcs interacted with both dsDNA and ssDNA ends (Hammarsten et al. 2000). We will return to the possible significance of this observation in a later section. Interestingly, DNA-PKcs can also be activated by the RNA component of telomerase (hTR) (Ting et al. 2009, 2005). Since M13 ss circular DNA also supports DNA-PK kinase activity (Soubeyrand et al. 2001), it seems likely that DNA-PKcs can be activated by secondary structure elements in nucleic acids, however the significance of this observation is not known.

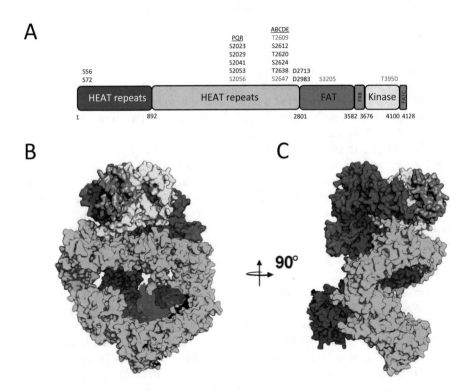

Fig. 12.3 Domain architecture and structure of DNA-PKcs. (**a**) Domain architecture of DNA-PKcs indicating the relative positions of the PQR and ABCDE phosphorylation clusters (see text for details). The residues noted are known phosphorylation sites following ionising radiation, and those highlighted in red are also phosphorylated in mitosis. (**b** and **c**) The x-ray crystal structure of DNA-PKcs at 4.3 Å as reported in (Sibanda et al. 2017), coloured to match the domain diagram. The PI3K-like domain (yellow) sits prominently at the head of DNA-PKcs, with the FRB domain adjacent (orange). The head region is cradled by the FAT domain (purple). The central cavity ring domain formed of HEAT repeats has a bowed shape (**c**), and contacts the N-terminal HEAT repeat region (blue) at the 'back' of the protein. PDB code 5LUQ

12.5 Structure of DNA-PKcs

Early bioinformatics analysis revealed that, like other members of the PIKK family, DNA-PKcs is composed of a large N-terminal helical domain, a region of conservation in the PIKK family members termed the FAT (FRAP, ATM TRRAP) domain, the kinase domain and a C-terminal region termed the FAT-C domain (Shiloh 2003; Bosotti et al. 2000; Lempiainen and Halazonetis 2009) (Fig. 12.3a). The N-terminal domain is composed of multiple HEAT (Huntingtin, Elongation factor 3, Protein Phosphatase 2A and Target Of Rapamycin 1) and armadillo domains (Perry and Kleckner 2003), and the kinase domain shares structural similarities with the catalytic domain of mTOR and the ePKs, with the FAT and FATC domains interacting directly with and supporting the kinase domain (Yang et al. 2013). As discussed below, DNA-PKcs also contains a number of functionally important phosphorylation sites including the ABCDE and PQR clusters (Fig. 12.3 and discussed further below).

The first clues to the structure of purified DNA-PKcs came from cryo-electron microscopy (cryo-EM) studies. The protein was shown to have an overall globular shape with a defined head and base and a central region with a low electron density region, suggesting the presence of a large channel of approximately 45 Å that was suitable in size for binding of dsDNA (Chiu et al. 1998; Williams et al. 2008; Leuther et al. 1999). The overall dimensions of DNA-PKcs are 120 Å in width and 150 Å in height. It was also suggested that the head domain might contained a smaller channel suitable for binding ssDNA (Williams et al. 2008). Similar regions of low electron density were observed by small angle X-ray scattering (SAXS); corresponding to a larger channel in the base and a smaller one in the head domain (Hammel et al. 2010; Dobbs et al. 2010). While it is tempting to speculate that this smaller channel might indeed interact with ssDNA, supporting biochemical studies that show that DNA-PKcs can be activated by dsDNA with ssDNA ends (Hammarsten et al. 2000; Leuther et al. 1999; DeFazio et al. 2002), direct evidence for this interaction is lacking.

A problem with these early low-resolution structures was that it was difficult to determine which part of the kinase corresponded to the kinase domain and which to the N-terminal domain (Dore et al. 2004). This critical issue was resolved by Blundell and colleagues with the resolution of the structure of DNA-PKcs (in complex with the C-terminal region of Ku80, described below) at 6.6 Å in 2010 (Sibanda et al. 2010), and then updated with a new 4.3 Å model in 2017 (Sibanda et al. 2017). The structure revealed that the head of the protein is composed of two lobes of the kinase domain which are encircled by the FAT and FAT-C domains, while the N-terminal HEAT repeats create a hollow double ring formation (Fig. 12.3b, c) (Sibanda et al. 2017). Rotated by 90°, the structure shows the bowed shape of the two distinct regions of HEAT repeats, similar to other HEAT domain containing proteins such as the A subunit of protein phosphatase PP2A (Grinthal et al. 2010; Groves et al. 1999). The 4.3 Å structure improves on the original by providing positions for amino acids (the PQR cluster can be found at the foot of the model, for example), and by including electron density for regions that were previously in question, such as confirming that the central cavity in DNA-PKcs is fully enclosed rather than with an opening (Sibanda et al. 2017). Additionally, the new DNA-PKcs crystal structure agrees with observations made using the information from the earlier, high-resolution structure of mTOR in complex with Lst8 (Yang et al. 2013). Like mTOR and members of the ePK family, the kinase domain of DNA-PKcs was predicted to consist of a small N-terminal lobe and a larger C-terminal lobe separated by a flexible hinge. In mTOR, the helical FAT domain forms an α-solenoid that wraps around and clamps onto the kinase domain (Yang et al. 2013). The structure of the FAT-C domain is integral to the kinase domain and it is likely that this arrangement is conserved in other PIKKs, and indeed in DNA-PKcs it is found to protect the active site (Yang et al. 2013; Sibanda et al. 2017). The mTOR structure contains a 4-helical bundle called the FKBP-rapamycin binding (FRB) domain that inserts into the N-terminal kinase lobe, and overhangs the ATP binding pocket (Yang et al. 2013). The recent DNA-PKcs structure confirms the presence of this FRB domain, but finds that it is positioned further into the active cleft than in the mTOR structure, and likely requires DNA-PKcs to undergo significant conformational changes in order for proteins to be presented to the active site (Sibanda et al. 2017). This FRB-like domain is not thought to be present in ATM or ATR, suggesting similarities in the mechanisms of action of mTOR and DNA-PKcs and perhaps explaining why some inhibitors target both mTOR and DNA-PKcs (Gil del Alcazar et al. 2014).

12.6 Mechanism of Activation of DNA-PKcs

Early studies showed that, in the presence of ends of dsDNA, the protein kinase activity of DNA-PKcs was enhanced five- to tenfold by the presence of the Ku heterodimer (Gottlieb and Jackson 1993; Chan et al. 1996). Moreover, DNA-PKcs and Ku were shown to form a stable structure only in the presence of dsDNA (Suwa et al. 1994). As described above, this led to the idea that DNA-PKcs and Ku assemble on dsDNA ends to form the active catalytic holoenzyme, DNA-PK. Biochemical studies have shown that the C-terminal 12 amino acids of Ku80, which is located at the extreme end of the flexible Ku80 CTR (Hammel et al. 2010) interacts directly with DNA-PKcs (Gell and Jackson 1999). Interestingly, this region is conserved in Nbs1 and ATRIP, which activate ATM and ATR, respectively, suggesting a common mechanism of activation for the PIKKs (Falck et al. 2005). Although one study cast doubt on the role of the Ku80CTR in activation of DNA-PKcs (Weterings et al. 2009), we and others recently showed unambiguously that Ku80CTR is required for activation of DNA-PKcs when discrete dsDNA molecules were used to assemble the complex (Radhakrishnan and Lees-Miller 2017; Woods et al. 2015), rather than a crude mixture of sonicated calf thymus DNA as used in the earlier study (Weterings et al. 2009). The requirement for the Ku80CTR for interaction with and activation of DNA-PKcs has now been confirmed by the structure of the Ku-DNA-PKcs complex as described below (Sibanda et al. 2017; Yin et al. 2017).

Concerted efforts in structural biology have finally begun to unravel the region of DNA-PKcs that is required for interaction with Ku. The recent crystal structure of DNA-PKcs included an α-helical bundle from the C-terminus of Ku80, which was found to bind at the foot of the DNA-PKcs structure, proximal to the PQR cluster and also the extreme N-terminal HEAT repeats (Sibanda et al. 2017). A study using cryo-EM noted that when complexed with streptavidin bound DNA and DNA-PKcs, the Ku dimer was most likely bound to the 'base' of DNA-PKcs (Villarreal and Stewart 2014), and this is now confirmed by two more cryo-EM based investigations which both find that Ku70/80 interacts near the foot at the 'rear' of DNA-PKcs (as opposed to the 'front' view of the crystal structure in Fig. 12.3b) (Yin et al. 2017; Villarreal and Stewart 2014; Sharif et al. 2017). The latter of these two publications also included DNA in the DNA-PK holoenzyme, and the models suggest that the broken end of DNA is passed to DNA-PKcs from Ku70/80, and that additional contacts from the C-terminal tail of Ku80 could provide a steric block to prevent access to the DNA end for other proteins (Yin et al. 2017). A positively charged cavity between the two distinct regions of HEAT repeats (the two are distinguishable in Fig. 12.3c) is shown to accommodate the DNA helix, although direct DNA-protein interactions were not noted (Yin et al. 2017). By comparing the crystal structure to the 6.6 Å cryo-EM DNA-PK holoenzyme, Yin and colleagues observed a structural shift in the HEAT regions, most notably at the N-terminus, where the tail curves in more tightly to the double ring structure (Yin et al. 2017). The movements of the HEAT regions cause structural changes across the entire molecule, resulting in an altered catalytic cleft, with the FRB domain rescinding to allow greater access to the active site (Yin et al. 2017). These exciting new insights are finally allowing us to understand the details of DNA-PKcs structure and activation, and will be the new foundations for future research in understanding the catalytic cycle and regulation.

12.7 Function of DNA-PKcs

12.7.1 DNA-PKcs in NHEJ

Most studies to date have focused on the role of DNA-PKcs in DSB repair. Cells lacking DNA-PKcs are radiation sensitive due to DSB repair defects and animals lacking DNA-PKcs have severe combined immunodeficiency (SCID) due to defects in V(D)J recombination (Lees-Miller et al. 1995; Kirchgessner et al. 1995). Data from several labs including our own suggests that DNA-PKcs is recruited to DSBs through its interaction with the Ku heterodimer where it undergoes extensive autophosphorylation and/or phosphorylation by other PIKKs in two main clusters, ABCDE and PQR (Table 12.2), and that these modifications result in a conformational change that releases DNA-PKcs from DNA ends or remodels the DNA-PK complex such that the DNA ends are now accessible to processing enzymes

Table 12.2 Known phosphorylation sites on DNA-PKcs

Residue	Modifying protein kinase	*In vitro*	*In cells*	Mutagenesis	Reference
S56				X	(Neal et al. 2011)
S72	DNA-PKcs		X	X	(Neal et al. 2011)
S2023				X	(Cui et al. 2005)
S2029				X	(Cui et al. 2005)
S2041				X	(Cui et al. 2005)
S2053				X	(Cui et al. 2005)
S2056	DNA-PKcs	X	X	X	(Douglas et al. 2007; Cui et al. 2005; Chen et al. 2005; Yajima et al. 2009)
T2609	DNA-PKcs, ATM, ATR	X	X	X	(Douglas et al. 2002; Chen et al. 2005; Yajima et al. 2009; Chan et al. 2002)
S2612	DNA-PKcs	X	X	X	(Douglas et al. 2002; Neal et al. 2014)
T2620	DNA-PKcs	X		X	(Douglas et al. 2002; Neal et al. 2014)
S2624	DNA-PKcs	X		X	(Douglas et al. 2002; Neal et al. 2014)
T2638	DNA-PKcs, ATR	X	X	X	(Douglas et al. 2002; Neal et al. 2014; Yajima et al. 2006; Soubeyrand et al. 2003)
T2647	DNA-PKcs, ATR	X	X	X	(Douglas et al. 2002; Neal et al. 2014; Yajima et al. 2006; Soubeyrand et al. 2003)
S2655				X	(Neal et al. 2014)
T2671				X	(Neal et al. 2014)
S2672				X	(Neal et al. 2014)
S2674				X	(Neal et al. 2014)
S2675				X	(Neal et al. 2014)
S2677				X	(Neal et al. 2014)
S3205	DNA-PKcs, ATM, PLK1	X	X	X	(Douglas et al. 2002, 2014; Neal et al. 2014)
S3821	DNA-PKcs	X			(Ma et al. 2005)
T3950	DNA-PKcs	X	X		(Douglas et al. 2007)
S4026	DNA-PKcs	X	X	X	(Ma et al. 2005; Bartlett and Lees Miller, unpublished observations)
S4102	DNA-PKcs	X			(Ma et al. 2005)

Known phosphorylation sites on DNA-PKcs, as described by phosphospecific antibodies and/or mass spectrometry *in vitro* (purified proteins) and/or in cells or by site directed mutagenesis *in vivo*. For updated reports on DNA-PKcs phosphorylation sites and other post-translational modifications, the reader is referred to the phosphosite web site (http://www.phosphosite.org/proteinAction.action?id=2072&showAllSites=true)

(Mahaney et al. 2009; Neal and Meek 2011; Wang and Lees-Miller 2013; Meek et al. 2008). This model is based on several observations. First, DNA-PKcs is highly phosphorylated *in vitro* (Douglas et al. 2002), autophosphorylated DNA-PKcs undergoes a large conformational change and interacts less efficiently with the Ku-DNA complex (Hammel et al. 2010), and DNA-PKcs in which several of the critical autophosphorylated residues are mutated to alanine is impaired in its ability to be released from DNA bound Ku both *in vitro* (Hammel et al. 2010; Block et al. 2004; Douglas et al. 2007; Jette and Lees-Miller 2015) and *in vivo* (Uematsu et al. 2007). In keeping with this model, cells expressing DNA-PKcs with ablation of the ABCDE cluster of phosphorylation sites are highly radiation sensitive due to inability to carry out NHEJ (Ding et al. 2003) and kinase-dead DNA-PKcs blocks end ligation (Jiang et al. 2015). Cells expressing alanine at the ABCDE cluster also have delayed Rad51 foci formation, indicating reduced initiation of homologous recombination (Shibata et al. 2011). Moreover, mice in which three of the ABCDE phosphorylation sites have been ablated die prematurely from hematopoietic bone marrow failure, defective DSB repair pathways, excessive DNA damage and p53-dependent apoptosis (Zhang et al. 2011), indicating the importance of phosphorylation of DNA-PKcs at these sites *in vivo*. Interestingly, alanine mutation of amino acids in the PQR cluster encourage increased processing of V(D)J coding ends, suggesting that the two phosphorylation clusters play opposite roles in the activation cycle of the kinase (Cui et al. 2005). However, it is important to note that whereas multiple sites in the ABCDE cluster have been verified *in vivo* (Douglas et al. 2007; Meek et al. 2007), *in vivo* evidence for phosphorylation of PQR sites other than S2056 is currently lacking.

12.7.2 DNA-PK Substrates

As described, early studies identified a number of *in vitro* substrates for DNA-PK and showed that the main consensus site was serine or threonine followed by glutamine (an SQ or TQ motif) (Bannister et al. 1993; Lees-Miller and Anderson 1989b; Lees-Miller et al. 1992). The preference for SQ/TQ sites was confirmed by combinatorial chemistry assays using small peptides (O'Neill et al. 2000). However, it quickly became apparent that *in vitro*, DNA-PK could phosphorylate many protein substrates on serines or threonines that were followed by amino acids other than glutamine, indicating that the phosphorylation consensus might be less restricted than originally defined. Identified DNA-PK phosphorylation sites on *in vitro* substrates along with potential *in vivo* substrates are listed in Table 12.3. What becomes clear from this list is that there are very few clear *in vivo* substrates of DNA-PKcs. Although scaffold attachment factor A (SAF-A, also known as heterogenous nucleoprotein U, hnRNP U) was reported to be phosphorylated on serine 59 (an SL site) by DNA-PKcs after DNA damage (Britton et al. 2009; Berglund and Clarke 2009), this site is not exclusive to DNA-PKcs as it is also phosphorylated by PLK1 in mitosis (Douglas et al. 2015). Accordingly, autophosphorylation of DNA-PKcs on S2056 is widely used as a marker of DNA-PKcs activity when suitable *in vivo* targets are absent.

Table 12.3 Reported substrates of DNA-PKcs. Experimentally determined substrates of DNA-PKcs, either by in vitro or in vivo experiments, as described in the references. See also (Dobbs et al. 2010)

Protein target	Reference
Artemis	(Goodarzi et al. 2006; Ma et al. 2005)
Beta-casein	(Carter et al. 1990, 1988)
C1D	(Erdemir et al. 2002)
c-Abl	(Kharbanda et al. 1997)
c-fos, c-jun	(Bannister et al. 1993; Lees-Miller and Anderson 1991)
CHK2	(Douglas et al. 2014; Tu et al. 2013; Shang et al. 2014)
c-myc	(Iijima et al. 1992)
eIF-2	(Ting et al. 1998)
GOLPH3	(Farber-Katz et al. 2014)
H2AX	(Park et al. 2003)
hnRNP A1	(Ting et al. 2009; Sui et al. 2015)
hnRNP U (Scaffold Attachment Factor-A/SAF-A)	(Britton et al. 2009; Berglund and Clarke 2009; Douglas et al. 2015)
HSP90α	(Walker et al. 1985; Lees-Miller et al. 1990; Lees-Miller and Anderson 1989b)
Interleukin enhancer-binding factor 2 and 3	(Ting et al. 1998)
Ku70, Ku80	(Lees-Miller et al. 1990; Gell and Jackson 1999; Chan et al. 1999; Douglas et al. 2005; Chu 1997)
Oct-1	(Schild-Poulter et al. 2003)
p53	(Lees-Miller et al. 1992; Mayo et al. 1997; Shieh et al. 1997)
PARP1	(Ariumi et al. 1999)
PNKP	(Zolner et al. 2011)
RPA	(Brush et al. 1994; Oakley et al. 2003; Block et al. 2004)
RNA Helicase A	(Zhang et al. 2004)
RNA Polymerase I and II	(Dvir et al. 1992, 1993; Kuhn et al. 1995; Labhart 1995; Peterson et al. 1995; Michaelidis and Grummt 2002; Chibazakura et al. 1997)
Sp1	(Jackson et al. 1990)
SV40 T Antigen	(Chen et al. 1991)
Vimentin	(Kotula et al. 2013)
WRN	(Yannone et al. 2001; Karmakar et al. 2002; Li and Comai 2002)
XLF	(Yu et al. 2008)
XRCC4	(Yu et al. 2003; Leber et al. 1998; Hsu et al. 2002)

12.7.3 DNA-PK Inhibitors and DNA-PKcs as an Anticancer Target

The development of DNA-PKcs inhibitors such as NU7441 (Zhao et al. 2006; Leahy et al. 2004) has been instrumental in identification of proteins that are phosphorylated by DNA-PK *in vivo*, and, more importantly, paved the way to evaluate the therapeutic potential of DNA-PKcs as a target for sensitizing tumour cells to radiation and DSB inducing drugs (Harnor et al. 2017; Collis et al. 2005; Cano 2017). Accordingly, other selective inhibitors for DNA-PKcs have been described (Morrison et al. 2016; Ihmaid et al. 2017; Ma et al. 2014; Pospisilova et al. 2017) and several, including a dual mTOR/DNA-PKcs inhibitor (denoted CC-115), the DNA-PKcs selective inhibitor VX-984 (Boucher et al. 2016) and the Merck Serono compound M3814 are currently in clinical trials for a variety of malignancies (Mortensen et al. 2015) (see also NCT02316197 and NCT02644278 on clinicaltrials.gov).

12.7.4   DNA-PKcs in V(D)J Recombination

In V(D)J recombination, lack of DNA-PKcs results in accumulation of unopened hairpins at DNA coding ends (Roth et al. 1992). A similar defect is observed in cells lacking the nuclease Artemis (Moshous et al. 2001), and DNA-PKcs was shown to be required for activation of the hairpin opening activity of Artemis (Ma et al. 2002). Initially this was thought to occur through DNA-PKcs-mediated phosphorylation of Artemis (Ma et al. 2002), however, later studies suggest that autophosphorylation-dependent release of DNA-PKcs from DNA ends is required for Artemis nuclease activity (Goodarzi et al. 2006). Recent investigations suggest that the presence of DNA-PKcs protein, but not kinase activity, is required for the recruitment of Artemis to hairpin ends, but this process requires phosphorylation of DNA-PKcs by ATM (Jiang et al. 2015). This study, using kinase dead DNA-PKcs, suggested that the inactive protein could recruit Artemis and allow for hairpin opening, but prevented DNA end ligation. The authors argue that ATM or DNA-PKcs-mediated phosphorylation of the ABCDE cluster is sufficient for end processing, but that strict trans-autophosphorylation of the PQR cluster is necessary for end ligation. The role of DNA-PKcs in V(D)J is becoming well understood, but agreement on whether the kinase also functions in the Class Switch Recombination (CSR) pathway is elusive. A recent publication comparing CSR function in cells from human patients with distinct mutations in DNA-PKcs showed that alternative end joining became the predominant pathway following NHEJ failure and that CSR defects were detected (Bjorkman et al. 2015).

Human patients with inherited *PRKDC* gene mutations are exceedingly rare, and only four cases have been described to date. These patients all have hypomorphic mutations and present with severe combined immune deficiency (SCID), depleted T and B cells and radiosensitivity (van der Burg et al. 2009; Woodbine et al. 2013; Mathieu et al. 2015), as expected from observations in murine systems (Taccioli et al. 1998). One patient had heterozygous mutations in *PRKDC*, with one gene copy found to produce an inactive enzyme and the other with only residual function. In addition to the expected SCID phenotype the patient also suffered abnormal growth, microcephaly and profound neurological defects (Woodbine et al. 2013). It is interesting to note that even in these rare cases, some residual activity of DNA-PKcs function is detected, suggesting that complete loss of the protein from birth in humans, unlike mice, could be lethal. Indeed, somatic deletion of DNA-PKcs in human cells has been shown to be lethal (Ruis et al. 2008).

12.8 Emerging Roles of DNA-PKcs in Transcription

Although DNA-PKcs was originally discovered as a factor that bound to promoter DNA and phosphorylated the C-terminal domain (CTD) of RNA polymerase (Dvir et al. 1992, 1993), its potential role in transcription was largely eclipsed by studies into its emerging roles in NHEJ and V(D)J recombination. However, recently roles for DNA-PKcs in transcription have re-emerged. DNA-PKcs is found in complex with poly-ADP ribose polymerase (PARP1) and topoisomerase II beta at estrogen response elements and is required for efficient transcription from estrogen responsive genes (Ju et al. 2006). Indeed, a complex of DNA-PKcs in complex with PARP-1 has been solved by cryo-EM (Spagnolo et al. 2012). Furthermore, DNA-PKcs-dependent phosphorylation of upstream stimulating factor (USF) has been linked to transcription of lipogenic genes (Wong et al. 2009; Wong and Sul 2010), and DNA-PK and DSBs have been implicated in broader aspects of transcription (Bunch et al. 2015; Calderwood 2016). The transcriptional activity of DNA-PKcs was recently found to be responsible for upregulating genes required for cell migration, invasion and metastasis with loss or inhibition of DNA-PKcs inhibiting metastasis in prostate cancer cells (Goodwin et al. 2015). DNA-PKcs has emerged as both a target and a modulator of the androgen response (AR) signalling pathway, with AR binding to the regulatory region of the *PRKDC* gene, and the DNA-PKcs protein interacting with the transcriptional machinery, and it is through this process that DNA-PKcs is observed to exert a pro-metastatic influence (Goodwin et al. 2015). While more work is required to elucidate the roles of DNA-PKcs in transcription and metastasis (see below), these studies indicate that DNA-PKcs could be an attractive therapeutic target in advanced malignancies.

12.9 Emerging Roles of DNA-PKcs in Mitosis

In addition to its well-studied phosphorylation in response to DNA damage, DNA-PKcs has been shown to be autophosphorylated on S2056 and T2609 during normal cellular mitosis (Lee et al. 2011). Mitotic phosphorylation of DNA-PKcs was observed at centrosomes and kinetochores and depletion of DNA-PKcs protein or inhibition of DNA-PKcs kinase activity resulted chromosome misalignment, abnormal nuclear morphologies and delayed progression through mitosis (Lee et al. 2011). Subsequently we, and others, confirmed these results and reported that DNA-PKcs fractionates with mitotic spindles (Douglas et al. 2014), interacts with polo like kinase (PLK1) (Douglas et al. 2014; Huang et al. 2014), is phosphorylated by PLK1 in mitosis (Douglas et al. 2014) and that DNA-PKcs phosphorylates CHK2 on T68 during mitosis (Douglas et al. 2014; Tu et al. 2013; Shang et al. 2014).

Moreover, recent reports indicate that DNA-PKcs regulates CDK1 activity and cyclin B stability, clearly implicating DNA-PKcs in regulation of entry into mitosis (Shang et al. 2015; Lee et al. 2015). Another link between DNA-PKcs and mitosis is its interaction with protein phosphatase 6 (PP6). DNA-PKcs interacts with PP6 in interphase (Mi et al. 2009; Douglas et al. 2010) and in mitosis (Douglas et al. 2014) and PP6 dephosphorylates and regulates Aurora A in mitosis (Zeng et al. 2010). PP6 also dephosphorylates DNA-PKcs S3205, a site phosphorylated by PLK1 in mitosis (Douglas et al. 2014). For a recent review of the emerging roles of DNA-PKcs in mitosis please refer to (Jette and Lees-Miller 2015).

12.10   Other Roles for DNA-PKcs

12.10.1   At Telomeres

Telomeres, the ends of chromosomes, can be regarded as endogenous DSBs, and are prevented from undergoing unscheduled NHEJ-dependent ligation by a complex of proteins that includes the shelterin complex and many members of the DNA damage response (Doksani and de Lange 2014; Feuerhahn et al. 2015). One of these proteins is DNA-PKcs, where it contributes to efficient telomere replication and end-capping, possibly through phosphorylation of heterogenous nuclear ribonuclear protein (hnRNP) A1 (Gauthier et al. 2012; Le et al. 2013; Sui et al. 2015; Williams et al. 2009). Interestingly, Ku70/80 binds to the RNA component of telomerase, hTR, and hTR supports phosphorylation of hnRNP A1 by DNA-PKcs (Ting et al. 2009, 2005).

12.10.2   In the Golgi

Another recently reported role for DNA-PKcs is in maintaining integrity of the Golgi body after DNA damage. DNA-PKcs phosphorylates GOLPH3 (Golgi phosphoprotein 3), resulting in increased interaction with MYO18A (unconventional myosin 18A), causing dispersal of the Golgi in response to DNA damage (Farber-Katz et al. 2014; Buschman et al. 2015). Other potential roles for DNA-PKcs outside DNA double strand break repair have recently been discussed (Goodwin and Knudsen 2014).

12.10.3   With the Cytoskeleton

Surprisingly, DNA-PKcs has also been implicated in regulation of the cell cytoskeleton and protein excretion. Kotula et al. reported that DNA-PKcs phosphorylates vimentin, a cytoskeletal network protein, in response to a DNA damage analog stimulus, and that in migrating cells this phosphorylation is associated with reduced cell adhesion and migration (Kotula et al. 2013). How these observations reconcile with findings that DNA-PKcs activity promotes metastasis through its transcriptional activity, and that over expression of DNA-PKcs protein is observed in invasive tumours (Hsu et al. 2012) remains to be determined. Other investigations demonstrate that DNA-PKcs regulates the secretion of a number of proteins in the cell microenvironment, and that these processes have also pro-metastatic effect (Kotula et al. 2015). Further, experiments in head and neck squamous cell carcinoma cell lines found that inhibition of DNA-PKcs reduced the invasive phenotype of the cells in culture (Romick-Rosendale et al. 2015). The reasons why DNA-PKcs activity and over-expression both correlate with reduced motility and migration and pro-metastatic activities are not clear, these contradictions may depend on the cell type, or other defects in genetically unstable cells. Certainly, this burgeoning area of research suggests that a more complete understanding of the activities of DNA-PKcs and its chemical inhibition may prove valuable for a variety of cancer treatments.

12.11   The Future for DNA-PKcs

DNA-PKcs has always presented as an enigma. It is one of the largest known human proteins kinases and its primary substrate in DSB repair appeared to be itself. However, over the past few years, it has emerged that DNA-PKcs plays a number of additional roles in the cell, from transcriptional and mitotic regulation to signalling in Golgi body dispersal and that it may phosphorylate additional targets, outside the DNA damage response. The recent identification of human patients with defective DNA-PKcs have underscored the importance of the kinase in immuno-competency and DNA repair, and also potentially in development. When considered alongside tantalizing links to metastasis, DNA-PKcs appears an attractive target for chemical inhibition in some cancer types, and indeed we await the results of clinical trials of dual and specific DNA-PKcs inhibitors.

Acknowledgments Work in the authors laboratory is supported by the Canadian Institute of Health Research, the Cancer Research Society and the Engineered Air Chair in Cancer Research. EB was supported by a University of Calgary Eyes High Post-Doctoral Fellowship.

References

Ariumi Y, Masutani M, Copeland TD, Mimori T, Sugimura T, Shimotohno K, Ueda K, Hatanaka M, Noda M (1999) Suppression of the poly(ADP-ribose) polymerase activity by DNA-dependent protein kinase in vitro. Oncogene 18:4616–4625

Banin S, Moyal L, Shieh S, Taya Y, Anderson CW, Chessa L, Smorodinsky NI, Prives C, Reiss Y, Shiloh Y et al (1998) Enhanced phosphorylation of p53 by ATM in response to DNA damage. Science 281:1674–1677

Bannister AJ, Gottlieb TM, Kouzarides T, Jackson SP (1993) c-Jun is phosphorylated by the DNA-dependent protein kinase in vitro; definition of the minimal kinase recognition motif. Nucleic Acids Res 21:1289–1295

Bartlett EJ, Lees Miller SP. unpublished observations

Berglund FM, Clarke PR (2009) hnRNP-U is a specific DNA-dependent protein kinase substrate phosphorylated in response to DNA double-strand breaks. Biochem Biophys Res Commun 381:59–64

Bjorkman A, Du L, Felgentreff K, Rosner C, Pankaj Kamdar R, Kokaraki G, Matsumoto Y, Davies EG, van der Burg M, Notarangelo LD et al (2015) DNA-PKcs Is involved in Ig class switch recombination in human B cells. J Immunol 195(12):5608–5615

Block WD, Lees-Miller SP (2005) Putative homologues of the DNA-dependent protein kinase catalytic subunit (DNA-PKcs) and other components of the non-homologous end joining machinery in Dictyostelium discoideum. DNA Repair 4:1061–1065

Block WD, Yu Y, Lees-Miller SP (2004) Phosphatidyl inositol 3-kinase-like serine/threonine protein kinases (PIKKs) are required for DNA damage-induced phosphorylation of the 32 kDa subunit of replication protein A at threonine 21. Nucleic Acids Res 32:997–1005

Block WD, Yu Y, Merkle D, Gifford JL, Ding Q, Meek K, Lees-Miller SP (2004) Autophosphorylation-dependent remodeling of the DNA-dependent protein kinase catalytic subunit regulates ligation of DNA ends. Nucleic Acids Res 32:4351–4357

Bosotti R, Isacchi A, Sonnhammer EL (2000) FAT: a novel domain in PIK-related kinases. Trends Biochem Sci 25:225–227

Boucher D, Hillier S, Newsome D, Wang Y, Takemoto D, Gu Y, Markland W, Hoover R, Arimoto R, Maxwell J et al (2016) Preclinical characterization of the selective DNA-dependent protein kinase (DNA-PK) inhibitor VX-984 in combination with chemotherapy. Ann Oncol 27:382P

Britton S, Froment C, Frit P, Monsarrat B, Salles B, Calsou P (2009) Cell nonhomologous end joining capacity controls SAF-A phosphorylation by DNA-PK in response to DNA double-strand breaks inducers. Cell Cycle 8:3717–3722

Brush GS, Anderson CW, Kelly TJ (1994) The DNA-activated protein kinase is required for the phosphorylation of replication protein A during simian virus 40 DNA replication. Proc Natl Acad Sci U S A 91:12520–12524

Bunch H, Lawney BP, Lin YF, Asaithamby A, Murshid A, Wang YE, Chen BP, Calderwood SK (2015) Transcriptional elongation requires DNA break-induced signalling. Nat Commun 6:10191

Buschman MD, Rahajeng J, Field SJ (2015) GOLPH3 links the Golgi, DNA damage, and cancer. Cancer Res 75:624–627

Calderwood SK (2016) A critical role for topoisomerase IIb and DNA double strand breaks in transcription. Transcription 7:75–83

Canman CE, Lim DS, Cimprich KA, Taya Y, Tamai K, Sakaguchi K, Appella E, Kastan MB, Siliciano JD (1998) Activation of the ATM kinase by ionizing radiation and phosphorylation of p53. Science 281:1677–1679

Cano C, Harnor SJ (2017) Targeting DNA-PK for cancer therapy. ChemMedChem 12(12):895–900

Carter TH, Kopman CR, James CB (1988) DNA-stimulated protein phosphorylation in HeLa whole cell and nuclear extracts. Biochem Biophys Res Commun 157:535–540

Carter T, Vancurova I, Sun I, Lou W, DeLeon S (1990) A DNA-activated protein kinase from HeLa cell nuclei. Mol Cell Biol 10:6460–6471

Chan DW, Chen BP, Prithivirajsingh S, Kurimasa A, Story MD, Qin J, Chen DJ (2002) Autophosphorylation of the DNA-dependent protein kinase catalytic subunit is required for rejoining of DNA double-strand breaks. Genes Dev 16:2333–2338

Chan DW, Mody CH, Ting NS, Lees-Miller SP (1996) Purification and characterization of the double-stranded DNA-activated protein kinase, DNA-PK, from human placenta. Biochem Cell Biol 74:67–73

Chan DW, Ye R, Veillette CJ, Lees-Miller SP (1999) DNA-dependent protein kinase phosphorylation sites in Ku 70/80 heterodimer. Biochemistry 38:1819–1828

Checkley S, MacCallum L, Yates J, Jasper P, Luo H, Tolsma J, Bendtsen C (2015) Bridging the gap between in vitro and in vivo: dose and schedule predictions for the ATR inhibitor AZD6738. Sci Rep 5:13545

Chen BP, Chan DW, Kobayashi J, Burma S, Asaithamby A, Morotomi-Yano K, Botvinick E, Qin J, Chen DJ (2005) Cell cycle dependence of DNA-dependent protein kinase phosphorylation in response to DNA double strand breaks. J Biol Chem 280:14709–14715

Chen YR, Lees-Miller SP, Tegtmeyer P, Anderson CW (1991) The human DNA-activated protein kinase phosphorylates simian virus 40 T antigen at amino- and carboxy-terminal sites. J Virol 65:5131–5140

Chibazakura T, Watanabe F, Kitajima S, Tsukada K, Yasukochi Y, Teraoka H (1997) Phosphorylation of human general transcription factors TATA-binding protein and transcription factor IIB by DNA-dependent protein kinase--synergistic stimulation of RNA polymerase II basal transcription in vitro. Eur J Biochem 247:1166–1173

Chiu CY, Cary RB, Chen DJ, Peterson SR, Stewart PL (1998) Cryo-EM imaging of the catalytic subunit of the DNA-dependent protein kinase. J Mol Biol 284:1075–1081

Chu G (1997) Double strand break repair. J Biol Chem 272:24097–24100

Collis SJ, DeWeese TL, Jeggo PA, Parker AR (2005) The life and death of DNA-PK. Oncogene 24:949–961

Cui X, Yu Y, Gupta S, Cho YM, Lees-Miller SP, Meek K (2005) Autophosphorylation of DNA-dependent protein kinase regulates DNA end processing and may also alter double-strand break repair pathway choice. Mol Cell Biol 25:10842–10852

Davidson D, Amrein L, Panasci L, Aloyz R (2013) Small molecules, inhibitors of DNA-PK, targeting DNA repair, and beyond. Front Pharmacol 4:5

DeFazio LG, Stansel RM, Griffith JD, Chu G (2002) Synapsis of DNA ends by DNA-dependent protein kinase. EMBO J 21:3192–3200

Ding Q, Reddy YV, Wang W, Woods T, Douglas P, Ramsden DA, Lees-Miller SP, Meek K (2003) Autophosphorylation of the catalytic subunit of the DNA-dependent protein kinase is required for efficient end processing during DNA double-strand break repair. Mol Cell Biol 23:5836–5848

Dobbs TA, Tainer JA, Lees-Miller SP (2010) A structural model for regulation of NHEJ by DNA-PKcs autophosphorylation. DNA Repair 9:1307–1314

Doksani Y, de Lange T (2014) The role of double-strand break repair pathways at functional and dysfunctional telomeres. Cold Spring Harb Perspect Biol 6:a016576

Dore AS, Drake AC, Brewerton SC, Blundell TL (2004) Identification of DNA-PK in the arthropods. Evidence for the ancient ancestry of vertebrate non-homologous end-joining. DNA Repair 3:33–41

Douglas P, Cui X, Block WD, Yu Y, Gupta S, Ding Q, Ye R, Morrice N, Lees-Miller SP, Meek K (2007) The DNA-dependent protein kinase catalytic subunit is phosphorylated in vivo on threonine 3950, a highly conserved amino acid in the protein kinase domain. Mol Cell Biol 27:1581–1591

Douglas P, Gupta S, Morrice N, Meek K, Lees-Miller SP (2005) DNA-PK-dependent phosphorylation of Ku70/80 is not required for non-homologous end joining. DNA Repair 4:1006–1018

Douglas P, Sapkota GP, Morrice N, Yu Y, Goodarzi AA, Merkle D, Meek K, Alessi DR, Lees-Miller SP (2002) Identification of in vitro and in vivo phosphorylation sites in the catalytic subunit of the DNA-dependent protein kinase. Biochem J 368:243–251

Douglas P, Ye R, Morrice N, Britton S, Trinkle-Mulcahy L, Lees-Miller SP (2015) Phosphorylation of SAF-A/hnRNP-U serine 59 by polo-like kinase 1 is required for mitosis. Mol Cell Biol 35:2699–2713

Douglas P, Ye R, Trinkle-Mulcahy L, Neal JA, De Wever V, Morrice NA, Meek K, Lees-Miller SP (2014) Polo-like kinase 1 (PLK1) and protein phosphatase 6 (PP6) regulate DNA-dependent protein kinase catalytic subunit (DNA-PKcs) phosphorylation in mitosis. Biosci Rep 34:e00113

Douglas P, Zhong J, Ye R, Moorhead GB, Xu X, Lees-Miller SP (2010) Protein phosphatase 6 interacts with the DNA-dependent protein kinase catalytic subunit and dephosphorylates gamma-H2AX. Mol Cell Biol 30:1368–1381

Dvir A, Peterson SR, Knuth MW, Lu H, Dynan WS (1992) Ku autoantigen is the regulatory component of a template-associated protein kinase that phosphorylates RNA polymerase II. Proc Natl Acad Sci U S A 89:11920–11924

Dvir A, Stein LY, Calore BL, Dynan WS (1993) Purification and characterization of a template-associated protein kinase that phosphorylates RNA polymerase II. J Biol Chem 268:10440–10447

Edwards SR, Wandless TJ (2007) The rapamycin-binding domain of the protein kinase mammalian target of rapamycin is a destabilizing domain. J Biol Chem 282:13395–13401

Erdemir T, Bilican B, Cagatay T, Goding CR, Yavuzer U (2002) Saccharomyces cerevisiae C1D is implicated in both non-homologous DNA end joining and homologous recombination. Mol Microbiol 46:947–957

Falck J, Coates J, Jackson SP (2005) Conserved modes of recruitment of ATM, ATR and DNA-PKcs to sites of DNA damage. Nature 434:605–611

Farber-Katz SE, Dippold HC, Buschman MD, Peterman MC, Xing M, Noakes CJ, Tat J, Ng MM, Rahajeng J, Cowan DM et al (2014) DNA damage triggers Golgi dispersal via DNA-PK and GOLPH3. Cell 156:413–427

Feuerhahn S, Chen LY, Luke B, Porro A (2015) No DDRama at chromosome ends: TRF2 takes centre stage. Trends Biochem Sci 40:275–285

Gauthier LR, Granotier C, Hoffschir F, Etienne O, Ayouaz A, Desmaze C, Mailliet P, Biard DS, Boussin FD (2012) Rad51 and DNA-PKcs are involved in the generation of specific telomere aberrations induced by the quadruplex ligand 360A that impair mitotic cell progression and lead to cell death. Cell Mol Life Sci 69:629–640

Gell D, Jackson SP (1999) Mapping of protein-protein interactions within the DNA-dependent protein kinase complex. Nucleic Acids Res 27:3494–3502

Gil del Alcazar CR, Hardebeck MC, Mukherjee B, Tomimatsu N, Gao X, Yan J, Xie XJ, Bachoo R, Li L, Habib AA et al (2014) Inhibition of DNA double-strand break repair by the dual PI3K/mTOR inhibitor NVP-BEZ235 as a strategy for radiosensitization of glioblastoma. Clin Cancer Res 20:1235–1248

Golding SE, Rosenberg E, Valerie N, Hussaini I, Frigerio M, Cockcroft XF, Chong WY, Hummersone M, Rigoreau L, Menear KA et al (2009) Improved ATM kinase inhibitor KU-60019 radiosensitizes glioma cells, compromises insulin, AKT and ERK prosurvival signaling, and inhibits migration and invasion. Mol Cancer Ther 8:2894–2902

Goodarzi AA, Yu Y, Riballo E, Douglas P, Walker SA, Ye R, Harer C, Marchetti C, Morrice N, Jeggo PA et al (2006) DNA-PK autophosphorylation facilitates Artemis endonuclease activity. EMBO J 25:3880–3889

Goodwin JF, Knudsen KE (2014) Beyond DNA repair: DNA-PK function in cancer. Cancer Discov 4:1126–1139

Goodwin JF, Kothari V, Drake JM, Zhao S, Dylgjeri E, Dean JL, Schiewer MJ, McNair C, Jones JK, Aytes A et al (2015) DNA-PKcs-mediated transcriptional regulation drives prostate cancer progression and metastasis. Cancer Cell 28:97–113

Gottlieb TM, Jackson SP (1993) The DNA-dependent protein kinase: requirement for DNA ends and association with Ku antigen. Cell 72:131–142

Grinthal A, Adamovic I, Weiner B, Karplus M, Kleckner N (2010) PR65, the HEAT-repeat scaffold of phosphatase PP2A, is an elastic connector that links force and catalysis. Proc Natl Acad Sci U S A 107:2467–2472

Groves MR, Hanlon N, Turowski P, Hemmings BA, Barford D (1999) The structure of the protein phosphatase 2A PR65/A subunit reveals the conformation of its 15 tandemly repeated HEAT motifs. Cell 96:99–110

Hammarsten O, DeFazio LG, Chu G (2000) Activation of DNA-dependent protein kinase by single-stranded DNA ends. J Biol Chem 275:1541–1550

Hammel M, Yu Y, Mahaney BL, Cai B, Ye R, Phipps BM, Rambo RP, Hura GL, Pelikan M, So S et al (2010) Ku and DNA-dependent protein kinase dynamic conformations and assembly regulate DNA binding and the initial non-homologous end joining complex. J Biol Chem 285:1414–1423

Harnor SJ, Brennan A, Cano C (2017) Targeting DNA-dependent protein kinase for cancer therapy. ChemMedChem 12:895–900

Hartley KO, Gell D, Smith GC, Zhang H, Divecha N, Connelly MA, Admon A, Lees-Miller SP, Anderson CW, Jackson SP (1995) DNA-dependent protein kinase catalytic subunit: a relative of phosphatidylinositol 3-kinase and the ataxia telangiectasia gene product. Cell 82:849–856

Hickson I, Zhao Y, Richardson CJ, Green SJ, Martin NM, Orr AI, Reaper PM, Jackson SP, Curtin NJ, Smith GC (2004) Identification and characterization of a novel and specific inhibitor of the ataxia-telangiectasia mutated kinase ATM. Cancer Res 64:9152–9159

Hsu DW, Gaudet P, Hudson JJ, Pears CJ, Lakin ND (2006) DNA damage signaling and repair in dictyostelium discoideum. Cell Cycle 5:702–708

Hsu HL, Yannone SM, Chen DJ (2002) Defining interactions between DNA-PK and ligase IV/XRCC4. DNA Repair 1:225–235

Hsu FM, Zhang S, Chen BP (2012) Role of DNA-dependent protein kinase catalytic subunit in cancer development and treatment. Transl Cancer Res 1:22–34

Huang B, Shang ZF, Li B, Wang Y, Liu XD, Zhang SM, Guan H, Rang WQ, Hu JA, Zhou PK (2014) DNA-PKcs associates with PLK1 and is involved in proper chromosome segregation and cytokinesis. J Cell Biochem 115:1077–1088

Hudson JJ, Hsu DW, Guo K, Zhukovskaya N, Liu PH, Williams JG, Pears CJ, Lakin ND (2005) DNA-PKcs-dependent signaling of DNA damage in Dictyostelium discoideum. Curr Biol 15:1880–1885

Hunter T (1995) When is a lipid kinase not a lipid kinase? When it is a protein kinase. Cell 83:1–4

Ihmaid S, Ahmed HEA, Al-Sheikh Ali A, Sherif YE, Tarazi HM, Riyadh SM, Zayed MF, Abulkhair HS, Rateb HS (2017) Rational design, synthesis, pharmacophore modeling, and docking studies for identification of novel potent DNA-PK inhibitors. Bioorg Chem 72:234–247

Iijima S, Teraoka H, Date T, Tsukada K (1992) DNA-activated protein kinase in Raji Burkitt's lymphoma cells. Phosphorylation of c-Myc oncoprotein. Eur J Biochem 206:595–603

Jackson SP, MacDonald JJ, Lees-Miller S, Tjian R (1990) GC box binding induces phosphorylation of Sp1 by a DNA-dependent protein kinase. Cell 63:155–165

Jette N, Lees-Miller SP (2015) The DNA-dependent protein kinase: a multifunctional protein kinase with roles in DNA double strand break repair and mitosis. Prog Biophys Mol Biol 117:194–205

Jiang W, Crowe JL, Liu X, Nakajima S, Wang Y, Li C, Lee BJ, Dubois RL, Liu C, Yu X et al (2015) Differential phosphorylation of DNA-PKcs regulates the interplay between end-processing and end-ligation during nonhomologous end-joining. Mol Cell 58:172–185

Ju BG, Lunyak VV, Perissi V, Garcia-Bassets I, Rose DW, Glass CK, Rosenfeld MG (2006) A topoisomerase IIbeta-mediated dsDNA break required for regulated transcription. Science 312:1798–1802

Karmakar P, Piotrowski J, Brosh RM Jr, Sommers JA, Lees-Miller SP, Cheng WH, Snowden CM, Ramsden DA, Werner BVA (2002) protein is a target of DNA-dependent protein kinase in vivo and in vitro, and its catalytic activities are regulated by phosphorylation. J Biol Chem 277:18291–18302

Kharbanda S, Pandey P, Jin S, Inoue S, Bharti A, Yuan ZM, Weichselbaum R, Weaver D, Kufe D (1997) Functional interaction between DNA-PK and c-Abl in response to DNA damage. Nature 386:732–735

Kirchgessner CU, Patil CK, Evans JW, Cuomo CA, Fried LM, Carter T, Oettinger MA, Brown JM (1995) DNA-dependent kinase (p350) as a candidate gene for the murine SCID defect. Science 267:1178–1183

Kotula E, Berthault N, Agrario C, Lienafa MC, Simon A, Dingli F, Loew D, Sibut V, Saule S, Dutreix M (2015) DNA-PKcs plays role in cancer metastasis through regulation of secreted proteins involved in migration and invasion. Cell Cycle 14:1961–1972

Kotula E, Faigle W, Berthault N, Dingli F, Loew D, Sun JS, Dutreix M, Quanz M (2013) DNA-PK target identification reveals novel links between DNA repair signaling and cytoskeletal regulation. PLoS One 8:e80313

Kuhn A, Gottlieb TM, Jackson SP, Grummt I (1995) DNA-dependent protein kinase: a potent inhibitor of transcription by RNA polymerase I. Genes Dev 9:193–203

Labhart P (1995) DNA-dependent protein kinase specifically represses promoter-directed transcription initiation by RNA polymerase I. Proc Natl Acad Sci U S A 92:2934–2938

Lavin MF, Khanna KK, Beamish H, Spring K, Watters D, Shiloh Y (1995) Relationship of the ataxia-telangiectasia protein ATM to phosphoinositide 3-kinase. Trends Biochem Sci 20:382–383

Le PN, Maranon DG, Altina NH, Battaglia CL, Bailey SM (2013) TERRA, hnRNP A1, and DNA-PKcs interactions at human telomeres. Front Oncol 3:91

Leahy JJ, Golding BT, Griffin RJ, Hardcastle IR, Richardson C, Rigoreau L, Smith GC (2004) Identification of a highly potent and selective DNA-dependent protein kinase (DNA-PK) inhibitor (NU7441) by screening of chromenone libraries. Bioorg Med Chem Lett 14:6083–6087

Leber R, Wise TW, Mizuta R, Meek K (1998) The XRCC4 gene product is a target for and interacts with the DNA-dependent protein kinase. J Biol Chem 273:1794–1801

Lee KJ, Lin YF, Chou HY, Yajima H, Fattah KR, Lee SC, Chen BP (2011) Involvement of DNA-dependent protein kinase in normal cell cycle progression through mitosis. J Biol Chem 286:12796–12802

Lee KJ, Shang ZF, Lin YF, Sun J, Morotomi-Yano K, Saha D, Chen BP (2015) The catalytic subunit of DNA-dependent protein kinase coordinates with polo-like kinase 1 to facilitate mitotic entry. Neoplasia 17:329–338

Lees-Miller SP, Anderson CW (1989a) Two human 90-kDa heat shock proteins are phosphorylated in vivo at conserved serines that are phosphorylated in vitro by casein kinase II. J Biol Chem 264:2431–2437

Lees-Miller SP, Anderson CW (1989b) The human double-stranded DNA-activated protein kinase phosphorylates the 90-kDa heat-shock protein, hsp90 alpha at two NH2-terminal threonine residues. J Biol Chem 264:17275–17280

Lees-Miller SP, Anderson CW (1991) The DNA-activated protein kinase, DNA-PK: a potential coordinator of nuclear events. Cancer Cells 3:341–346

Lees-Miller SP, Chen YR, Anderson CW (1990) Human cells contain a DNA-activated protein kinase that phosphorylates simian virus 40 T antigen, mouse p53, and the human Ku autoantigen. Mol Cell Biol 10:6472–6481

Lees-Miller SP, Godbout R, Chan DW, Weinfeld M, Day RS 3rd, Barron GM, Allalunis-Turner J (1995) Absence of p350 subunit of DNA-activated protein kinase from a radiosensitive human cell line. Science 267:1183–1185

Lees-Miller SP, Sakaguchi K, Ullrich SJ, Appella E, Anderson CW (1992) Human DNA-activated protein kinase phosphorylates serines 15 and 37 in the amino-terminal transactivation domain of human p53. Mol Cell Biol 12:5041–5049

Lempiainen H, Halazonetis TD (2009) Emerging common themes in regulation of PIKKs and PI3Ks. EMBO J 28:3067–3073

Leuther KK, Hammarsten O, Kornberg RD, Chu G (1999) Structure of DNA-dependent protein kinase: implications for its regulation by DNA. EMBO J 18:1114–1123

Li B, Comai L (2002) Displacement of DNA-PKcs from DNA ends by the Werner syndrome protein. Nucleic Acids Res 30:3653–3661

Ma CC, Li H, Wan RZ, Liu ZP (2014) Developments of DNA-dependent protein kinase inhibitors as anticancer agents. 2014 Oct 13. [Epub ahead of print]. PMID:25307307

Ma Y, Lu H, Schwarz K, Lieber MR (2005) Repair of double-strand DNA breaks by the human nonhomologous DNA end joining pathway: the iterative processing model. Cell Cycle 4:1193–1200

Ma Y, Pannicke U, Lu H, Niewolik D, Schwarz K, Lieber MR (2005) The DNA-dependent protein kinase catalytic subunit phosphorylation sites in human Artemis. J Biol Chem 280:33839–33846

Ma Y, Pannicke U, Schwarz K, Lieber MR (2002) Hairpin opening and overhang processing by an Artemis/DNA-dependent protein kinase complex in nonhomologous end joining and V(D)J recombination. Cell 108:781–794

Mahaney BL, Meek K, Lees-Miller SP (2009) Repair of ionizing radiation-induced DNA double-strand breaks by non-homologous end-joining. Biochem J 417:639–650

Manning G, Whyte DB, Martinez R, Hunter T, Sudarsanam S (2002) The protein kinase complement of the human genome. Science 298:1912–1934

Mathieu AL, Verronese E, Rice GI, Fouyssac F, Bertrand Y, Picard C, Chansel M, Walter JE, Notarangelo LD, Butte MJ et al (2015) PRKDC mutations associated with immunodeficiency, granuloma, and autoimmune regulator-dependent autoimmunity. J Allergy Clin Immunol 135:1578–88.e5

Mayo LD, Turchi JJ, Berberich SJ (1997) Mdm-2 phosphorylation by DNA-dependent protein kinase prevents interaction with p53. Cancer Res 57:5013–5016

Meek K, Dang V, Lees-Miller SP (2008) DNA-PK: the means to justify the ends? Adv Immunol 99:33–58

Meek K, Douglas P, Cui X, Ding Q, Lees-Miller SP (2007) trans Autophosphorylation at DNA-dependent protein kinase's two major autophosphorylation site clusters facilitates end processing but not end joining. Mol Cell Biol 27:3881–3890

Mi J, Dziegielewski J, Bolesta E, Brautigan DL, Larner JM (2009) Activation of DNA-PK by ionizing radiation is mediated by protein phosphatase 6. PLoS One 4:e4395

Michaelidis TM, Grummt I (2002) Mechanism of inhibition of RNA polymerase I transcription by DNA-dependent protein kinase. Biol Chem 383:1683–1690

Morrison R, Al-Rawi JM, Jennings IG, Thompson PE, Angove MJ (2016) Synthesis, structure elucidation, DNA-PK and PI3K and anti-cancer activity of 8- and 6-aryl-substituted-1-3-benzoxazines. Eur J Med Chem 110:326–339

Mortensen DS, Perrin-Ninkovic SM, Shevlin G, Elsner J, Zhao J, Whitefield B, Tehrani L, Sapienza J, Riggs JR, Parnes JS et al (2015) Optimization of a series of triazole containing mammalian target of rapamycin (mTOR) kinase inhibitors and the discovery of CC-115. J Med Chem 58:5599–5608

Moshous D, Callebaut I, de Chasseval R, Corneo B, Cavazzana-Calvo M, Le Deist F, Tezcan I, Sanal O, Bertrand Y, Philippe N et al (2001) Artemis, a novel DNA double-strand break repair/V(D)J recombination protein, is mutated in human severe combined immune deficiency. Cell 105:177–186

Munck JM, Batey MA, Zhao Y, Jenkins H, Richardson CJ, Cano C, Tavecchio M, Barbeau J, Bardos J, Cornell L et al (2012) Chemosensitization of cancer cells by KU-0060648, a dual inhibitor of DNA-PK and PI-3K. Mol Cancer Ther 11:1789–1798

Neal JA, Dang V, Douglas P, Wold MS, Lees-Miller SP, Meek K (2011) Inhibition of homologous recombination by DNA-dependent protein kinase requires kinase activity, is titratable, and is modulated by autophosphorylation. Mol Cell Biol 31:1719–1733

Neal JA, Meek K (2011) Choosing the right path: does DNA-PK help make the decision? Mutat Res 711:73–86

Neal JA, Sugiman-Marangos S, VanderVere-Carozza P, Wagner M, Turchi J, Lees-Miller SP, Junop MS, Meek K (2014) Unraveling the complexities of DNA-dependent protein kinase autophosphorylation. Mol Cell Biol 34:2162–2175

Oakley GG, Patrick SM, Yao J, Carty MP, Turchi JJ, Dixon K (2003) RPA phosphorylation in mitosis alters DNA binding and protein-protein interactions. Biochemistry 42:3255–3264

O'Neill T, Dwyer AJ, Ziv Y, Chan DW, Lees-Miller SP, Abraham RH, Lai JH, Hill D, Shiloh Y, Cantley LC et al (2000) Utilization of oriented peptide libraries to identify substrate motifs selected by ATM. J Biol Chem 275:22719–22727

Park EJ, Chan DW, Park JH, Oettinger MA, Kwon J (2003) DNA-PK is activated by nucleosomes and phosphorylates H2AX within the nucleosomes in an acetylation-dependent manner. Nucleic Acids Res 31:6819–6827

Perry J, Kleckner N (2003) The ATRs, ATMs, and TORs are giant HEAT repeat proteins. Cell 112:151–155

Peterson SR, Jesch SA, Chamberlin TN, Dvir A, Rabindran SK, Wu C, Dynan WS (1995) Stimulation of the DNA-dependent protein kinase by RNA polymerase II transcriptional activator proteins. J Biol Chem 270:1449–1454

Pospisilova M, Seifrtova M, Rezacova M (2017) Small molecule inhibitors of DNA-PK for tumor sensitization to anticancer therapy. J Physiol Pharmacol 68:337–344

Radhakrishnan SK, Lees-Miller SP (2017) DNA requirements for interaction of the C-terminal region of Ku80 with the DNA-dependent protein kinase catalytic subunit (DNA-PKcs). DNA Repair 57:17–28

Reaper PM, Griffiths MR, Long JM, Charrier JD, Maccormick S, Charlton PA, Golec JM, Pollard JR (2011) Selective killing of ATM- or p53-deficient cancer cells through inhibition of ATR. Nat Chem Biol 7:428–430

Romick-Rosendale LE, Hoskins EE, Privette Vinnedge LM, Foglesong GD, Brusadelli MG, Potter SS, Komurov K, Brugmann SA, Lambert P, Kimple RJ et al (2015) Defects in the Fanconi anemia pathway in head and neck cancer cells stimulate tumor cell invasion through DNA-PK and Rac1 signaling. Clin Cancer Res 22(8):2062–2073

Roth DB, Menetski JP, Nakajima PB, Bosma MJ, Gellert M (1992) V(D)J recombination: broken DNA molecules with covalently sealed (hairpin) coding ends in scid mouse thymocytes. Cell 70:983–991

Ruis BL, Fattah KR, Hendrickson EA (2008) The catalytic subunit of DNA-dependent protein kinase regulates proliferation, telomere length, and genomic stability in human somatic cells. Mol Cell Biol 28:6182–6195

Savitsky K, Bar-Shira A, Gilad S, Rotman G, Ziv Y, Vanagaite L, Tagle DA, Smith S, Uziel T, Sfez S et al (1995) A single ataxia telangiectasia gene with a product similar to PI-3 kinase. Science 268:1749–1753

Schild-Poulter C, Shih A, Yarymowich NC, Hache RJ (2003) Down-regulation of histone H2B by DNA-dependent protein kinase in response to DNA damage through modulation of octamer transcription factor 1. Cancer Res 63:7197–7205

Shang ZF, Tan W, Liu XD, Yu L, Li B, Li M, Song M, Wang Y, Xiao BB, Zhong CG et al (2015) DNA-PKcs negatively regulates cyclin B1 protein stability through facilitating its ubiquitination mediated by Cdh1-APC/C pathway. Int J Biol Sci 11:1026–1035

Shang Z, Yu L, Lin YF, Matsunaga S, Shen CY, Chen BP (2014) DNA-PKcs activates the Chk2-Brca1 pathway during mitosis to ensure chromosomal stability. Oncogene 3:e85

Sharif H, Li Y, Dong Y, Dong L, Wang WL, Mao Y, Wu H (2017) Cryo-EM structure of the DNA-PK holoenzyme. Proc Natl Acad Sci U S A 114:7367–7372

Shibata A, Conrad S, Birraux J, Geuting V, Barton O, Ismail A, Kakarougkas A, Meek K, Taucher-Scholz G, Lobrich M et al (2011) Factors determining DNA double-strand break repair pathway choice in G2 phase. EMBO J 30:1079–1092

Shieh SY, Ikeda M, Taya Y, Prives C (1997) DNA damage-induced phosphorylation of p53 alleviates inhibition by MDM2. Cell 91:325–334

Shiloh Y (2003) ATM and related protein kinases: safeguarding genome integrity. Nat Rev Cancer 3:155–168

Sibanda BL, Chirgadze DY, Ascher DB, Blundell TL (2017) DNA-PKcs structure suggests an allosteric mechanism modulating DNA double-strand break repair. Science 355:520–524

Sibanda BL, Chirgadze DY, Blundell TL (2010) Crystal structure of DNA-PKcs reveals a large open-ring cradle comprised of HEAT repeats. Nature 463:118–121

Sipley JD, Menninger JC, Hartley KO, Ward DC, Jackson SP, Anderson CW (1995) Gene for the catalytic subunit of the human DNA-activated protein kinase maps to the site of the XRCC7 gene on chromosome 8. Proc Natl Acad Sci U S A 92:7515–7519

Soubeyrand S, Pope L, Pakuts B, Hache RJ (2003) Threonines 2638/2647 in DNA-PK are essential for cellular resistance to ionizing radiation. Cancer Res 63:1198–1201

Soubeyrand S, Torrance H, Giffin W, Gong W, Schild-Poulter C, Hache RJ (2001) Activation and autoregulation of DNA-PK from structured single-stranded DNA and coding end hairpins. Proc Natl Acad Sci U S A 98:9605–9610

Spagnolo L, Barbeau J, Curtin NJ, Morris EP, Pearl LH (2012) Visualization of a DNA-PK/PARP1 complex. Nucleic Acids Res 40:4168–4177

Sui J, Lin YF, Xu K, Lee KJ, Wang D, Chen BP (2015) DNA-PKcs phosphorylates hnRNP-A1 to facilitate the RPA-to-POT1 switch and telomere capping after replication. Nucleic Acids Res 43:5971–5983

Suwa A, Hirakata M, Takeda Y, Jesch SA, Mimori T, Hardin JA (1994) DNA-dependent protein kinase (Ku protein-p350 complex) assembles on double-stranded DNA. Proc Natl Acad Sci U S A 91:6904–6908

Taccioli GE, Amatucci AG, Beamish HJ, Gell D, Xiang XH, Torres Arzayus MI, Priestley A, Jackson SP, Marshak Rothstein A, Jeggo PA et al (1998) Targeted disruption of the catalytic subunit of the DNA-PK gene in mice confers severe combined immunodeficiency and radiosensitivity. Immunity 9:355–366

Tavecchio M, Munck JM, Cano C, Newell DR, Curtin NJ (2012) Further characterisation of the cellular activity of the DNA-PK inhibitor, NU7441, reveals potential cross-talk with homologous recombination. Cancer Chemother Pharmacol 69:155–164

Ting NS, Kao PN, Chan DW, Lintott LG, Lees-Miller SP (1998) DNA-dependent protein kinase interacts with antigen receptor response element binding proteins NF90 and NF45. J Biol Chem 273:2136–2145

Ting NS, Pohorelic B, Yu Y, Lees-Miller SP, Beattie TL (2009) The human telomerase RNA component, hTR, activates the DNA-dependent protein kinase to phosphorylate heterogeneous nuclear ribonucleoprotein A1. Nucleic Acids Res 37:6105–6115

Ting NS, Yu Y, Pohorelic B, Lees-Miller SP, Beattie TL (2005) Human Ku70/80 interacts directly with hTR, the RNA component of human telomerase. Nucleic Acids Res 33:2090–2098

Tu WZ, Li B, Huang B, Wang Y, Liu XD, Guan H, Zhang SM, Tang Y, Rang WQ, Zhou PK (2013) gammaH2AX foci formation in the absence of DNA damage: mitotic H2AX phosphorylation is mediated by the DNA-PKcs/CHK2 pathway. FEBS Lett 587:3437–3443

Uematsu N, Weterings E, Yano K, Morotomi-Yano K, Jakob B, Taucher-Scholz G, Mari PO, van Gent DC, Chen BP, Chen DJ (2007) Autophosphorylation of DNA-PKCS regulates its dynamics at DNA double-strand breaks. J Cell Biol 177:219–229

van der Burg M, van Dongen JJ, van Gent DC (2009) DNA-PKcs deficiency in human: long predicted, finally found. Curr Opin Allergy Clin Immunol 9:503–509

Villarreal SA, Stewart PL (2014) CryoEM and image sorting for flexible protein/DNA complexes. J Struct Biol 187:76–83

Walker AI, Hunt T, Jackson RJ, Anderson CW, Double-stranded DNA (1985) induces the phosphorylation of several proteins including the 90 000 mol. wt. heat-shock protein in animal cell extracts. EMBO J 4:139–145

Wang C, Lees-Miller SP (2013) Detection and repair of ionizing radiation-induced DNA double strand breaks: new developments in nonhomologous end joining. Int J Radiat Oncol Biol Phys 86:440–449

Weterings E, Verkaik NS, Keijzers G, Florea BI, Wang SY, Ortega LG, Uematsu N, Chen DJ, van Gent DC (2009) The Ku80 carboxy terminus stimulates joining and artemis-mediated processing of DNA ends. Mol Cell Biol 29:1134–1142

Williams ES, Klingler R, Ponnaiya B, Hardt T, Schrock E, Lees-Miller SP, Meek K, Ullrich RL, Bailey SM (2009) Telomere dysfunction and DNA-PKcs deficiency: characterization and consequence. Cancer Res 69:2100–2107

Williams DR, Lee KJ, Shi J, Chen DJ, Stewart PL (2008) Cryo-EM structure of the DNA-dependent protein kinase catalytic subunit at subnanometer resolution reveals alpha helices and insight into DNA binding. Structure 16:468–477

Wong RH, Chang I, Hudak CS, Hyun S, Kwan HY, Sul HS (2009) A role of DNA-PK for the metabolic gene regulation in response to insulin. Cell 136:1056–1072

Wong RH, Sul HS (2010) Insulin signaling in fatty acid and fat synthesis: a transcriptional perspective. Curr Opin Pharmacol 10:684–691

Woodbine L, Neal JA, Sasi NK, Shimada M, Deem K, Coleman H, Dobyns WB, Ogi T, Meek K, Davies EG et al (2013) PRKDC mutations in a SCID patient with profound neurological abnormalities. J Clin Invest 123:2969–2980

Woods DS, Sears CR, Turchi JJ (2015) Recognition of DNA termini by the C-Terminal region of the Ku80 and the DNA-dependent protein kinase catalytic subunit. PLoS One 10:e0127321

Yajima H, Lee KJ, Chen BP (2006) ATR-dependent phosphorylation of DNA-dependent protein kinase catalytic subunit in response to UV-induced replication stress. Mol Cell Biol 26:7520–7528

Yajima H, Lee KJ, Zhang S, Kobayashi J, Chen BP (2009) DNA double-strand break formation upon UV-induced replication stress activates ATM and DNA-PKcs kinases. J Mol Biol 385:800–810

Yang H, Rudge DG, Koos JD, Vaidialingam B, Yang HJ, Pavletich NP (2013) mTOR kinase structure, mechanism and regulation. Nature 497:217–223

Yannone SM, Roy S, Chan DW, Murphy MB, Huang S, Campisi J, Chen DJ (2001) Werner syndrome protein is regulated and phosphorylated by DNA-dependent protein kinase. J Biol Chem 276:38242–38248

Yin X, Liu M, Tian Y, Wang J, Xu Y (2017) Cryo-EM structure of human DNA-PK holoenzyme. Cell Res 27(11):1341–1350

Yu Y, Mahaney BL, Yano K, Ye R, Fang S, Douglas P, Chen DJ, Lees-Miller SP (2008) DNA-PK and ATM phosphorylation sites in XLF/Cernunnos are not required for repair of DNA double strand breaks. DNA Repair 7:1680–1692

Yu Y, Wang W, Ding Q, Ye R, Chen D, Merkle D, Schriemer D, Meek K, Lees-Miller SP (2003) DNA-PK phosphorylation sites in XRCC4 are not required for survival after radiation or for V(D)J recombination. DNA Repair 2:1239–1252

Zeng K, Bastos RN, Barr FA, Gruneberg U (2010) Protein phosphatase 6 regulates mitotic spindle formation by controlling the T-loop phosphorylation state of Aurora A bound to its activator TPX2. J Cell Biol 191:1315–1332

Zhang S, Schlott B, Gorlach M, Grosse F (2004) DNA-dependent protein kinase (DNA-PK) phosphorylates nuclear DNA helicase II/RNA helicase A and hnRNP proteins in an RNA-dependent manner. Nucleic Acids Res 32:1–10

Zhang S, Yajima H, Huynh H, Zheng J, Callen E, Chen HT, Wong N, Bunting S, Lin YF, Li M et al (2011) Congenital bone marrow failure in DNA-PKcs mutant mice associated with deficiencies in DNA repair. J Cell Biol 193:295–305

Zhao Y, Thomas HD, Batey MA, Cowell IG, Richardson CJ, Griffin RJ, Calvert AH, Newell DR, Smith GC, Curtin NJ (2006) Preclinical evaluation of a potent novel DNA-dependent protein kinase inhibitor NU7441. Cancer Res 66:5354–5362

Zolner AE, Abdou I, Ye R, Mani RS, Fanta M, Yu Y, Douglas P, Tahbaz N, Fang S, Dobbs T et al (2011) Phosphorylation of polynucleotide kinase/ phosphatase by DNA-dependent protein kinase and ataxia-telangiectasia mutated regulates its association with sites of DNA damage. Nucleic Acids Res 39:9224–9237

Chapter 13
Targeting DNA-PK as a Therapeutic Approach in Oncology

Celine Cano, Suzannah J. Harnor, Elaine Willmore, and Stephen R. Wedge

Abstract DNA-dependent protein kinase (DNA-PK) is a nuclear serine/threonine protein kinase member of the phosphatidylinositol 3-kinase-related kinase (PIKK) family of enzymes and, once activated, is a key participant in the repair of DNA-double strand breaks (DSBs), playing a central role in non-homologous end joining (NHEJ).

There have been significant efforts to identify small molecule catalytic inhibitors of DNA-PK, predominantly as an approach to induce chemo- and radio-sensitisation. The catalytic inhibitors described to date, differ in their potency, selectivity and the reversibility of inhibition. These inhibitors have been established from varied chemical structures that includes use of arylmorpholine, benzaldehde, chromen-4-one and indolin-2-one scaffolds. Clinical exploitation of DNA-PK inhibition in combination with DNA-damaging therapies may require strategies to maximize the likelihood of attaining an increased therapeutic index, such as the use of appropriate biomarker strategies to guide inhibitor dose and schedule, localisation of genotoxin treatment, or the elucidation of additional determinants of tumour sensitivity. M-3814 and VX-984 (M-9831) are examples of DNA-PK catalytic inhibitors that have advanced into clinical development, and which may help to determine whether such an approach represents a plausible therapeutic strategy for cancer therapy.

Keywords DNA-PK · DNA-repair · NHEJ · Inhibitor · Kinase · Chemopotentiation · Radiopotentiation

C. Cano · S. J. Harnor
Northern Institute for Cancer Research, Newcastle University, School of Chemistry, Newcastle upon Tyne, UK
e-mail: celine.cano@newcastle.ac.uk; suzannah.harnor@newcastle.ac.uk

E. Willmore · S. R. Wedge (✉)
Northern Institute for Cancer Research, Newcastle University, Medical School, Newcastle upon Tyne, UK
e-mail: elaine.willmore@newcastle.ac.uk; steve.wedge@newcastle.ac.uk

© Springer International Publishing AG, part of Springer Nature 2018   339
J. Pollard, N. Curtin (eds.), *Targeting the DNA Damage Response for Anti-Cancer Therapy*, Cancer Drug Discovery and Development, https://doi.org/10.1007/978-3-319-75836-7_13

13.1 Introduction

DNA-dependent protein kinase (DNA-PK) plays a major role in the cellular response to DNA damage, mediating the rapid repair of double strand breaks (DSB). DNA-PK is activated by both endogenous DSB (such as that arising from oxidative damage occurring during metabolic processes) and by exogenous agents that induce DSB, including clinically-used chemotherapeutics and radiotherapy. DNA-PK comprises a catalytic subunit (DNA-PKcs) and a dimeric complex of the Ku70 and Ku80 subunits, which have high affinity for DSB ends and thereby recruit the catalytic subunit to the site of the DNA lesion (Smith and Jackson 1999; Hill and Lee 2010).

Mammalian cells have evolved two main pathways to resolve DSBs, which prove highly toxic if unrepaired (Jackson and Bartek 2009). Homologous recombination (HR) promotes highly accurate repair by using homologous templates on sister chromatids and therefore occurs during S and G2 phases of the cell cycle (West 2003). In contrast, non-homologous end joining (NHEJ) (Jackson and Bartek 2009; Khanna and Jackson 2001; Collis et al. 2005) has evolved primarily to allow cells to rapidly repair DSB during any phase of the cell cycle (though preferentially during G1) (Chapman et al. 2012). A third repair pathway, referred to as alternative non-homologous end-joining (Alt-NHEJ) or microhomology-mediated endjoining (MMEJ), can also be engaged as a backup to canonical NHEJ but is used less frequently, being particularly error-prone and leading to the induction of deletion mutations and gene translocations (Simsek and Jasin 2010).

Both the kinase activity of the catalytic subunit and the DNA binding activity of Ku70 and Ku80 are required for NHEJ. Recent evidence, guided by structural analysis of DNA-PKcs in complex with a Ku80 peptide, suggests that an allosteric mechanism is involved in kinase activation (Sibanda et al. 2017). Importantly, these data also reveal a putative mechanism responsible for directing the cell to either HR or NHEJ, resulting from competition between Ku80 and BRCA1 DNA binding. This conformational change also stimulates DNA-PKcs enzyme activity (Hammarsten and Chu 1998; West et al. 1998). Although kinase activity is known to be essential for repair by NHEJ, the exact sequence of critical phosphorylation events is unclear. Activated DNA-PKcs is itself heavily phosphorylated (via *trans*-autophosphorylation and by the activity of other proteins), with two particular clusters of phosphorylated residues at Ser2056 and Thr2609, thought to be involved in the restriction of DNA processing and the dissociation of DNA-PKcs from the Ku heterodimer respectively (Uematsu et al. 2007; Cui et al. 2005). DNA-PKcs activity can also promote phosphorylation of proteins responsible for DNA ligation (e.g., XRCC4 and DNA ligase IV) (Leber et al. 1998; Wang et al. 2004), and of other signaling proteins such as Akt (Bozulic et al. 2008).

The catalytic activity of DNA-PKcs is also required for its function in V(D)J recombination, which is central to adaptive immunity, with loss of DNA-PK being known to result in a severely immunocompromised phenotype (Blunt et al. 1995). Other biological processes reportedly influenced by DNA-PKcs activity, include a role in metabolic control where it can influence the activity of AMPK, a key energy sensor involved in the regulation of glucose uptake (Amatya et al. 2012; Park et al. 2017), and an ability to regulate a number of transcriptional responses, such as those induced by particular nuclear hormone receptors (Goodwin et al. 2015).

DNA-PKcs expression at both the protein and mRNA level varies among tumour types. In chronic lymphocytic leukaemia (CLL), high DNA-PKcs correlated with DNA-PK activity, and is associated with chemoresistance and a reduced treatment-free interval in patients (Muller et al. 1998; Willmore et al. 2008). Increased expression of DNA-PKcs has also been reported in gastric cancer (Li et al. 2013) and correlates with poor clinical outcome in ovarian cancer (Abdel-Fatah et al. 2014) and hepatocellular cancer (HCC) (Cornell et al. 2015). Whilst a prognostic association between DNA-PKcs and poor disease outcome does not necessarily confirm that the tumour has a dependency on the protein's kinase activity, this has been demonstrated experimentally in castrate-resistant prostate cancer, where DNA-PK catalytic function is found to be a driver of metastatic disease (Goodwin et al. 2015). Given the role of DNA-PK in chemo- and radio-resistance, and its potential role as a driver of other tumorigenic processes, there has been significant interest in identifying inhibitors of the catalytic subunit. However, DNA-PK has proven to be a significantly challenging target for structural biology, the holoenzyme structure only recently being resolved to 5.8 Å with the development of cryo-electron microscopy (Sharif et al. 2017). Consequently, the discovery of inhibitors has been driven by screening approaches with subsequent optimisation using medicinal chemistry expertise. The majority of inhibitors have been designed to occupy the ATP-binding site, however, given the homology between the kinase domains of the phosphatidylinositol 3-kinase (PI-3K) related kinase (PIKK) family members (including ATM (Ataxia telangiectasia mutated kinase), ATR (ATM and Rad3-related kinase) and mTOR (Mammalian Target of Rapamycin)) (Khanna and Jackson 2001; Collis et al. 2005), development of selective inhibitors has been challenging. The design of inhibitors with confirmed target specificity and potency, is essential to enable the potential of DNA-PK inhibition to be evaluated accurately in preclinical studies and clinical applications.

13.2 Small Molecule Inhibitors of DNA-PK Catalytic Activity

The development of small molecule DNA-PK inhibitors has been studied extensively over the past two decades, transitioning from early non-specific compounds to highly selective, potent inhibitors that have entered into clinical trials (Fig. 13.1).

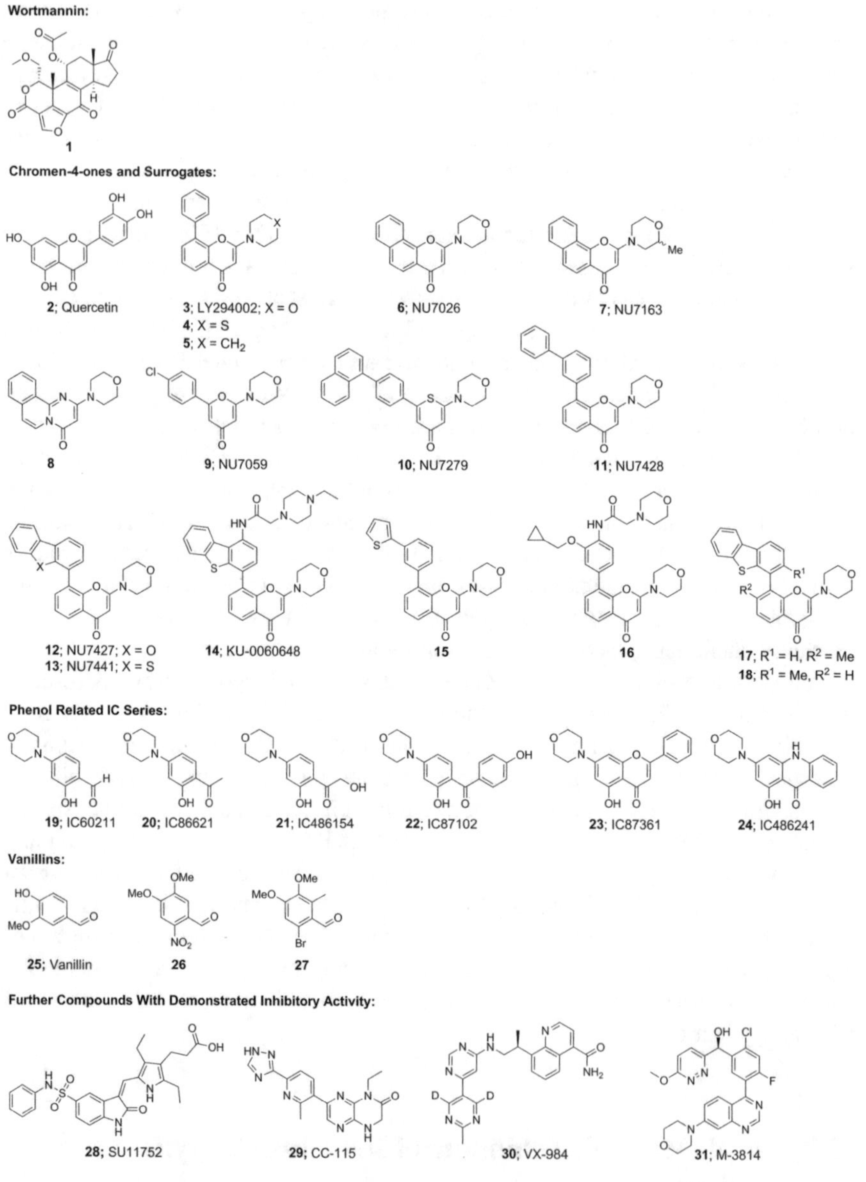

Wortmannin:

Chromen-4-ones and Surrogates:

2; Quercetin   3; LY294002; X = O   6; NU7026   7; NU7163
                4; X = S
                5; X = CH₂

8   9; NU7059   10; NU7279   11; NU7428

12; NU7427; X = O   14; KU-0060648   15   16   17; R¹ = H, R² = Me
13; NU7441; X = S   18; R¹ = Me, R² = H

Phenol Related IC Series:

19; IC60211   20; IC86621   21; IC486154   22; IC87102   23; IC87361   24; IC486241

Vanillins:

25; Vanillin   26   27

Further Compounds With Demonstrated Inhibitory Activity:

28; SU11752   29; CC-115   30; VX-984   31; M-3814

Fig. 13.1 Small molecule inhibitors of DNA-PK catalytic activity

13.3 Wortmannin

Originally found to have antifungal and anti-inflammatory properties, wortmannin (**1**), is a metabolite of the fungi *Penicillium wortmannii K*. This sterol-like compound was subsequently found to be a potent and selective inhibitor of PI-3K family kinases, including inhibition of purified bovine brain PI-3K activity with an IC_{50} of 4.2 nM (Powis et al. 1994). Walker *et al.* verified non-competitive irreversible inhibition with co-crystallographic studies of the resulting covalent complex in the ATP-binding pocket of PI3Kγ (Wymann et al. 1996; Walker et al. 2000). By forming covalent adducts with DNA-PKcs lysine 3751 in the region of the molecule harbouring its kinase domain, wortmannin inhibits DNA-PK at higher concentrations (Ki = 120 nM) via a non-competitive mechanism (Izzard et al. 1999). Despite being an interesting early tool compound, the relative structural complexity of wortmannin presents some challenges for synthetic chemistry and its poor selectively limit its potential. Despite these caveats, a three to five-fold enhancement of IR-induced cytotoxicity and an inhibition of IR-induced DSB repair in Chinese hamster ovary cells was determined using wortmannin (Boulton et al. 1996).

13.4 Chromen-4-ones and Surrogates: LY2094002, NU7441 and KU-0060648

With the aim of developing PI3K-specific inhibitors, Lilly pharmaceuticals undertook a screen of compounds derived from the polyphenol compound quercetin (**2**). In 1994, the chromen-4-one structure LY294002 (**3**) was reported as an inhibitor of PI3K (Vlahos et al. 1994). Further profiling of **3** showed that the compound was an equipotent inhibitor of DNA-PK, mTOR and PI3K (Table 13.1) (Vlahos et al. 1994; Griffin et al. 2005).

The importance of the oxygen of the morpholine of LY294002 was assessed by replacing the oxygen with either a sulfur or a carbon. Interestingly, replacement by sulphur, to provide thio derivative **4** (IC_{50} = 1.61 μM), was tolerated, whilst piperidine analogue **5** exhibited reduced potency (IC_{50} = 4.67 μM). When the structure of LY294002 is in complex with human PI-3Kγ, X-ray crystallography verifies that within the ATP-binding domain of the kinase, the morpholine oxygen makes a hydrogen bond interaction with the backbone amide group of Val-882. This further substantiates the key role of the morpholine substituent (Fig. 13.2) (Walker et al. 2000).

Table 13.1 Inhibitory activity (IC_{50} μM) of DNA-PK inhibitors against different PIKK family members

	DNA-PK	PI-3K (p110α)	ATM	ATR	mTOR
LY294002	1.5±0.2[a]	2.3±0.8[a] (1.4)[b]	>100[a]	>100[a]	2.5±0.2[a]
NU7026	0.23[b]	13[b]	>100[b]	>100[b]	6.4[b]
NU7163	0.19[b]	2.4[b]	>100[b]	>100[b]	4.8[b]
8	0.28[b]	>100[b]	>100[b]	>100[b]	5.3[b]
NU7441	0.014[c]	5[c]	>100[c]	<100[c]	1.7[c]

Values taken from references Vlahos et al. 1994[a], Griffin et al. 2005[b] and Leahy et al. 2004[c]

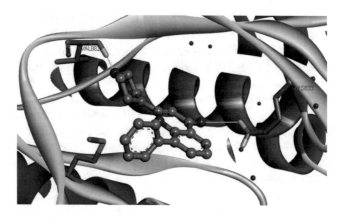

Fig. 13.2 Crystal structure of LY294002 (**3**) in complex with the ATP-binding domain of PI-3Kγ. The figure was prepared from PDB file 1E7V using Discovery Studio 4.1

Although LY294002 suffered from rapid metabolic clearance and induced toxicity *in vivo*, the compound guided the design of derivatives with improved potency and selectivity against DNA-PK. The first analogues investigated were benzopyranone and pyrimidoisoquinolinone derivatives, in studies undertaken by the Newcastle University Drug Discovery Group in collaboration with KuDOS Pharmaceuticals (Griffin et al. 2005). Incorporation of a fused ring on the chromen-4-one, led to an increase in potency against DNA-PK (NU7026 (**6**); $IC_{50} = 0.23 \, \mu M$) (Table 13.1). Variation of the fused phenyl ring around the chromenon-4-one structure gave slightly less active compounds than NU7026. In contrast, substituting the morpholine moiety with a methyl group improved potency (NU7163 (**7**); $IC_{50} = 0.19 \, \mu M$) (Table 13.1). It is worth noting that adding an additional methyl group at the morpholine 2 or 6-position resulted in reduced inhibitory activity (Griffin et al. 2005; Hardcastle et al. 2005). Interestingly, these early LY294002 derivatives demonstrated a better selectivity profile for DNA-PK over other PIKK family members, as exemplified with NU7026, reported to be 60-fold more potent against DNA-PK than PI-3K (p110α) (Table 13.1). Introducing a pyrimidoisoquinolinone scaffold as an isosteric replacement of the chromen-4-one also led to an equipotent compound (**8**; $IC_{50} = 0.28 \, \mu M$) (Table 13.1) (Cano et al. 2010a).

In vitro experiments demonstrated that NU7026 acts as a radiosensitiser, giving a 2-fold dose enhancement in mouse embryonic fibroblast cells (Veuger et al. 2003). Because of the known ability of topoisomerase II (TOP2) inhibitor-induced DSBs to activate DNA-PK, chemosensitisation by NU7026 was explored using a panel of TOP2 poisons in K562 and ML-1 human leukaemia cell lines. NU7026 (10 μM) was found to increase sensitivity to TOP2 poisons by 2–19 fold, by retarding DNA DSB repair and exacerbating the G2 cell cycle block (Willmore et al. 2004).

With a view to truncating the chromenone core, synthesis of substituted monocyclic pyran-2-one, pyran-4-one, thiopyran-4-one and pyridin-4-one derivatives was undertaken (Hollick et al. 2007). Structure-activity relationship (SAR) studies around

6-substituted-2-morpholino-pyran-4-ones and 6-substituted-2-morpholinothiopyran-4-ones led to the identification of NU7059 (9; DNA-PK; IC_{50} = 0.18 μM) and NU7279 (10; DNA-PK IC_{50} = 0.19 μM), both exhibiting a tenfold increase in potency against DNA-PK (Hollick et al. 2007; Hollick et al. 2003). A multi-parallel library approach was also conducted to synthesise 6-, 7-, and 8-aryl substituted chromen-4-ones. Encouragingly, substitution at the 8-position provided a group of inhibitors with activity comparable to NU7026. NU7428 (11; IC_{50} = 0.11 μM) showed a ten fold increase in potency compared with LY294002, and the dibenzofuranyl derivative NU7427 (12) demonstrated further improved inhibitory activity (IC_{50} = 0.04 μM). The incorporation of a dibenzothiophenyl group increased the potency by 100-fold when compared with LY294002 (NU7441 (13); IC_{50} = 0.02 μM), along with excellent selectivity over other PIKK family members (Table 13.1) (Leahy et al. 2004).

NU7441 (8-dibenzothiophen-4-yl-2-morpholin-4-yl-chromen-4-one) has been used in over 70 studies in the literature to date. NU7441 was characterised using the SW620 and LoVo cell lines and it was found that 1μM NU7441 enhanced the cytotoxicity of etoposide (2–12 fold), doxorubicin (2–10 fold) and IR (2–4 fold). (Zhao et al. 2006) Importantly, *in vivo* studies showed that despite its relatively poor solubility, which can limit bioavailability following oral administration, NU7441 increased etoposide-induced tumour growth delay in an SW620 human colon carcinoma xenograft model (Zhao et al. 2006). As well as the effects on cell growth and cytotoxicity, the ability of NU7441 to inhibit repair of DSBs was analysed. In breast cancer (Cowell et al. 2005) and HCC cell lines (Cornell et al. 2015). NU7441 delayed the disappearance of IR- and TOP2 poison-induced γH2AX foci, indicating that the mechanism by which NU7441 enhanced cytotoxicity of these agents was due at least in part to inhibition of DNA-PK-mediated DSB repair.

The potency and selectivity of NU7441 provided an opportunity to explore the translational potential of inhibiting DNA-PK activity. In a panel of 54 patient-derived CLL tumours, 1 μM NU7441 potentiated the cytotoxicity of cholorambucil and fludarabine (drugs used to treat CLL) from 2 to 20-fold, increased drug-induced DSB and γH2AX foci and inhibited the drug-stimulated autophosphorylation of DNA-PK (Ser2056) (Willmore et al. 2008). This study illustrates the concept of using a DNA-PK inhibitor to enhance the cytotoxicity of DNA damaging agents in a defined clinical indication. Additional data denoted that NU7441 was particularly effective at enhancement of TOP2 poison-induced cytotoxicity in multidrug resistant (MDR) cell lines (Mould et al. 2014), and since TOP2 poisons are good substrates for the MDR1 drug efflux pump, the effect of NU7441 on drug efflux was examined. Studies conducted in 4 paired cell lines, each comprising a sensitive (parental) and drug-resistant (MDR1-expressing) counterpart, showed that as well as inhibiting DNA-PK, NU7441 resulted in a small but significant increase in intracellular accumulation of doxorubicin and vincristine in MDR1 expressing cells. For example, in CCRF-CEM VCR/R cells, NU7441 (1 μM for 8 h) increased levels of vincristine by 2.1-fold, which was similar to the increase achieved following exposure to verapamil, a known MDR1 modulator. These data indicate that in MDR1 over-expressing cells, NU7441 can act as a dual DNA-PK and MDR1 inhibitor

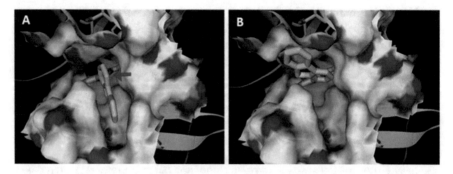

Fig. 13.3 Homology model of the ATP-binding site of the DNA-Dependent Protein Kinase (DNA-PK) used to guide inhibitor design (Clapham et al. 2012). The 3D model was constructed on the basis of the known X-ray crystal structure of PI3Kγ from RCSB protein data bank (PDB ID: 1E7V) as a template, and with DNA-PK sequence from Swiss-Port (ID: PRKDC_DICDI) using Prime in Maestro molecular modelling program (licensed from Schrödinger, LGG). NU7441 (**13**) is represented in (**a**) an orthogonal, and (**b**) "in plane" pose

(Mould et al. 2014). However, further studies to fully assess the potential of NU7441 as an inhibitor of the MDR1 drug efflux pump is merited since in a second study using a panel of HCC cell lines verapamil increased the nuclear accumulation of doxorubicin but NU7441 did not (Cornell et al. 2015).

A PI-3Kγ-derived homology model of the ATP-binding site of DNA-PK was used to guide further inhibitor design (Fig. 13.3) (Clapham et al. 2012).

According to this model, the dibenzothiophene 1-position of NU7441 is pointing towards solvent and therefore predicted to accommodate water-soluble side chains that can be used to increase compound solubility (Fig. 13.3a, arrow). A multi-parallel library approach was undertaken to investigate improvements in compound potency and physicochemical properties based on this hypothesis. The newly synthesised inhibitors all possessed polar substituents at the dibenzothiophene 1-position (Cano et al. 2013). Several compounds were highly potent against DNA-PK and potentiated the cytotoxicity of IR *in vitro* tenfold or more (e.g., KU-0060648 (**14**); DNA-PK $IC_{50} = 5.0 \pm 1$ nM, IR dose modification ratio = 13). In addition, KU-0060648 was shown to potentiate not only IR *in vitro*, but also DNA-damage inducing TOP2 poisons (doxorubicin, etoposide) both *in vitro* and *in vivo* (Cano et al. 2013). In addition to the promising biological activity and improved drug-like properties of KU-0060648 compared to NU7441, acceptable plasma protein binding, combined with weak activity against the hERG ion channel (involved in cardiac repolarisation) and a panel of CYP450 drug metabolizing enzymes was now evident (Table 13.2). However, a number of these compounds, including KU-0060648, were discovered in a counter screen against other PIKK family members, to be potent mixed DNA-PK and PI-3K inhibitors (Cano et al. 2013; Munck et al. 2012). Nonetheless, KU-0060648 demonstrated chemosensitisation effects that were dependent upon DNA-PK expression: the compound enhanced doxorubicin cytotoxicity significantly (up to 32-fold) in MO59-Fus-1 DNA-PK proficient cells but did not affect the cytotoxicity in MO59J DNA-PK deficient cells which were intrinsically more sensitive to doxorubicin

Table 13.2 Properties of NU7441 (**13**) and KU-0060648 (**14**) (Data are the mean ± the standard deviation or individual values; adapted from reference Cano et al. 2013)

Assay		NU7441	KU-0060648
Enzyme	DNA-PK IC_{50} (nM)	42 ± 2	5.0 ± 1
Cellular (HeLa)	pDNA-PK EC_{50} (nM)	212, 339	136 ± 17
	IR-DMR (0.1 µM DNA-PK inhibitor)	2.2 ± 0.2	4.0 ± 0.4
	IR-DMR (0.5 µM DNA-PK inhibitor)	2.8 ± 0.1	13 ± 2
Other	Log$D$ (pH = 7.4)	>4.3	3.05
	hERG IC_{50} (µM)	14, 19	>20
	Solubility at pH 7.4 (µM)	<0.3, <0.2	161 ± 103[a]
	Human plasma protein binding (% Free)	0.04, 0.17	6.2, 3.6
	CYP_{450} inhibition (µM)[b]	-	> 10

[a]Amorphous material (crystalline solubility at pH7.4 buffer = 6.0 µM)
[b]Tested in CYP 3A4, 2D6, 2C9, 2C19 and 1A2 (IR-DMR, the dose modification ratio, defined as the percentage of cell survival in the absence of compound with 2 Gy treatment divided by that in the presence of compound plus 2Gy treatment as determined in 6 – 8 day clonogenic assays; logD, the distribution coefficient calculated as the ratio for the sum of all species of a compound in 1-octanol *versus* that in water at equilibrium; hERG, the human ether-a-go-go-related gene)

(Munck et al. 2012). Importantly, this study also quantified potent cellular inhibition of DNA-PK activity by KU-0060648 (inhibition of IR-induced DNA-PKcs autophosphorylation at Ser2056) demonstrating an IC_{50} of 0.02 µM in MCF-7 breast tumour cells and 0.136 µM in HeLa cells (Table 13.2) (Cano et al. 2013; Munck et al. 2012).

Additional SAR studies around LY294002 and NU7441 have been conducted and have led to the identification of 8-biarylchromenon-4-one derivatives (e.g. **15**; IC_{50} = 18 nM) and *O*-alkoxyphenylchromen-4-one analogues (e.g. **16**; IC_{50} = 8 nM) (Desage-El Murr et al. 2008; Clapham et al. 2011).

Stable pairs of resolvable atropisomers, due to restricted rotation between the chromen-4-one and dibenzothiophene rings, were also generated via substitution of a methyl group at either the chromenone 7-position (**17**) (DNA PK; IC_{50} = 0.005 µM) or dibenzothiophene 3-position (**18**) (DNA PK; IC_{50} = 1.7 µM) of parent compound NU7441 (Clapham et al. 2012; Cano et al. 2010b). Interestingly, in comparison with NU7441, substitution at the chromenone 7-position gave an improvement in potency against DNA-PK, whereas substitution at the dibenzothiophene 3-position resulted in a reduction in potency. Following chiral resolution, each pair of atropisomers was evaluated and the conclusion made that DNA-PK inhibitory activity resided exclusively in the (−)-atropisomer enantiomer, with the antipodal (+)-atropisomer proving inactive (Mould et al. 2014; Clapham et al. 2012).

13.5   Phenol Related IC Series

Benzaldehyde derivative, 2-hydroxy-4-morpholin-4-yl-benzaldehyde (IC60211, IC_{50} = 400 nM) (**19**), is a representative example of a new series of morpholine containing DNA-PK inhibitors reported by the ICOS Corporation and Array

Table 13.3 Inhibitory activity (IC_{50} nM) of representative DNA-PK inhibitors against various PI-3Ks (adapted from references Knight et al. 2004 and Kashishian et al. 2003)

	DNA-PK	p110α	p110β	p110δ	p110γ
IC60211	400	10000	2800	5100	37000
IC86621	120	1400	135	880	1000
IC486154	44	890	42	490	180
IC87102	35	2700	400	1800	5000
IC87361	34	3800	1700	2800	7900

Biopharma. Optimisation of IC60211 led to DNA-PK selective inhibitors (**20–24**), all of which maintained the arylmorpholine substructure, which was found to be critical for kinase inhibitory activity. IC86621 (**20**) is chemically stable and despite not being the most potent compound in the series (IC_{50} = 120 nM), was found to act as a selective and reversible ATP-competitive inhibitor, exhibiting high selectivity against other kinases such as PI-3 K family members (Table 13.3) (Knight et al. 2004; Kashishian et al. 2003). IC86621 (**20**) and IC486154 (**21**) are selective with respect to PI-3K subunit (p110) α, γ and δ, but are equipotent with p110β. The more highly developed morpholino-flavanoid, IC87361 (**23**) is 50-fold more selective for DNA-PK than for p110β (Kashishian et al. 2003).

In vitro, the arylmorpholine compounds IC86621, IC87102 (**22**) and IC87361 are radio- and chemosensitisers and delay repair of DNA DSBs (Kashishian et al. 2003). These compounds also radiosensitise *in vivo* and display superior pharmacokinetic profiles in comparison to other specific DNA-PK inhibitors (Shinohara et al. 2005).

The small-molecule DNA-PK inhibitor IC486241 (**24**) (IC_{50} < 100 μM) differs structurally by way of possessing an acridinone core and is relatively non-toxic as monotherapy (IC_{50} ≥ 29 μM in both HCT-116 and HT-29 cell lines) and found to synergize with 7-ethyl-10-hydroxy-camptothecin (irinotecan, SN38) to enhance killing of colon cancer cells *in vitro* (Davidson et al. 2012a). Additionally, IC486241 was shown to sensitise three genetically diverse breast cancer cell lines to the TOP2 inhibitor doxorubicin (Davidson et al. 2012b). Furthermore, IC486241 decreased doxorubicin-induced DNA-PKcs autophosphorylation on Ser2056 and increased doxorubicin-induced DNA fragmentation (Davidson et al. 2012b).

13.6   Vanillins

It has been demonstrated that members of the vanillin family are simple and relatively specific inhibitors of DNA-PK (Durant and Karran 2003). Even though the activity of vanillin (**25**) (IC_{50} = 1.5 mM) was estimated to be 1000-fold lower than wortmannin, the simple low molecular weight structure presented the opportunity to synthesise further derivatives. A screen of approximately 53,000 organic drug-like compounds was carried out, which aimed to discover structurally related benzaldehyde derivatives. Two compounds that exhibited DNA-PK inhibition at a concentration of 100 μM were 4,5-dimethoxy-2-nitrobenzaldehyde (**26**) (IC_{50} = 15 μM) and 2-bromo-4,5-dimethoxybenzaldehyde (**27**) (IC_{50} = 30 μM), 100-fold and 50-fold more potent than vanillin respectively. Interestingly, non-aldehyde analogues were ineffectual, indicating that the aldehyde group is essential for inhibitory activity (Durant and Karran 2003). Vanillin interacts preferentially with protein lysine residues in the catalytic centre of PI-3K, via Schiff base formation (Chobpattana et al. 2000). The simplicity of vanillin-based molecules makes them attractive initial compounds for structure-based chemistry optimisation, but to enable them to be useful tools for assessing the biochemical mechanism of DNA-PK and the contribution of pathways to DSB repair, the solubility and selectivity would have to be significantly enhanced (Durant and Karran 2003).

13.7 SU11752 (Sugen Incorporated)

SU11752 (**28**) was identified by library screening of three-substituted indolin-2-ones, as an ATP-competitive DNA-PK inhibitor (IC_{50} = 0.13 ± 0.028 μM) with comparable potency to wortmannin (IC_{50} = 0.10 μM) (Izzard et al. 1999), but with selectivity for DNA-PK over PI-3K (p110γ; IC_{50} = 1.10 μM) (Ismail et al. 2004). SU11752 also does not inhibit ATM kinase activity in cells, at concentrations that result in inhibition of DSB repair (12 μM). SU11752 sensitised cells to ionising radiation but lacked sufficient potency for *in vivo* studies (Ismail et al. 2004).

13.8 CC-115 (Celgene)

CC-115 (**29**) is an orally bioavailable equipotent inhibitor of the kinase activities of both DNA-PK (IC_{50} = 0.013 μM) and mammalian target of rapamycin (mTOR) (IC_{50} = 0.021 μM) (Mortensen et al. 2015). By virtue of the latter activity, CC-115 will inhibit both the raptor-mTOR (TORC1) and rictor-mTOR (TORC2) complexes that transduce responses downstream of the PI-3K and Akt signalling pathway. Selective inhibition of mTOR has been pursued by others as a therapeutic strategy in oncology, and the entry of CC-115 into patient trials in 2011 (NCT01353625) as a monotherapy treatment in a range of tumour settings (prostate cancer, multiple myeloma, Ewing's osteosarcoma, lymphoma, CLL) suggests that these clinical studies have been developed to examine the compound's unique dual pharmacology. Whether having additional activity against mTOR will limit the dose of CC-115 that can be administered and hence limit the magnitude of DNA-PK inhibition that can be achieved clinically, remains to be determined, however early results from the trial have shown partial responses in 8 CLL patients, including those with ATM loss (Thijssen et al. 2016).

13.9 VX-984 (M-9831, Merck KGaA and Vertex Pharmaceuticals Incorporated)

Vertex Pharmaceuticals discovered VX-984 also known as M-9831 (**30**) as a DNA-PK inhibitor for clinical development and initiated a phase I combination study with pegylated liposomal doxorubicin in the USA in December 2015 (NCT02644278), in patients with advanced solid tumours or lymphomas. In isolated enzyme studies VX-984 (M-9831) is reported to demonstrate selectivity for DNA-PK in comparison to all Class I PI-3 K isoforms, ranging from 80-fold selectivity *versus* PI-3Kα to 1300-fold for PI-3Kβ (Boucher et al. 2016). The compound was also reported to have an IC_{50} of 88 ± 64 nM for inhibition of DNA-PKcs autophosphorylation (Ser2056) in A549 lung cancer cells (Boucher et al. 2016). VX-984 (M-9831) is administered orally and augments the efficacy of radiotherapy in lung tumour models *in vivo* when administered at 50–100 mg/kg twice-daily (Boucher et al. 2016). As part of a licensing deal, Merck KGaA acquired the rights to VX-984 in January 2017 and are continuing to develop it for the treatment of solid tumours.

13.10 M-3814 (Merck KGaA)

Merck KGaA are known to be developing an orally-administered inhibitor of DNA-PK called M-3814 (**31**) (Zenke et al. 2016; Fuchss et al. 2017). In December 2014, M-3814 entered phase I clinical development in Germany (NCT02316197) in patients with solid tumours who had DNA repair deficiencies, such as loss of ATM or BRCA function, or in patients with CLL. In this study the compound was administered orally as monotherapy, chronically in continuous 21 day cycles (once- or twice-daily). M3814 was tolerated up to 400 mg twice-daily, with further dose-escalation being prohibited by an impurity issue. This dose resulted in stable disease in 6 patients (20% of those examined) for 18 weeks, but there was no evidence of any partial responses. Plasma pharmacokinetic analyses also revealed highly variable exposure (Van Bussel et al. 2017).

In July 2015, M-3814 entered a phase I trial in the USA and Germany (NCT02516813) in combination with radiotherapy. This included a Phase 1a in patients with solid tumours receiving palliative radiotherapy, involving compound administration 1.5 h prior to each 3Gy dose of radiotherapy, with a total of 10 fractions of radiotherapy (up to five fractions per week). In January 2017, seven patients had been treated and two of these had local tumour control, however, plasma pharmacokinetic analyses again demonstrated significant variability (Van Triest et al. 2017). In the Phase 1b, M-3814 is being combined with a more conventional 60 Gy total dose of radiotherapy, given as 2Gy fractions (5 fractions per week) in patients with advanced non-small cell lung cancer or head and neck squamous cell carcinoma. The trial also incorporates a proof-of-principle study to examine the pharmacodynamic and mechanistic consequences of drug treatment, whereby patients with at least two solid tumour lesions, will have one lesion irradiated with a 10–25 Gy single dose of radiotherapy and samples taken for comparison with those from a second lesion treated the following day with an equivalent dose of radiotherapy but 1.5 h after the patient has received a single dose of M-3814.

13.11 Clinical Application of a DNA-PK Inhibitor

DNA-PK has all the potential hallmarks of an attractive target for cancer therapy, given its role in chemo- and radio-resistance and implication in tumourigenesis, that the protein possesses a druggable kinase domain that is critical for DSB repair, that there are potential markers for assessing the pharmacodynamic activity of an inhibitor such as the Ser2056 autophosphorylation site, and that additional markers of DSB repair (e.g., γH2AX) are available to provide direct proof-of-mechanism. The clinical use of a DNA-PK catalytic activity inhibitor for cancer treatment however, still requires further definition. The profound synthetic lethality observed between PARP inhibitors and a tumour cell HR deficiency such as loss of BRCA-1 or BRCA-2 (Bryant et al. 2005; Farmer et al. 2005), has created an expectation that similar genetically defined vulnerabilities will be identified for inhibitors of other DNA-repair processes. ATM, another DSB-activated signaling kinase, is one candidate gene whose loss may confer sensitivity to DNA-PK inhibitors, particularly since ATM and DNA-PK participate in complementary DSB repair pathways. ATM-deficient cancer cells have been found to rely on DNA-PK for survival after DNA damage, and inhibition or knock-down of DNA-PK can re-sensitise drug-resistant ATM-null tumors to the TOP2 poison, doxorubicin (Jiang et al. 2009). It has been proposed that this strategy would be effective where loss of ATM occurs with high frequency in drug-resistant tumours, such as in CLL (Knittel et al. 2015). Whilst there is some experimental evidence to support this concept (Riabinska et al. 2013), these data (including data with the dual PI3K and DNA-PK inhibitor, KU60648) are somewhat limited to date. Additional preclinical work and ongoing clinical studies, which aim to examine the activity of M-3814 in patients with ATM loss or CC-115 treatment in CLL, may help to clarify whether this is an attractive therapeutic strategy.

In addition to trying to identify a genetic susceptibility for monotherapy treatment based upon a deficiency in DNA repair, a DNA-PK inhibitor could also conceivably be used as a therapy in prostate cancer through its ability to suppress defined transcriptional responses. Activation of the androgen receptor (AR) which is known to drive prostate cancer progression, simulates transcription of *PRKDC*, which encodes DNA-PKcs, and DNA-PKcs is also able to bind directly to AR and act as a transcriptional co-activator (Goodwin et al. 2015). Treatment with NU7441 has been shown to perturb this regulatory signaling loop and reduce activated AR-gene transcription (Goodwin et al. 2015). DNA-PKcs has also been found to interact directly with the AR splice variant AR-V7, which can be expressed in late-stage disease and contributes to the development of castrate-resistant prostate cancer (Goodwin et al. 2015). TMPRSS2-ERG gene rearrangements are also found in approximately 50% of prostate cancers (Tomlins et al. 2005) and known to drive cancer progression, in part by inducing the transcription of of a subset of genes involved invasion and metastasis (Tian et al. 2014). DNA-PKcs has been reported to interact directly with TMPRSS2-ERG and inhibition of its enzyme activity by treatment with NU7026 claimed to inhibit prostate cancer cell invasion (Brenner et al. 2011). Collectively these findings indicate that there may be a rationale for inhibition of DNA-PKcs activity in prostate cancer which is independent of an interaction with free DNA ends. Although sustained inhibition of the target would be required in this setting which may to lead to immunosuppression and have consequences on the maintenance of genomic fidelity, these side-effects may be permissible in the treatment of advanced cancer patients.

As a combination therapy, the ability of a DNA-PK inhibitor to augment the tumour cell killing of DNA DSB inducing TOP2 chemotherapy or radiotherapy is clear. However, such a strategy will require careful consideration of how to minimize normal tissue toxicities. At present, a rationale for being able to achieve an improved therapeutic index is not entirely obvious, although differences in tumour cell *versus* normal tissue responses may feasibly exist. Encouragingly, strong augmentation of the antitumour response to radiotherapy has been observed in mice (Fuchss et al. 2017) and clinically this approach may benefit further from advances in radiotherapy technologies that aim to limit broader effects upon the host. Well-characterised selective inhibitors of DNA-PK will be invaluable in assessing the translational potential of this approach.

13.12   Summary

DNA-PK is an exciting therapeutic target and catalytic inhibitors are effective at sensitising tumour cells to DSB-inducing agents. Current challenges in the development of these inhbitors include the development of strategies to maximize the therapeutic index when used in combination with genotoxic agents and the identification of patient populations that will particularly benefit from treatment. Ongoing clinical trials with novel DNA-PK catalytic inhibitors, as monotherapy and in combination with chemotherapy or radiotherapy, may begin to inform on whether this approach represents a promising strategy for cancer treatment.

References

Abdel-Fatah TM, Arora A, Moseley P, Coveney C, Perry C, Johnson K, Kent C, Ball G, Chan S, Madhusudan S (2014) ATM, ATR and DNA-PKcs expressions correlate to adverse clinical outcomes in epithelial ovarian cancers. BBA Clin 2:10–17

Amatya PN, Kim HB, Park SJ, Youn CK, Hyun JW, Chang IY, Lee JH, You HJ (2012) A role of DNA-dependent protein kinase for the activation of AMP activated protein kinase in response to glucose deprivation. Biochim Biophys Acta 1823:2099–2108

Blunt T, Finnie NJ, Taccioli GE, Smith GC, Demengeot J, Gottlieb TM, Mizuta R, Varghese AJ, Alt FW, Jeggo PA, Jackson SP (1995) Defective DNA-dependent protein kinase activity is linked to V(D)J recombination and DNA repair defects associated with the murine scid mutation. Cell 80:813–823

Boucher D, Hoover R, Wang Y, Gu Y, Newsome D, Ford P, Moody C, Damagnez V, Arimoto R, Hillier S, Wood M, Markland W, Eustace B, Cottrell K, Penney M, Furey B, Tanner K, Maxwell J, Charifson P (2016) Potent radiation enhancement with VX-984, a selective DNA-PKcs inhibitor for the treatment of NSCLC. Proc Amer Assoc Cancer Res. https://doi.org/10.1158/1538-7445.AM2016-3716. Abstract 3716

Boulton S, Kyle S, Yalçintepe L, Durkacz BW (1996) Wortmannin is a potent inhibitor of DNA double strand break but not single strand break repair in Chinese hamster ovary cells. Carcinogenesis 17:2285–2290

Bozulic L, Surucu B, Hynx D, Hemmings BA (2008) PKBalpha/Akt1 acts downstream of DNA-PK in the DNA double-strand break response and promotes survival. Mol Cell 30:203–213

Brenner JC, Ateeq B, Li Y, Yocum AK, Cao Q, Asangani IA, Patel S, Wang X, Liang H, Yu J, Palanisamy N, Siddiqui J, Yan W, Cao X, Mehra R, Sabolch A, Basrur V, Lonigro RJ, Yang J, Tomlins SA, Maher CA, Elenitoba-Johnson KS, Hussain M, Navone NM, Pienta KJ, Varambally S, Feng FY, Chinnaiyan AM (2011) Mechanistic rationale for inhibition of poly(ADP-ribose) polymerase in ETS gene fusion-positive prostate cancer. Cancer Cell 19:664–678

Bryant HE, Schultz N, Thomas HD, Parker KM, Flower D, Lopez E, Kyle S, Meuth M, Curtin NJ, Helleday T (2005) Specific killing of BRCA2-deficient tumours with inhibitors of poly(ADP-ribose) polymerase. Nature 434:913–917

Cano C, Barbeau RO, Bailey C, Cockcroft X, Curtin N, Duggan H, Frigerio M, Golding BT, Hardcastle IR, Hummersone MG, Knights C, Menear KA, Newell DR, Richardson C, Smith GCM, Spittle B, Griffin RJ (2010a) DNA-dependent protein kinase (DNA-PK) inhibitors; synthesis and biological activity of quinolin-4-one and pyridopyrimidin-4-one surrogates for the chromen-4-one chemotype. J Med Chem 53:8498–8507

Cano C, Golding BT, Haggerty K, Hardcastle IR, Peacock M, Griffin RJ (2010b) Atropisomeric 8-arylchromen-4-ones exhibit enantioselective inhibition of the DNA-dependent protein kinase (DNA-PK). Org Biomol Chem 8:1922–1928

Cano C, Saravanan K, Bailey C, Bardos J, Curtin NJ, Frigerio M, Golding BT, Hardcastle IR, Hummersone MG, Menear KA, Newell DR, Richardson CJ, Shea K, Smith GCM, Thommes P, Ting A, Griffin RJ (2013) 1-substituted (Dibenzo[b,d]thiophen-4-yl)-2-morpholino-4H-chromen-4-ones endowed with dual DNA-PK PI3-K inhibitory activity. J Med Chem 56:6386–6401

Chapman JR, Taylor MR, Boulton SJ (2012) Playing the end game: DNA double-strand break repair pathway choice. Mol Cell 47:497–510

Chobpattana W, Jeon IJ, Smith JS (2000) Kinetics of interaction of vanillin with amino acids and peptide in model systems. J Agric Food Chem 48:3885–3889

Clapham K, Bardos J, Finlay R, Golding BT, Hardcastle IR, Menear KA, Newell DR, Turner P, Young G, Griffin RJ, Cano C (2011) DNA-dependent protein kinase (DNA-PK) inhibitors: structure-activity relationships for O-alkoxyphenylchromen-4-one probes of the ATP-binding domain. Bioorg Med Chem Lett 21:966–970

Clapham KM, Rennison T, Jones G, Craven F, Bardos J, Golding BT, Griffin RJ, Haggerty K, Hardcastle IR, Thommes P, Cano C (2012) Potent enantioselective inhibition of DNA-dependent protein kinase (DNA-PK) by atropisomeric chromenone derivatives. Org Biomol Chem 10:6747–6757

Collis SP, DeWeese TL, Jeggo PA, Parker AR (2005) The life and death of DNA-PK. Oncogene 24:949–961

Cornell L, Munck JM, Alsinet C, Villanueva A, Ogle L, Willoughby CE, Televantou D, Thomas HD, Jackson J, Burt AD, Newell D, Rose J, Manas DM, Shapiro GI, Curtin NJ, Reeves HL

(2015) DNA-PK - a candidate driver of hepatocarcinogenesis and tissue biomarker that predicts response to treatment and survival. Clin Cancer Res 21:925–933

Cowell IG, Durkacz BW, Tilby MJ (2005) Sensitization of breast carcinoma cells to ionizing radiation by small molecule inhibitors of DNA-dependent protein kinase and ataxia telangiectsia mutated. Biochem Pharmacol 71:13–20

Cui X, Yu Y, Gupta S, Cho YM, Lees-Miller SP, Meek K (2005) Autophosphorylation of DNA-dependent protein kinase regulates DNA end processing and may also alter double-strand break repair pathway choice. Mol Cell Biol 25:10842–10852

Davidson D, Coulombe Y, Martinez-Marignac VL, Amrein L, Grenier J, Hodkinson K, Masson J, Aloyz R, Panasci L (2012a) Irinotecan and DNA-PKcs inhibitors synergize in killing of colon cancer cells. Investig New Drugs 30:1248–1256

Davidson D, Grenier J, Martinez-Marignac VL, Amrein L, Shawi M, Tokars M, Aloyz R, Panasci L (2012b) Effects of the novel DNA dependent protein kinase inhibitor, IC486241, on the DNA damage response to doxorubicin and cisplatin in breast cancer cells. Investig New Drugs 30:1736–1742

Desage-El Murr M, Cano C, Golding BT, Hardcastle IR, Hummersone MG, Menear KA, Frigerio M, Curtin NJ, Richardson C, Smith GCM, Griffin RJ (2008) 8-Biarylchromen-4-one Inhibitors of the DNA-Dependent Protein Kinase (DNA-PK). Bioorg Med Chem Lett 18:4885–4890

Durant S, Karran P (2003) Vanillins- a novel family of DNA-PK inhibitors. Nucleic Acids Res 31:5501–5512

Farmer H, McCabe N, Lord CJ, Tutt AN, Johnson DA, Richardson TB, Santarosa M, Dillon KJ, Hickson I, Knights C, Martin NM, Jackson SP, Smith GC, Ashworth A (2005) Targeting the DNA repair defect in BRCA mutant cells as a therapeutic strategy. Nature 434:917–921

Fuchss T, Mederski WW, Emde U, Buchstallter H-P, Zenke F, Zimmermann A, Sirrenberg C, Vassilev L, Damstrup L, Urbahns K, Blaukat A (2017) Highly potent and selective DNA-PK inhibitor M3814 with sustainable anti-tumor activity in combination with radiotherapy. Proc Amer Assoc Cancer Res. https://doi.org/10.1158/1538-7445.AM2017-4198. Abstract 4198

Goodwin JF, Kothari V, Drake JM, Zhao S, Dylgjeri E, Dean JL, Schiewer MJ, McNair C, Jones JK, Aytes A, Magee MS, Snook AE, Zhu Z, Den RB, Birbe RC, Gomella LG, Graham NA, Vashisht AA, Wohlschlegel JA, Graeber TG, Karnes RJ, Takhar M, Davicioni E, Tomlins SA, Abate-Shen C, Sharifi N, Witte ON, Feng FY, Knudsen KE (2015) DNA-PKcs-mediated transcriptional regulation drives prostate cancer progression and metastasis. Cancer Cell 28:97–113

Griffin RJ, Fontana G, Golding BT, Guiard S, Hardcastle IR, Leahy JJ, Martin N, Richardson C, Rigoreau L, Stockley M, Smith GCM (2005) Selective benzopyranone and pyrimido[2,1-a] isoquinolin-4-one inhibitors of DNA-dependent protein kinase: synthesis, structure-activity studies, and radiosensitization of a human tumor cell line in vitro. J Med Chem 48:569–585

Hammarsten O, Chu G (1998) DNA-dependent protein kinase: DNA binding and activation in the absence of Ku. Proc Natl Acad Sci U S A 95:525–530

Hardcastle IR, Cockcroft X, Curtin NJ, Desage-El Murr M, Leahy JJJ, Stockley M, Golding BT, Rigoreau L, Richardson C, Smith GCM, Griffin RJ (2005) Discovery of potent chromen-4-one inhibitors of the DNA-dependent protein kinase (DNA-PK) using a small-molecule library approach. J Med Chem 48:7829–7846

Hill R, Lee PWK (2010) The DNA-dependent protein kinase (DNA-PK). Cell Cycle 9:3460–3469

Hollick JJ, Golding BT, Hardcastle IR, Martin N, Richardson C, Rigoreau L, Smith GC, Griffin RJ (2003) 2,6-Disubstituted pyran-4-one and thiopyran-4-one inhibitors of DNA-Dependent protein kinase (DNA-PK). Bioorg Med Chem Lett 13:3083–3086

Hollick JJ, Rigoreau JM, Cano-Soumillac C, Cockcroft X, Curtin N, Frigerio M, Golding BT, Guiard S, Hardcastle IR, Hickson I, Hummersone MG, Menear KA, Martin N, Matthews I, Newell DR, Ord R, Richardson C, Smith GC, Griffin RJ (2007) Pyranone, thiopyranone and pyridone inhibitors of phosphatidylinositol 3-kinase related kinases (PIKKs). Structure-activity relationships for DNA-dependent protein kinase (DNA-PK) inhibition, and identification of the first potent and selective inhibitor of the ataxia telangiectasia mutated (ATM) kinase. J Med Chem 503:1958–1972

Ismail IH, Martensson S, Moshinsky D, Rice A, Tang C, Howlett A, McMahon G, Hammarsten O (2004) SU11752 inhibits the DNA-dependent protein kinase and DNA double-strand break repair resulting in ionizing radiation sensitization. Oncogene 23:873–882

Izzard RA, Jackson SP, Smith GC (1999) Competitive noncompetitive inhibition of the DNA-dependent protein kinase. Cancer Res 59:2581–2586

Jackson SP, Bartek J (2009) The DNA-damage response in human biology and disease. Nature 461:1071–1078

Jiang H, Reinhardt HC, Bartkova J, Tommiska J, Blomqvist C, Nevanlinna H, Bartek J, Yaffe MB, Hemann MT (2009) The combined status of ATM and p53 link tumor development with therapeutic response. Genes Dev 23:1895–1909

Kashishian A, Douangpanya H, Clark D, Schlachter ST, Eary CT, Schiro JG, Huang H, Burgess LE, Kesicki EA, Halbrook J (2003) DNA-dependent protein kinase inhibitors as drug candidates for the treatment of cancer. Mol Cancer Ther 2:1257–1264

Khanna KK, Jackson SP (2001) DNA double-strand breaks: signaling, repair and the cancer connection. Nat Genet 27:247–254

Knight ZA, Chiang GG, Alaimo RJ, Kenski DM, Ho CB, Coan K, Abraham RT, Shokat KM (2004) Isoform-specific phosphoinositide-3-kinase inhibitors from an arylmorpholine scaffold. Bioorg Med Chem 12:4749–4759

Knittel G, Liedgens P, Reinhardt HC (2015) Targeting ATM-deficient CLL through interference with DNA repair pathways. Front Genet 6(Article 207):1–9

Leahy JJJ, Golding BT, Griffin RJ, Hardcastle IR, Richardson C, Rigoreau L, Smith GC (2004) Identification of a highly potent and selective DNA-dependent protein kinase (DNA-PK) inhibitor (NU7441) by screening of chromenone libraries. Bioorg Med Chem Lett 14:6083–6087

Leber R, Wise TW, Mizuta R, Meek K (1998) The XRCC4 gene product is a target for and interacts with the DNA-dependent protein kinase. J Biol Chem 273:1794–1801

Li W, Xie C, Yang Z, Chen J, Lu NH (2013) Abnormal DNA-PKcs and Ku 70/80 expression may promote malignant pathological processes in gastric carcinoma. World J Gastroenterol 19:6894–6901

Mortensen DS, Perrin-Ninkovic SM, Shevlin G, Elsner J, Zhao J, Whitefield B, Tehrani L, Sapienza J, Riggs JR, Parnes JS, Papa P, Packard G, Lee BG, Harris R, Correa M, Bahmanyar S, Richardson SJ, Peng SX, Leisten J, Khambatta G, Hickman M, Gamez JC, Bisonette RR, Apuy J, Cathers BE, Canan SS, Moghaddam MF, Raymon HK, Worland P, Narla RK, Fultz KE, Sankar S (2015) Optimization of a series of triazole containing mammalian target of rapamycin (mTOR) kinase inhibitors and the discovery of CC-115. J Med Chem 58:5599–5608

Mould E, Berry P, Jamieson D, Hill C, Cano C, Tan N, Elliott S, Durkacz B, Newell D, Willmore E (2014) Identification of dual DNA-PK MDR1 inhibitors for the potentiation of cytotoxic drug activity. Biochem Pharmacol 88:58–65

Muller C, Chistodoulopoulos G, Salles B, Panasci L (1998) DNA-dependent protein kinase activity correlates with clinical and in vitro sensitivity of chronic lymphocytic leukemia lymphocytes to nitrogen mustards. Blood 92:2213–2219

Munck JM, Batey MA, Zhao Y, Jenkins H, Richardson CJ, Cano C, Tavecchio M, Barbeau J, Bardos J, Griffin RJ, Menear K, Thommes P, Martin NMB, Newell DR, Smith GC, Curtin NJ (2012) Chemosensitisation of cancer cells by KU-0060648; a dual inhibitor of DNA-PK and PI-3K. Mol Cancer Ther 11:1789–1798

Park S-J, Gavrilova O, Brown AL, Soto JE, Bremner S, Kim J, Xu X, Yang S, Um J-H, Koch LG, Britton SL, Lieber RL, Philip A, Baar K, Kohama SG, Abel ED, Kim MK, Chung JH (2017) DNA-PK promotes the mitochondrial, metabolic and physical decline that occurs during aging. Cell Metab 25:1135–1146

Powis G, Bonjouklian R, Breggren MM, Gallegos A, Abraham R, Ashendel C, Zalkow L, Matter WF, Dodge J, Grindey G, Vlahos CJ (1994) Wortmannin a potent and selective inhibitor of phosphatidylinositol-3-kinase. Cancer Res 54:2419–2423

Riabinska A, Daheim M, Herter-Sprie GS, Winkler J, Fritz C, Hallek M, Thomas RK, Kreuzer KA, Frenzel LP, Monfared P, Martins-Boucas J, Chen S, Reinhardt HC (2013) Therapeutic targeting of a robust non-oncogene addiction to PRKDC in ATM-defective tumors. Sci Transl Med 5:189 ra78

Sharif H, Li Y, Dong L, Wang WL, Mao Y, Wu H (2017) Cryo-EM structure of the DNA-PK holoenzyme. Proc Natl Acad Sci U S A 114:7367–7372

Shinohara ET, Geng L, Tan J, Chen H, Shir Y, Edwards E, Halbrook J, Kesicki EA, Kashishian A, Hallahan DE (2005) DNA-dependent protein kinase is a molecular target for the development of noncytotoxic rediation-sensitizing drugs. Cancer Res 65:4987–4992

Sibanda BL, Chirgadze DY, Ascher DB, Blundell TL (2017) DNA-PKcs structure suggests an allosteric mechanism modulating DNA-double strand break repair. Science 355:520–524

Simsek D, Jasin M (2010) Alternative end-joining is suppressed by the canonical NHEJ component Xrcc4/ligase IV during chromosomal translocation formation. Nat Struct Mol Biol 17:410–416

Smith GCM, Jackson SP (1999) The DNA-dependent protein kinase. Genes Dev 13:916–934

Thijssen R, Ter Burg J, Garrick B, van Bochove GG, Brown JR, Fernandes SM, Rodríguez MS, Michot JM, Hallek M, Eichhorst B, Reinhardt HC, Bendell J, Derks IA, van Kampen RJ, Hege K, Kersten MJ, Trowe T, Filvaroff EH, Eldering E, Kater AP (2016) Dual TORK/DNA-PK inhibition blocks critical signaling pathways in chronic lymphocytic leukaemia. Blood 128:574–583

Tian TV, Tomavo N, Huot L, Flourens A, Bonnelye E, Flajollet S, Hot D, Leroy X, de Launoit Y, Duterque-Coquillaud M (2014) Identification of novel TMPRSS2:ERG mechanisms in prostate cancer metastasis: involvement of MMP9 and PLXNA2. Oncogene 33:2204–2214

Tomlins SA, Rhodes DR, Perner S, Dhanasekaran SM, Mehra R, Sun XW, Varambally S, Cao X, Tchinda J, Kuefer R, Lee C, Montie JE, Shah RB, Pienta KJ, Rubin MA, Chinnaiyan AM (2005) Recurrent fusion of TMPRSS2 and ETS transcription factor genes in prostate cancer. Science 310:644–648

Uematsu N, Weterings E, Yano K, Morotomi-Yano K, Jakob B, Taucher-Scholz G, van Gent DC, Chen BP, Chen DJ (2007) Autophosphorylation of DNA-PKCS regulates its dynamics at DNA double-strand breaks. J Cell Biol 177:219–229

Van Bussel M, Mau-Soerensen M, Damstrup L, Nielsen D, Verheul HMW, Aftimos PG, De Jonge MJ, Berghoff K, Schellens JHM (2017) A multicenter phase I trial of the DNA-dependent protein kinase (DNA-PK) inhibitor M3814 in patients with solid tumors. J Clin Oncol 35. https://doi.org/10.1200/JCO.2017.35.15_suppl.2556. Abstract 2556

Van Triest B, Damstrup L, Falkenius J, Budach V, Troost E, Samuels M, Goddemeier T, Geertsen PF (2017) A phase Ia/Ib trial of the DNA-dependent protein kinase inhibitor (DNA-PKi) M3814 in combination with radiotherapy in patients with advanced solid tumors. J Clin Oncol 35. https://doi.org/10.1200/JCO.2017.35.15_suppl.e14048. Abstract e14048

Veuger SJ, Curtin NJ, Richardson CJ, Smith GC, Durkacz BW (2003) Radiosensitization DNA repair inhibition by the combined use of novel inhibitors of DNA-dependent protein kinase and poly(ADP-ribose) polymerase-1. Cancer Res 63:6008–6015

Vlahos CJ, Matter WF, Hui KY, Brown RF (1994) A specific inhibitor of phosphatidylinositol 3-kinase, 2-(4-morpholinyl)-8-phenyl-4H-1-benzopyran-4-one (LY294002). J Biol Chem 269:5241–5248

Walker EH, Pacold ME, Perisic O, Stephens L, Hawkins PT, Wymann MP, Williams RL (2000) Structural determinants of phosphoinositide 3-kinase inhibition by wortmannin, LY294002, quercetin, myricetin and staurosporine. Mol Cell 6:909–919

Wang YG, Nnakwe C, Lane WS, Modesti M, Frank KM (2004) Phosphorylation and regulation of DNA ligase IV stability by DNA-dependent protein kinase. J Biol Chem 279:37282–37290

West SC (2003) Molecular views of recombination proteins and their control. Nat Rev Mol Cell Biol 4:435–445

West RB, Yaneva M, Lieber MR (1998) Productive and nonproductive complexes of Ku and DNA-dependent protein kinase at DNA termini. Mol Cell Biol 18:5908–5920

Willmore E, de Caux S, Sunter NJ, Tilby MJ, Jackson GH, Austin CA, Durkacz BW (2004) A novel DNA-dependent protein kinase inhibitor, NU7026, potentiates the cytotoxicity of topoisomerase II poisons used in the treatment of leukemia. Blood 103:4659–4665

Willmore E, Elliott SL, Mainou-Fowler T, Summerfield GP, Jackson GH, O'Neill F, Lowe C, Carter A, Harris R, Pettitt AR, Cano-Soumillac C, Griffin RJ, Cowell IG, Austin CA, Durkacz BW (2008) DNA-dependent protein kinase is a therapeutic target and an indicator of poor prognosis in B-cell chronic lymphocytic leukemia. Clin Cancer Res 14:3984–3992

Wymann MP, Bulgarelli-Leva G, Zvelebil MJ, Pirola L, Vanhaesebroeck B, Waterfield MD, Panayotou G (1996) Wortmannin inactivates phosphoinositide 3-kinase by covalent modification of Lys-802, a residue involved in the phosphate transfer reaction. Mol Cell Biol 16:1722–1733

Zenke FT, Zimmermann A, Sirrenberg C, Dahmen H, Vassilev L, Pehl U, Fuchss T, Blaukat A (2016) M3814, a novel investigational DNA-PK inhibitor: enhancing the effect of fractionated radiotherapy leading to complete regression of tumors in mice. In: Proceedings of the 107th Annual Meeting of the American Association for Cancer Research 2016 Apr 16–20. AACR, New Orleans, LA. Philadelphia (PA). Cancer Res., 76(14 Suppl):Abstract nr 1658

Zhao Y, Thomas HD, Batey M, Cowell I, Richardson C, Griffin RJ, Calvert AH, Newell DR, Smith GC, Curtin N (2006) Preclinical evaluation of a potent novel DNA-dependent protein kinase inhibitor NU7441. Cancer Res 66:5354–5362

Chapter 14
Dbait: A New Concept of DNA Repair Pathways Inhibitor from Bench to Bedside

Marie Dutreix, Flavien Devun, Nirmitha Herath, and Patricia Noguiez-Hellin

Abstract Biological systems need to be robust, both for survival of individuals under stress and for plasticity required for adaptation and evolution. In principle, networks can achieve robustness through redundancy. The most direct mechanism is simple substitutional redundancy, if a protein or a pathway are inactive another protein or pathway can substitute to perform the same function. Functional plasticity and redundancy are essential mechanisms underlying the ability to survive and maintain genome integrity. However, it is the cause of failure of many targeted therapies as alternative pathways can replace the function inactivated by the hit of the targeted enzyme.

Keywords Dbait · DNA damage repair · DT101 · AsiDNA · Genotoxic drug · Radiation

14.1 DNA Repair Robustness and Redundancy

One of the main drawbacks of the DNA repair network is that it is principally designed to restore the integrity of the DNA molecule whatever the cost in degrading the genetic information, hence repair of DNA damage may be associated with mutations, ranging from single-base substitutions to chromosomal rearrangements. These changes are

M. Dutreix (✉)
Institut Curie, PSL Research University, CNRS, INSERM, UMR 3347, Orsay, France

Université Paris Sud, Université Paris-Saclay, CNRS, INSERM, UMR 3347, Orsay, France
e-mail: marie.dutreix@curie.fr

F. Devun · N. Herath · P. Noguiez-Hellin
Institut Curie, PSL Research University, CNRS, INSERM, UMR 3347, Orsay, France

Université Paris Sud, Université Paris-Saclay, CNRS, INSERM, UMR 3347, Orsay, France

DNA Therapeutics, Genopole, Evry, France

© Springer International Publishing AG, part of Springer Nature 2018   359
J. Pollard, N. Curtin (eds.), *Targeting the DNA Damage Response for Anti-Cancer Therapy*, Cancer Drug Discovery and Development,
https://doi.org/10.1007/978-3-319-75836-7_14

used by some important biological activities such as the immune response, development and evolution to generate required genetic diversity. Alterations of DNA repair are thought to be often initiation events in cancer development and could be the Achilles' heel of aggressive tumors.

The importance of DNA repair is evident from the large investment that cells make in DNA repair enzymes. For example, several percent of the coding capacity of bacteria and yeast is devoted solely to DNA repair functions. The importance of DNA repair is also demonstrated by the increased rate of mutation that follows the inactivation of a DNA repair gene. To counteract DNA damage, repair mechanisms specific for many types of lesion have evolved (Fig. 14.1). It has been demonstrated that they operate in most living organisms including humans. Double-strand breaks (DSBs) are the most toxic form of DNA damage and one single DSB left unrepaired is sufficient to lead to cell death by loss of genetic material in the daughter cell (Paques and Haber 1999). Therefore DSBs are the only damage structures to be addressed by several pathways. DSBs are repaired by at least three independent pathways: non homologous end joining (NHEJ) promotes the re-ligation of DSBs in an efficient but potentially inaccurate manner, homologous recombination (HR) (West 2003; Caldecott 2008) precisely restores the genomic sequence of the broken DNA ends by utilizing sister chromatids as template for repair and, when NHEJ is

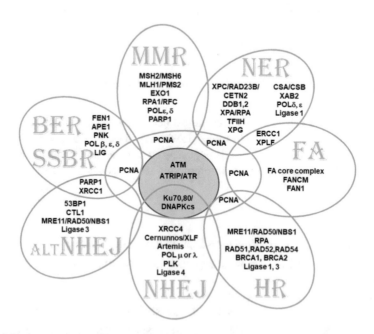

Fig. 14.1 Non exhaustive list of genes involved in main repair pathways: *BER* Base Excusion Repair, *MMR* Mismatch Repair, *NER* Nucleotide Excision Repair, *FA* Fanconi Anemia DNA repair, *HR* Homologous Recombination, *NHEJ* Non Homologous End Joining, *Alt-NHEJ* alternative Non Homologous End Joining

inactive and HR cannot proceed as sister chromatids are not present an alternative pathway called alt-NHEJ takes place. DSBs can occur directly as a consequence of radiation or chemotherapy drugs (as some topoisomerase inhibitors) or more frequently as a consequence of replication or transcription errors as a result of other dedicated repair pathways failing to eliminate the initial damage event. The critical role of DSB repair in living system evolution is not only revealed by the redundancy of the pathways but also by the lack of common enzymes where inactivation could lead to a general defect in DSB repair (Fig. 14.1).

The repair activities must be precisely regulated, since each in its own right can wreak havoc on the integrity of DNA if misused or allowed to access DNA at the inappropriate time or place. Thus, eukaryotic cells have developed strategies to recruit and activate the right factors in the right place at the right time. The cellular mechanisms that coordinate the choice of which pathways to employ for efficient DNA repair act by regulating the recruitment of DNA repair enzymes to sites of DNA damage, where they become activated.

14.2 The Dbait Concept: A Pathway Inhibitor

Over the last decade, numerous laboratories or pharmaceutical companies developed drug molecules targeting the main DNA repair proteins to modulate the DNA repair activity (Bianchi et al. 1986; Chikamori et al. 2010; Fortini and Dogliotti 2007; Jalal et al. 2011; Kuzminov 2001; Lord and Ashworth 2012; Lundin et al. 2002; Wyman and Kanaar 2006). Currently, the most advanced inhibitors are the poly (ADP-ribose) polymerase (PARP) inhibitors (PARPi) with the recent approvals of olaparib (Lynparza), rucaparib (Rubraca) and niriparib (Zejula). PARPi target tumour cells that are HR deficient because their mechanism of action is based on exploiting synthetic lethality (Shaheen et al. 2011; Aly and Ganesan 2011). This HR deficiency generally consists of BRCA1 mutations. However such enzyme-targeted therapies face emergent resistance resulting from target mutations or redundant repair pathway hyperactivation. Many tumors that initially responded to PARPi treatments finally relapsed through compensatory mutations restoring DNA repair capacity (Aly and Ganesan 2011; Peng et al. 2014).

A majority of cancers are today treated by agents causing DNA damage such as chemotherapy (CT) and the radiotherapy (RT). However the therapeutic index of CT and RT is limited due to the intrinsic or acquired resistance of tumors and toxicity of treatments on healthy tissues which limits the using dose (Moding et al. 2013). The efficiency of RT and CT is, in the majority of these cases, directly linked to their capacity to induce damage in the DNA. Cancer cells are commonly very capable of repairing this damage, so allowing the cells to survive to the DNA damaging treatments (Oliver et al. 2010; Willers et al. 2013). It is thus essential to develop new therapeutic agents targeting the pathways of DNA repair specifically to restore sensitivity to DNA damaging agents.

To efficiently inhibit DNA repair and prevent emergence of resistance, new strategies have been developed. One of these strategies is represented by Dbait which is designed to globally inhibit the DSB repair machinery, by preventing recruitment of enzymes involved in DSB and SSB break repair at the damage site. Indeed, one of the early events in DNA repair is the recruitment of the different enzymes at the damage site. This recruitment is promoted by modification of the chromatin (mainly phosphorylation of the H2AX histone variant) by the phosphatidylinositol 3-kinase (PI3K) like kinase family members, ATM, ATR or DNA-PK (Durocher and Jackson 2001). At single-strand breaks (SSBs) and some residual DSBs, the recruitment of BER enzymes and alternative NHEJ is promoted by the production of poly-ADP-ribose polymers (PAR) by the activated PARP (Beck et al. 2014). As repair of the breaks is essential for the life of the cell, these PI3K kinases and PARP polymerases together play a very important role in maintaining genome integrity and are extremely abundant in the cell. Inhibiting the recruitment and / or activation of this system by conventional small molecules is almost impossible. An alternative original approach is to use ectopic (out of the damage site) activation of damage signaling by small molecules mimicking DNA damage structures to prevent recognition of the location of the endogenous DNA damage on the chromosomes. These molecules called AsiDNA (also known as DT01) induce the phosphorylation of H2AX and the production of PAR in the absence of damage, generating a false signal that hides the signal at the sites of chromosomal DNA damage induced by the DNA damage treatment. As a result the repair enzymes are no longer recruited at the damage site and the formation of repair foci is inhibited.

14.2.1   Selection of the Dbait Molecule Active Compound

Short double stranded DNA molecules were screened for their ability to activate DNA-PK and PARP1 using enzymatic assays. Molecules of varying in length, sequence and end structure were tested (Quanz et al. 2009a, b; Croset et al. 2013). Only molecules with at least one blunt end and a length greater than 32 bp were able to activate both DNA-PK and PARP1. Shorter molecules, molecules with no end, or molecules with single-strand extremity showed lower capacity to activate both enzymes. The DNA sequence had no effect on the activation of DNA-PK or PARP1, indicating that the structure of the molecule is the active property of the siDNA.

14.2.2   AsiDNA Signaling Activity

The Dbait molecules were modified to be used in living cells (organisms). The two strands were tethered by a non-nucleic acid polymer at one end to prevent dissociation and the blunt extremity was protected by adding three phosphorotioate modifications at the extremity of both strands (Fig. 14.2a). In addition, DNA has very poor cell penetration, which was addressed by covalently binding a cholesterol motif to the 5′ strand end to promote cellular uptake via cholesterol trafficking mechanisms. The resulting molecule (called AsiDNA) was highly soluble (up to 80 mg/ml in water). Similar data were obtained in cell culture using either AsiDNA or Dbait with polyethylenimine (PEI) or superfect as transfection vectors (Berthault

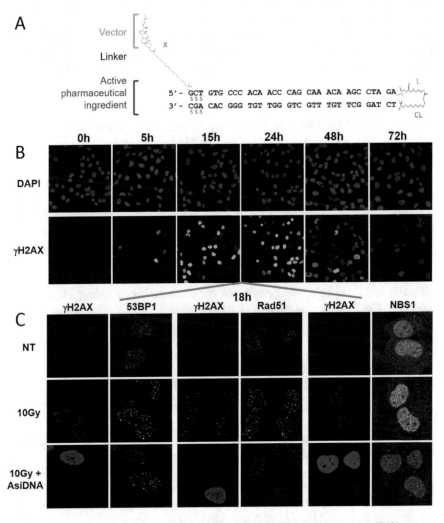

Fig. 14.2 Kinetics of signaling induced by AsiDNA in MRC5-SV fibrosblasts. (**a**) AsiDNA strucuture, L is an amino linker, X a cholesteryl tetraethyleneglycol, CL a carboxylic (Hydroxyundecanoic) acid Linker and s a phosphorothioate linkage; (**b**) Kinetics of Pan-nuclear phosphorylation of H2AX (red staining) treated 24 h with AsiDNA, washed and observed up to 72 h (maximal effect was observed between 15 and 24 h). (**c**) Inhibition of 53BP1, NBS1 and RAD51 repair enzyme recruitment in cells treated with AsiDNA, irradiated 10 Gy and observed 2 h after irradiation

et al. 2011). In animal studies and the clinic, AsiDNA was exclusively used to avoid transfection vector associated toxicity.

Treating cells with Dbait/PEI (Quanz et al. 2009a) or AsiDNA induces pan-nuclear phosphorylation of the serine 139 of the histone H2AX on the chromatin (Fig. 14.2b). The activation of the phosphorylation lasts for 2–3 days according to the cell type involved. Tumor cells keep dividing while their chromatin is highly modified. Cells with a high level of spontaneous damage die after several days from necrotic death (mitotic catastrophy). Furthermore, all the cells treated with Dbait or AsiDNA show a defect in the formation of repair foci after irradiation. Specifically, the proteins 53BP1, Nbs1 (Quanz et al. 2009b), RAD51 (Quanz et al. 2009a), BRCA1, PCNA and XRCC1 (Croset et al. 2013) do not form foci at sites of damage induced by irradiation (Fig. 14.2c). This inhibition lasts as long as the modification of the chromatin.

14.2.3 AsiDNA Inhibits Repair of DNA Damage Induced by Radiation and Genotoxic Drugs

Analysis of DNA repair after irradiation and treatment with AsiDNA, using single cell comet assays, indicates that repair is inhibited in radioresistant cells leading to a significant decrease of their survival after irradiation (Quanz et al. 2009b; Biau et al. 2014). The sensitizing effect of AsiDNA is not restricted to damage induced by irradiation as similar decreases in DNA repair and the related cell survival were observed with different DNA damaging drugs such as camptothecin (Devun et al. 2012),5-FU (Devun et al. 2012; Herath et al. 2016), oxaliplatin (Croset et al. 2013), temozolomide, cisplatin, carboplatin and doxorubicin, (unpublished). In all cases, the induced cell death was essentially mitotic death occurring asynchronously with cell growth and with no significant apoptotic events.

14.3 Micronuclei as a Predictive Biomarker of Sensitivity to AsiDNA

Large-scale chromosomal rearrangements (LST) reflect tumor genetic instability and have been proposed to be predictive of response to DNA damage repair inhibitors. Sensitivity to AsiDNA,was associated with a high level of LST and a high spontaneous frequency of cells with micronuclei (MN) (Jdey et al. 2017; Fenech 1993). MN result from chromosomal breakage or spindle damage. They can be easily detected in biopsies with hematoxylin and eosin staining (HES) (Jadhav et al. 2011). This makes this biomarker cheap and readily adoptable in most cancer hospitals. The finding that low basal levels of LSTs and MN could be biomarkers of resistance to AsiDNA suggests that aggressive tumors with high genetic instability (frequently with a poor prognosis) may be the preferential indication for AsiDNA treatment.

14.4 AsiDNA and Hyperthermia

Numerous studies demonstrated that hyperthermia can sensitize cells to DNA damaging agents. Its combination with various chemotherapies or radiotherapy has been shown to be cytotoxic and to inhibit tumor growth in animal models (Braun and Hahn 1975; Hill and Denekamp 1979; Hazan et al. 1984). Clinical trials have confirmed that hyperthermia significantly improves radiotherapy efficacy in numerous malignancies (Franckena and van der Zee 2010; Hurwitz et al. 2011; De Haas-Kock et al. 2009). This synergistic effect might be due to the accumulation of DNA double-strand breaks (DSBs), the most lethal type of DNA damage, in cells treated with mild hyperthermia. Based on *in vitro* studies, it was speculated that hyperthermia could induce DNA damage directly (Warters and Henle 1982; Anai et al. 1988; Wong et al. 1995). It was reported that mild hyperthermia induces phosphorylation of histone H2AX, similar to the formation of the radiation induced repair foci at DSBs (Wong et al. 1995; Rogakou et al. 1999). Recently, it has been suggested that this phenomenon is the result of hyperthermia-induced homologous recombination (HR) inhibition (Krawczyk et al. 2011). Nevertheless, the effects of hyperthermia on DNA repair/damage are still not fully elucidated probably due to the variations in different heating protocols used in the different studies.

Regardless of the mechanism of hyperthermia on the formation of DNA damage, its use with AsiDNA treatment may prevent repair and could be of therapeutic interest. One way to induce hyperthermia in patient tumors is through radiofrequency ablation (RFA). RFA involves delivering a high-frequency alternating current with an electrode placed percutaneously or surgically in the tumor. Tumor cells are killed rapidly in the tumor center due to high temperatures while there is cellular damage at the tumor periphery where temperatures are lower. However the rapid drop in temperature at the periphery of large tumors limits the amount of damage and may lead to tumor recurrence (Itoh et al. 2002). Inhibiting the main DSB repair pathways, could enhance mild hyperthermia-induced cytotoxicity.

Pretreating the cells with Dbait/PEI sensitized all tested human adenocarcinoma cell lines to mild hyperthermia. The efficacy of sublethal-RFA (SL-RFA) with and without AsiDNA administration was assessed on human HT29 colorectal xenografted tumors. Combining AsiDNA administrations with SL-RFA delayed tumor growth and significantly improved median survival compared to SL-RFA alone. This efficacy was further strengthened when the AsiDNA was administered after RFA suggesting that the schedule is a critical parameter for such targeted therapies. Efficacy was confirmed by pathological analysis. The ablated lesion is often described as having distinct zones. Necrotic tissue with structurally damaged tumor cells is found in the central zone. The transition zone, surrounding the central zone, is exposed to lower temperatures, inducing eosinophilic cells with condensed chromatin representing ongoing necrosis (Itoh et al. 2002). The outermost zone includes normal tissue surrounding the transition zone (Bhardwaj et al. 2012). AsiDNA and RFA significantly increased the size of the central and transition zones, i.e. necrosis and ongoing necrosis. Tumors that received combined treatment showed significantly larger areas of necrosis and ongoing necrosis than those treated with SL-RFA. Some specimens that were treated with SL-RFA and AsiDNA showed no viable tumor cells while others presented small areas of viable cells, with lower mitosis than that found in tumors treated with SL-RFA. This was confirmed by Ki67 immuno-staining which showed a decrease in the Ki67 index in tumors receiving combined treatment compared to those treated with SL-RFA alone.

14.5   AsiDNA and Chemotherapy

In different preclinical tumor models, including patient derived xenografts (PDX), it has been demonstrated that either with local administration (intratumoraly or subcutaneously adjacent to the tumor) or with systemic administration (intravenously, IV or intraperitoneally, IP) AsiDNA increases the efficacy of chemotherapy (Devun et al. 2012; Herath et al. 2016; Herath et al. 2017) AsiDNA molecules accumulate in tumors following systemic injection (IP or IV) regardless of the tumor localization (e.g., skin, liver, brain). They enter cells and trigger activation of DNA-PK that can be revealed by high phosphorylation of H2AX in tumor tissues. AsiDNA administration sensitizes the tumors to chemotherapy treatment such as platinum salt (carboplatin/cisplatin), anthracycline antitumor antibiotic (doxorubicin) and topoisomerase II poison (etoposide).

Intrinsic resistance to AsiDNA was not detected in many cases but where it was, changing the chemotherapy or replacing it by radiotherapy usually was sufficient to render cells sensitive to the AsiDNA. This was particularly observed when the chemotherapy resistance was due to rapid repair via a pathway insensitive to DSB DNA damage signaling such as direct repair by MGMT, which responds to damage induced by monofunctional methylating agents. For example, the SK28Mel melanoma model is highly resistant to the alkylating drug dacarbazine via overexpression of the MGMT repair enzyme and is also resistant to radiotherapy. However, whereas addition of AsiDNA does not improve the tumor response to dacarbazine (data not published) it strongly stimulates the response to radiotherapy (Biau et al. 2014).

Intraperitoneal administration was used to demonstrate that systemic administration of AsiDNA improves tumor control and is well tolerated in the chemotherapy resistant triple negative breast tumor model, MDA-MB231. A protocol with carboplatin similar to the clinical protocol was used with 3 cycles of carboplatin administered as s single injection followed by 2 weeks of rest per cycle. AsiDNA was administered daily for 5 days the week of chemotherapy treatment. Combination treatment showed a better tumor growth control compared to standalone treatments (Fig. 14.3). Whereas single treatments did not stabilize or cure tumors, among the seven animals treated with the combination, one was cured (with no recurrence) and two others were stable during the year of observation.

No increase of carboplatin toxicity was observed in animals after the three cycles of treatment. Interestingly, the bone marrow depletion induced by the carboplatin was not increased by the AsiDNA administration.

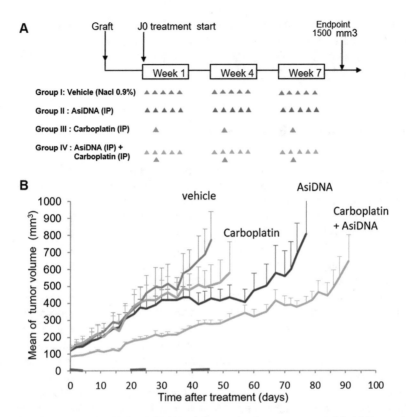

Fig. 14.3 Tumor growth of MDA-MB-231 triple negative breast cancer model. (**a**) Protocol of treatment: (6–10 mice/group) received 3 cycles of treatment by systemic administration of DT01 alone (5 mg/day) or in combination with carboplatin (1 × 50 mg/kg/cycle) administered by intraperitoneal injection (IP). (**b**) Mean tumor growth, errors bars represent the standard error of the mean (SEM)

14.6 AsiDNA and PARP Inhibitors

The most advanced drugs in the class of the DNA repair inhibitors are the PARP inhibitors, with clinical trials showing significant benefits in patients with *BRCA* mutated ovarian cancer. Essentially, cells deficient in HR are 100- to 1000-fold more sensitive to PARP inhibitors than HR proficient cell lines. AsiDNA inhibits HR by preventing recruitment of the Nbs1/Mre11 complex, BRCA1 and RAD51 to the DNA damage site (Fig. 14.2). Combination of AsiDNA with PARPi increases the accumulation of unrepaired damage, resulting in cell death in all tumor cells independent to their ability to perform HR. (Jdey et al. 2017) In contrast, non-tumor cells do not show an increase of DNA damage nor lethality. Analysis of multi-level omics data from breast cancer cells highlighted that resistance to AsiDNA or olaparib was associated with differential DNA repair and cell cycle molecular profiles, which supports the broad activity of the combination. Treatment synergy was confirmed with the 6 PARPi that have been approved or are in development (Jdey et al. 2017). These data support the notion that synthetic lethality can be achieved by the combination of two targeted agents.

14.7   AsiDNA and Radiotherapy

Since the discovery of the DNA damaging properties of ionizing radiation and the first observation of their toxic effects on proliferative tissues, radiotherapy has become a standard treatment for many cancers. The curative effect of this treatment is impaired by the high capacity some tumour cells have to recover from the induced damage and thus become resistant to treatment. DNA repair has been identified as the main mechanism of radioresistance. Many laboratories have demonstrated the potential of using inhibitors of DNA repair to enhance radiotherapy efficiency (Helleday et al. 2008; Thoms and Bristow 2010; Begg et al. 2011). AsiDNA molecules were tested with radiotherapy in rodent brain tumors recapitulating glioblastoma features. Their local administration in brain was well tolerated and did not increase radiation toxicity. Radiotherapy (two sessions of 6 Gy in 2 weeks) increased the median survival of animals with brain tumors by 40% and the addition of AsiDNA administration before each radiotherapy increased median by 60% (Coquery et al. 2012).

Cutaneous melanoma is another tumor type known to be highly resistant to radiation. A mouse melanoma xenograft was used to assess the efficacy of AsiDNA administration in combination with external radiotherapy or internal radiotherapy. Mice were treated with 10 fractions of radiotherapy over 2 weeks with AsiDNA given 6 times just prior to every other dose of radiation. Treatment with RT alone increased median survival by 17%, while the combination with AsiDNA increased median survival by 200%. No in-field skin toxicity was observed (Biau et al. 2014). The radiosensitising effect of AsiDNA was dose dependent. Doubling the treatment time to 4 weeks increased the efficacy but still did not show any associated toxicity. Interestingly the lack of radiosensitising effects on healthy tissues was confirmed in a mouse experiment in which Dbait was combined with internal radiotherapy from iodine 131 coupled to the melanin targeting agent ICF01012. In this experiment anti-tumor activity was observed for the combination but Dbait did not enhance normal tissue toxicity from [^{131}I]-ICF01012 treatment (Viallard et al. 2016).

14.8   AsiDNA First-in-Human Clinical Application

Taken together the mouse data suggest AsiDNA can provide a beneficial effect on tumor growth with no toxicity or radiosensitisation of normal tissue (specifically skin). Nevertheless it is essential to confirm this in clinical studies. Therefore a specific trial was designed to monitor the radio-sensitising effects of AsiDNA in healthy skin and in skin metastasis of melanoma (melanoma in transit). The metastatic spread of melanoma to large areas on the skin requires the irradiation of considerable areas of healthy skin between tumor nodes, which facilitate the monitoring of adverse events in healthy irradiated tissue. Conventional therapies such as chemotherapy and RT display poor antitumor activities in melanoma skin metastasis (Kim et al. 2010; Kirkwood et al. 2012). In fact, RT (≤ 5 Gy per fraction) provides complete responses in less than 10% of the patients (Konefal et al. 1987; Olivier et al. 2007).

The first-in-human, phase I trial using AsiDNA, was an open label, non-randomized, multi-centre study. Patients were assigned sequentially to escalating daily total doses of AsiDNA (DT01) (from 16 to 96 mg), plus RT following a traditional 3+3 design. The primary objective was to evaluate the safety and tolerability profiles of AsiDNA in combination with RT. The secondary objectives were to determine the dose-limiting toxicities (DLTs), the pharmacokinetic (PK) parameters of AsiDNA, pharmacodynamic biomarkers, and to identify preliminary signs of efficacy. AsiDNA was administered three times a week (every other day) over 2 weeks (six administrations of AsiDNA in total) by intratumoral (IT) injection and also in healthy skin in the periphery of two tumors (PT). RT was administered to the entire area with metastatic spread to a total dose of 30 Gy in ten fractions over 2 weeks.

Similar to the results obtained in the animal models AsiDNA was well tolerated and none of the patients displayed DLT. The drug was rapidly absorbed into plasma in all patients. The time to reach peak plasma concentrations varied across patients and became longer with increasing doses. The amount of drug absorbed expressed as Cmax and AUC varied between patients however it increased approximately proportional with the dose. The half-life was around 5 h at the highest dose (i.e. 96 mg). It is reasonable to assume that the observed PK variability is mainly driven by the administration of the compound into tissue in and around the tumor. One would expect much lower PK variability and dose proportional exposure after intravenous administration as observed in rats and monkeys (Schlegel et al. 2012). Patient response was evaluated by considering all target lesions from each patient. Of the 21 evaluable patients, 5% displayed a complete response (CR) to treatment, and 62% had a partial response (PR), resulting in an overall response rate (ORR) of 67% (Fig. 14.4). Overall, 86% had no local disease progression at exit. There was a significant correlation between DT01 systemic exposure and efficacy (Le Tourneau et al. 2016).

In conclusion, this phase I trial demonstrates that local administration of AsiDNA in combination with RT is safe. It confirms the lack of radiosensitisation of healthy tissues and suggests a possible antitumor effect in patients with metastatic skin of melanoma.

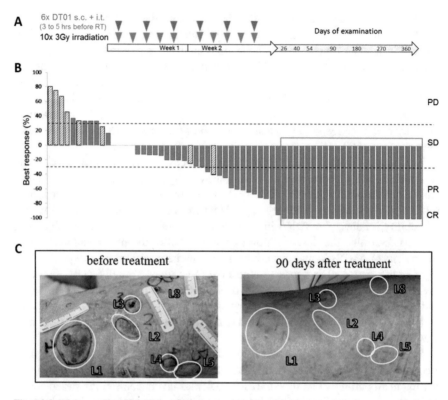

Fig. 14.4 Main results of DRIIM trial. Patients with skin melanoma metastasis were treated with radiotherapy and AsiDNA; (**a**) protocol of treatment: all patients received radiotherapy on the area of the metastasis and two tumors were treated by intratumoral and peripheric injection of AsiDNA at doses of 16, 32, 48, 64, 96 mg per cohort; (**b**) Waterfall plot of best overall response for 64 lesions according to modified RECIST; (**c**) Illustration of the complete response of a patient from the cohort treated with 48 mg AsiDNA, photographs of the irradiated area were taken before begining of treatment and 90 days later. No recurrence was observed during the survey time

14.9 Perspectives

Inhibition of DSB DNA repair pathways seem to be a promising approach to treat tumors that have developed resistance to conventional genotoxic treatment. The high specificity of the AsiDNA molecules for tumor cells is an interesting observation. Though the mechanism underlying this differential activity is still unclear, one can postulate that defects in the DNA damage response that accumulate during the evolution of a tumor may render the cancer cells dependent on their remaining DNA repair capacity for survival. The double burden of increasing damage with genotoxic agents and decreasing the repair capacity by AsiDNA could be sufficient to shift the surviving status of the tumour cells to death by mitotic catastrophe. Extensive studies are ongoing to identify the cell properties that protect healthy cells and allow some low grade tumors to be resistant to AsiDNA combinations.

References

Aly A, Ganesan S (2011) BRCA1, PARP, and 53BP1: conditional synthetic lethality and synthetic viability. J Mol Cell Biol 3(1):66–74

Anai H, Maehara Y, Sugimachi K (1988) In situ nick translation method reveals DNA strand scission in HeLa cells following heat treatment. Cancer Lett 40(1):33–38

Beck C, Robert I, Reina-San-Martin B, Schreiber V, Dantzer F (2014) Poly(ADP-ribose) polymerases in double-strand break repair: focus on PARP1, PARP2 and PARP3. Exp Cell Res 329(1):18–25

Begg AC, Stewart FA, Vens C (2011) Strategies to improve radiotherapy with targeted drugs. Nat Rev Cancer 11(4):239–253

Berthault N, Maury B, Agrario C et al (2011) Comparison of distribution and activity of nanoparticles with short interfering DNA (Dbait) in various living systems. Cancer Gene Ther 18(10):695–706

Bhardwaj N, Dormer J, Ahmad F et al (2012) Heat shock protein 70 expression following hepatic radiofrequency ablation is affected by adjacent vasculature. J Surg Res 173(2):249–257

Bianchi V, Pontis E, Reichard P (1986) Changes of deoxyribonucleoside triphosphate pools induced by hydroxyurea and their relation to DNA synthesis. J Biol Chem 261(34):16037–16042

Biau J, Devun F, Jdey W et al (2014) A preclinical study combining the DNA repair inhibitor Dbait with radiotherapy for the treatment of melanoma. Neoplasia 16(10):835–844

Braun J, Hahn GM (1975) Enhanced cell killing by bleomycin and 43 degrees hyperthermia and the inhibition of recovery from potentially lethal damage. Cancer Res 35(11 Pt 1):2921–2927

Caldecott KW (2008) Single-strand break repair and genetic disease. Nat Rev Genet 9(8):619–631

Chikamori K, Grozav AG, Kozuki T, Grabowski D, Ganapathi R, Ganapathi MK (2010) DNA topoisomerase II enzymes as molecular targets for cancer chemotherapy. Curr Cancer Drug Targets 10(7):758–771

Coquery N, Pannetier N, Farion R et al (2012) Distribution and radiosensitizing effect of cholesterol-coupled Dbait molecule in rat model of glioblastoma. PLoS One 7(7):e40567

Croset A, Cordelieres FP, Berthault N et al (2013) Inhibition of DNA damage repair by artificial activation of PARP with siDNA. Nucleic Acids Res 41(15):7344–7355

De Haas-Kock DF, Buijsen J, Pijls-Johannesma M et al (2009) Concomitant hyperthermia and radiation therapy for treating locally advanced rectal cancer. Cochrane Database Syst Rev 3:CD006269

Devun F, Bousquet G, Biau J et al (2012) Preclinical study of the DNA repair inhibitor Dbait in combination with chemotherapy in colorectal cancer. J Gastroenterol 47(3):266–275

Durocher D, Jackson SP (2001) DNA-PK, ATM and ATR as sensors of DNA damage: variations on a theme? Curr Opin Cell Biol 13(2):225–231

Fenech M (1993) The cytokinesis-block micronucleus technique and its application to genotoxicity studies in human populations. Environ Health Perspect 101(Suppl 3):101–107

Fortini P, Dogliotti E (2007) Base damage and single-strand break repair: mechanisms and functional significance of short- and long-patch repair subpathways. DNA Repair (Amst) 6(4):398–409

Franckena M, van der Zee J (2010) Use of combined radiation and hyperthermia for gynecological cancer. Curr Opin Obstet Gynecol 22(1):9–14

Hazan G, Lurie H, Yerushalmi A (1984) Sensitization of combined cis-platinum and cyclophosphamide by local hyperthermia in mice bearing the Lewis lung carcinoma. Oncology 41(1):68–69

Helleday T, Petermann E, Lundin C, Hodgson B, Sharma RA (2008) DNA repair pathways as targets for cancer therapy. Nat Rev Cancer 3(8):193–204

Herath NI, Devun F, Lienafa MC et al (2016) The DNA repair inhibitor DT01 as a novel therapeutic strategy for chemosensitization of colorectal liver metastasis. Mol Cancer Ther 15(1):15–22

Herath NI, Devun F, Herbette A et al (2017) Potentiation of doxorubicin efficacy in hepato-cellular carcinoma by the DNA repair inhibitor DT01 in preclinical models. Eur Radiol 27(10):4435–4444

Hill SA, Denekamp J (1979) The response of six mouse tumours to combined heat and X rays: implications for therapy. Br J Radiol 52(615):209–218

Hurwitz MD, Hansen JL, Prokopios-Davos S et al (2011) Hyperthermia combined with radiation for the treatment of locally advanced prostate cancer: long-term results from Dana-Farber Cancer Institute study 94-153. Cancer 117(3):510–516

Itoh T, Orba Y, Takei H et al (2002) Immunohistochemical detection of hepatocellular carcinoma in the setting of ongoing necrosis after radiofrequency ablation. Mod Pathol 15(2):110–115

Jadhav K, Gupta N, Ahmed MB (2011) Micronuclei: an essential biomarker in oral exfoliated cells for grading of oral squamous cell carcinoma. J Cytol 28(1):7–12

Jalal S, Earley JN, Turchi JJ (2011) DNA repair: from genome maintenance to biomarker and therapeutic target. Clin Cancer Res 17(22):6973–6984

Jdey W, Thierry S, Russo C et al (2017) Drug-driven synthetic lethality: bypassing tumor cell genetics with a combination of AsiDNA and PARP inhibitors. Clin Cancer Res 23(4):1001–1011

Kim C, Lee CW, Kovacic L, Shah A, Klasa R, Savage KJ (2010) Long-term survival in patients with metastatic melanoma treated with DTIC or temozolomide. Oncologist 15(7):765–771

Kirkwood JM, Bastholt L, Robert C et al (2012) Phase II, open-label, randomized trial of the MEK1/2 inhibitor selumetinib as monotherapy versus temozolomide in patients with advanced melanoma. Clin Cancer Res 18(2):555–567

Konefal JB, Emami B, Pilepich MV (1987) Malignant melanoma: analysis of dose fractionation in radiation therapy. Radiology 164(3):607–610

Krawczyk PM, Eppink B, Essers J et al (2011) Mild hyperthermia inhibits homologous recom-bination, induces BRCA2 degradation, and sensitizes cancer cells to poly (ADP-ribose) poly-merase-1 inhibition. Proc Natl Acad Sci U S A 108(24):9851–9856

Kuzminov A (2001) Single-strand interruptions in replicating chromosomes cause double-strand breaks. Proc Natl Acad Sci U S A 98(15):8241–8246

Le Tourneau C, Dreno B, Kirova Y et al (2016) First-in-human phase i study of the DNA-repair inhibitor DT101 in combination with radiotherapy in patients with skin metastases from mela-noma. Brit J Cancer 114:1199–1205

Lord CJ, Ashworth A (2012) The DNA damage response and cancer therapy. Nature 481(7381):287–294

Lundin C, Erixon K, Arnaudeau C et al (2002) Different roles for nonhomologous end joining and homologous recombination following replication arrest in mammalian cells. Mol Cell Biol 22(16):5869–5878

Moding EJ, Kastan MB, Kirsch DG (2013) Strategies for optimizing the response of cancer and normal tissues to radiation. Nat Rev Drug Discov 12(7):526–542

Oliver TG, Mercer KL, Sayles LC et al (2010) Chronic cisplatin treatment promotes enhanced dam-age repair and tumor progression in a mouse model of lung cancer. Genes Dev 24(8):837–852

Olivier KR, Schild SE, Morris CG, Brown PD, Markovic SN (2007) A higher radiotherapy dose is associated with more durable palliation and longer survival in patients with metastatic mela-noma. Cancer 110(8):1791–1795

Paques F, Haber JE (1999) Multiple pathways of recombination induced by double-strand breaks in Saccharomyces cerevisiae. Microbiol Mol Biol Rev 63(2):349–404

Peng G, Chun-Jen Lin C, Mo W et al (2014) Genome-wide transcriptome profiling of homologous recombination DNA repair. Nat Commun 5:3361

Quanz M, Chassoux D, Berthault N, Agrario C, Sun JS, Dutreix M (2009a) Hyperactivation of DNA-PK by double-strand break mimicking molecules disorganizes DNA damage response. PLoS One 4(7):e6298

Quanz M, Berthault N, Roulin C et al (2009b) Small-molecule drugs mimicking DNA damage: a new strategy for sensitizing tumors to radiotherapy. Clin Cancer Res 15(4):1308–1316

Rogakou EP, Boon C, Redon C, Bonner WM (1999) Megabase chromatin domains involved in DNA double-strand breaks in vivo. J Cell Biol 146(5):905–916

Schlegel A, Buhler C, Devun F et al (2012) Pharmacokinetics and toxicity in rats and monkeys of coDbait: a therapeutic double-stranded DNA oligonucleotide conjugated to cholesterol. Mol Ther Nucleic Acids 1:e33

Shaheen M, Allen C, Nickoloff JA, Hromas R (2011) Synthetic lethality: exploiting the addiction of cancer to DNA repair. Blood 117(23):6074–6082

Thoms J, Bristow RG (2010) DNA repair targeting and radiotherapy: a focus on the therapeutic ratio. Semin Radiat Oncol 20(4):217–222

Viallard C, Chezal JM, Mishellany F et al (2016) Targeting DNA repair by coDbait enhances melanoma targeted radionuclide therapy. Oncotarget 7(11):12927–12936

Warters RL, Henle KJDNA (1982) degradation in chinese hamster ovary cells after exposure to hyperthermia. Cancer Res 42(11):4427–4432

West SC (2003) Molecular views of recombination proteins and their control. Nat Rev Mol Cell Biol 4(6):435–445

Willers H, Azzoli CG, Santivasi WL, Xia F (2013) Basic mechanisms of therapeutic resistance to radiation and chemotherapy in lung cancer. Cancer J 19(3):200–207

Wong RS, Dynlacht JR, Cedervall B, Dewey WC (1995) Analysis by pulsed-field gel electrophoresis of DNA double-strand breaks induced by heat and/or X-irradiation in bulk and replicating DNA of CHO cells. Int J Radiat Biol 68(2):141–152

Wyman C, Kanaar R (2006) DNA double-strand break repair: all's well that ends well. Annu Rev Genet 40:363–383

Chapter 15
Alternative Non-homologous End-Joining: Mechanisms and Targeting Strategies in Cancer

Pratik Nagaria and Feyruz V. Rassool

Abstract Repair of DNA double-strand breaks (DSB)s is essential to the growth and survival of normal as well as cancer cells. Alteration of DSB repair properties in cancer cells can not only drive genomic instability, but also confer increased sensitivity to DSB-inducing agents. Development of agents that selectively inhibit DSB repair pathways will facilitate the design of therapeutic strategies that exploit the differences in DSB repair properties between normal and cancer cells. While mechanisms for classic non-homologous end joining (C-NHEJ) and Homologous recombination (HR) DSB repair pathways have been well studied in cancer, less is known about the alternative and highly error-prone, ALT-NHEJ pathway. Here, we discuss the mechanisms for ALT-NHEJ, alterations in this repair pathway in cancer, inhibition of ALT-NHEJ and future directions for cancer therapies that target this pathway.

Keywords Alternative non-homologous end-joining · Microhomology-mediated end joining · PARP1 · Double-strand break repair · Cancer therapeutics · Genomic instability

15.1 Introduction

Cells have evolved a complex network of pathways that function in response to DNA damage. DNA double-strand breaks (DSB)s are potentially lethal events caused by external agents, such as ionizing radiation (IR) or internally, when DNA

P. Nagaria
Department of Radiation Oncology and Marlene and Stewart Greenebaum Comprehensive Cancer Center, University of Maryland School of Medicine, Baltimore, MD, USA

BioReliance Corporation, A MilliporeSigma Company, Rockville, MD, USA

F. V. Rassool (✉)
Department of Radiation Oncology and Marlene and Stewart Greenebaum Comprehensive Cancer Center, University of Maryland School of Medicine, Baltimore, MD, USA
e-mail: frassool@som.umaryland.edu

© Springer International Publishing AG, part of Springer Nature 2018
J. Pollard, N. Curtin (eds.), *Targeting the DNA Damage Response for Anti-Cancer Therapy*, Cancer Drug Discovery and Development, https://doi.org/10.1007/978-3-319-75836-7_15

polymerases encounter an unrepaired nick in DNA. The cytotoxicity of these lesions results from the fact that they are very difficult to repair, as there is no template strand to guide the repair. If DSBs are incorrectly repaired, they can cause a wide range of genetic alterations, including large DNA deletions and gross chromosomal rearrangements that are a characteristic feature of cancer cells. Abnormalities in the DSB response, including defects in DSB repair, have been identified as the underlying cause of hereditary forms of breast cancer (Farmer et al. 2005). Since genomic instability is a common characteristic of both inherited and sporadic forms of cancer cells, it appears likely that abnormalities in the DNA damage and repair response also contribute to the development and progression of sporadic cancers (Rassool and Tomkinson 2010). In addition, oncogenes may also impact the repair and mutagenic consequences of DNA damage by altering the relative activities of DSB repair pathways that repair the same lesion, presumably by genetic and epigenetic mechanisms (Negrini et al. 2010). Given that cancer cells rely on altered regulation of DSBs for genomic instability and disease progression, these same pathways may be selectively targeted as a therapetic strategy. While mechanisms for HR and C-NHEJ are well known, far less is understood about ALT-NHEJ. This chapter will focus on the current mechanisms for ALT-NHEJ and prospects for targeting this pathway in therapeutic strategies in cancer.

15.2　DSB Repair

The repair of DSBs occurs via two mechanistically distinct pathways, HR and DNA dependent protein kinase (DNA-PKcs)-dependent NHEJ (also referred as classical or C-NHEJ) pathways. However, in the recent decade, studies indicate that NHEJ can also function in a DNA-PKcs-independent manner, which is particularly deleterious (Rassool and Tomkinson 2010). This alternative pathway, referred to as ALT-NHEJ, does not require DNA-PK or other C-NHEJ factors. The repair events mediated by ALT-NHEJ frequently involve large DNA deletions and often, but not always, involve short stretches of sequence homologies at the respective break-point junctions. Thus, this pathway is sometimes referred to as microhomology-mediated end-joining (MMEJ), and the extensive presence of microhomologous sequences can lead to significant increases in chromosomal abnormalities, including chromosomal translocations (Rassool and Tomkinson 2010).

15.2.1　Homologous Recombination

The predominant pathway that repairs replication-associated DSBs is characterized by the invasion of a single-strand DNA (ssDNA) into a homologous duplex (Arnaudeau et al. 2001; Khanna and Jackson 2001). This repair pathway, which is active in the late S and G2 phase of the cell cycle, utilizes the undamaged sister chromatid as the template for repair. Because the sister chromatid is identical in

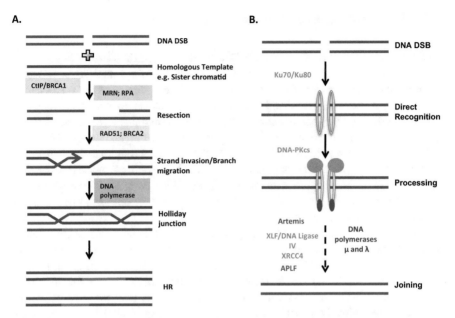

Fig. 15.1 Simplified model of HR and C-NHEJ. Error-free repair by homologous recombination (HR) pathway requires a homologous template (e.g. sister chromatid) for activation. DNA end-resection is the key initiating stage of HR. Faithful recombination requires coordination of several proteins and protein complexes (e.g. BRCA1, BRCA2, RAD51, MRN). Classical non-homologous end-joining (C-NHEJ), which is activated upon the recognition of DSB by binding of Ku70/Ku80 heterodimer protein complex, requires the activity of catalytic subunit of DNA protein-kinase (DNA-PKcs). C-NHEJ does not require DNA end-resection or a homologous template, and is thus error-prone

sequence to the damaged DNA strand, the repair reaction faithfully restores the genetic information of the damaged chromosome and is thus viewed as being error-free. HR is initiated by DNA end-resection in a $5'–3'$ manner that involves the human MRE11-RAD50-NBS1 (MRN) complex, and CtBP interacting protein (CtIP, encoded by the *RBBP8* gene), the endonuclease activity of which facilitates a DNA strand with $3'$-single-stranded overhangs (ssO's) (Yun and Hiom 2009; Sartori et al. 2007). The $3'$-overhang is rapidly bound by ssDNA-binding replication protein A (RPA), which is replaced by the DNA strand invasion of the RAD51-ssDNA complex on the template duplex DNA to search for homology, a process facilitated by BRCA2 interaction with RAD51 (Petalcorin et al. 2006) (Fig. 15.1a) (for further details on HR refer to Hartlerode and Scully (2009)).

Notably, many chemotherapeutic agents block DNA replication, leading to the stalling and/or collapse of replication forks and the generation of lesions that are repaired by HR (Keller et al. 2001; Saleh-Gohari et al. 2005). If the HR pathway is inactivated, for example through deletions or mutations of BRCA genes in hereditary breast cancer, there are back-up pathways that can repair DSBs. These pathways, which include ALT-NHEJ, are error-prone, generating deletions and chromosomal translocations (Rassool and Tomkinson 2010).

15.2.2 Non-homologous End-Joining

In the repair of DSBs by C-NHEJ, the DNA ends are brought together in a reaction that is independent of extensive DNA sequence homology and so is prone to introducing errors ranging from small insertions and deletions at the break site to the joining of previously unlinked DNA ends (Lieber 2008). In addition to repairing DSBs caused by endogenous and exogenous DNA damaging agents, the C-NHEJ proteins also participate in immunoglobulin gene rearrangements (Lieber et al. 2006). While the repair of DSBs by C-NHEJ occurs throughout the cell cycle, C-NHEJ is the major DSB repair pathway in G0, G1 and early S phase (Lieber et al. 2003). Most DSBs are rapidly repaired by C-NHEJ but there is a slower phase that reflects the repair of a subset of DSBs that are either more complex DSB lesions or occur in condensed chromatin.

The C-NHEJ pathway is initiated by the Ku70/Ku86 heterodimer, a ring shaped complex that binds to and encircles DNA ends (Fig. 15.1b) (Lieber et al. 2003). This serves to protect the DNA ends from degradation and to recruit the catalytic sub-unit of DNA-PK (DNA-PKcs) to form the activated DNA-PK holoenzyme (Gottlieb and Jackson 1993). The kinase activity of DNA-PK is critical for C-NHEJ with a key substrate being DNA-PKcs itself. The key step in C-NHEJ is the physical juxtaposition of DNA ends. This end-bridging occurs via interactions between DNA-bound DNA-PKcs molecules (Yaneva et al. 1997; DeFazio et al. 2002). If C-NHEJ is inactivated, end-resection of DSBs will allow for repair by either HR or other resection dependent pathways [i.e. single-strand annealing (SSA), synthesis-dependent strand annealing (SDSA)] or ALT-NHEJ, as discussed in the next section (Fig. 15.2).

15.3 Alternative Non-homologous End-Joining (ALT-NHEJ)

15.3.1 Identification

Historically, ALT-NHEJ was identified as a pathway that comes to the fore in somatic cells that are depleted of C-NHEJ activity. In S. Cerevisiae, analysis of DSB junctions from ku70 mutant strains demonstrated deletions of several hundred base pairs at DSB junctions, presenting the first evidence that an alternative end-joining mechanism in cells could be mutagenic in nature (Boulton and Jackson 1996a, b). This pathway was shown to function at lower efficiency (25- to 100-fold), compared with the C-NHEJ pathway. Moreover, it was observed that ku70 inhibited this alternative end-joining pathway (Critchlow and Jackson 1998). Further studies indicated widespread utilization of this alternative end-joining in DNA-PKcs, LIG4 or Ku70/80 deficient human and mouse cells (Lee et al. 1997; Gao et al. 1998; Wang et al. 2003, 2006). Additionally, in hamster cells, V(D)J recombination products demonstrated large deletions in terminal sequences when C-NHEJ was defective

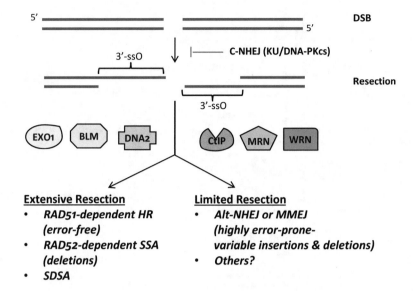

Fig. 15.2 DSB repair pathway choice driven by end-resection. DNA end-resection helicases and endonucleases (e.g. EXO1, BLM, DNA2, CtIP, MRN, WRN) regulate the switch between error-free and error-prone DSB repair pathways in normal non-tumorigenic cells and malignant tumorigenic cells. While extensive resection favors repair via HR, limited end-resection could expose microhomologies leading to mutagenic ALT-NHEJ mediated repair

(Pergola et al. 1993). When both HR and C-NHEJ activity were depleted by genetic depletion of Rad54 and Ku70 in the DT40 chicken B-cell line, cells displayed several fold greater levels of chromosomal aberrations and cell death (Takata et al. 1998). Notably, repair defects in C-NHEJ deficient backgrounds were not only characterized by large DNA deletions, but these abnormalities were often associated with short sequences of homology or microhomology (Kabotyanski et al. 1998; Roth and Wilson 1986; Feldmann et al. 2000).

While most of these early studies on ALT-NHEJ described it as a back-up mechanism for C-NHEJ, conclusions were often based on studies using extrachromosomal plasmid repair substrates (Wang et al. 2003; Verkaik et al. 2002). However, more recent studies using intra-chromosomally integrated plasmid reporters have demonstrated that ALT-NHEJ is functional in C-NHEJ proficient cells as well (Truong et al. 2013).

15.3.2 ALT-NHEJ Mechanism

While functional activities of ALT-NHEJ were identified in the absence of C-NHEJ, the protein players involved in this pathway had not been identified. Audebert et al. demonstrated that in the absence of DNA-PKcs/XRCC4/Ligase IV dependent

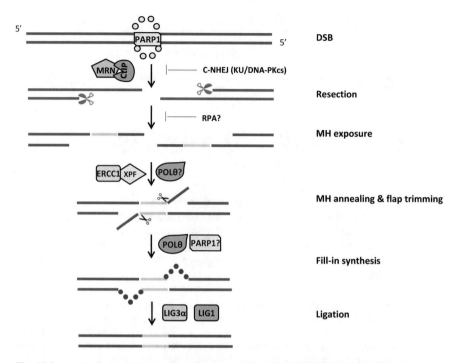

Fig. 15.3 Model of alternative non-homologous end-joining (ALT-NHEJ). ALT-NHEJ is initiated upon recognition and tethering of DSB ends by PARP1. Binding of PARP1 to DSBs displaces KU70/KU80 and vice-versa. Thus, C-NHEJ and ALT-NHEJ mechanisms are inhibitory with respect to each other. Next, DNA end-resection exposes microhomologous sequences, facilitating the error-prone annealing of breaks, polymerase-mediated fill-in synthesis and ligation. This series of reactions are postulated to occur via the coordinated activities of POLθ, ERCC1-XPF and LIG3α

NHEJ or C-NHEJ, cells utilized end-joining which required the synaptic activity of PARP1 and the ligation activity of the XRCC1-DNA LIG3α (LIG3) complex (Audebert et al. 2004), proteins that had heretofore been implicated in single-strand break repair (SSBR). Moreover, their studies and that of others suggested that ALT-NHEJ operates independently of the nature of DSB sequence (Audebert et al. 2008). Precise mechanisms through which ALT-NHEJ function are not well understood and are the subject of intense research. Nonetheless, studies in the last decade have identified key stages of ALT-NHEJ, which can be divided into four distinct steps discussed below (Fig. 15.3—**Schematic of ALT-NHEJ**).

15.3.2.1 DNA end Recognition and Tethering

The first step in ALT-NHEJ is the recognition and tethering of DSB ends. PARP1, which has a high affinity for binding to ssDNA nicks and blunt DS ends, plays a critical role in the tethering process (Menissier-de Murcia et al. 1989). Structural studies indicate that PARP1 uses specialized zinc-finger domains to sense and bind to DNA SSBs and DSBs, supporting the evidence of its DNA tethering functions in

ALT-NHEJ (Langelier and Pascal 2013). Moreover, by accounting for ~80% of the cell's total PARylation activity, PARP1 catalyzes the activation and recruitment of repair proteins, including the ligation complex XRCC1/LIG3 (Kim et al. 2005). The role of PARP1 in DSB repair was further supported by independent observations showing that Ku directly competes with PARP1 for binding to DSBs (Wang et al. 2006) and impedes PARP1's mobilization to damaged chromatin (Cheng et al. 2011). In addition, conditional expression of Ku in human fibrosarcoma cell lines also decreases PAR synthesis and ssDNA production in damaged chromatin (Cheng et al. 2011). Mansour et al. further demonstrated that depletion of PARP1, pharmacologically or genetically, abolished Ku-independent end-joining in cells (Mansour et al. 2010). These studies present strong evidence for PARP1 in tethering DSBs and initiating ALT-NHEJ.

15.3.2.2 Processing of DSBs

DNA end-resection as a decision point for the type of DSB repair—DNA end-resection is a critical early step that commits cells to the type of DSB repair. Typically, C-NHEJ machinery can work with high fidelity when the DSB ends are compatible or when small deletions of 1–4 bp form incompatible DSB ends (Guirouilh-Barbat et al. 2004). However, when DNA ends are truly incompatible (or lack 3′-OH/5′-P), additional processing is required. This processing reaction is known as end-resection, and is initiated by nucleolytic degradation of 5′-strands to yield 3′-single strand oligomers (ssO). ssO's also serve as substrates for strand invasion of RAD51 onto homologous duplex DNA during HR, highlighting this step as a critical juncture of DSB repair outcome. Interestingly, a recent study demonstrates that ssO's, by binding to Ku and preventing its assembly on dsDNA ends, inhibits C-NHEJ and promotes AL-NHEJ (Yuan et al. 2015). Moreover, when short sequence microhomologies are exposed following resection, cells may choose to complete ligation and repair via ALT-NHEJ (Yuan et al. 2015). Resection, thus represents a junction of regulatory switch between HR, C-NHEJ and alternative repair pathways [i.e. single-strand annealing (SSA), synthesis-dependent strand annealing (SDSA), reviewed in Mehta and Haber (2014)] and ALT-NHEJ. Roles of resection in dictating the DSB repair choice will be discussed in more detail below (Fig. 15.2).

Mechanism of DNA end-resection—Studies by Mimitou et al. suggest a two-step mechanism for DSB end-resection processing involving MRE11/RAD50/NBS1 (MRN) and C-terminal binding protein (CTBP) interacting protein (CtIP) (Mimitou and Symington 2008). CtIP promotes dsDNA-specific endonuclease activity by the Mre11 subunit and preferentially cleaves 5′-terminated dsDNA ends (Mimitou and Symington 2008). Depletion of CtIP leads to decreased ALT-NHEJ activity (Yun and Hiom 2009; Bennardo et al. 2008), and pharmacological depletion of MRE11 decreases intra-chromosomal end-joining as well as end-resection in both C-NHEJ competent XRCC4-wild-type (WT) and -deficient cells (Xie et al. 2009).

In the first step of end-resection, MRN and CtIP remove small oligonucleotides from the DNA ends to form an early DNA strand intermediate (Mimitou and

Symington 2008). Small base pair sequences are processed (~20 bp in mammalian cells) in this initial resection step, making ends available for ALT-NHEJ. Using HR and MMEJ competitive reporter substrates, it was demonstrated that the initial short end-resection step is shared between HR and ALT-NHEJ pathways. In fact, ALT-NHEJ accounts for 10–20% of total DSB repair activity when both pathways are intact (Truong et al. 2013).

In the second step of end-resection, MRE11 nuclease activity promotes the retention of exonuclease 1 (EXO1), and several DNA helicases and exonucleases (i.e. DNA2, BLM, WRN, CtIP and EXO1) at the DSB end, which co-operate to generate extensive tracts of single-stranded DNA that serve as excellent substrates for either HR or SSA (Truong et al. 2013; Krasner et al. 2015; Sturzenegger et al. 2014). Interestingly, longer ssDNA overhangs favor RPA binding and further resection (Krasner et al. 2015). RPA also competes with Ku in binding DNA ends and influences the timing and efficiency of resection (Chen et al. 2013). RPA also protects these ssOs from nucleolytic cleavage. Additionally, RPA facilitates DNA2 recruitment by direct interaction and promotes extensive resection *in vivo*, channeling repair towards ALT-NHEJ (Chen et al. 2013). However, it is still unclear how cells limit mutagenic ALT-NHEJ upon generation of resected ends, or how cells mediate the decision of repair pathway utilization for annealing the resected ends. Deng et al. recently demonstrated that RPA may have an essential function in channeling the resected ends to HR instead of ALT-NHEJ (Deng et al. 2014a, b). Mutations in *rfa1*, the yeast homolog of human RPA, not only leads to a reduced ability to interact with ssDNA molecules but also causes greater than 100-fold increase in ALT-NHEJ. Biochemically, the mutant *rfa* complexes were defective in SSA and also failed to remove ssDNA structures (Deng et al. 2014a, b). These findings present strong evidence that RPA either has a direct or indirect role in suppressing intermolecular annealing reactions at microhomologies and thus suppress ALT-NHEJ by channeling reactions towards HR.

DSB end-resection, processing and cell cycle—CtIP is activated in a cell cycle phase specific manner. Activation of CtIP's role in DSB processing requires phosphorylation, which is mediated by multiple kinases including ATM, ATR and cyclin dependent kinases (CDKs) (Wang et al. 2013; Peterson et al. 2013). Phosphorylation-mediated activation mainly occurs in S/G2 cell-cycle phase. Nonphosphorylated CtIP mutants fail in initiating DSB resection and processing. Independent studies by Wang et al. and Peterson et al. suggest that T859 phosphorylation in CtIP is essential for its activity in resection and DSB repair (Wang et al. 2013; Peterson et al. 2013).

In contrast, Polo-like kinase 3 (PLK3) phosphorylate CtIP in the G1 phase of the cell cycle in a damage-inducible fashion. Phosphorylation of serine at position 327 of the CtIP protein activates end-resection in G1 phase, and can promote complex rearrangements resulting from ALT-NHEJ (Barton et al. 2014). Moreover, studies with recombinant CtIP found that there are 36 phosphorylation sites on CtIP and besides the nuclease activity that promotes resection, CtIP also has 5'-flap endonuclease activity which is essential in promoting activities in DSB processing (Makharashvili et al. 2014).

15.3.2.3 Annealing at Microhomologies and Polymerase-Mediated Fill-In Synthesis

Annealing of microhomologous DNA sequences—The next step in ALT-NHEJ is annealing of complementary microhomologous DNA sequences and polymerase-mediated fill-in synthesis. The exact mechanisms through which complementary base pairing occurs in ALT-NHEJ are still not understood, but RPA binding to ssOs represents a critical juncture inhibiting the annealing of complementary base pairs *in vitro* (Deng et al. 2014b). An alternative mechanism available for annealing the resected DSB is single-strand annealing (SSA). This mechanism requires the exposure of long tracts of repeat sequences, which are derived from extensive resection. Rad52 is a key protein implicated in SSA (New et al. 1998), but does not appear to be required for ALT-NHEJ (Deng et al. 2014b).

Fill-in synthesis—*In vitro* and *in vivo* evidence has recently implicated polymerase theta (POLθ, encoded by the *POLQ* gene) in facilitating fill-in synthesis during ALT-NHEJ (Kent et al. 2015; Ceccaldi et al. 2015; Mateos-Gomez et al. 2015). POLθ was initially described as an open reading frame in humans with homology to *E. coli* DNA polymerase I (Sharief et al. 1999), and subsequent studies demonstrated its polymerase activity (Seki et al. 2003). Interestingly, POLθ can function in a template-independent mechanism, supporting efficient extension of ssDNA as well as dsDNA (Hogg et al. 2012). Ceccaldi et al. demonstrated that POLθ interacts with RAD51 and inhibits HR by limiting RAD51 accumulation at resected DNA ends. Notably, POLθ-mediated ALT-NHEJ is required to promote the survival of cells with a compromised HR repair pathway. Consistent with this, while mice with loss of *Polq* alone are viable, loss of HR and *Polq* leads to embryonic lethality (Ceccaldi et al. 2015). These results suggest that ALT-NHEJ may provide a critical outlet that promotes cell survival in HR deficient cancer cells. POLθ's ability to perform these essential functions can be attributed to its unique structure. For example, the DNA-dependent ATPase domain in POLθ suppresses the RAD51-ssDNA nucleofilament assembly (Ceccaldi et al. 2015; Seki et al. 2003). The polymerase domain of POLθ contains a conserved loop domain, known as insertion loop 2, which is essential for extending resected ends using the opposing overhang as a template (Kent et al. 2015). These studies support a critical role of POLθ in ALT-NHEJ, especially for resected DNA containing 2–6 bp of microhomology. Besides ALT-NHEJ, POLθ is also implicated in low-fidelity DNA synthesis (Seki et al. 2004), 5'-dRP lyase activity similar to Polβ in BER (Prasad et al. 2009).

15.3.2.4 Ligation of DSBs in ALT-NHEJ

The functions of LIGIV (LIG4) in C-NHEJ are well documented (Rassool and Tomkinson 2010). Besides LIG4, the only other known mammalian ligases are LIGI (LIG1) and LIGIII (LIG3) (Tomkinson and Levin 1997). LIG1 is the major ligase activity in proliferating cells and has an essential role in base excision repair (BER) as part of the multi-protein complex, which includes XRCC1.

However, in the absence of LIG1, LIG3α provides backup function and is essential during DNA replication and BER. In contrast, joining of DNA ends in ALT-NHEJ is facilitated by LIG3α, while LIG1 provides a backup function (Simsek et al. 2011a; Soni et al. 2014). Thus, there are redundancies in the functions of LIG1 and LIG3α. Whether the role of LIG3 is essential in ALT-NHEJ is unclear. While both LIG1 and LIG3 deficiency cause cell lethality, the mitochondrial isoform of LIG3α, but not the nuclear isoform, is essential for cell viability (Simsek et al. 2011b). Moreover, LIG1 can efficiently backup LIG3α functions in all nuclear processes including DNA repair (Oh et al. 2014). Structural studies have provided more insights into the mechanism by which LIG3α maintains a robust intermolecular DNA end joining activity. These activities are dependent upon the unique Zn-finger domain and DNA-binding domain of LIG3α (Simsek et al. 2011b; Cotner-Gohara et al. 2008, 2010).

Until recently, the consensus in the literature from biochemical as well as biological studies indicated that XRCC1 works as a scaffold protein that guides LIG3α to the nuclei and co-ordinates the association of DNA repair protein complex (Ellenberger and Tomkinson 2008). However, recent studies suggest that XRCC1 functions are dispensable in ALT-NHEJ (Soni et al. 2014; Zha et al. 2011). Interestingly, PARP1 also performs a key function in the multi-protein ligation complex. Both XRCC1 and LIG3α can interact with PAR(ylated) PARP1 *in vitro*, which guides its recruitment to the sites of DNA damage (Masson et al. 1998). LIG3α and XRCC1 also demonstrate increased association with MRN, particularly in context of DNA damage in C-NHEJ deficit conditions (Della-Maria et al. 2011). Thus, these multi-protein interactions drive joining of resected products in ALT-NHEJ.

15.4 Pathological Consequences of DSB Repair by ALT-NHEJ

A significant number of studies implicate ALT-NHEJ in a highly mutagenic pathway, leading to an increased frequency of cancers. Absence of LIG4 in human cell lines substantially decreases the fidelity of end-joining repair *in vivo* (Smith et al. 2003). Haploinsufficiency of *Lig4* in mice leads to increased transformation of non-lymphoid tissues and cultured fibroblasts and sensitizes these cells to DNA damage (Sharpless et al. 2001). Furthermore, mice lacking both p53 and C-NHEJ components *DNA-PKcs* (Guidos et al. 1996; Nacht et al. 1996), *Ku80* (Difilippantonio et al. 2000; Lim et al. 2000), *Xrcc4* (Gao et al. 2000), or *Lig4* (Frank et al. 2000), succumb in early postnatal life to progenitor B-cell lymphomas with IgH-Myc translocations and amplifications.

Notably, there is also evidence that the steady state levels of key factors in C-NHEJ are frequently reduced in cancer cell lines (Sharpless et al. 2001; Sallmyr et al. 2008; Tobin et al. 2012, 2013). In chronic myeloid leukemia (CML), classical end-joining factors, Artemis and LIG4 are downregulated, whereas expression of

WRN and LIG3 are upregulated (Sallmyr et al. 2008). These expression changes drive genomic instability through increased utilization of ALT-NHEJ in cancer cells (Sallmyr et al. 2008). LIG4 is also reduced in colon, cervical and breast cancer cell lines (Chen et al. 2008). Compared to normal cell counterparts, repair activity from cellular extracts of bladder cancers and urothelial carcinoma cell lines show an extensive use of microhomologies in repair of DSBs (Bentley et al. 2004; Windhofer et al. 2008). Importantly, knockdown of LIG3α reduces DSB repair by NHEJ in CML but not normal myeloid cells (Sallmyr et al. 2008). Simsek et al. (2010) demonstrated that *Xrcc4/Lig4* suppresses translocation events in mice. Moreover, in their studies, translocation breakpoint junctions from expression of DSB-inducing *I-SceI* endonuclease displayed similar characteristics in wild-type and Xrcc4/Lig4-deficient mouse cells, including a similar bias to microhomology use, indicating ALT-NHEJ is the primary mediator of translocation formation in murine cells (Simsek and Jasin 2010). Together these studies suggest that ALT-NHEJ is upregulated in a variety of cancers and is likely to contribute to the deletions and translocations that drive cancer progression and is a potential therapeutic target.

While repair by ALT-NHEJ is implicated in development of genetic instability in cancer, the role of C-NHEJ in this process has been reexamined. Analysis of endonuclease-induced DSB junctions in human cells showed lower microhomology usage in translocations with decreasing frequency in absence of LIG4 (Ghezraoui et al. 2014). Another study that utilized inducible systems to generate experimental inter-chromosomal translocations in human stem cells, observed a low frequency of ALT-NHEJ (Brunet et al. 2009). Next-generation sequencing analyses of human cancer patients showed that balanced chromosomal translocations frequently involve sequence from multiple chromosomes and that only a few of these breakpoint junctions showed microhomologies (Chiang et al. 2012). These studies suggest that C-NHEJ repair may play a more profound role in generating chromosome translocations than previously anticipated.

15.5   ALT-NHEJ as a Novel Targeted Therapeutic Strategy in Cancers

As discussed above, ALT-NHEJ represents a prime target for chemo- and radiosensitization in particular in cancer cells that demonstrate deficiencies in classical DSB repair pathways i.e. HR and C-NHEJ (Fig. 15.4—**Positive and Negative Regulators of ALT-NHEJ**). Interestingly, several factors required for basic function of ALT-NHEJ, such as PARP1, XRCC1, LIG3α, were originally identified as components of BER. Moreover, drugs targeting these pathways, their pharmacodynamics and pharmacokinetics have either been tested pre-clinically or are currently under evaluation.

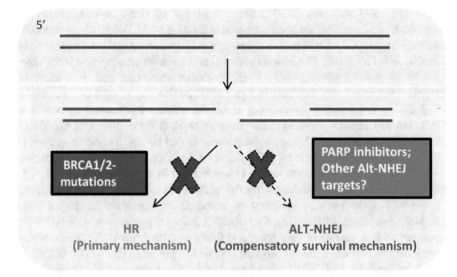

Fig. 15.4 ALT-NHEJ targets for inducing synthetic lethality. DSB repair pathways (C-NHEJ, ALT-NHEJ, SSA) serve as backup mechanisms in HR-deficient cancer cells exposed to genotoxic insults, such as chemotherapy. Recent studies highlight the possibility that these back-up mechanisms esp. ALT-NHEJ serve as a compensatory survival mechanism. Thus, co-inhibition of ALT-NHEJ in HR-deficient cancers, e.g. using PARP inhibitors, POLθ or LIG3α inhibitors etc. represents a novel strategy to induce synthetic lethality in these cells

In this next section, we will discuss potential targets of ALT-NHEJ for cancer therapy. We will also discuss strategies that may lead to further therapeutic opportunities in combination with other therapies.

15.5.1 PARP Inhibitors (PARPis)

PARP1 is historically known as a DNA nick sensor, and through this it appears to function in the surveillance of overall DDR that includes recognition of SSBs and coordination of BER, and regulating choices between HR, C-NHEJ and ALT-NHEJ. Therefore, it is not surprising that PARPs are considered as prime therapeutic targets in cancers exhibiting DNA repair abnormalities.

PARPis are particularly effective against BRCA1- and BRCA2-defective tumors by inducing synthetic lethality in these cells. The mechanisms of PARP inhibitor action involve the following: (1) Disrupting SSB repair and inducing the formation of stalled replication forks, which require adequate DSB repair processes (Hochegger et al. 2006; Sugimura et al. 2008). (2) In conditions of HR deficiency, inhibition of PARP1 induces activation of DNA-PKcs-dependent NHEJ, leading to formation of non-viable errors and cell death (Patel et al. 2011; De Lorenzo et al. 2013). (3) Trapping of PARP1 at SSB repair intermediates formed during BER (Murai et al. 2012).

Trapped PARP1 protein provides hindrance to access by proteins involved in BER. Moreover, multiple repair pathways recognize trapped PARP1-DNA structures including Fanconi Anemia (FA), SSA, HR, NHEJ, SDSA (Murai et al. 2012, 2013). Hence, PARP1 inhibitors are proposed to be promising targets in cancers with DNA repair abnormalities involving these pathways as well and would be candidates for a BRCAness phenotype, which describes features in certain sporadic tumors that are similar to *BRCA1/BRCA2* mutant tumors e.g. HR deficiencies (Lupo and Trusolino 2014).

Pre-clinically, PARPis show a degree of cytotoxicity as a mono-therapy agent against human and murine cancer cell lines *in vitro* and *in vivo*. In combination therapies, PARP inhibitors appear to potentiate synergistically or additively the toxic effects of several drugs utilized in standard chemotherapy regimen including temozolomide (Plummer et al. 2013), DNA intercalating agents (e.g. cisplatin) (Michels et al. 2014), topoisomerase inhibitors (Sonnenblick et al. 2015; Znojek et al. 2014) and even epigenetic therapies (Orta et al. 2014).

Clinically, PARPis have been found to be relatively non-toxic in normal cells when compared to traditional chemotherapeutics. PARPis are particularly effective when administered to BRCA-deficient cells (Sonnenblick et al. 2015), forming the premise of synthetic lethality of HR deficient cancers to PARP inhibitors. A synthetic lethality model predicts that combined depletion of BRCA1 or BRCA2 concomitantly with PARP in combination is toxic to the cells whereas loss of the single gene is not. Indeed, both pre-clinical and clinical data in BRCA-*mut* breast and ovarian cancers have provided widespread evidence of the effectiveness of this approach. Of note, Olaparib is the first PARP inhibitor approved first by European Medicines Agency (EMA) and then by U.S. Food and Drug Administration (FDA) for patients with advanced ovarian cancer with germline mutation in *BRCA* (Kim et al. 2015). In one of the early clinical Phase II trials, olaparib showed encouraging results with more than 18 months of disease free survival in metastatic BRCA1 or BRCA2 mutated breast cancers (Fong et al. 2009). Olaparib showed an overall response period of 8 months in hereditary BRCA negative ovarian cancer. In 2014, Olaparib was the first PARP inhibitor to receive FDA approval for germline BRCA mutated ovarian cancers that have received prior chemotherapy. There are now three PARPi approved by the FDA, all for ovarian cancer second line/maintenance therapy: olaparib (Lynparza), rucaparib (Rubraca) and niraparib (Zejula).

More recently, the development of ultra-potent PARPis, such as talazoparib has renergized the PARPi therapy landscape (Shen et al. 2013). Talazoparib traps PARP in chromatin in the low nanomolar range, which correlates with its cytotoxic effects. Increased binding of unmodified PARP1 to chromatin, which could very well be the premise of PARP trapping, was first demonstrated by Satoh and Lindahl (1992). Upon modification via auto PARylation (poly ADP-ribosylation), increased negative charge on PARP1 increases its dissociation from DNA, leading to increased accessibility of the repair factors. Murai et al. demonstrated that talazoparib shows significantly higher efficacy at trapping PARP1 in chromatin in comparison to Veliparib and Olaparib, implying that PARP trapping is a primary mechanism driving PARP inhibitor lethality (Murai et al. 2012, 2013; Shen et al. 2015). Clinical studies are currently ongoing and results will determine whether PARP entrapment on damaged chromatin increases its therapeutic efficacy in patients with breast and ovarian cancer.

15.5.2 LIG3 Inhibitors in Combination with PARPis

Tobin et al. demonstrated that relative to a non-tumorigenic breast epithelial cell line, MCF10a, breast cancer cell lines that include tamoxifen- and aromatase-resistant derivatives of MCF7 and triple-negative breast cancer cells have higher steady-state levels of LIG3 and PARP1, concomitant with reduced steady-state levels of DNA LIG4 (Tobin et al. 2012). This results in increased dependence upon ALT-NHEJ to repair DSBs and the accumulation of chromosomal deletions. Moreover, biopsies from hormone insensitive tumors also showed elevated levels of ALT-NHEJ (Tobin et al. 2012). Importantly, cell lines exhibiting increased ALT-NHEJ also showed significantly higher sensitivity to a combination of PARP and DNA ligase III inhibitors. In findings similar to those in breast cancers, albeit in a completely different cancer model, Sallmyr et al. reported that chronic myeloid leukemia (CML) cell lines expressing constitutively active tyrosine kinase (TK) fusion protein BCR-ABL1 utilize ALT-NHEJ to repair DSBs (Sallmyr et al. 2008). Of note, these cells are driven by increased expression of DNA LIG3α and the end-resection nuclease implicated in Werner Syndrome (WRN). BCR-ABL1 cells are also driven by a significant increase in reactive oxygen species (ROS) and ROS-induced DSB formation. Inhibition of ALT-NHEJ activity by siRNA-knockdown of DNA LIG3α or WRN, leads to increased accumulation of unrepaired DSBs indicating that BCR-ABL1 driven CML may utilize ALT-NHEJ as a survival mechanism and ALT-NHEJ presents a novel therapeutic target (Sallmyr et al. 2008). Following up, Tobin et al. demonstrated that the range of CML cells that could benefit from inhibition of ALT-NHEJ includes TK inhibitor (TKI)-resistant CML, which particularly show an increase in PARP1 and LIG3 (Tobin et al. 2013). Incubation of these cell lines with a combination of DNA ligase and PARP inhibitors inhibited ALT-NHEJ and selectively decreased survival with the effect being greater in the TKI-resistant derivative. Importantly, analysis of clinical samples from CML patients confirmed that the expression levels of PARP1 and DNA LIG3α correlated with the sensitivity to the DNA repair inhibitor combination. Overall, these studies show that the sensitivity of breast cancer and leukemia cell lines to a combination of DNA ligase and PARP inhibitors correlates with the steady state levels of PARP1 and DNA LIG3α, and ALT-NHEJ activity. Importantly, these studies demonstrate that increased ALT-NHEJ could represent a novel biomarker for expansion of PARP-targeted therapeutics and that the strategy of targeting ALT-NHEJ may also be applicable to a wide range of solid tumors. Furthermore, targeting PARP1-driven DSB repair in BRCA-deficient tumors may extend the synthetic lethality paradigm to include alterations in ALT-NHEJ (Figs. 15.4 and 15.5).

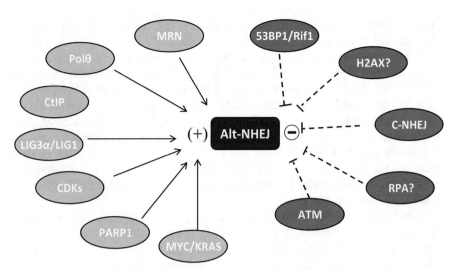

Fig. 15.5 Positive and Negative Regulators of ALT-NHEJ. Regulators of ALT-NHEJ that are potential therapeutic targets

15.5.3 POLQ (POLθ)

As discussed above, POLθ plays an essential role in gap filling during ALT-NHEJ and while mice lacking POLθ are viable, they show an increased level of micronuclei in red blood cells in response to oxidative stress and ionizing radiation (Shima et al. 2004; Goff et al. 2009). Bone marrow stromal cells from the *Polq−/−* mice, and *Polq*-null mouse cell lines are hypersensitive to IR and other DSB-inducing agents (Goff et al. 2009; Li et al. 2011). Additionally, depletion of POLθ in HeLa cells also sensitized the cells to γ-irradiation (Higgins et al. 2010a). Double knockout of DNA damage response gene *Atm* and *Polq^chaos1* in mice led to a synergistic increase in chromosomal instability (Shima et al. 2004). ATM kinase is recruited to DSBs by the MRN complex and begins a signaling cascade to facilitate HR and its functions are also implicated in other DSB repair mechanisms. In their study, Shima et al. show that pharmacological inhibition of ATM increases IR-sensitivity in wild-type but not in *Polq−/−* cells, indicating overlapping functions. Loss of both *Atm* and *Polq^chaos1* was semi-lethal and the surviving mice suffered from growth retardation. These observations indicate that at least in mice, *Polq* has a role recognizing the DSBs and attempting to repair it, that complements the recombination machinery regulated by ATM. Recent studies have presented significant evidence that POLθ participates in ALT-NHEJ and cells utilize this as a survival mechanism when subjected to genotoxic stresses or under HR deficiency (Kent et al. 2015; Mateos-Gomez et al. 2015). Using *in vitro* biochemical studies, Kent et al. showed that the polymerase domain of POLθ is critical in processing breaks via MMEJ. Further, following annealing POLθ uses the opposing overhang as a template to stabilize the DNA synapse and displaces annealed ssDNA during template extension (Kent et al. 2015). Yousefzadeh et al. showed that

Polq-null murine cells are selectively hypersensitive to DNA strand breaking agents, and presented evidence that damage resistance requires the DNA polymerase activity of POLθ (Yousefzadeh et al. 2014). An independent study also recently presented strong evidence supporting POLθ function in ALT-NHEJ. Authors demonstrate that loss of POLθ leads to significant increase in translocations involving CRISPR/Cas9 induced DSBs and that POLθ-mediated EJ is utilized heavily at deprotected telomeres, which could have consequences in genomic instability (Mateos-Gomez et al. 2015). In addition, it was found that loss of *Polq* in mice results in increased rates of HR, as indicated by accumulation of RAD51 at DSBs. Moreover, depletion of *Polq* decreased the colony formation capacity of BRCA-deficient cells. Interestingly, the authors also show that PARP1 facilitates the recruitment of POLQ to DSBs (γH2AX) (Mateos-Gomez et al. 2015).

Data presented by Fernandez-Vidal et al. suggest that POLθ has a role in replication origin firing (Fernandez-Vidal et al. 2014). The authors demonstrate that POLθ binds to chromatin during early G1, and interacts with the Orc2 and Orc4, which are components of the replication origin recognition complex. Although POLθ-depleted cells exhibit a normal density of activated origins in S phase, irregular shifts in replication origin firing are observed at a number of replication domains. POLθ over-expression, on the other hand, causes delayed replication (Fernandez-Vidal et al. 2014). Interestingly, oncogenes such as MYC are also closely involved in DNA replication and genomic stress associated with replication (Herold et al. 2009). Consistent with this, results from a study conducted in colorectal cancer suggest that overexpression of POLθ is more strongly associated with poor patient survival when replication and origin firing factors are upregulated (Pillaire et al. 2010). These results imply that POLθ-mediated repair is indeed utilized during DNA replication when DNA damage levels are high, as is often found in many cancers or when tumors are subjected to chemo or radiotherapy. Overall, studies above suggest that combined DNA repair-dependent and independent functions of POLθ in make it a viable target in cancers.

Biological expression of POLθ in very low in normal tissues and is limited to embryonic cell, testis, and lymphoid tissues, where it is implicated in Class Switch Recombination (CSR) (Shima et al. 2004). However, POLQ is often overexpressed in several cancers including breast, lung and oral cancers (Higgins et al. 2010b; Lemee et al. 2010; Kawamura et al. 2004). Moreover, triple negative breast cancer tumors, which often exhibit several DNA repair abnormalities (Tobin et al. 2012), are most frequently associated with high POLθ levels, accompanied by DNA damage, checkpoint activation and genetic instability (Lemee et al. 2010). Additionally, POLQ overexpression has been linked to a poorer clinical outcome compared with tumors that expressed low POLQ levels (Kawamura et al. 2004).

Based on the presented evidence, it appears that POLθ-targeted therapy could be beneficial in cancers exhibiting high ALT-NHEJ (Fig. 15.4), however more studies in human cells that distinguish its function in DNA replication, error-prone DSB repair and cancer progression would be needed to support this proposition. Regardless, POLθ could be a useful biomarker for PARP-inhibitor response, and is a potential therapeutic target for overcoming resistance to these drugs (Ceccaldi et al. 2015; Mateos-Gomez et al. 2015).

15.5.4 Oncogenic Modulators of ALT-NHEJ

Recent studies demonstrate that oncogenes such as KRAS or MYC may mediate ALT-NHEJ directly or indirectly. Muvarak et al. (2015) demonstrated that the oncogene MYC plays a key role in transcriptional activation of LIG3 and PARP1, contributing to the increased ALT-NHEJ activity in TK-activated leukemia. Notably, MYC's effect on ALT-NHEJ are not only transcriptional but also post-transcriptional, through negative regulation of miRNAs (miR-150 and miR-22). Inhibition of MYC and overexpression of miR-150 and -22 decreased ALT-NHEJ activity and the expression patterns were correlated in human patient samples of CML (Muvarak et al. 2015). Interestingly, the role of MYC in driving defects in DSB repair has been demonstrated previously (Karlsson et al. 2003). Overexpression of MYC in MEFs disrupts the repair of DSBs, both by HR and C-NHEJ, resulting in a several-magnitude increase in chromosomal breaks and translocations. Moreover, expression of MYC promotes cell growth and DNA replication even in the presence of limiting growth factors (Eilers et al. 1991). Also, MYC can induce reactive oxygen species (ROS) and DNA damage in normal and cancer cells, accelerating tumor progression (Vafa et al. 2002). Despite significant effects of MYC expression on DDR, activation of MYC induces cyclin E-CDK2 and E2F1 activity thereby promoting DNA replication (Vlach et al. 1996). MYC is thus linked to promoting DNA replication under genotoxic stress, a mechanism that is implicated in aiding MYC-induced tumorigenesis. In an independent study in T-cell acute lymphoblastic leukemia (T-ALL), Hahnel et al. demonstrate that activating K-RAS mutations in cancers is associated with increased expression of XRCC1, LIG3 and PARP1 and concomitant increase in ALT-NHEJ activity (Hahnel et al. 2014). The authors demonstrate that KRAS-mutated cells, which activate its oncogenic activities, rely on the ALT-NHEJ repair pathway for cell survival upon genotoxic stress. Depletion of LIG3 abolishes the resistance of T-ALL cells to apoptotic cell death (Hahnel et al. 2014). The above results indicate that MYC and K-RAS oncogene-driven cancers rely on ALT-NHEJ for survival by direct or indirect mechanisms (Fig. 15.5).

Targets of oncogenic modulators such as cell-cycle proteins have presented problems in drug development because of lack of specificity. However, we propose that inhibitors of ALT-NHEJ, such as PARPis, could be a useful strategy in cancers with activation of MYC or K-RAS (Table 15.1).

15.6 ALT-NHEJ as a Negative Consequence of DNA Repair Inhibitor Therapy?

As discussed earlier, ALT-NHEJ is a highly mutagenic DSB repair pathway associated with genomic instability and cancer progression (Rassool and Tomkinson 2010). Some studies suggest that inhibition of ATM, the predominant kinase responsible for the activation of multiple cell cycle checkpoints following DSB induction, can lead to increased ALT-NHEJ and genomic instability, as a secondary

Table 15.1 MYC-driven cancers that could potentially benefit from ALT-NHEJ targeted therapy

Cancer	MYC status	References
Breast cancer	Amplification (20–50% total; 80–90% ductal and TNBC)	Berns et al. (1992a, b); Harada et al. (1994); Horiuchi et al. (2012)
Ovarian cancer	Amplification (30–50%)	Chen et al. (2005); Baker et al. (1990)
Lung cancer	Amplification; C-MYC, L-MYC and MYCN	Little et al. (1983); Mitani et al. (2001)
Thyroid cancer	Overexpression; MYCN	Boultwood et al. (1988); Roncalli et al. (1994)
Prostate cancer	Amplification (20–60%)	Jenkins et al. (1997); Fleming et al. (1986); Varambally et al. (2005)
Colon cancer	Amplification (~30%)	Kozma et al. (1994); Augenlicht et al. (1997)
Liver cancer	Amplification (20–50%)	Takahashi et al. (2007)
Leukemia/lymphoma	Amplification	Nesbit et al. (1999); Thomas et al. (2004)

and unintended consequence (Bennardo and Stark 2010; Gunn et al. 2011). ATM-deficient cells are exquisitely sensitive to ionizing radiation and therefore inhibitors of ATM should potentiate the cytotoxicity of ionizing radiation and chemotherapeutic drugs that cause DSBs.

A potential problem with using ATM inhibitors as cancer therapeutics is that they may also sensitize normal tissues to DNA damage. In this scenario, the inhibitor of the DNA damage response will not preferentially enhance killing of the cancer cell and so there will be no therapeutic gain. Since cancer cells are presumed to have abnormalities in the DNA damage response, a subset of cancers with a particular DNA repair abnormality may be uniquely sensitive to ATM inhibition. Interestingly, Bennardo et al. report that ATM suppresses chromosomal rearrangements by limiting the incorrect end utilization during EJ between DSB repeats in an intra-chromosomal reporter. EJ caused by ATM disruption is ALT-NHEJ-like and is dependent on C-NHEJ factors, specifically DNA-PKcs, XRCC4, and XLF (Bennardo and Stark 2010). Thus, the authors postulate that a therapeutic strategy of ATM inhibition may also disrupt faithful end utilization in non-tumor cells, which could lead to therapy-related secondary malignancies. Conversely, ATM/DNA-PKcs inhibition could also make cells more dependent on PARP-dependent ALT-NHEJ for survival and more amenable to ALT-NHEJ therapy. Additionally, ATM/DNA-PKcs inhibitors in combination with POLQ inhibitors may be an attractive therapeutic strategy in tumors that over express POLQ and exhibit increased ALT-NHEJ activity.

15.7 Conclusions and Future Directions

Here, we have discussed the latest concepts of ALT-NHEJ pathway and how it functions in the context of other DSB repair pathways in normal and cancer cells. While upregulation of this highly mutagenic pathway was initially observed in cells deficient in C-NHEJ, ALT-NHEJ activity is also expressed in normal cells and increased in cancer cells, in particular those resistant to therapy. Moreover, ALT-NHEJ is closely associated with the generation of genomic changes that are the drivers of disease progression. Cancer cells with DNA repair deficiencies, such as HR, are also dependent on ALT-NHEJ to repair DSBs and survive genotoxic insults. Therefore, PARP1, LIG3, POLQ and other key components of ALT-NHEJ could be attractive therapeutic targets in these cancers.

Unfortunately, a potential deleterious result of long-term treatment with DNA repair or DNA damage response inhibitors (such as ATM inhibitors) could be increased ALT-NHEJ activity that may further cause generation of secondary malignancies associated with the highly error prone nature of repair by ALT-NHEJ. Further insights and discoveries of factors (such as end-resection factors, pro-oncogenic factors etc.) that regulate the switch between error-prone and error-free DSB repair pathways in normal cells would help in the development of specific cancer-targeted ALT-NHEJ therapeutics. Future studies should focus on the role of ALT-NHEJ in driving these devastating diseases and the development of ALT-NHEJ inhibitors is eagerly awaited as a potential treatment strategy in cancer.

References

Arnaudeau C, Lundin C, Helleday T (2001) DNA double-strand breaks associated with replication forks are predominantly repaired by homologous recombination involving an exchange mechanism in mammalian cells. J Mol Biol 307(5):1235–1245

Audebert M, Salles B, Calsou P (2004) Involvement of poly(ADP-ribose) polymerase-1 and XRCC1/DNA ligase III in an alternative route for DNA double-strand breaks rejoining. J Biol Chem 279(53):55117–55126

Audebert M, Salles B, Calsou P (2008) Effect of double-strand break DNA sequence on the PARP-1 NHEJ pathway. Biochem Biophys Res Commun 369(3):982–988

Augenlicht LH, Wadler S, Corner G, Richards C, Ryan L, Multani AS et al (1997) Low-level c-myc amplification in human colonic carcinoma cell lines and tumors: a frequent, p53-independent mutation associated with improved outcome in a randomized multi-institutional trial. Cancer Res 57(9):1769–1775

Baker VV, Borst MP, Dixon D, Hatch KD, Shingleton HM, Miller D (1990) c-myc amplification in ovarian cancer. Gynecol Oncol 38(3):340–342

Barton O, Naumann SC, Diemer-Biehs R, Kunzel J, Steinlage M, Conrad S et al (2014) Polo-like kinase 3 regulates CtIP during DNA double-strand break repair in G1. J Cell Biol 206(7):877–894

Bennardo N, Stark JM (2010) ATM limits incorrect end utilization during non-homologous end joining of multiple chromosome breaks. PLoS Genet 6(11):e1001194

Bennardo N, Cheng A, Huang N, Stark JM (2008) Alternative-NHEJ is a mechanistically distinct pathway of mammalian chromosome break repair. PLoS Genet 4(6):e1000110

Bentley J, Diggle CP, Harnden P, Knowles MA, Kiltie AE (2004) DNA double strand break repair in human bladder cancer is error prone and involves microhomology-associated end-joining. Nucleic Acids Res 32(17):5249–5259

Berns EM, Klijn JG, van Putten WL, van Staveren IL, Portengen H, Foekens JA (1992a) c-myc amplification is a better prognostic factor than HER2/neu amplification in primary breast cancer. Cancer Res 52(5):1107–1113

Berns EM, Klijn JG, van Staveren IL, Portengen H, Noordegraaf E, Foekens JA (1992b) Prevalence of amplification of the oncogenes c-myc, HER2/neu, and int-2 in one thousand human breast tumours: correlation with steroid receptors. Eur J Cancer 28(2–3):697–700

Boulton SJ, Jackson SP (1996a) Identification of a Saccharomyces cerevisiae Ku80 homologue: roles in DNA double strand break rejoining and in telomeric maintenance. Nucleic Acids Res 24(23):4639–4648

Boulton SJ, Jackson SP (1996b) Saccharomyces cerevisiae Ku70 potentiates illegitimate DNA double-strand break repair and serves as a barrier to error-prone DNA repair pathways. EMBO J 15(18):5093–5103

Boultwood J, Wyllie FS, Williams ED, Wynford-Thomas D (1988) N-myc expression in neoplasia of human thyroid C-cells. Cancer Res 48(14):4073–4077

Brunet E, Simsek D, Tomishima M, DeKelver R, Choi VM, Gregory P et al (2009) Chromosomal translocations induced at specified loci in human stem cells. Proc Natl Acad Sci U S A 106(26):10620–10625

Ceccaldi R, Liu JC, Amunugama R, Hajdu I, Primack B, Petalcorin MI et al (2015) Homologous-recombination-deficient tumours are dependent on Poltheta-mediated repair. Nature 518(7538):258–262

Chen CH, Shen J, Lee WJ, Chow SN (2005) Overexpression of cyclin D1 and c-Myc gene products in human primary epithelial ovarian cancer. Int J Gynecol Cancer 15(5):878–883

Chen X, Zhong S, Zhu X, Dziegielewska B, Ellenberger T, Wilson GM et al (2008) Rational design of human DNA ligase inhibitors that target cellular DNA replication and repair. Cancer Res 68(9):3169–3177

Chen H, Lisby M, Symington LS (2013) RPA coordinates DNA end resection and prevents formation of DNA hairpins. Mol Cell 50(4):589–600

Cheng Q, Barboule N, Frit P, Gomez D, Bombarde O, Couderc B et al (2011) Ku counteracts mobilization of PARP1 and MRN in chromatin damaged with DNA double-strand breaks. Nucleic Acids Res 39(22):9605–9619

Chiang C, Jacobsen JC, Ernst C, Hanscom C, Heilbut A, Blumenthal I et al (2012) Complex reorganization and predominant non-homologous repair following chromosomal breakage in karyotypically balanced germline rearrangements and transgenic integration. Nat Genet 44(4):390–397. S1

Cotner-Gohara E, Kim IK, Tomkinson AE, Ellenberger T (2008) Two DNA-binding and nick recognition modules in human DNA ligase III. J Biol Chem 283(16):10764–10772

Cotner-Gohara E, Kim IK, Hammel M, Tainer JA, Tomkinson AE, Ellenberger T (2010) Human DNA ligase III recognizes DNA ends by dynamic switching between two DNA-bound states. Biochemistry 49(29):6165–6176

Critchlow SE, Jackson SP (1998) DNA end-joining: from yeast to man. Trends Biochem Sci 23(10):394–398

De Lorenzo SB, Patel AG, Hurley RM, Kaufmann SH (2013) The elephant and the blind men: making sense of PARP inhibitors in homologous recombination deficient tumor cells. Front Oncol 3:228

DeFazio LG, Stansel RM, Griffith JD, Chu G (2002) Synapsis of DNA ends by DNA-dependent protein kinase. EMBO J 21(12):3192–3200

Della-Maria J, Zhou Y, Tsai MS, Kuhnlein J, Carney JP, Paull TT et al (2011) Human Mre11/human Rad50/Nbs1 and DNA ligase IIIalpha/XRCC1 protein complexes act together in an alternative nonhomologous end joining pathway. J Biol Chem 286(39):33845–33853

Deng SK, Chen H, Symington LS (2014a) Replication protein A prevents promiscuous annealing between short sequence homologies: implications for genome integrity. BioEssays 37(3):305–313

Deng SK, Gibb B, de Almeida MJ, Greene EC, Symington LS (2014b) RPA antagonizes microhomology-mediated repair of DNA double-strand breaks. Nat Struct Mol Biol 21(4):405–412

Difilippantonio MJ, Zhu J, Chen HT, Meffre E, Nussenzweig MC, Max EE et al (2000) DNA repair protein Ku80 suppresses chromosomal aberrations and malignant transformation. Nature 404(6777):510–514

Eilers M, Schirm S, Bishop JM (1991) The MYC protein activates transcription of the alpha-prothymosin gene. EMBO J 10(1):133–141

Ellenberger T, Tomkinson AE (2008) Eukaryotic DNA ligases: structural and functional insights. Annu Rev Biochem 77:313–338

Farmer H, McCabe N, Lord CJ, Tutt AN, Johnson DA, Richardson TB et al (2005) Targeting the DNA repair defect in BRCA mutant cells as a therapeutic strategy. Nature 434(7035):917–921

Feldmann E, Schmiemann V, Goedecke W, Reichenberger S, Pfeiffer P (2000) DNA double-strand break repair in cell-free extracts from Ku80-deficient cells: implications for Ku serving as an alignment factor in non-homologous DNA end joining. Nucleic Acids Res 28(13):2585–2596

Fernandez-Vidal A, Guitton-Sert L, Cadoret JC, Drac M, Schwob E, Baldacci G et al (2014) A role for DNA polymerase theta in the timing of DNA replication. Nat Commun 5:4285

Fleming WH, Hamel A, MacDonald R, Ramsey E, Pettigrew NM, Johnston B et al (1986) Expression of the c-myc protooncogene in human prostatic carcinoma and benign prostatic hyperplasia. Cancer Res 46(3):1535–1538

Fong PC, Boss DS, Yap TA, Tutt A, Wu P, Mergui-Roelvink M et al (2009) Inhibition of poly(ADP-ribose) polymerase in tumors from BRCA mutation carriers. N Engl J Med 361(2):123–134

Frank KM, Sharpless NE, Gao Y, Sekiguchi JM, Ferguson DO, Zhu C et al (2000) DNA ligase IV deficiency in mice leads to defective neurogenesis and embryonic lethality via the p53 pathway. Mol Cell 5(6):993–1002

Gao Y, Chaudhuri J, Zhu C, Davidson L, Weaver DT, Alt FW (1998) A targeted DNA-PKcs-null mutation reveals DNA-PK-independent functions for KU in V(D)J recombination. Immunity 9(3):367–376

Gao Y, Ferguson DO, Xie W, Manis JP, Sekiguchi J, Frank KM et al (2000) Interplay of p53 and DNA-repair protein XRCC4 in tumorigenesis, genomic stability and development. Nature 404(6780):897–900

Ghezraoui H, Piganeau M, Renouf B, Renaud JB, Sallmyr A, Ruis B et al (2014) Chromosomal translocations in human cells are generated by canonical nonhomologous end-joining. Mol Cell 55(6):829–842

Goff JP, Shields DS, Seki M, Choi S, Epperly MW, Dixon T et al (2009) Lack of DNA polymerase theta (POLQ) radiosensitizes bone marrow stromal cells in vitro and increases reticulocyte micronuclei after total-body irradiation. Radiat Res 172(2):165–174

Gottlieb TM, Jackson SP (1993) The DNA-dependent protein kinase: requirement for DNA ends and association with Ku antigen. Cell 72(1):131–142

Guidos CJ, Williams CJ, Grandal I, Knowles G, Huang MT, Danska JS (1996) V(D)J recombination activates a p53-dependent DNA damage checkpoint in scid lymphocyte precursors. Genes Dev 10(16):2038–2054

Guirouilh-Barbat J, Huck S, Bertrand P, Pirzio L, Desmaze C, Sabatier L et al (2004) Impact of the KU80 pathway on NHEJ-induced genome rearrangements in mammalian cells. Mol Cell 14(5):611–623

Gunn A, Bennardo N, Cheng A, Stark JM (2011) Correct end use during end joining of multiple chromosomal double strand breaks is influenced by repair protein RAD50, DNA-dependent protein kinase DNA-PKcs, and transcription context. J Biol Chem 286(49):42470–42482

Hahnel PS, Enders B, Sasca D, Roos WP, Kaina B, Bullinger L et al (2014) Targeting components of the alternative NHEJ pathway sensitizes KRAS mutant leukemic cells to chemotherapy. Blood 123(15):2355–2366

Harada Y, Katagiri T, Ito I, Akiyama F, Sakamoto G, Kasumi F et al (1994) Genetic studies of 457 breast cancers. Clinicopathologic parameters compared with genetic alterations. Cancer 74(8):2281–2286

Hartlerode AJ, Scully R (2009) Mechanisms of double-strand break repair in somatic mammalian cells. Biochem J 423(2):157–168

Herold S, Herkert B, Eilers M (2009) Facilitating replication under stress: an oncogenic function of MYC? Nat Rev Cancer 9(6):441–444

Higgins GS, Prevo R, Lee YF, Helleday T, Muschel RJ, Taylor S et al (2010a) A small interfering RNA screen of genes involved in DNA repair identifies tumor-specific radiosensitization by POLQ knockdown. Cancer Res 70(7):2984–2993

Higgins GS, Harris AL, Prevo R, Helleday T, McKenna WG, Buffa FM (2010b) Overexpression of POLQ confers a poor prognosis in early breast cancer patients. Oncotarget 1(3):175–184

Hochegger H, Dejsuphong D, Fukushima T, Morrison C, Sonoda E, Schreiber V et al (2006) Parp-1 protects homologous recombination from interference by Ku and ligase IV in vertebrate cells. EMBO J 25(6):1305–1314

Hogg M, Sauer-Eriksson AE, Johansson E (2012) Promiscuous DNA synthesis by human DNA polymerase theta. Nucleic Acids Res 40(6):2611–2622

Horiuchi D, Kusdra L, Huskey NE, Chandriani S, Lenburg ME, Gonzalez-Angulo AM et al (2012) MYC pathway activation in triple-negative breast cancer is synthetic lethal with CDK inhibition. J Exp Med 209(4):679–696

Jenkins RB, Qian J, Lieber MM, Bostwick DG (1997) Detection of c-myc oncogene amplification and chromosomal anomalies in metastatic prostatic carcinoma by fluorescence in situ hybridization. Cancer Res 57(3):524–531

Kabotyanski EB, Gomelsky L, Han JO, Stamato TD, Roth DB (1998) Double-strand break repair in Ku86- and XRCC4-deficient cells. Nucleic Acids Res 26(23):5333–5342

Karlsson A, Deb-Basu D, Cherry A, Turner S, Ford J, Felsher DW (2003) Defective double-strand DNA break repair and chromosomal translocations by MYC overexpression. Proc Natl Acad Sci U S A 100(17):9974–9979

Kawamura K, Bahar R, Seimiya M, Chiyo M, Wada A, Okada S et al (2004) DNA polymerase theta is preferentially expressed in lymphoid tissues and upregulated in human cancers. Int J Cancer 109(1):9–16

Keller KL, Overbeck-Carrick TL, Beck DJ (2001) Survival and induction of SOS in Escherichia coli treated with cisplatin, UV-irradiation, or mitomycin C are dependent on the function of the RecBC and RecFOR pathways of homologous recombination. Mutat Res 486(1):21–29

Kent T, Chandramouly G, McDevitt SM, Ozdemir AY, Pomerantz RT (2015) Mechanism of microhomology-mediated end-joining promoted by human DNA polymerase theta. Nat Struct Mol Biol 22(3):230–237

Khanna KK, Jackson SP (2001) DNA double-strand breaks: signaling, repair and the cancer connection. Nat Genet 27(3):247–254

Kim MY, Zhang T, Kraus WL (2005) Poly(ADP-ribosyl)ation by PARP-1: 'PAR-laying' NAD+ into a nuclear signal. Genes Dev 19(17):1951–1967

Kim G, Ison G, McKee AE, Zhang H, Tang S, Gwise T et al (2015) FDA approval summary: olaparib monotherapy in patients with deleterious germline BRCA-mutated advanced ovarian cancer treated with three or more lines of chemotherapy. Clin Cancer Res 21(19):4257–4261

Kozma L, Kiss I, Szakall S, Ember I (1994) Investigation of c-myc oncogene amplification in colorectal cancer. Cancer Lett 81(2):165–169

Krasner DS, Daley JM, Sung P, Niu H (2015) Interplay between Ku and replication protein A in the restriction of Exo1-mediated DNA break end resection. J Biol Chem 290(30):18806–18816

Langelier MF, Pascal JM (2013) PARP-1 mechanism for coupling DNA damage detection to poly(ADP-ribose) synthesis. Curr Opin Struct Biol 23(1):134–143

Lee SE, Mitchell RA, Cheng A, Hendrickson EA (1997) Evidence for DNA-PK-dependent and -independent DNA double-strand break repair pathways in mammalian cells as a function of the cell cycle. Mol Cell Biol 17(3):1425–1433

Lemee F, Bergoglio V, Fernandez-Vidal A, Machado-Silva A, Pillaire MJ, Bieth A et al (2010) DNA polymerase theta up-regulation is associated with poor survival in breast cancer, perturbs DNA replication, and promotes genetic instability. Proc Natl Acad Sci U S A 107(30):13390–13395

Li Y, Gao X, Wang JY (2011) Comparison of two POLQ mutants reveals that a polymerase-inactive POLQ retains significant function in tolerance to etoposide and gamma-irradiation in mouse B cells. Genes Cells 16(9):973–983

Lieber MR (2008) The mechanism of human nonhomologous DNA end joining. J Biol Chem 283(1):1–5

Lieber MR, Ma Y, Pannicke U, Schwarz K (2003) Mechanism and regulation of human non-homologous DNA end-joining. Nat Rev Mol Cell Biol 4(9):712–720

Lieber MR, Yu K, Raghavan SC (2006) Roles of nonhomologous DNA end joining, V(D)J recombination, and class switch recombination in chromosomal translocations. DNA Repair (Amst) 5(9–10):1234–1245

Lim DS, Vogel H, Willerford DM, Sands AT, Platt KA, Hasty P (2000) Analysis of ku80-mutant mice and cells with deficient levels of p53. Mol Cell Biol 20(11):3772–3780

Little CD, Nau MM, Carney DN, Gazdar AF, Minna JD (1983) Amplification and expression of the c-myc oncogene in human lung cancer cell lines. Nature 306(5939):194–196

Lupo B, Trusolino L (2014) Inhibition of poly(ADP-ribosyl)ation in cancer: old and new paradigms revisited. Biochim Biophys Acta 1846(1):201–215

Makharashvili N, Tubbs AT, Yang SH, Wang H, Barton O, Zhou Y et al (2014) Catalytic and noncatalytic roles of the CtIP endonuclease in double-strand break end resection. Mol Cell 54(6):1022–1033

Mansour WY, Rhein T, Dahm-Daphi J (2010) The alternative end-joining pathway for repair of DNA double-strand breaks requires PARP1 but is not dependent upon microhomologies. Nucleic Acids Res 38(18):6065–6077

Masson M, Niedergang C, Schreiber V, Muller S, Menissier-de Murcia J, de Murcia G (1998) XRCC1 is specifically associated with poly(ADP-ribose) polymerase and negatively regulates its activity following DNA damage. Mol Cell Biol 18(6):3563–3571

Mateos-Gomez PA, Gong F, Nair N, Miller KM, Lazzerini-Denchi E, Sfeir A (2015) Mammalian polymerase theta promotes alternative NHEJ and suppresses recombination. Nature 518(7538):254–257

Mehta A, Haber JE (2014) Sources of DNA double-strand breaks and models of recombinational DNA repair. Cold Spring Harb Perspect Biol 6(9):a016428

Menissier-de Murcia J, Molinete M, Gradwohl G, Simonin F, de Murcia G (1989) Zinc-binding domain of poly(ADP-ribose)polymerase participates in the recognition of single strand breaks on DNA. J Mol Biol 210(1):229–233

Michels J, Vitale I, Saparbaev M, Castedo M, Kroemer G (2014) Predictive biomarkers for cancer therapy with PARP inhibitors. Oncogene 33(30):3894–3907

Mimitou EP, Symington LS (2008) Sae2, Exo1 and Sgs1 collaborate in DNA double-strand break processing. Nature 455(7214):770–774

Mitani S, Kamata H, Fujiwara M, Aoki N, Tango T, Fukuchi K et al (2001) Analysis of c-myc DNA amplification in non-small cell lung carcinoma in comparison with small cell lung carcinoma using polymerase chain reaction. Clin Exp Med 1(2):105–111

Murai J, Huang SY, Das BB, Renaud A, Zhang Y, Doroshow JH et al (2012) Trapping of PARP1 and PARP2 by clinical PARP Inhibitors. Cancer Res 72(21):5588–5599

Murai J, Huang SY, Renaud A, Zhang Y, Ji J, Takeda S et al (2013) Stereospecific PARP trapping by BMN 673 and comparison with olaparib and rucaparib. Mol Cancer Ther 13(2):433–443

Muvarak N, Kelley S, Robert C, Baer MR, Perrotti D, Gambacorti-Passerini C et al (2015) c-MYC generates repair errors via increased transcription of alternative-NHEJ fdactors, LIG3 and PARP1, in tyrosine kinase-activated leukemias. Mol Cancer Res 13(4):699–712

Nacht M, Strasser A, Chan YR, Harris AW, Schlissel M, Bronson RT et al (1996) Mutations in the p53 and SCID genes cooperate in tumorigenesis. Genes Dev 10(16):2055–2066

Negrini S, Gorgoulis VG, Halazonetis TD (2010) Genomic instability—an evolving hallmark of cancer. Nat Rev Mol Cell Biol 11(3):220–228

Nesbit CE, Tersak JM, Prochownik EV (1999) MYC oncogenes and human neoplastic disease. Oncogene 18(19):3004–3016

New JH, Sugiyama T, Zaitseva E, Kowalczykowski SC (1998) Rad52 protein stimulates DNA strand exchange by Rad51 and replication protein A. Nature 391(6665):407–410

Oh S, Harvey A, Zimbric J, Wang Y, Nguyen T, Jackson PJ et al (2014) DNA ligase III and DNA ligase IV carry out genetically distinct forms of end joining in human somatic cells. DNA Repair (Amst) 21:97–110

Orta ML, Hoglund A, Calderon-Montano JM, Dominguez I, Burgos-Moron E, Visnes T et al (2014) The PARP inhibitor Olaparib disrupts base excision repair of 5-aza-2′-deoxycytidine lesions. Nucleic Acids Res 42(14):9108–9120

Patel AG, Sarkaria JN, Kaufmann SH (2011) Nonhomologous end joining drives poly(ADP-ribose) polymerase (PARP) inhibitor lethality in homologous recombination-deficient cells. Proc Natl Acad Sci U S A 108(8):3406–3411

Pergola F, Zdzienicka MZ, Lieber MR (1993) V(D)J recombination in mammalian cell mutants defective in DNA double-strand break repair. Mol Cell Biol 13(6):3464–3471

Petalcorin MI, Sandall J, Wigley DB, Boulton SJ (2006) CeBRC-2 stimulates D-loop formation by RAD-51 and promotes DNA single-strand annealing. J Mol Biol 361(2):231–242

Peterson SE, Li Y, Wu-Baer F, Chait BT, Baer R, Yan H et al (2013) Activation of DSB processing requires phosphorylation of CtIP by ATR. Mol Cell 49(4):657–667

Pillaire MJ, Selves J, Gordien K, Gourraud PA, Gentil C, Danjoux M et al (2010) A 'DNA replication' signature of progression and negative outcome in colorectal cancer. Oncogene 29(6):876–887

Plummer R, Lorigan P, Steven N, Scott L, Middleton MR, Wilson RH et al (2013) A phase II study of the potent PARP inhibitor, Rucaparib (PF-01367338, AG014699), with temozolomide in patients with metastatic melanoma demonstrating evidence of chemopotentiation. Cancer Chemother Pharmacol 71(5):1191–1199

Prasad R, Longley MJ, Sharief FS, Hou EW, Copeland WC, Wilson SH (2009) Human DNA polymerase theta possesses 5′-dRP lyase activity and functions in single-nucleotide base excision repair in vitro. Nucleic Acids Res 37(6):1868–1877

Rassool FV, Tomkinson AE (2010) Targeting abnormal DNA double strand break repair in cancer. Cell Mol Life Sci 67(21):3699–3710

Roncalli M, Viale G, Grimelius L, Johansson H, Wilander E, Alfano RM et al (1994) Prognostic value of N-myc immunoreactivity in medullary thyroid carcinoma. Cancer 74(1):134–141

Roth DB, Wilson JH (1986) Nonhomologous recombination in mammalian cells: role for short sequence homologies in the joining reaction. Mol Cell Biol 6(12):4295–4304

Saleh-Gohari N, Bryant HE, Schultz N, Parker KM, Cassel TN, Helleday T (2005) Spontaneous homologous recombination is induced by collapsed replication forks that are caused by endogenous DNA single-strand breaks. Mol Cell Biol 25(16):7158–7169

Sallmyr A, Tomkinson AE, Rassool FV (2008) Up-regulation of WRN and DNA ligase IIIalpha in chronic myeloid leukemia: consequences for the repair of DNA double-strand breaks. Blood 112(4):1413–1423

Sartori AA, Lukas C, Coates J, Mistrik M, Fu S, Bartek J et al (2007) Human CtIP promotes DNA end resection. Nature 450(7169):509–514

Satoh MS, Lindahl T (1992) Role of poly(ADP-ribose) formation in DNA repair. Nature 356(6367):356–358

Seki M, Marini F, Wood RD (2003) POLQ (Pol theta), a DNA polymerase and DNA-dependent ATPase in human cells. Nucleic Acids Res 31(21):6117–6126

Seki M, Masutani C, Yang LW, Schuffert A, Iwai S, Bahar I et al (2004) High-efficiency bypass of DNA damage by human DNA polymerase Q. EMBO J 23(22):4484–4494

Sharief FS, Vojta PJ, Ropp PA, Copeland WC (1999) Cloning and chromosomal mapping of the human DNA polymerase theta (POLQ), the eighth human DNA polymerase. Genomics 59(1):90–96

Sharpless NE, Ferguson DO, O'Hagan RC, Castrillon DH, Lee C, Farazi PA et al (2001) Impaired nonhomologous end-joining provokes soft tissue sarcomas harboring chromosomal translocations, amplifications, and deletions. Mol Cell 8(6):1187–1196

Shen Y, Rehman FL, Feng Y, Boshuizen J, Bajrami I, Elliott R et al (2013) BMN 673, a novel and highly potent PARP1/2 inhibitor for the treatment of human cancers with DNA repair deficiency. Clin Cancer Res 19(18):5003–5015

Shen Y, Aoyagi-Scharber M, Wang B (2015) Trapping Poly(ADP-Ribose) Polymerase. J Pharmacol Exp Ther 353(3):446–457

Shima N, Munroe RJ, Schimenti JC (2004) The mouse genomic instability mutation chaos1 is an allele of Polq that exhibits genetic interaction with Atm. Mol Cell Biol 24(23):10381–10389

Simsek D, Jasin M (2010) Alternative end-joining is suppressed by the canonical NHEJ component Xrcc4-ligase IV during chromosomal translocation formation. Nat Struct Mol Biol 17(4):410–416

Simsek D, Brunet E, Wong SY, Katyal S, Gao Y, McKinnon PJ et al (2011a) DNA ligase III promotes alternative nonhomologous end-joining during chromosomal translocation formation. PLoS Genet 7(6):e1002080

Simsek D, Furda A, Gao Y, Artus J, Brunet E, Hadjantonakis AK et al (2011b) Crucial role for DNA ligase III in mitochondria but not in Xrcc1-dependent repair. Nature 471(7337):245–248

Smith J, Riballo E, Kysela B, Baldeyron C, Manolis K, Masson C et al (2003) Impact of DNA ligase IV on the fidelity of end joining in human cells. Nucleic Acids Res 31(8):2157–2167

Soni A, Siemann M, Grabos M, Murmann T, Pantelias GE, Iliakis G (2014) Requirement for Parp-1 and DNA ligases 1 or 3 but not of Xrcc1 in chromosomal translocation formation by backup end joining. Nucleic Acids Res 42(10):6380–6392

Sonnenblick A, de Azambuja E, Azim HA Jr, Piccart M (2015) An update on PARP inhibitors—moving to the adjuvant setting. Nat Rev Clin Oncol 12(1):27–41

Sturzenegger A, Burdova K, Kanagaraj R, Levikova M, Pinto C, Cejka P et al (2014) DNA2 cooperates with the WRN and BLM RecQ helicases to mediate long-range DNA end resection in human cells. J Biol Chem 289(39):27314–27326

Sugimura K, Takebayashi S, Taguchi H, Takeda S, Okumura K (2008) PARP-1 ensures regulation of replication fork progression by homologous recombination on damaged DNA. J Cell Biol 183(7):1203–1212

Takahashi Y, Kawate S, Watanabe M, Fukushima J, Mori S, Fukusato T (2007) Amplification of c-myc and cyclin D1 genes in primary and metastatic carcinomas of the liver. Pathol Int 57(7):437–442

Takata M, Sasaki MS, Sonoda E, Morrison C, Hashimoto M, Utsumi H et al (1998) Homologous recombination and non-homologous end-joining pathways of DNA double-strand break repair have overlapping roles in the maintenance of chromosomal integrity in vertebrate cells. EMBO J 17(18):5497–5508

Thomas L, Stamberg J, Gojo I, Ning Y, Rapoport AP (2004) Double minute chromosomes in monoblastic (M5) and myeloblastic (M2) acute myeloid leukemia: two case reports and a review of literature. Am J Hematol 77(1):55–61

Tobin LA, Robert C, Nagaria P, Chumsri S, Twaddell W, Ioffe OB et al (2012) Targeting abnormal DNA repair in therapy-resistant breast cancers. Mol Cancer Res 10(1):96–107

Tobin LA, Robert C, Rapoport AP, Gojo I, Baer MR, Tomkinson AE et al (2013) Targeting abnormal DNA double-strand break repair in tyrosine kinase inhibitor-resistant chronic myeloid leukemias. Oncogene 32(14):1784–1793

Tomkinson AE, Levin DS (1997) Mammalian DNA ligases. BioEssays 19(10):893–901

Truong LN, Li Y, Shi LZ, Hwang PY, He J, Wang H et al (2013) Microhomology-mediated end joining and homologous recombination share the initial end resection step to repair DNA double-strand breaks in mammalian cells. Proc Natl Acad Sci U S A 110(19):7720–7725

Vafa O, Wade M, Kern S, Beeche M, Pandita TK, Hampton GM et al (2002) c-Myc can induce DNA damage, increase reactive oxygen species, and mitigate p53 function: a mechanism for oncogene-induced genetic instability. Mol Cell 9(5):1031–1044

Varambally S, Yu J, Laxman B, Rhodes DR, Mehra R, Tomlins SA et al (2005) Integrative genomic and proteomic analysis of prostate cancer reveals signatures of metastatic progression. Cancer Cell 8(5):393–406

Verkaik NS, Esveldt-van Lange RE, van Heemst D, Bruggenwirth HT, Hoeijmakers JH, Zdzienicka MZ et al (2002) Different types of V(D)J recombination and end-joining defects in DNA double-strand break repair mutant mammalian cells. Eur J Immunol 32(3):701–709

Vlach J, Hennecke S, Alevizopoulos K, Conti D, Amati B (1996) Growth arrest by the cyclin-dependent kinase inhibitor p27Kip1 is abrogated by c-Myc. EMBO J 15(23):6595–6604

Wang H, Perrault AR, Takeda Y, Qin W, Iliakis G (2003) Biochemical evidence for Ku-independent backup pathways of NHEJ. Nucleic Acids Res 31(18):5377–5388

Wang M, Wu W, Rosidi B, Zhang L, Wang H, Iliakis G (2006) PARP-1 and Ku compete for repair of DNA double strand breaks by distinct NHEJ pathways. Nucleic Acids Res 34(21):6170–6182

Wang H, Shi LZ, Wong CC, Han X, Hwang PY, Truong LN et al (2013) The interaction of CtIP and Nbs1 connects CDK and ATM to regulate HR-mediated double-strand break repair. PLoS Genet 9(2):e1003277

Windhofer F, Krause S, Hader C, Schulz WA, Florl AR (2008) Distinctive differences in DNA double-strand break repair between normal urothelial and urothelial carcinoma cells. Mutat Res 638(1–2):56–65

Xie A, Kwok A, Scully R (2009) Role of mammalian Mre11 in classical and alternative nonhomologous end joining. Nat Struct Mol Biol 16(8):814–818

Yaneva M, Kowalewski T, Lieber MR (1997) Interaction of DNA-dependent protein kinase with DNA and with Ku: biochemical and atomic-force microscopy studies. EMBO J 16(16):5098–5112

Yousefzadeh MJ, Wyatt DW, Takata K, Mu Y, Hensley SC, Tomida J et al (2014) Mechanism of suppression of chromosomal instability by DNA polymerase POLQ. PLoS Genet 10(10):e1004654

Yuan Y, Britton S, Delteil C, Coates J, Jackson SP, Barboule N et al (2015) Single-stranded DNA oligomers stimulate error-prone alternative repair of DNA double-strand breaks through hijacking Ku protein. Nucleic Acids Res 43(21):10264–10276

Yun MH, Hiom K (2009) CtIP-BRCA1 modulates the choice of DNA double-strand-break repair pathway throughout the cell cycle. Nature 459(7245):460–463

Zha S, Guo C, Boboila C, Oksenych V, Cheng HL, Zhang Y et al (2011) ATM damage response and XLF repair factor are functionally redundant in joining DNA breaks. Nature 469(7329):250–254

Znojek P, Willmore E, Curtin NJ (2014) Preferential potentiation of topoisomerase I poison cytotoxicity by PARP inhibition in S phase. Br J Cancer 111(7):1319–1326

About the Editors

John Pollard is Principal Research Fellow and Head of Biological Sciences at Vertex Pharmaceuticals' UK research site. John joined Vertex in 1999 following a PhD at Southampton University and Postdoctoral positions at St. Andrews and Birmingham Universities in bioorganic chemistry. During his tenure at Vertex, John has led a series of oncology research and development projects across cell cycle control, survival and growth, and most recently DNA damage, which together have yielded multiple clinical candidates. John has served as global research lead for Vertex's oncology effort and led numerous collaborations with academic groups and pharma companies.

Nicola Curtin is Professor of Experimental Cancer Therapeutics at Newcastle University, UK. After obtaining her PhD in hepatocarcinogenesis from the University of Surrey she started working at Newcastle University, initially exploring novel therapies for liver cancer, then the cytotoxic mechanisms of novel antifolates and the role of nucleoside transport. Prof. Curtin was a founding member of the Newcastle Anticancer Drug Discovery Initiative and contributed to the development of PARP inhibitors, including the identification of their synthetic lethality in cells lacking homologous recombination function. Her work focusses on the DNA damage response in general, and she has also worked on the preclinical development of ATM, ATR and DNA-PK inhibitors for the treatment of cancer. In addition, she undertakes translational studies to identify pharmacodynamic biomarkers and those predictive of response to DDR inhibitor therapy in cultured cells and patient material. She's also the co-editor of PARP Inhibitors for Cancer Therapy in this series.

© Springer International Publishing AG, part of Springer Nature 2018
J. Pollard, N. Curtin (eds.), *Targeting the DNA Damage Response for Anti-Cancer Therapy*, Cancer Drug Discovery and Development, https://doi.org/10.1007/978-3-319-75836-7

Printed in the United States
By Bookmasters